Emergency Psychiatry

PRIMERS ON PSYCHIATRY

Stephen M. Strakowski, MD, Series Editor

Published and Forthcoming Titles

Emergency Psychiatry

Edited by

TONY THRASHER, DO, MBA, DFAPA

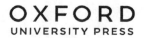

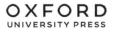

Oxford University Press is a department of the University of Oxford. It furthers
the University's objective of excellence in research, scholarship, and education
by publishing worldwide. Oxford is a registered trade mark of Oxford University
Press in the UK and certain other countries.

Published in the United States of America by Oxford University Press
198 Madison Avenue, New York, NY 10016, United States of America.

Library of Congress Cataloging-in-Publication Data
Names: Thrasher, Tony, editor.
Title: Emergency psychiatry / [edited by] Tony Thrasher.
Other titles: Emergency psychiatry (Thrasher) | Primer on.
Description: New York : Oxford University Press, [2023] |
Series: Primer on series |
Includes bibliographical references and index.
Identifiers: LCCN 2023006089 (print) | LCCN 2023006090 (ebook) |
ISBN 9780197624005 (paperback) | ISBN 9780197624029 (epub) |
ISBN 9780197624036 (online)
Subjects: MESH: Emergency Services, Psychiatric—methods |
Mental Disorders—diagnosis | Mental Disorders—therapy
Classification: LCC RC480.6 (print) | LCC RC480.6 (ebook) |
NLM WM 401 | DDC 616.89/025—dc23/eng/20230323
LC record available at https://lccn.loc.gov/2023006089
LC ebook record available at https://lccn.loc.gov/2023006090

DOI: 10.1093/med/9780197624005.001.0001

Printed in Canada by Marquis Book Printing

Contents

SECTION I. THE APPROACH TO EMERGENCY PSYCHIATRIC EVALUATION

SECTION II. SPECIFIC DISORDERS, DIAGNOSES, AND SYMPTOMS FREQUENTLY ENCOUNTERED AS PSYCHIATRIC EMERGENCIES

Acknowledgments

My significant gratitude toward the finest group of physicians I have ever worked with—the Psychiatric Crisis Service of Milwaukee County. Love and appreciation to Amy, Noah, and Owen for their patience, support, and enthusiasm for not only our mission but also my passion.

Tony Thrasher, DO, MBA, DFAPA

Contributors

Arpit Aggarwal, MD
Associate Professor of Clinical Psychiatry
Department of Psychiatry
University of Missouri, Columbia
Columbia, MO, USA

Margaret E. Balfour, MD, PhD
Associate Professor of Psychiatry
Chief of Quality and Clinical Innovation
Connections Health Solutions
University of Arizona
Tucson, AZ, USA

Laura W. Barnett, DO
Clinical Assistant Professor
Department of Psychiatry
The Ohio State University Wexner
    Medical Center
Columbus, OH, USA

Jennifer Baumhauer, MD
Clinical Assistant Professor
Department of Psychiatry
University of Michigan
Ann Arbor, MI, USA

Bernard Biermann, MD, PhD
University of Michigan Medical School
Ann Arbor, MI, USA

Joseph B. Bond, MD, MPH
Child, Adolescent, & Adult Psychiatrist
Department of Psychiatry
Massachusetts General Hospital & Harvard
    Medical School
Boston, MA, USA

Sara Brady, MD
Physician
Department of Psychiatry and Behavioral
    Medicine
Medical College of Wisconsin
Milwaukee, WI, USA

Heidi Burns, MD
Assistant Professor
Department of Child and Adolescent
    Psychiatry
University of Michigan
Ann Arbor, MI, USA

Daniel Cho, MD
Assistant Professor
Department of Psychiatry
University of Hawaii,
Honolulu, HI, USA

Claire Drom, MD
Staff Psychiatrist
Department of Psychiatry and
    Behavioral Health
CentraCare Clinic
St. Cloud, MN, USA

Matthew L. Goldman, MD, MS
Medical Director, Comprehensive
    Crisis Services
San Francisco Department of Public
    Health
San Francisco, CA, USA

Ishmael Gomes
Department of Psychiatry
University of Hawaii
Honolulu, HI, USA

Thomas W. Heinrich, MD
Professor of Psychiatry and Family
    Medicine
Department of Psychiatry and
    Behavioral Medicine
Medical College of Wisconsin
Milwaukee, WI, USA

Earl Hishinuma, PhD
Adjunct Professor
Department of Psychiatry
University of Hawaii at Manoa
Honolulu, HI, USA

Victor Hong, MD
Associate Clinical Professor
Department of Psychiatry
University of Michigan
Ann Arbor, MI, USA

Victor Huynh, DO
Resident Physician
Department of Psychiatry
University of Hawaii
Honolulu, HI, USA

Justin Kuehl, PsyD
Chief Psychologist
Milwaukee County Behavioral Health
    Division
Milwaukee, WI, USA

Kristie Ladegard, MD
Assistant Professor and Clinical Director of
    School Based Psychiatry
Department of Psychiatry
University of Colorado
Denver, CO, USA

Stephen Leung, MD
Assistant Clinical Professor
Department of Psychiatry and Behavioral
    Sciences
University of California, San Francisco
San Francisco, CA, USA

Shafi Lodhi, MD
Psychiatric Emergency Services
Department of Psychiatry and Behavioral
    Neuroscience
University of Cincinnati
Cincinnati, OH, USA

Nasuh Malas, MD, MPH
Associate Professor
Department of Psychiatry and Department
    of Pediatrics
University of Michigan
Ann Arbor, MI, USA

Katherine Maloy, MD
Assistant Clinical Professor
Department of Psychiatry
New York University
New York, NY, USA

Anna K. McDowell, MD
Mental Health Service
Rocky Mountain Regional Veterans Affairs
    Medical Center
Aurora, CO, USA

Benjamin Merotto, MD
Behavioral Health Services
Denver Health and Hospital Authority
Denver, CO, USA

Julie Ruth Owen, MD, MBA
Assistant Professor; Medical Director,
    Emergency Department Psychiatry
    Service
Department of Psychiatry & Behavioral
    Medicine; Department of Emergency
    Medicine
Medical College of Wisconsin
Milwaukee, WI, USA

Oluwole Popoola, MD, MPH
Assistant Clinical Professor
Department of Psychiatry
University of Missouri
Columbia, MO, USA

Richard Rhoads, MD
Medical Director
Connections Health Solutions
Phoenix, AZ, USA

Janet Richmond
McLean Hospital
Boston, MA, USA

John S. Rozel, MD, MSL
Professor of Psychiatry/Adjunct Professor
    of Law
University of Pittsburgh
Pittsburgh, PA, USA

Eileen P. Ryan, DO
Professor
Department of Psychiatry and
    Behavioral Health
The Ohio State University Wexner
    Medical Center
Columbus, OH, USA

Megan B. Schabbing, MD
System Medical Director
Department of Psychiatric Emergency
    Services
OhioHealth
Columbus, OH, USA

Annaliese Koller Shumate, BA, DO
Staff Psychiatrist
Milwaukee County Crisis Services
Milwaukee County
Milwaukee, WI, USA

Scott A. Simpson, MD, MPH
Medical Director, Psychiatric Emergency
    Services
Behavioral Health Services
Denver Health
Denver, CO, USA

Sarah Slocum, MD
Psychiatry Service Line Physician Lead
Exeter Health Resources
Exeter, NH, USA

Nicole R. Smith, MD
Psychiatrist
Prism Psychiatry Practice
Washington, DC, USA

Layla Soliman
Dept of Psychiatry
Atrium Health/Wake Forest University
    School of Medicine
Charlotte, NC, USA

Ian Steele, MD
Assistant Professor
Department of Psychiatry and Behavioral
    Medicine
Medical College of Wisconsin
Milwaukee, WI, USA

Junji Takeshita, MD
Professor and Associate Chair, Clinical
    Services
Geriatric Psychiatry Program Director
Department of Psychiatry
John A. Burns School of Medicine
University of Hawai'i at Mānoa
Honolulu, HI, USA

Seth Thomas, MD
Director of Quality and Performance
Emergency Medicine
Vituity
Emeryville, CA, USA

Jessica Tse, DO
Child and Adolescent Psychiatry Fellow
Department of Psychiatry
University of Utah
Salt Lake City, UT, USA

Helena Winston, MD
Assistant Professor
Department of Psychiatry
Denver Health and the University of Colorado
    Anschutz Medical Campus
Denver and Aurora, CO, USA

Chelsea Wolf, MD, MA
Assistant Professor and Medical Director,
    Adult Inpatient Psychiatry
Department of Psychiatry
Denver Health Medical Center
Denver, CO, USA

SECTION I
THE APPROACH TO EMERGENCY PSYCHIATRIC EVALUATION

1

An Initial Approach to the Emergency Evaluation

Pitfalls, Pearls, and Notice of Countertransference

Janet Richmond

Introduction

This chapter introduces the new clinician to techniques used to engage and evaluate the psychiatric patient in the emergency setting. The goal of the examination is to quickly establish rapport, contain affect, and gather enough information to arrive at a differential diagnosis that informs stabilization and disposition. An effective interview should be trauma-informed, collaborative, noncoercive, and have a treatment component.[1-5] The evaluation is rapid and focused rather than a complete workup as is done in an outpatient intake. In the emergency psychiatric evaluation, attention is paid to the chief complaint, the history of the present illness, the mental status examination, a safety assessment, and the patient's request.[3,6-8] A biopsychosocial understanding of the patient's situation is also necessary to inform treatment and disposition. The objective is to elicit as much information as needed, focusing more on how to elicit the information rather than asking a list of actuarial questions that frequently give only limited information. The exam is a process of generating hypotheses that change over the course of the interview as new information is elicited. For example, is the patient psychotic because he stopped his antipsychotic medication? The patient appears psychotic; is he truly psychotic or just terribly anxious? Or is he in the middle of a thyroid storm? Although this type of interviewing may appear to be inefficient, it is a systematic way of interviewing that elicits information organically yet is not lengthy to conduct. Finally, this model of interviewing draws on psychoanalytic[1,9] and object relations theory.

The Biopsychosocial Model

Lazare[10] developed a framework for clinical decision-making by using a biopsychosocial framework (Table 1.1). In this model, "the clinician must learn to elicit specific data to confirm or refute clinical hypotheses rather than gather a complete history." He used George Engel's biopsychosocial model[11] to develop his interviewing method. Lazare states that using this model ensures that the clinician does not come to a premature closure in the examination and "provide(s) a stimulus for the exploration of relevant but neglected clinical questions" during the interview.

Table 1.1 Lazare's Hypotheses in the Biopsychosocial Model

Psychological	Social Impact	Biological	Consider First Conditions That Are
Precipitating event	Change in the social environment		Probable
Personality style	Cultural factors	Axis I disorders	Serious
Unresolved grief	Religious and spiritual factors	Medical/neurological illness	Treatable
Developmental crisis	Social isolation	Alcohol or drug use	Resource availability
Coping skills/ego defenses	Social interactions		Patient's behavior
Interpersonal conflicts/attachment problems	Inability to get what one wants or needs from others		
History of traumatic events	External events (suicide, violence, traumatic events)		

Adapted from Lazare.[10]

In the first few minutes of the interview, the clinician generates hypotheses, which the clinician rules in or out. Then, based on further information, the clinician generates more hypotheses. More serious conditions, such as acute medical illness, psychosis, or homicidal or suicidal ideation/intent, are first on the list of hypotheses to rule in or out.

As noted above, performing an emergency psychiatric examination can be done without a preset list of questions and can elicit more information than a reductionistic checklist. Interviewing techniques include the use of open-ended questions interwoven with more focused, closed-ended questions; sitting in silence; and paying attention to one's own countertransference feelings, both physiologic and emotional.[3,12]

Most patients are not seeking a diagnosis in the emergency department (ED), but clinicians strive to make one and then believe that the assessment is complete. Lazare and Engel argue that there are more elements to take into consideration. In my clinical work, this type of formulation has been useful even in the evaluation of potentially suicidal patients. It has often obviated the need for hospitalization, even when multiple risk factors superficially indicated that the patient was imminently lethal and in need of involuntary hospitalization. The following case illustrates a biopsychosocial evaluation.

Case Example

A 40-year-old male with no known prior psychiatric or medical history is brought to the ED after becoming agitated at work. He is dressed in a suit and tie and is neat and clean except for excessive sweating and a haphazardly undone tie. He reports feeling agitated and believes he is having "flashbacks" to the terrorist attacks on September 11, 2001 (9/11), when he was in one of the towers of the World Trade Center in New York City but escaped unharmed. At the time, he had nightmares and exaggerated startle responses, but these remitted within the first month after the event. His primary care doctor had diagnosed insomnia and had prescribed a sleeping aid (zolpidem), which the patient used for only 2 weeks. He does not drink, use drugs, or take supplements. He is an attorney, and he is embarrassed that he was so upset in front of his partners, one of whom took him to the ED. His wife corroborates the history. From a *biomedical* framework, the change in mental status could stem from an array of new-onset medical illnesses, including an acute cardiac event, thyroid storm, hyperglycemia, or impairment of the hypothalamic–pituitary–adrenal axis. A full medical workup is completely negative. The medical diagnosis is panic attack. The next step is to generate hypotheses, the first being whether the diagnosis of panic attack is accurate or due to another psychiatric illness or an occult medical illness that the medical examination did not pick up.

Is there a family history of psychiatric illness such as bipolar disorder that could now be emerging in the patient? Is this a delayed post-traumatic stress disorder reaction and, if so, what precipitated it? Is the patient's report that he does not use substances accurate?

As he speaks, the clinician listens for clues as to what may have precipitated these "flashbacks" (which are actually intrusive memories of the event and not actual flashback phenomena). From the *social* component, are the patient's marriage and job secure? Is he worried about finances? From the psychological frame, what might be triggering these intense memories? What happened to disrupt his usual coping skills?

During the interview, the clinician listens for data to confirm or refute hypotheses, asking focused questions when necessary and generating further hypotheses, exploring each thoroughly. The patient's marriage, job, and finances are secure. There are no recent life cycle events and no family psychiatric or substance abuse history. Once again, the patient denies personal use of substances and is convincing. He reviews his reactions to 9/11 and, when asked, goes into some detail about the specific traumatic event that he is reexperiencing today. The clinician then asks the patient to "walk me through your day" (up to and including the onset of today's symptoms) to determine a precipitant. Almost immediately the patient pauses, is shocked, and "remembers" that while on his way to work that morning, he was delayed by a serious traffic accident in which a car caught on fire and a father and two young children were rescued unharmed. At the time of 9/11, the patient's two children were school aged, and as he watched the towers blazing, he remembered seeing two children approximately the same age as his children being hurried by their mother to safety. Throughout the day (of 9/11), he had had intrusive thoughts that his children could have been in the rubble, but his wife had kept them back home due to a stomach flu. While retelling his story, the patient had an upsurge in adrenergic symptoms that resolved as he was able to understand his reaction. Despite generating all these hypotheses and doing so in a nonstructured format, the entire evaluation took 20 minutes. An additional 10 minutes was spent helping the patent reintegrate his experiences and reequilibrate.

The Interview

The best interview does not feel like an interview to the patient, nor does it look like one to the casual observer. Instead, it looks like a conversation dedicated to learning about the patient, their illness, their ability to cope, and what the patient would like to see happen in the ED. This method of interviewing builds rapport.

It is current practice to use a trauma-informed approach for all patients. The emergency room environment may be threatening or trigger memories or reactions from past traumatic events. These may have occurred in a previous emergency room visit or with previous medical providers. Listen and observe for any signs that the patient may be tentative, agitated, or even hostile. Chapter 22 discusses trauma-informed care in detail.

Structure of the Interview

The Environment

Attention to the physical environment as well as the clinician's initial nonverbal behavior sets the tone. General principles for safety in the environment include the removal of large and small items such as pens and paper clips that can be thrown. When indicated, have Security readily available. Friendly but not intense eye contact is preferred. Keep your hands visible. Both patient and clinician should have equal access to the door, and if the patient appears volatile or unpredictable, stand or sit far enough away so that you are not punched or kicked.[3] In all interviews, try to sit at or below the patient's eye level. If possible, avoid standing over the patient; it makes for a symbolic imbalance of power.

Observation

Even before entering the room, there is a wealth of information to be gleaned from simply observing the patient, first in the waiting room and then in the exam room. What the patient is wearing, their level of neatness and hygiene, as well as their psychomotor activity can be diagnostic tools and generate hypotheses. The well-dressed and groomed patient in Vignette 1.1 was diaphoretic with his collar and tie loosened. These two factors should lead a clinician to generate questions about any acute medical illnesses or the patient's level of orientation and cognitive functioning.

Verbal Engagement

Introduce yourself, ask the patient's name and how they would like to be addressed. Consider addressing the patient by their last name because using their first name might appear overly personal or infantilizing, creating an imbalance of power. Other patients prefer to be called by their first name, despite the risk of overfamiliarity.

Establishing Rapport and Building an Alliance

Establishing rapport allows for the development of a therapeutic alliance. Alliance is a psychotherapeutic concept whereby the patient and clinician enter into a relationship built on the tacit or stated agreement that the clinician will partner with the patient to help solve the patient's problem. In turn, a successful alliance allows the patient to believe that they can trust the clinician. Alliances result in better clinical outcomes.[12,13] Alliances are built from the patient's past experiences with authority figures, including parents and medical providers (police and other persons in authority). Patients come with an a priori transference, either positive or negative. A patient who admires medical providers may be cooperative and appropriate. Another patient might be overly solicitous or seductive. A fearful or suspicious patient might be hostile or wary. These patients may be difficult to engage or be uncooperative because of their past experiences that are then projected onto the clinician, even though the patient may never have met the clinician. Later, this chapter introduces interviewing skills to deal with such scenarios.

Often, beginning clinicians assume an alliance prematurely[12] and move in too quickly with focused questions or comments that may break or thwart the alliance. Those types of inquiries may be perceived as challenging or confrontational. Other clinicians, particularly trainees, try to establish rapport when it is already there. When the clinician dwells too long on building the alliance, this can have the opposite effect, breaking down rapport and even angering the patient.[12] The goal of the interview is to provide enough support so that more challenging areas of exploration do not seem so threatening.[13] Another principle is to stabilize the patient before exploration.[2] This means attending to real-life concerns (e.g., ensuring that their children or belongings are safe)[14] and that acute issues such as pain or agitation are addressed.[3] If a patient asks for a particular medication, it may be best to give it to them. This is akin to the patient who comes in with a chief concern of crushing chest pain and asks for pain relief. Even if there is a suspicion of drug abuse, this is not the time to argue with the patient. Similarly, the emergency psychiatric clinician cannot insist on conducting a complete evaluation before stabilizing and rendering treatment, including pharmacotherapy.[2] Often, beginners believe they must explore before stabilization, which is a mistake in the ED.[2,3,15]

Presenting Problem and the Patient's Request

Patients come to the ED with many underlying wishes and longings. These "requests"[8] are different from the chief complaint and are frequently not verbalized. They can sometimes be communicated through body language or affective tone. For example, a patient whose chief complaint is "I'm suicidal" might have the underlying wish that the clinician uses their authority to muster up a change in the patient's situation. The *request* is "I wouldn't be suicidal if my girlfriend came back to me. Could you call her and talk to her?" (really, "persuade her to change her mind since she'll listen to you because you're the doctor"). The request may or may not be realistic or possible, but it is still important to uncover. Otherwise, the interview may reach an impasse or at the end of the exam the patient may be dissatisfied with the outcome and either leave in a huff or delay the end of the visit. Asking "What would you like to see happen here today?" early in the interview allows the clinician to address these requests. If the patient replies "I don't know," the clinician can respond that "often people have an idea of what they want accomplished in the visit. I'd like to hear what it is [even if it's not easy to talk about]" or "As we continue to talk, let's both try to figure out what it is."

The History of Present Illness and Precipitant

Using open-ended questions establishes rapport because it communicates to the patient that you want to listen to what the patient says, unlike many others in the patient's life who may not. The precipitant is useful, even necessary, to understand: Why did the patient need the emergency room *today* rather than yesterday or next week? If the patient glosses over the content too quickly or shows no affect, slow them down and develop a timeline: "First you came home, and then your daughter walked into the kitchen, etc." Watch for emerging affect, the patient's thought process and cognition. If the patient floods with affect and cannot contain themself, slow the patient down and ask about content and objective facts. If too much content is without affect, ask about the patient's feelings. Sometimes it is helpful to verbalize them for the patient: "If that happened to me, I'd be terribly upset."

Once the alliance is established, the clinician can then explore more deeply and use focused, specific questions. If you wonder whether the patient is psychotic, asking focused questions such as "Do you ever have the feeling that others are following you?" is a risk if the alliance is not adequately established. A less challenging entry to the question might be, "Do you tend to be a cautious person?" Focused questions are essential, but timing is crucial. Moving in with that type of question too soon can challenge, offend, or frighten the patient. If that happens, apologize, reestablish rapport, and resume building the alliance. Rehabilitate the interview and then later return to that question.[2]

The Rest of the Story: History of Relevance

Other elements of the psychiatric examination, such as past psychiatric, medical, family, military, and social history, may be useful to understand the current presentation. Again, collecting this information for completion sake is not the goal of the emergency evaluation. Whatever extraneous information you gather is "free information."[3]

Other interviewing techniques include summarization, clarification, interpretation, and confrontation. The latter are to be used judiciously but can be very effective. An example of an interpretation might be, "You mentioned that your mother died from stomach cancer, and you're here today with a stomachache. Do you see a connection?" Another example is, "Your boss said something so hurtful and humiliating that you wanted to disappear, so you thought about killing yourself." (This interpretation actually helped a patient reconstitute. She was no longer suicidal, realized how outrageous the boss had been, became appropriately angry, and was successfully followed in outpatient care.) The following is an example of an interpretation and a confrontation: "You had a disagreement with your boss, and now you're here having an argument with me when your beef is really with the boss. You're trying to get under my skin the way he [your boss] got under yours."

Mental Status

Aside from the patient's request, history of present illness, and collateral information, the most essential piece of the emergency exam is the mental status examination, which can also be done through careful listening, followed by a focus on areas needing clarification or exploration. For example, elements that could potentially be gathered without asking specific questions are level of arousal, motor, speech, cognition, orientation, attitude, thought process, affect, and overall mood. A nonfocused interview might even reveal the presence or absence of hallucinations, delusions, and suicidal or homicidal ideation. If not, these areas can be quickly explored.

The following case presents an interview using a biopsychosocial framework and demonstrating many of the interviewing techniques noted above.

Case Example

A 78-year-old previously healthy and active female is brought to the ED by her son, who reports an insidious decline in functioning for the past 2 months. Her husband of 52 years died from a long-term illness 8 months ago. The couple had been very devoted to each other, and the patient had cared for her husband at home. She had help, but she felt strength and purpose helping him through his last days. Following his death, the patient seemed to go through the grieving process uneventfully and after 3 months had resumed her usual activities—visiting with friends, going to the theater, and playing tennis twice a week. Although episodes of sadness and longing surfaced occasionally, they were short-lived and occurred on anniversary dates. Most of the patient's memories of her husband brought comfort and a smile. The hypotheses generated were whether there was some occult difficulty grieving the loss of her husband (psychological) or a problematic social impact (change in status to a widow, financial problems, etc.).

Approximately 2 months ago, the patient had stopped playing tennis and reported feeling too tired to join her friends for evening theater. She began sleeping more and had gained approximately 10 pounds, which she attributed to "sitting around all day." Usually a meticulous and stylish dresser, she began wearing old sweatshirts with stains. "I'm not going anywhere, so why should I dress up?" Her appetite was poor, and she complained about decreased concentration. Based on what he had read about early signs of cognitive impairment, the son was concerned that the patient was experiencing the beginning of dementia. The patient was anhedonic and anergic but was not suicidal.

The interview went as follows:

CLINICIAN: Hello Ms. Boston, I'm Sarah Brown from the Psychiatry Department. What brings you in today?
PATIENT: I've been feeling down lately. My son thought I should come in.
CLINICIAN: You've been feeling down, could you say more?
PATIENT: Not really; just don't feel like doing anything. I just sit around the house all day.
CLINICIAN: And what do you do in the house?
PATIENT: Just sit, watch television.
CLINICIAN: I understand that's very different from how you normally are. Is that right?

The patient goes on with sparse speech, but she is cooperative with the interviewer. She describes most of her neurovegetative symptoms by saying more about her day: Does she cook? No, no appetite. How's her sleep? Can't fall asleep. The interviewer asks more focused questions to fill in the information:

CLINICIAN: When you're watching television, can you keep track of the story or do you drift off?" *(The clinician is asking about concentration.)* Are there any shows that are your favorites?" (If the patient perks up and lists her favorite show, she is not pervasively anhedonic, which might rule out depression.)

Then the interviewer explores the question of complicated grief:

CLINICIAN: Your husband died 8 months ago. I'm so sorry. How has the adjustment been going?"

Again, the interviewer gleans what she can from the patient while still attending to the patient's motor activity, eye contact, production of thoughts, and affect. She listens for any psychotic material and for any memory issues as the patient tells her story in her own words.

If the patient has not mentioned particular areas that the interviewer deems relevant, the interviewer can then ask focused questions: "Did you ever think about joining him [in death]?" This question comes later in the interview so that rapport has been achieved and sustained, and the question is in context. It could have been asked in the section on neurovegetative signs ("Is the depression ever so bad that you think about killing yourself?"), but knowing that many bereaved persons consider joining their loved ones, the interviewer waited until this area was explored. The clinician can ask directly about any social fallout from the husband's death—financial problems or concerns about selling her house. Are couples' friends pulling away now that she is single? The psychosocial aspects of this patient's presentation have been carefully explored, as well as the biological component of a clinical depression. Thus far, the patient appears to have a clinical depression. The bereavement has been unremarkable without evidence of avoidance or impaired functioning, and there are no financial or other social issues that concern the patient. She has ample funds, is comfortable in her current home, and has maintained her friendships.

The interviewer also considers other potential medical possibilities, not yet accepting the conclusion that this patient has a clinical depression. She has noticed that the patient's skin is dry and flaky, and her face is plethoric. The patient has little psychomotor movement, except for an occasional rubbing of her arms because she is cold. Her unwashed hair is also sparse. Is there an underlying medical condition that has not been picked up in the medical clearance? The interviewer thus asks about her medical history and family medical history. The patient has no active medical problems other than well-controlled hypertension for which she has taken the same antihypertensive for years. Her son interrupts and says that the patient also has hypothyroidism, but there is no mention of this medication on the triage note. The son states that this is an example of the patient's forgetfulness. The patient suddenly looks up and says,

> Oh, I forgot to refill my thyroid prescription! I noticed that I was running low and had a reminder to call my doctor, but that was the day the patio deck collapsed. I was so focused on that, that I never called the doctor for the refill. I've been off my thyroid medication for the past 3 months. Could that be the problem?

A thyroid-stimulating hormone test confirmed hypothyroidism, and the patient was restarted on levothyroxine.

The patient's mental status change was a result of hypothyroidism. She indeed sounded as though she was grieving her husband appropriately. A biopsychosocial emergency evaluation was complete. Estimated time: 20 minutes.

Types of Patients: Interviewing Techniques and Tips

The Overtalkative Patient

For the overtalkative patient, displaying circumstantial or tangential thinking, the interviewer needs to focus more. For example, "Before you talk about Y, let's go back to X." This tells the patient that you have been listening and want to help them organize the information. This may have to be done several times until you either have the information needed or determine that the patient cannot provide it. For example, "Let's go back to what you said about your experience with [X medication]. What were the side effects?" If the patient goes off in another area, "It all started when I went to the doctor" (who prescribed the medication, etc.), the interviewer can interrupt and say, "But I was asking specifically about side effects? Did you have nausea?" Hypotheses can be generated about the reason for the circumstantial thinking: Is there some cognitive decline? Is there a thought disorder? Is this an example of an obsessional style or distancing way of relating? Is the patient purposely being vague?

If the patient rushes through the narrative—"I had a fight with my mother, and she called the cops"—slow it down and get the time sequence. This helps both you and the patient see the event more objectively and helps you determine if the patient can think in temporal sequence. "Let's go back; walk me through what happened. I want a picture in my head as to what happened."

The Silent Patient

The patient may be silent out of fear, suspicion, defiance, or deference to authority figures. If mute, consider dissociation or catatonia, which can suddenly burst into catatonic excitement. You will need to quickly sense what the problem is by gaining clues from collateral information and nursing staff who have already seen the patient.

Comment on their silence and ask, "What is going on?" You can think out loud and suggest that "silence has many meanings—fear . . . anger . . . defiance . . . shock . . . or exhaustion. Do any of them fit your situation?" If the patient continues to be silent, ask if they would like juice or food. Asking about sleep, or whether they are cold or too warm, can break the ice. Would they like some medication? These are nonthreatening questions that good mothers and good doctors ask. If the patient continues to be silent, excuse yourself and tell the patient when you will return. You may need to return several times, but something will declare itself at some point.

For the suspicious or fearful patient, tell them that you are there to help. Do not make any quick motions and tell them exactly what you are doing, even if you are just sitting down. "I'm going to sit here; you can have a seat over there. We're both going to have access to the door. . . . You look frightened; can you tell me if that's the case?" If you do not want to give the patient the impression that you can "read their mind," you can share your feelings: "I'm feeling uneasy/nervous/frightened in here?" If you are truly in fear, appeal to the patient's wish to be in control: "I'm feeling frightened; should I leave the room? Should I be worried about my safety in here?" Even a suspicious patient might well relax more if the interviewer shares the patient's feelings. I have often seen a curious glance after I have said this to a patient. If the patient tells you to get out, do so. Do not try to exercise your authority now. The patient is telling you that they have tenuous control, and this is a warning to you. Leave and get help. You can go back with help and ask the patient if there is something you can do to help them feel calmer. "Perhaps some medication? What has worked for you in the past?" This tells the patient that you are not going to use your authority to control them but to collaborate with them and value their recommendations. If the patient reassures you that you are safe, you need to determine if you believe it. If not, you may state, "I still don't feel comfortable. I'm going to leave the room right now" (and get out of the room quickly, but do not turn your back because the patient might attack from behind). If you believe the patient, then you can gently begin the interview, trying to build rapport and an alliance. "Can you tell me what you're feeling? Can you tell me what happened that you're here?" or "My notes say that the police brought you in after your mother called 911; what happened?"

The Paranoid or Psychotic Patient

Paranoid patients may interpret empathic or sympathetic statements as pity. They fear that their power will be diminished. They are frightened and offended by this level of intimacy. They are not used to people being kind to them unless there is a price to pay. Staying neutral yet kindly is the best strategy. A paranoid patient also has a strong grandiose streak: Why else would aliens choose him over others? You can speak to that with a less challenging question, "Wow, that's quite a burden to be chosen and to receive all this negative attention." You are allying with both the grandiosity and the undesired attention. "How did these people land on you [to be] the brunt of their anger?" It can diffuse tension and help build the alliance.

The Suicidal Patient

If the patient has been talking about all the stress in their life, you can determine the patient's state of hopelessness by reflecting and asking, "You've been dealing with so much, how do you keep going? What gives you hope?" Or ask, "What matters to you most?"[16] Here, you are assessing protective factors without having to resort to pat questions such as "Who's your support?" That type of question can be off-putting: "Don't pull that shrink talk on me!" Instead, ask, "What has kept you from actually getting the pills [for an overdose]?" This will assess the patient's impulse control. Sometimes there is another affect underneath the suicidal urge: "I see how despairing you are, but I'm wondering if you're also angry about this?" If the patient can mobilize their anger and see that they are not trapped without any other options but suicide, it might obviate the need for hospitalization. Another example: "With all this stress, do you ever think of ending it all? Or "Some people in your situation would feel trapped and think about suicide. . . . How about you? Have you thought about it?" These questions can glean more than the cryptic "Are you suicidal?" that may not be answered truthfully.

For the patient who cannot express their feelings, sharing one's own reaction can normalize feelings and teach the patient that these are human emotions. "When you're talking about what you've been through, I feel very sad. . . . Is that how you feel? Is it possible that I'm feeling the sadness that you can't [aren't]?"

The Grandiose Manic Patient

Underlying the grandiosity of a manic patient is one who unconsciously believes that he has little merit. You need to ally with the grandiosity. Allow them to tell you how grand they are. "How do you sleep doing all the [creative/important] things you are doing? You sound quite [energetic/busy/productive/pressured] to work as fast as you can/in need of getting your ideas out quickly because of their importance."

Manic patients dislike an interviewer who is not as fast as they are. They may be perturbed that the interviewer is not following their train of thought quickly enough and may accuse the interviewer of being "stupid." Acknowledge this: "'I'm sorry I'm not keeping up with you, and it is frustrating when I'm so slow, but please try to put up with me, OK?"

The Personality Disordered Patient

The personality disordered patient has ingrained patterns of behavior that the patient uses to get what they needs or wants.[3] The patient does not know any other way of behaving. It is worth remembering this because the personality disordered patient can seem as irrational as a psychotic patient and test the patience of even the most skilled interviewer.

Narcissistic patients have a lack of self-esteem, but it is difficult to sympathize with that part of them when you are being assaulted by their narcissism. Ally with the narcissism as best you can:

> I understand that you have reasons to believe that [an opiate] is what you need right now, and that you are in tremendous pain, but unfortunately I don't agree with your conclusion so I will not be able to prescribe that. But how about [Y]?

If the patient tries to wear you down, repeat your decision one last time and then (with Security if necessary) back out of the room. Do not get pulled into the patient's attempts to wear you down and pressure or frighten you into giving them something that is not warranted.

The borderline patient in crisis may be hostile or agitated. Interviewing techniques for the agitated patient are discussed below. It is worth remembering that their emotional dysregulation is often the result of impaired attachment due to childhood neglect or trauma. Knowing this can help the clinician feel sympathy for the patient, which helps the clinician be more empathic.

The Agitated, Hostile, or Uncooperative Patient

Much has been written about verbal de-escalation of the agitated patient and the different presentations of agitation.[3,17] Agitation falls on a spectrum that can move from anxiety all the way to violence. The patient's attitude toward the examiner can become the whole focus of engagement and makes establishing rapport and understanding the problem challenging.

A patient must be cooperative for the evaluation to take place. To calm a patient, offer creature comforts such as food, a drink, or blankets. Ask the patient if there is a medication they use when this upset. This gives the patient control. Listen for real-life issues that can be solved: calling a friend to care for a pet or securing the patient's belongings before they are discarded.[3] Acknowledge and normalize feelings. Agree with what you can and agree to disagree with what you cannot. An example is the patient who is angry because he needed to wait a long time to be seen. Without getting into explanations, a simple "I don't like to wait either" acknowledges the patient's grievance and normalizes the feeling. Keeping the interview brief, taking time-outs, and returning for another short exchange even several times may be preferable.[3] Emergency work requires flexibility and creativity.

Another approach is to reveal one's own emotional reaction in a judicious manner. (See Vignette 1.3.) The patient who is perturbing the clinician should be met with an interpretation or even a confrontation, which needs to be said without any trace of a punitive or angry tone: "I feel like I'm being dragged into a fight with you. Is this what happened this morning when you tried to drive the other car off the road?" Another approach might be, "I'm feeling annoyed by this conversation, and need to step out to calm down so that we don't end up arguing." The patient might be surprised and sometimes aghast that the clinician is impacted by what the patient is saying. Many boisterous or argumentative patients believe that loudness and pushiness are the only way they can have impact; otherwise, it is as though they do not exist, let alone being taken into consideration. This self-disclosure models appropriate management of feelings. If the patient is aghast and says, "You're the doctor, you're not supposed to get mad," the response can be that you are human and have feelings too. Self-disclosure can be extremely useful in the emergency interview and does not have to compromise the clinician's authority. It must be used judiciously. None of these techniques are useful when the clinician has already become furious with the patient. Recognizing when one is *becoming* or *on the way* to being annoyed or angry is when to use these techniques.

Fishkind[3-5] outlines 10 rules or "domains" that go into an interaction with a volatile patient to de-escalate the situation. They are summarized in Box 1.1.

Box 1.1 Fishkind's Principles of Verbal De-Escalation

Respect the patient's personal space.
Don't be provocative or authoritarian.
Establish verbal contact.
Be concise.
Identify wants and feelings; the patient's "request."
Listen closely to what the patient is saying.
Agree with what you can or agree to disagree.
"Lay down the law" and set clear limits in neutral tone.
Offer choices and optimism.
Debrief the patient and staff.

Adapted from Fishkind.[4,5]

Vignettes 1.1–1.3 provide examples of interviews with an agitated, hostile patient that demonstrate some skills to use to diffuse a tense situation.

Vignette 1.1

Security is outside patient's room.

CLINICIAN: Hi, I'm Doctor Green from Psychiatry.
PATIENT: Oh great, now the shrinks are here. You new here? Never seen you before.
CLINICIAN: Yeah new to this ER, but not new to psychiatry or emergency rooms. *(Clinician is not threatened by the patient's hostility and implication that the clinician is a beginner. She briefly responds to the question and then moves to the issue at hand.)* So why don't we talk about what happened that you ended up here. It doesn't look like you wanted to be here.

Vignette 1.2

Another potential scenario, same patient.

PATIENT: I don't want to see shrinks you're not coming near me get the F out of here!*(The patient is shrieking, waving his hands. Security is on standby. The clinician attempts to establish verbal contact, but it is not possible. The clinician asks what he would like to see happen in the ED.)*
PATIENT: None of your business.
CLINICIAN: Really? But you're angry here in the emergency room so it is my business.
PATIENT: Then I just don't want to talk to you. But if I did, I would tell you to get away from me. I would tell you that I'll never talk to you! I'll never say a word in this place! I want out of here! You hear me you *x*x. *(The patient escalates with insults but remains in behavioral control.)*
CLINICIAN: Is there anything that would help you feel calmer? Some juice? A blanket? Is there any medication that might help take the edge off?
PATIENT: No.
CLINICIAN: Well, let's take a break and I'll come back and hopefully you can talk to me. *(The clinician does not suspect psychosis; the patient appears to be able to remain in behavioral control. Taking breaks can be useful as long as the patient is being watched. Breaks help decrease the potential for argument between clinician and patient, and they give some time for the patient to cool down and perhaps then be able to put into words what he is so intensely feeling.)*

Vignette 1.3

Another scenario, same patient. The patient draws the interviewer into an argument.

CLINICIAN: We really do need to take a break I'm getting annoyed.

PATIENT: What d'ya mean *you're* getting annoyed? *You're* the doctor! You're not supposed to get mad!

CLINICIAN: Yeah, I'm the doctor but I've got feelings too. I want to be treated with respect the same way you want to be treated with respect.

Clinician returns.

CLINICIAN: Any calmer?

PATIENT: Yeah, How about you? *(Note patient is curious how the clinician feels.)*

CLINICIAN: Yeah, I'm fine. I'm fine now. I was getting annoyed earlier. [And no, I'm not angry anymore because I had a chance to cool down. That was a useful way of dealing with anger.]

PATIENT: Yeah sometimes I do that to people. You know, you're the first doctor who ever told me that [I was annoying them]. *(Alliance formed through clinician's earlier self-disclosure.)*

CLINICIAN: Really? Why do you think so? *(The clinician can now explore.)*

PATIENT: They're scared of me.

CLINICIAN: Oh, what do you do that's so scary? *(Further exploration but now the patient is not defensive.)*

The patient tells the interviewer that he scared his sister by threatening to set the house on fire.

CLINICIAN: Ahh, she thought you might actually do it? Do you think that was a possibility? *(Clinician can ask about the patient's impulsivity and likelihood of doing harm.)*

In this scenario, the clinician is flexible but at the same time firm and respectful. She tells the patient the conditions with which she will continue to engage with him (her "working conditions")[18] or "laying down the law."[4,5] She has set these conditions in a respectful but firm manner. She is clear about the need for safety and civility; she is willing to be flexible and take breaks yet remains firm regarding acceptable behavior. She uses self-disclosure to facilitate alliance building and to help the patient feel that he is among other humans—not at the mercy of rigid authority.

Countertransference: When the Patient Pushes Your Buttons—Pitfalls and Mistakes

Working with patients in behavioral or emotional emergencies inevitably gives rise to countertransference reactions.[2,3,13,15] Countertransference feelings are important and should not be ignored. This helps the clinician avoid acting out and also to better understand the patient. Although unchecked countertransference feelings need to be contained, countertransference can be a good diagnostic tool and working within it is useful.

Some patients are provocative. They may project their hostility onto the clinician by insulting, bullying, threatening, or questioning the clinician's authority, credentials, competence, age, or even personality, appearance, gender, or race. Some may be seductive and attempt to ingratiate or bully the clinician to give them something that they want. Other patients may touch on the therapist's own losses or reawaken memories of one's own traumas. At these times, the clinician needs to feel the affect, empathize with the patient, acknowledge their own feelings, and then pull back and reengage the intellect: "What hypothesis does this information generate?" "How can I use this information and my feelings to better understand and respond to the patient appropriately?" There is also the need to be aware of both implicit and overt bias that all clinicians bring to clinical encounters.[19]

It is worth noting that countertransference responses are not always negative. One can identify with a patient, and that can help build rapport. At other times, overidentification is problematic. Whatever the response, recognizing the feelings and being able to use them effectively increases the chance of an alliance.

Avoiding Interviewing Mistakes

Mistakes happen to the best clinicians. Patients do forgive us when they sense that we have their best interests in mind. Hilfiker[20] poignantly discusses a case in which a terrible mistake was made and the parents of a lost pregnancy forgave the doctor when he could not forgive himself.

Perhaps the biggest fear of the psychiatric clinician is that a patient released from the ED will commit suicide. No clinician or screening scale can predict suicide. However, a climate of total risk aversion infantilizes the patient and can create iatrogenic dependency on the emergency and hospital system. It teaches patients that they are not in charge of their own lives but that clinicians are in charge. Kernberg reminds us that good treatment comes with risk. The goal is to minimize that risk, not eliminate it. Chapter 4 discusses the suicidal patient in greater detail, and Chapter 21 focuses on high-acuity risk assessment.

As noted above, interpreting prematurely, not setting limits, and insufficient backup are problematic. Confrontation can be a useful technique but must be used judiciously.

Impatience and lack of time usually disrupt the alliance. Rushing in too quickly with focused questions may cause the patient to feel challenged or accused. Apologize, pull back to less affect-laden topics, and then later return to the charged area to determine if the patient is now willing to talk about it. "Can we go back to . . .?" As noted previously, the opposite is also true: Dwelling too long on building an alliance when one has already been formed can annoy the patient and have the opposite effect.

Interpreting prematurely or assuming that you know how the patient is feeling can also be problematic. Thus, "you must feel very sad about the death of your mother" might be met with "Are you crazy? I hated her! You're not listening to me!" This is an example of an empathic failure.

Emergency rooms or any medical encounter can induce shame.[21] Patients who feel ashamed or humiliated will not easily form an alliance. It is my view that humiliation can be as traumatic as any tangible event and can severely decenter a person. Again, a trauma-informed approach helps decrease the likelihood that such an error will occur.

Confrontation can be a useful technique but must be used judiciously so as not to be punitive or humiliating. When the patient has successfully managed to anger you, there

---

Box 1.2 Avoiding Interviewing Mistakes

Safety
Lack of adequate backup staff
Trying to engage the patient when the patient tells you to get out of the room
Alliance
Failing to be trauma-informed
Assuming an alliance prematurely
Asking direct questions that may be challenging too soon in the interview
Dwelling too long on establishing an alliance when one already exists
Trying to dissuade a fixed belief or a delusion
Inadvertently humiliating the patient
Making assumptions/empathic failures
Clinician's Attitude and Behavior
Arguing with the patient
Being judgmental, provocative, or argumentative
Setting limits when one is angry/being punitive or threatening
Impatience and time pressure

Adapted from Richmond.[7]

---

is a tendency to lapse into irrational thinking along with the patient. A neutral tone is best, as is having Security behind you to enforce the limit: "If you try to leave the ED, Security will stop you."[2,3]

Box 1.2 outlines some common interviewing mistakes.

Secondary Traumatization and Burnout

Emergency work can be exhilarating, but much trauma and loss pass through the average ED. Witnessing and experiencing chronic exposure to trauma can bruise any clinician, even experienced ones. Identifying with a patient's grief or sense of horror can also be painful for the clinician. The more exposure to trauma, the more potential for the development of stress-related disorders. It is referred to in the literature as secondary traumatization, vicarious traumatization, or compassion fatigue.[22]

The skilled clinician understands this type of constant exposure is an occupational hazard; it can be treated, leading to increased resiliency and empathy. Decreasing exposure by having some designated time for administrative or other clinical duties outside of the ED is recommended. Debriefings with other ED staff about difficult patients is a good idea, despite the inherent time problems. It is well worth it to carve out a regular time to meet, even over lunch.

Secondary traumatization is different from burnout because it is not the result of excessive exposure to traumatic events but, rather, to medical systems that do not support their staff, issue unreasonable demands on clinicians' time, and even make demands that the clinician may experiences as a "moral injury."[22,23] Whereas secondary traumatization includes a personal sense of failure, social isolation, intrusive thoughts of the traumatic event, and even a sense of moral injury, burnout leads to cynicism, disillusionment, irritability, and anger.[22]

A Word About Temperament

There is an emerging literature describing the unique skill sets and temperament best suited for emergency psychiatry work.[14,24,25] The temperament of the successful emergency psychiatric clinician is that of an authentic, flexible clinician who possesses advanced interviewing skills. The clinician should be nondefensive, able to use countertransference skillfully, spontaneous but judicious with self-disclosure, and able to tolerate ambiguity. The clinician must be comfortable making rapid and accurate clinical decisions with limited information and thrive in an environment that can be chaotic. In addition, the clinician needs to be authoritative without being authoritarian[2] and have a strong understanding of medical illnesses, particularly those that can present as behavioral emergencies.[14]

Although ED work is not the same as doing psychotherapy, psychotherapeutic theory is often called upon for diagnostic purposes and treatment of crises. A psychodynamic and object relations theoretical base can assist in alliance building. Understanding the underlying dynamics of the patient's situation can inform outcome and even risk assessments.

Conclusion

This chapter gives the beginning emergency psychiatry clinician theory and tools to conduct an effective emergency interview. The use of self is essential, and being direct and flexible enables the building and sustaining of an alliance. This chapter offers a different paradigm for the emergency interview by thinking less in terms of narrow diagnostic categories and using a broader, more comprehensive model that allows for establishing rapport and building alliances.

References

1. Thrasher T. The field as a master class in interviewing. *Psychiatric Times*. January 29, 2021.

2. Berlin JS. Collaborative de-escalation. In: Zeller SL, Nordstrom KD, Wilson MP, eds. *The Diagnosis and Management of Agitation*. Cambridge University Press; 2017:144–155.

3. Richmond JS, Berlin JS, Fishkind AB, et al. Verbal de-escalation of the agitated patient: Consensus statement of the American Association for Emergency Psychiatry Project BETA De-escalation Workgroup. *West J Emerg Med*. 2012;13(1):17–25.

4. Fishkind A. Agitation II: De-escalation of the aggressive patient and avoiding coercion. In: Glick RL, Berlin JS, Fishkind AB, Zeller SL, eds. *Emergency Psychiatry Principles and Practice*. Wolters Kluwer; 2008:125–136.

5. Fishkind A. Calming agitation with words not drugs. *Curr Psychiatry*. 2002;1(4):32–40.

6. Berlin JS. The modern emergency psychiatry interview. In: Zun LS, Nordstrom K, Wilson MP, eds. *Behavioral Emergencies for Healthcare Providers*. Springer; 2021:39–47. https://doi.org/10.1007/978-3-030-52520-0_3

7. Richmond JS. De-escalation in the emergency department. In: Zun LS, Nordstrom K, Wilson MP, eds. *Behavioral Emergencies for Healthcare Providers*. Springer; 2021:221–229. https://doi.org/10.1007/978-3-030-52520-0_21

8. Lazare A, Eisenthal S, Wasserman L. The customer approach to patienthood. Attending to patient requests in a walk-in clinic. *Arch Gen Psychiatry*. 1975;32(5):553–558.

9. Cardoso Zoppe EHC, Schoueri P, Castro M, Neto FL. Teaching psychodynamics to psychiatric residents through psychiatric outpatient interviews. *Acad Psychiatry*. 2009;33(1):51–55.

10. Lazare A. The psychiatric examination in the walk-in clinic. Hypothesis generation and hypothesis testing. *Arch Gen Psychiatry*. 1976;33(1):96–102.

11. Engel GL. The need for a new medical model: A challenge for biomedicine. *Science*. 1977;196(4286):129–136.

12. Kleespies P, Richmond JS. Evaluating behavior emergencies: The clinical interview. In: Kleespies P, ed. *Behavioral emergencies: An evidence-based resource for evaluating and managing risk of suicide, violence, and victimization*. American Psychological Association; 2009:33–55.

13. Rosenberg RC. Advanced interviewing techniques. In: Glick RL, Zeller S, Berlin JS, eds. 2nd ed. Wolters Kluwer; 2021:85–92.

14. Richmond JS, Dragatsi D, Stiebel V, Rozel JS, Rasimus JJ. American Association for Emergency Psychiatry Recommendations to Address Psychiatric Staff Shortages in Emergency Settings. *Psychiatr Serv*. 2021;72(4):437–443.

15. Berlin JS, Gudeman J. Interviewing for acuity and the acute precipitant. In: Glick RL, Berlin JS, Fishkind AB, Zeller SL, eds. *Emergency Psychiatry: Principles and Practice*. Lippincott Williams & Wilkins; 2008:100–102.

16. Meltzer B. 2020.

17. Zeller SL, Nordstrom K, Wilson MP. *The Diagnosis and Management of Agitation*. Cambridge University Press; 2017.

18. Pearlman CA. 1998.

19. Agboola IK, Coupet E Jr, Wong AH. "The coats that we can take off and the ones we can't": The role of trauma-informed care on race and bias during agitation in the emergency department. *Ann Emerg Med*. 2021;77(5):493–498.

20. Hilfiker D. Facing our mistakes. *N Engl J Med*. 1984;310(2):118–122.

21. Lazare A. Shame and humiliation in the medical encounter. *Arch Intern Med*. 1987;147(9):1653–1658.

22. Richmond JS. Loss and trauma. In: Glick RL, Zeller SL, Berlin JS, eds. *Emergency Psychiatry: Principles and Practice*. 2nd ed. Wolters Kluwer; 2021::287–298.

23. Litz BT, Stein N, Delaney E, et al. Moral injury and moral repair in war veterans: A preliminary model and intervention strategy. *Clin Psychol Rev*. 2009;29(8):695–706.

24. Brasch J, Glick RL, Cobb TG, Richmond J. Residency training in emergency psychiatry: A model curriculum developed by the Education Committee of the American Association for Emergency Psychiatry. *Acad Psychiatry*. 2004;28(2):95–103.

25. Richmond JS, Glick RL, Dragatsi DD. Supervision of ancillary personnel. In: Fitz-Gerald MJ, Takeshita J, eds. *Models of Emergency Psychiatric Services That Work: Integrating Psychiatry and Primary Care*. Springer; 2020:135–142. https://doi.org/10.1007/978-3-030-50808-1_13

2

Evaluating and Managing the Agitated Patient

Victor Hong, Jennifer Baumhauer, and Stephen Leung

Introduction

The management of agitation is one of the most challenging and stressful elements of psychiatric emergency care, both for trainees and for more experienced clinicians and staff. It is crucial to comprehend all the components of agitation because it may portend a life-threatening emergency and can lead to physical aggression and harm to self and others. There has been a significant evolution in the understanding and treatment of agitation that is briefly reviewed here. However, the primary goal of this chapter is to provide practical tools to utilize in the management of agitation, from early recognition to skills for handling severe aggression. Case vignettes are included to highlight various types of agitation, each with its own nuances and challenges. The chapter first provides background information about clinical agitation. Then it discusses how to optimally assess an agitated patient, and it offers a guide for verbal de-escalation, medication-based, and physical interventions. Because pediatric agitation necessitates its own specialized approach, see Chapter 15 for further details.

Background

Agitation is defined as a state of excessive psychomotor activity and irritability. It is best understood on a spectrum, from the initial phase of having a rising, uncomfortable feeling to overt physical aggression. Agitation is common (~2.6% prevalence)[1] in medical emergency settings, and it is even more prevalent in psychiatric emergency settings.[2]

The challenges associated with managing agitation result partly from the variety and complexity of its etiologies. As such, it is helpful to consider agitation as a symptom or collection of symptoms, which then shifts the clinical focus to identifying its cause rather than merely treating the symptom.[3] When a concerted effort was made to standardize the management of agitation for Project BETA (Best Practices in the Evaluation and Treatment of Agitation), it was discovered that traditionally, management of agitation was largely a one-size-fits-all approach, in which medications were the focus of treatment, typically a first-generation antipsychotic being utilized along with a benzodiazepine.[4] The majority of the time, the etiology of the agitation was not taken into account.

It has come into clearer focus that indeed etiology should inform the clinical approach to agitation. There can be psychiatric, medical, substance-related, psychosocial, and other causes of agitation, each requiring a specific approach grounded in some general underlying principles. For example, patients with borderline personality disorder may respond well to verbal de-escalation; those with acute psychosis may require medication management; those with delirium need an emergent medical workup; those with dementia may benefit from a reduction in stimulation; and so on.

Early Intervention

When discussing agitation, recommendations often bypass the pre-assessment—that is, what the clinician does prior to evaluating the patient. It is important, when possible, to gather information that could potentially be helpful, which means the assessment of agitation ideally begins before meeting the patient. Reviewing the medical record to understand a patient's medical and psychiatric history, use of substances, medication regimen, and allergies is a helpful preamble to evaluation. Knowledge of a past history of violent aggression is key to factor into your assessment of risk for violence. Communication with law enforcement personnel, outpatient clinicians, family members, and ambulance staff is crucial in developing an awareness of the context of the patient's visit. Were they physically aggressive in the community? Have they shown signs of delirium or intoxication? What is the timeline of events? A well-run, collaborative system helps enable these pre-discussions to occur, with the physical environment and layout of the emergency setting, staffing model, and workflow all geared toward the prevention and management of agitation. An ideal setting is quiet, with less intense lighting, a stable and comfortable temperature, and immobile furniture. Certainly, training staff in the management of acute agitation is crucial. System development or optimization, physical space design, and training methods are considerations beyond the scope of this chapter.

When available, the nursing triage assessment can provide valuable information, with vital signs, the nurse's observations, and chief complaint all illuminating the situation at hand. Initiating the assessment without first speaking to the nurse who conducted the triage is a common pitfall because the patient could be agitated to the point of presenting imminent danger, and one could miss crucial information to guide the interview.

Another aspect of the evaluation that is central to clinical management of patients with agitation is the garnering of information from collateral informants, whether parents or other loved ones, friends, roommates, nursing or group home staff, or outpatient providers. For the individual who is not adequately able or willing to communicate due to their mental state, these sources of information may prove more reliable than the patient.

Then comes the assessment of the patient, which certainly includes the clinical interview. Because those who are acutely agitated are often poor historians, the mental status exam emerges as a powerful tool and often is the crux of the evaluation. The patient's appearance can provide clues as to what they were doing before coming to the emergency setting or if they are aware of the weather. Their behavior affords the clinician a wealth of information before the individual even says a word, whether they are pacing or wildly gesticulating or have their fists clenched. Their speech can be pressured or loud. They can in some cases verbally express how angry, irritable, or agitated they are, and for others their mood can be inferred. Their affect can display their true emotions regardless of what is said. A disorganized thought process can be a window into the patient's inability to understand their environment, process what is being communicated to them, and control their impulses. If an individual has paranoia or is responding to internal stimuli, their risk of violence is significantly elevated.

Patients exhibiting signs of agitation should be evaluated as expeditiously as possible. Acute agitation must be triaged and treated as an emergency requiring immediate action. With each passing minute, agitation can worsen, safety can become more compromised, and the need for physical management becomes more likely. Delays to care can lead to patient or staff injuries, the inability to treat a potentially life-threatening condition, and increase the distress of all involved. It follows that early recognition of the signs of acute or impending agitation is central to early intervention (Figure 2.1).

Providers should recognize and manage their own emotions when approaching patients with symptoms of agitation. Fear and distress are common reactions and, if unchecked, can lead to hostility, avoidance, and the mismanagement of care. It is important to recognize that although some clinicians can tolerate interactions with agitated patients seemingly better than others, no one is entirely comfortable in these situations. It is normal to be scared, even traumatized by these incidents, and seeking support from colleagues and supervisors is highly recommended. This issue reinforces why an organized, collaborative approach is helpful, as are repetition and experience, which inform one's instincts and hone skills. With time, the ability to stay relatively calm and rationally process the ideal next steps can develop.

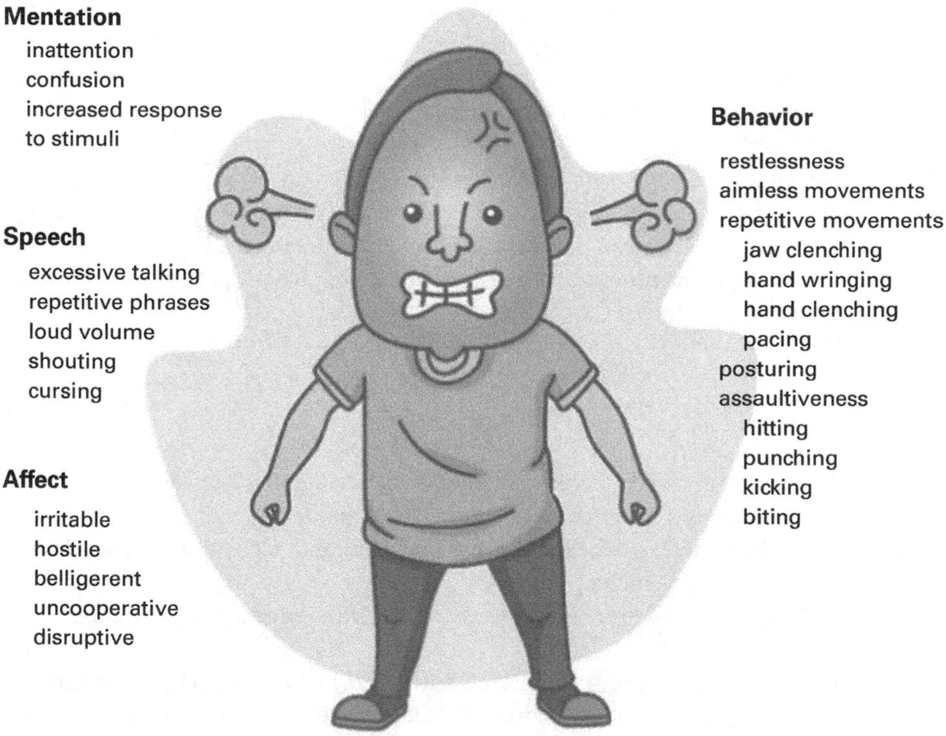

Mentation
   inattention
   confusion
   increased response
   to stimuli

Speech
   excessive talking
   repetitive phrases
   loud volume
   shouting
   cursing

Affect
   irritable
   hostile
   belligerent
   uncooperative
   disruptive

Behavior
   restlessness
   aimless movements
   repetitive movements
      jaw clenching
      hand wringing
      hand clenching
      pacing
      posturing
   assaultiveness
      hitting
      punching
      kicking
      biting

Figure 2.1 Signs and symptoms of agitation.

Maintenance of Safety

"Safety first" is a central tenet of optimal management of agitation. When indicated, and when available, utilizing trained security personnel as support during evaluation is strongly recommended. Clinicians' feelings of anxiety, shame, and fragility in requesting additional support, although common, must be managed and overcome in the emergency setting in favor of engaging in the safest possible practice. If security personnel are unavailable, an increased number of respondents, including other clinical staff members, may be indicated.

Giving the agitated individual adequate physical space significantly mitigates the potential for an assault to occur, with a general rule being two arm's length distance,[5] but in some cases, even more space is indicated. Scanning the room for any objects that could be used as a projectile or weapon is another important step, as is positioning yourself in a way such that either you as the evaluator or the patient can quickly exit the room if needed. Although these represent long-standing best practices, they require repetition and rehearsal because in the often chaotic acute emergency setting, one can be harried and distracted from these safety steps. If it is clear that the proposed area for the interview is not adequately safe, one should seek a more appropriate environment, if available, such as a room in which seclusion or restraint is possible. Because each emergency setting has variable availability of rooms/areas, the clinician must gain an awareness of all of the options and the unit's protocols.

How one behaves physically with an agitated patient can also contribute to optimizing safety. Maintaining an open posture with one's hands visible can help mitigate the potential of the patient believing something is being hidden from them, such as a weapon. Touching an agitated patient, even in a supportive manner, is rarely indicated and often can trigger a violent response. Eye contact needs to be causal and not too intense so as to avoid the nonverbal communication that this is a confrontation.

The issue of utilizing one's "gut feeling" has been raised, to sense impending danger. Although there is certainly not empirical evidence to support a practice of relying solely on one's intuition, it can be a valuable tool. If a clinician feels quite uncomfortable or scared, it may be time to change the approach or give the patient more time to de-escalate.

Verbal De-Escalation

Although identification of the etiology of the patient's agitation is a primary goal, verbal de-escalation remains a first-line intervention for agitation regardless of the cause. Verbal de-escalation skills can be learned and practiced, and they are critical to safe and productive clinical engagement.

Project BETA identified four main objectives in working with agitated patients:[5]

1. Ensuring the safety of the patient, staff, and others in the immediate environment
2. Empowering the patient to manage distress and emotions in an effort to regain control of their behavior
3. Avoiding usage of seclusion or restraint
4. Reducing the risk of further escalation of agitation

Although previous history of agitation and violence is pertinent to assessing the patient's propensity for further episodes of violence, the signs and symptoms actively displayed by the patient in real time are certainly most indicative of violent outcomes. Several objective scales, including the Behavioural Activity Rating Scale, have been increasingly employed by staff in emergency settings to assess the level agitation on presentation.[6] These scales utilize objective signs related to a point system, resulting in a score indicating mild, moderate, or severe agitation. Use of these tools helps standardize and reduce subjectivity of the assessment and can create a shared language among staff. Although ideal, verbal de-escalation may not always be an available choice if agitation is severe.

The optimal approach to verbal de-escalation requires preparation. The safety measures mentioned previously (e.g., ensuring that the physical space is as safe as possible, ensuring that adequate staffing support is present, conducting a multidisciplinary pre-discussion, and contingency planning) can offer a good context in which to initiate verbal de-escalation. Once environmental and personal safety has been optimized, the clinician can engage the patient, attempt to establish a collaborative relationship, and implement de-escalation techniques.

The following case illustrates core principles of successful verbal de-escalation.

Case Example

Mr. O is a 27-year-old male with a history of depression who presents for suicidal ideation. After careful evaluation, he is believed to warrant inpatient hospitalization for safety and stabilization despite his desire to go home. He has never been hospitalized before. Several minutes after being told of this decision, a nurse expresses concern about Mr. O's state, noting he is pacing the room, loudly mumbling to himself, and repeatedly requesting to speak with someone.

Observations from the nurse raise concern for escalating agitation in the setting of involuntary hospitalization. Behind the scenes, the team prepares for engagement, alerting appropriate support and security staff of the situation while choosing one individual to lead the encounter. They discuss potential scenarios, including what to do if Mr. O's agitation escalates. The chosen team leader then enters the patient's room, respecting Mr. O's personal space, maintaining appropriate distance, and aware of his own body language and tone of voice. The provider knows it is rarely helpful to raise one's own voice in such cases.

DR. X: Hello Mr. O, I'm Dr. X, the psychiatrist you spoke to earlier. Your nurse informed me that you wished to speak again.

MR. O: (pacing, wringing hands, speaking quickly) Yes, I need to go home, I came in for referrals, and now I'm being held here, I just need to go home, this isn't happening.

DR. X: I understand your preference is to leave the hospital, but at this time that is not an option due to concerns for your safety.

MR. O: (yelling) I can't, I'll be fine, I don't need to be in the hospital! I'm not going into the hospital!

DR. X: I know it must be frustrating to feel like your preferences aren't being heard. But our goal is the same as yours: to keep you safe, which is why we feel you need to spend some time in the hospital.

When verbally engaging an agitated patient, it is paramount to remember they can have difficulty processing information and become easily confused. The primary communicator should use basic, concise phrases and repeat themself when necessary to convey important points and set limits. Giving the patient sufficient time to process new information is also important. Throughout the interaction, Dr. X attempts to identify and reflect the patient's wants and feelings, listening actively to what the patient is saying and making supportive comments.

MR. O: (sits down, exasperated, still talking loudly) I can't believe this is happening to me, my friend came to the hospital with the same problems, and she left with a therapist! That's all I need, I should be able to leave too!

DR. X: I believe anyone who came in expecting referrals and finding they were being hospitalized would feel the same as you: upset and maybe even frightened. We do believe it is necessary for your safety at this time.

Although the patient and physician disagree on the intervention needed at this time (hospitalization), finding some agreement, whether through facts, principle, or odds of the situation, helps validate and enhance the therapeutic alliance. Note that Dr. X still maintains that hospitalization is necessary.

MR. O: (hitting his head with his hands, then jumping up and posturing towards the physician) I JUST DON'T WANT TO BE HOSPITALIZED!

DR. X: (backing away slightly) Mr. O., I understand this is upsetting for you, but your behavior now is scaring me and the other staff. We cannot let you leave the hospital at this time, but I would like to see if we can find a way to make you more comfortable now. Would you mind taking a seat so we can talk?

MR. O: (sits down, cautiously)

DR. X: Can I get you something to drink, some food, or a phone to call someone?

MR. O: I'm sorry, I'm sorry, I'm just very scared, and anxious, and don't know what to do. I'll take a water. And maybe a phone so I can let my parents know what's going on.

DR. X: I understand this is a difficult time for you. I am confident with the right care through hospitalization things will start to get better. Let me get you that water and a phone. If you feel your anxiety is getting too high, let us know and we can discuss a medication to help keep you calm while you're waiting.

As the patient continues to perseverate, he displays further signs of agitation. Dr. X uses this opportunity to convey the emotions elicited by the behavior, of which the patient is likely unaware. All the while, the physician sets clear limits while offering choices and optimism where possible to assist the patient in feeling some semblance of control. Ultimately, the patient is de-escalated out of the agitated state.

Utilization of verbal de-escalation can improve safety, reduce the use of force, and models nonviolent problem-solving. If time and circumstances permit, debriefing with the patient and other staff following the interaction can help with treatment planning and improving understanding and processes. Premature escalation to interventions such as utilization of medications can be perceived as dismissive, rejecting, or humiliating by patients.

Special Populations

Agitation Related to Substance Use

From 2006 to 2014, the rate of mental health and substance use-related emergency department (ED) visits increased 44.1%.[7] The primary diagnoses of alcohol-related disorders and substance-related disorders increased 76.3% and 73.7%, respectively. Patients with substance use disorders and psychiatric comorbidity are higher ED utilizers compared to patients with a substance use disorder but without psychiatric comorbidity.[8] The volume of presentations, as well as the fact that intoxication and withdrawal syndromes are frequently associated with agitation, demands that the emergency clinician must be adept at identifying and treating agitation secondary to substance use. For more information on the management of intoxication and withdrawal states, see Chapter 8.

Alcohol

Mr. B, a 42-year-old male with a history of depression and alcohol use disorder, voluntarily presents to the psychiatric emergency services for suicidal ideation and is seeking psychiatric hospitalization. His last drink was approximately 36 hours ago. He reveals that he has been drinking a "fifth" daily during the past few months and that he has been admitted to the intensive care unit in the past when he stopped drinking. Vital signs during his initial triage are notable for a blood pressure of 140/95 mmHg and heart rate of 110 beats per minute. He is slightly diaphoretic and tremulous. His blood alcohol level is zero, and urine drug screen is negative for all substances. While awaiting psychiatric hospitalization, he becomes progressively confused, agitated, and appears to be responding to internal stimuli.

Alcohol-related presentations are frequently associated with acute agitation in the ED.[1] An alcohol level, whether through blood alcohol concentration (BAC) or breathalyzer, should be obtained for any patient suspected of recent alcohol use upon arrival and potentially again as their BAC may continue to rise if the patient consumed alcohol shortly before arrival to the ED.

When the primary cause of agitation is likely alcohol intoxication, antipsychotics are often preferred over benzodiazepines due to the risk of respiratory suppression when benzodiazepines are combined with alcohol.[9] Haloperidol (with or without an anticholinergic), olanzapine, and droperidol are all reasonable options, with one large retrospective study demonstrating decreased length of stay with droperidol.[10] However, droperidol may not be widely available on formulary. Compared to haloperidol, olanzapine has a decreased risk of QTc prolongation—an important factor to consider because chronic alcohol use is associated with hypomagnesemia, which can elongate QTc.[11]

Alcohol withdrawal should be suspected among any patient who has abruptly stopped drinking after a significant period of heavy daily alcohol use. Common features of alcohol withdrawal include hypertension, tachycardia, diaphoresis, anxiety, hyperarousal, insomnia, and irritability.[12] Onset of severe complications of alcohol withdrawal, such as seizures and delirium tremens (DTs), can occur within 48–72 hours from the last drink. Because untreated or undertreated complicated alcohol withdrawal has a high mortality rate, vigilance is needed to prevent adverse outcomes. Predictors of complicated alcohol withdrawal (e.g., withdrawal seizures or DTs) include older age, prior history of complicated withdrawal, hypokalemia, and the presence of severe withdrawal symptoms despite high BAC.[12] Individuals with this history in addition to significant signs and symptoms of withdrawal require medical management.

ED clinicians will be responsible for initiating treatment because prompt control of withdrawal reduces the incidence of adverse events.[13] When agitation is associated with alcohol withdrawal, benzodiazepines are the preferred treatment, with lorazepam, diazepam, and chlordiazepoxide frequently used and no single benzodiazepine demonstrating superiority.[14] Diazepam and chlordiazepoxide are longer acting benzodiazepines and may provide a smoother detoxification; however, because both chlordiazepoxide and diazepam are hepatically metabolized, lorazepam may be preferred in patients with liver disease. All patients receiving benzodiazepines should have their vital signs serially monitored because instability can portend a worsening condition.

Benzodiazepines

Similar to alcohol intoxication and withdrawal in overall presentation, benzodiazepine intoxication or withdrawal can also be associated with agitation. Benzodiazepine withdrawal can be life-threatening, with some experts recommending hospitalization for withdrawal from very high doses ($\geq$100 mg of diazepam equivalents daily).[14] Benzodiazepine withdrawal is treated with large doses of benzodiazepines in the acute phase (and may be initiated in the ED), followed by a prolonged taper. Treatment of withdrawal from multiple benzodiazepines should be consolidated to monotherapy whenever possible, with some preference given toward longer acting benzodiazepines such as diazepam.[15]

Opioids

With the current opioid epidemic, patients who use prescribed and illicit opioids have become more prevalent in EDs. It is important to recognize opioid withdrawal as a potential factor that can exacerbate agitation. Opioid withdrawal can be extremely uncomfortable, with common physical symptoms of pain, hyperalgesia, insomnia, and gastrointestinal distress.[16] Psychiatric symptoms of opioid withdrawal include anxiety, agitation, dysphoria, and irritability. The chronology of opioid withdrawal is highly variable depending on the type of opioids used and the presence of adulterants, although withdrawal symptoms typically start within 12 hours of last usage and peak within 36–72 hours.[16] Although opioid withdrawal is rarely life-threatening,[17] it should be treated in order to keep the patient comfortable and reduce the risk of agitation. Treating a patient's opioid withdrawal may also help with alliance building and facilitate disposition to either psychiatric or substance use treatment.

Treatment of opioid withdrawal with either buprenorphine or methadone is quickly becoming the standard of care.[17] However, the logistics of providing medication-assisted treatment in the ED is complicated and largely dependent on addiction treatment services available within the hospital system. If buprenorphine or methadone are available treatments in the ED, these options should be pursued because there is evidence that ED-initiated medication-assisted treatment significantly increases engagement in addiction treatment.[18] Non-opioid pharmacologic treatments such as loperamide, metoclopramide, and ondansetron can be used to treat gastrointestinal distress associated with withdrawal.[17] Alpha-2 agonists such as clonidine and lofexidine can treat autonomic hyperactivity from withdrawal and may have an anxiolytic effect; patients should be monitored for signs of hypotension.[16] Pain-reducing medications such as ibuprofen can assist with headache and other types of pain, and in some cases, benzodiazepines can be utilized to calm agitation and anxiety.

Stimulants

Mrs. S is a 25-year-old female brought to the psychiatric emergency services by law enforcement in the middle of the night for evaluation of psychosis and agitation after she was found yelling at bystanders in a convenience store. She is unable to cooperate with initial triage assessment due to mood lability. She can be heard from a distance yelling about being abducted by aliens. She is visibly disheveled with poor dentition and is actively picking at her skin. She accuses the medical team of stealing $300,000 from her and tries to punch nursing staff before being physically restrained.

Acute and chronic use of stimulants, such as methamphetamine and cocaine, can lead to delusions, grandiosity, paranoia, and perceptual disturbances.[19] Compared to cocaine, methamphetamine may cause more severe psychotic symptoms, potentially due to neurotoxic effects and different mechanisms of action. A systematic review found that methamphetamine-related presentations were more likely to present with agitation, aggression, and homicidal behavior compared with other substance-related presentations.[20]

Benzodiazepines are considered a first-line treatment for stimulant-related agitation.[9] There is a dearth of quality studies on the treatment of stimulant-related psychosis, with some evidence supporting the use of haloperidol, olanzapine, and quetiapine.[21] Antipsychotics may be considered if psychotic symptoms are prominent or if benzodiazepines are ineffective.

Phencyclidine

Phencyclidine (PCP) is a synthetic compound with anesthetic and hallucinogenic properties and is frequently associated with agitation. A 2015 case series found that the most common presenting symptoms of PCP intoxication included horizontal and vertical nystagmus, agitation, and retrograde amnesia.[22] No high-quality studies have compared treatments for PCP-related agitation. Most patients only require supportive care and decreased stimuli (quiet room and dim lights), although the availability of a calm environment is limited in some settings. For more severe agitation requiring chemical and physical restraints, benzodiazepines (lorazepam or diazepam) are preferred and have the additional benefit of reducing PCP-induced hypertension and seizures.[23] There is evidence for using haloperidol for PCP-induced psychosis,[24] although it is recommended to utilize benzodiazepines as first-line and reserve antipsychotics for adjunctive purposes or for prominent psychotic symptoms.[25]

Cannabis and Synthetic Cannabinoids

Cannabis use alone is unlikely to result in severe agitation requiring intervention in the ED. Nonetheless, clinicians should be aware that in rare circumstances, it can cause agitation. Neuropsychiatric symptoms of cannabis use are generally self-limiting, require no treatment, and result in a short length of stay in the ED.[26] Synthetic cannabinoids, on the other hand, are more commonly associated with agitation and psychotic symptoms compared to cannabis.[27] Similar to other cases in which substance intoxication leads to agitation, benzodiazepines can reduce agitation here and antipsychotics can be used for acute psychosis.[28]

Nicotine

Nicotine withdrawal may cause agitation, and a thorough assessment of nicotine use should be included in the patient evaluation. It is important to assess the use of not only combustible cigarettes but also all forms of nicotine, including e-cigarettes, chewing tobacco, and nicotine replacement therapy (NRT). A randomized controlled trial found that smokers with schizophrenia demonstrated significantly less agitation if they were treated with NRT.[29] Being proactive in offering NRT to all patients who use nicotine is recommended because they will likely develop withdrawal symptoms if their visit to the ED is prolonged.

Personality Disorders

For individuals with a known or suspected personality disorder, the approach to agitation requires due consideration of what may be more or less effective, while maintaining general principles of agitation management. The focus here is on the two most prevalent types of personality disorders seen in the ED: antisocial personality disorder (ASPD) and borderline personality disorder (BPD).[30]

Antisocial Personality Disorder

Mr. B is a 47-year-old male with a reported history of alcohol use disorder, ASPD, and bipolar disorder. He has presented to the ED four times in the past month. The staff rushes over, saying, "He's back again! He needs to leave." When asked to identify his chief complaint, they say "the same as always, he wants three hots and a cot and is demanding about it." When evaluating the patient, he is sleeping and does not respond to your introduction. A staff member says loudly, "C'mon, get up!" and shakes his body. He wakes and explodes with anger.

When treating those with ASPD, several issues are crucial to consider. Recall that the diagnostic criteria for ASPD include impulsivity, aggressiveness, and disregard for the safety of others, all of which can be associated with violent behavior, necessitating keen attention to the safety measures previously discussed. Specific attention to optimal management of agitated individuals is needed.[31] Often, clinicians assume that patients with ASPD are malingering when they present to the ED. Although in some cases this may be true, it is dangerous to assume, because individuals with ASPD can present true safety risks. Moreover, when patients with ASPD are suspected of malingering, direct confrontation can increase agitation and necessitate more aggressive interventions, including physical management. It is generally more effective to attempt to align with the patient and determine their goals for the visit. If their wishes cannot be granted, this should be discussed in a direct but tactful manner, citing the limitations of what is possible in the ED. Escalation of behavior is certainly a potential outcome in these cases, and staff should be prepared for this possibility.

Borderline Personality Disorder

Mr. V is a 24-year-old male with a history of depression, post-traumatic stress disorder, and BPD. He presents with numerous cuts on his arms, and immediately upon being triaged by the nursing staff, he starts to raise his voice saying he wants to leave, that his visit was a mistake, and he starts pacing back and forth. Efforts are made to attempt to calm him down, and staff request that the physician order an injectable medication immediately. As the nurse approaches Mr. V with the medication, he becomes more agitated and begins to gesticulate wildly, saying this is all "triggering" him.

Given the prevalence of individuals with BPD presenting to EDs and the unique associated challenges, special considerations are necessary to optimize management.[32] Given that emotional dysregulation and self-harm behaviors are core features of the illness, staff often use benzodiazepines and antipsychotic medications to calm the patient.[31] These measures are sometimes necessary if a patient is so agitated or anxious that the evaluation cannot take place, but quite often, active validation and verbal de-escalation are effective and sufficient. Perhaps more than others, BPD patients can benefit from clinicians talking with them, helping them understand that the staff is there to help and validating their distress. In many cases, this approach can lead to rapid stabilization.

It is easy for staff to become dysregulated around BPD patients, particularly if the patient exhibits provocative behaviors. If these staff emotions go unchecked, it can lead to hostility or dismissiveness toward the patient that, due to the interpersonal hypersensitivity inherent in BPD, can undermine the therapeutic alliance and further complicate arriving at an ideal disposition.[33] Given that experiences of trauma are common in those with BPD, care must be taken not to retraumatize the patient with aggressive actions. A thoughtful and trauma-informed approach is crucial here, attending to elements such as allowing the patient to have choices to maintain a sense of control and attempting to understand what the patient needs to feel safe.

Delirium and Dementia

Mr. A is an 85-year-old male with Alzheimer's disease who is brought to the ED by his wife and daughter for a 1-week-long history of worsening confusion and irritability. His family became concerned today after he was unable to remember his wife's name and waved his cane at her in a threatening manner. He has also been talking about seeing his deceased brother in the home. His vital signs are notable for a low-grade fever. A brief neurologic exam appears normal. He appears anxious and afraid. While obtaining a medication list from his family, the physician discovers that the family has recently been administering diphenhydramine at bedtime to help with sleep.

Behavioral disturbances due to delirium and dementia are commonly associated with agitation. Distinguishing between chronic symptoms of dementia and more acute symptoms of delirium is crucial to a comprehensive emergency evaluation. It is important to note the time of symptom onset (hours to days in delirium and months in dementia) and level of arousal (often impaired in delirium and more stable in dementia), which may provide useful clues. Treatment strategies for agitation associated with delirium and dementia are reviewed here together because there is significant overlap and they often present concurrently with baseline cognitive impairment and superimposed mental status changes. The recognition of possible delirium is key, with specific attention to potential etiologies or precipitating factors including infection, trauma, pain, substance use, medication changes, and medication side effects. Physical exam, vital signs, and laboratory findings should augment the history-taking process. Life-threatening causes or those requiring further medical evaluation and/or intervention need to be ruled out. When the likely source or sources are found, then mitigating strategies can be implemented.

Nonpharmacologic interventions take precedence over pharmacologic interventions for treatment of agitation in delirium and dementia.[34] Guidelines include providing frequent reassurance and redirection, attempting to reorient the patient with calendars and clocks, minimizing overstimulation (quiet room, controlled lighting, and consistent caregivers), increasing family interactions with the patient, and clear and simple communication. Given the frailty of many individuals with dementia and delirium, use of physical restraints should be further minimized.[35]

Medications may be needed for severe agitation refractory to nonpharmacologic interventions. The benefits of using medications in elderly or medically compromised patients should be carefully weighed against the risks. For example, medications used to treat agitation may worsen other conditions or cause gait instability, leading to falls.[36] Other potential side effects of calming medications include sedation, extrapyramidal symptoms, and QTc prolongation. In addition, the therapeutic window of a particular medication may be narrower for elderly patients due to drug–drug interactions, alterations in drug metabolism, and medical comorbidities.

The use of antipsychotics for off-label treatment of behavioral disturbances in patients with dementia is associated with increased mortality.[37] There is limited evidence supporting the use of any particular antipsychotic over another, although a retrospective cohort study found that quetiapine may be associated with the lowest mortality risk, whereas haloperidol may be associated with the highest mortality risk. The U.S. Food and Drug Administration has issued black box warnings against the off-label use of both typical and atypical antipsychotics for treatment of dementia-related behavioral disturbances. However, expert consensus suggests that antipsychotics can be appropriate for patients with dementia, particularly in individuals with dangerous agitation or psychosis.[38] As with all medications for geriatric patients or those with underlying medical complexity or cognitive decline, medications should be started at low doses and titrated slowly to determine the minimum effective dose.

Similarly, guidelines for pharmacologic treatment of delirium recommend reserving use of antipsychotics and other sedating medications for treatment of severe agitation that poses risk of harm to patient or staff safety or threatens interruption of essential medical therapies.[39] For delirium-related agitation meeting this level of severity, suggestions include starting with a low dose of one of quetiapine, olanzapine, risperidone, or haloperidol and maintaining an effective dose for approximately 2 days before tapering. If there are sleep–wake cycle issues, melatonin or ramelteon can be administered, with avoidance of sedative–hypnotics. Unless there are issues such as alcohol or benzodiazepine withdrawal, benzodiazepines for agitation in the setting of dementia or delirium are to be avoided, given the risk of drug–drug interactions, further cognitive deficits, dizziness, disinhibition, and development of tolerance and dependence.[40,41]

Psychosis and Mania

Ms. T is a 54-year-old female with a history of schizophrenia who presents with police after being found walking aimlessly in the cold for several hours without shoes. During triage, she appears restless, wringing her hands and pacing, talking despite being alone in the room. When approached to check her vital signs, she stares intensely and takes prolonged periods of time to answer basic questions, irritably mumbling that she cannot stay as she "must get back to my research or they'll know." She attempts to leave the room mid-sentence several times.

Individuals with acute psychosis and mania represent a significant proportion of those presenting with agitation in the emergency setting.[42] Although many of these individuals have well-documented underlying thought and mood disorders, many also present to the ED in their first psychotic or manic episode and require careful evaluation of the source of their psychosis and subsequent agitation. It is important to remember that psychosis is a symptom, not a diagnosis, that can arise from many different etiologies, and rapidly escalate into agitated and aggressive behavior. Many of the characteristic symptoms of psychosis can contribute to agitation, such as the mistrust of others related to underlying paranoia and auditory or visual hallucinations causing distress. With limited insight into their current mental state, patients may feel angry and upset they have been involuntarily brought to the hospital. Manic patients' inherent emotional lability and racing thoughts can predispose them to agitated states, and their internal distress can become so overwhelming that it triggers psychomotor agitation. These individuals are often frightened, fragile, and vulnerable, warranting thoughtful engagement for de-escalation.

Although agitated patients in states of psychosis or mania are often disorganized, dysregulated, and labile and require intensive staffing resources, the principles of de-escalation apply just as with any other etiology of agitation. Every effort should be made to reduce stimuli for patients prior to engagement, promoting a calm, nonthreatening environment. Verbal de-escalation should be the initial intervention employed, with concise, simple language. Repetition may be necessary because manic and psychotic patients' cognitive state often limits their attention, memory, and ability to process information. Should medications be warranted, although benzodiazepines can reduce agitation, antipsychotics are preferred because they more precisely target the underlying etiology.[43]

Agitation in Pregnancy

Acute agitation in the pregnant patient should be treated as an emergency due to potential for obstetric complications.[44] The evaluation of the agitated pregnant woman should include a physical examination, vital signs, and basic labs to rule out medical etiologies. Discontinuation of psychiatric medications during pregnancy may increase the risk of relapse in mood disorders and schizophrenia.[45] An obstetrics consult may be prudent if the viability of the fetus is at risk. Further details on these topics are elaborated upon in Chapter 18.

Verbal de-escalation should be used whenever possible to prevent harm to the fetus from pharmacologic interventions or restraints. If the patient has a known psychiatric history, it may be reasonable to administer their prescribed medications.[44] For mild agitation, experts recommend diphenhydramine as safe to use in pregnancy.[45] For moderate to severe agitation, second-generation antipsychotics, such as olanzapine and ziprasidone, and quetiapine are also believed to be safe in pregnancy, although there is limited evidence to support their use. Benzodiazepines such as lorazepam are not contraindicated in pregnancy and can be used with close monitoring of respiratory rate.[44]

Physical restraints should only be used as a last resort with individuals who are pregnant, even more so than in other conditions. After 20 weeks of gestation, physical restraints may compromise placental blood flow, and the preferred positioning of the patient is in the left lateral decubitus position, with the right hip positioned 10–12 cm off the bed with pillows or blankets.[44] Vital signs should be frequently monitored, and as always, the patient should be assessed for removal of restraints as soon as it is safe to do so.

Psychopharmacological Management

If verbal de-escalation is inadequate or ineffective in controlling agitation and the patient continues to present danger to themself or others, or is unable to participate in the interview, medications may be necessary. When considering medications for agitation, it is important to recall that the goal of medications is to calm the patient as opposed to overly sedating them, which that can increase the likelihood of respiratory depression and falls, and it often delays the evaluation and disposition.[9] The medication choice, dose, and how often to repeat are key considerations in the psychopharmacological management of agitation.

Ideally, the patient would be agreeable to taking medications because this bodes well for the therapeutic alliance, reduces trauma or conflict, and empowers them as a partner in their treatment. However, when agitation is severe, involuntary medications are often necessary. When medication is required, the onset of efficacy, reliability of delivery, side effect profile, etiology of agitation, and patient preference are important factors. Table 2.1 outlines medication guidelines by severity of agitation. Refer to the section titled "Special Populations" for clinical management of specific etiologies of agitation.

Table 2.1 Summary of Pharmacologic Interventions for Undifferentiated Agitation[1,9,46–51]

Severity	Medications	Route	Clinical Pearls
Mild	Lorazepam 1–2 mg	PO	Relatively slow onset of action within 20–30 minutes. May repeat dose in 2 hours with maximum 12 mg per 24 hours. Avoid benzodiazepines if high suspicion for alcohol or benzodiazepine intoxication.
Moderate	Olanzapine 5–10 mg PO Haloperidol 5 mg + lorazepam 2 mg	PO PO	Available in ODT formulation. May repeat dose in 20 minutes with maximum 30 mg per 24 hours. Haloperidol is often administered in combination with lorazepam, promethazine, or diphenhydramine to minimize acute risk of EPS.
Severe	Olanzapine 5–10 mg Ziprasidone 20 mg Droperidol 5–10 mg IM Haloperidol 5 mg + Lorazepam 2 mg	IM IM IM IM	Avoid administering olanzapine in combination with benzodiazepines. Requires time for medication to reconstitute. FDA black box warning for reports of death associated with QTc prolongation and torsades de pointes.[52] Availability may be limited as a result. Lorazepam may be given with 25–50 mg diphenhydramine for EPS prophylaxis.

EPS, extrapyramidal symptoms; FDA, U.S. Food and Drug Administration; IM, intramuscular; IV, intravenous; ODT, orally disintegrating tablet; PO, by mouth.

Restraints and Seclusion

Despite utilization of verbal de-escalation and medications, a subset of agitated patients may continue to demonstrate self-destructive and violent behavior. The imminent likelihood of harm to themselves or others in this state is greatly heightened, and to ensure the safety of the patient and those around them, the use of seclusion or physical restraints may be warranted. The use of these measures has received significant attention given the risk of death or serious injury of individuals if the restraint/seclusion methods and monitoring are not appropriate.[53] Documented injuries from prospective studies of restraint include skin abrasions or lacerations, circulatory issues, positional asphyxia, aspiration, bone fractures/breaks, dehydration, incontinence, thrombosis, rhabdomyolysis, and loss of strength and mobility.[54] Especially at high risk for complications when in restraint and seclusion are patients with unstable medical conditions, such as a cardiac or respiratory illness, infection, or metabolic illness; those in a delirious state; those with neurologic conditions, including dementia; intoxicated patients, particularly in overdose; and pregnant patients.[55] Their use has been further contested because psychological trauma is a frequent adverse effect from these interventions, particularly for those with a history of previous trauma.[56] This underscores the use of seclusion and restraint as interventions of last resort, utilized only when all other less-restrictive measures have failed and were adequately documented.

When considering the use of seclusion or restraint, one must determine which form to use, attempting to balance least-restrictive measures with maintaining the safety of all those involved.[57] If the patient remains highly agitated yet does not appear at imminent risk of violence or self-harm, seclusion can be implemented. Seclusion is defined as confinement of an individual in a room alone where they are prevented from physically leaving. Spaces for seclusion can be locked or unlocked, and this choice should be related to the patient's willingness and likelihood to remain in seclusion. Prior to being placed in seclusion, the purpose and rationale for seclusion should be clearly stated, as well as stipulations for removal from seclusion. The space chosen for seclusion should be safe for the patient and staff, with removal of objects, including furniture, that can be weaponized. During seclusion, the patient should be continuously monitored to ensure that further harm is mitigated.

Should the patient be deemed to be highly agitated and at imminent risk of violence or self-harm, or if seclusion is inadequate to maintain safety of the patient or others, then the utilization of restraint is warranted. This state may develop at any point throughout the evaluation, and in some cases it can be present at the outset. Restraint is defined as the action of physically restricting an individual's body in the effort to limit physical activity for their protection and that of others. This is most frequently accomplished in the ED by two- or four-point limb locks on a stretcher, but belts, vests, hand mitts, or specialized chairs have also been utilized to varying degrees of success. Physical holds, such as laying hands on a patient during forced medication administration, are also generally considered a form of restraint. As with seclusion, prior to implementing a restraint, a clear statement of the purpose and rationale for restraint should be made, as well as stipulations for release. The importance of continuously monitoring the restrained patient cannot be overstated because this minimizes the possibility of injury to the patient and can inform a decision about when release may be safe. Monitoring in restraint includes close observation of vital signs and physical characteristics, particularly deviations from normal ranges, which may signal exacerbations of underlying medical disorders predisposing an individual to rapid decompensation and subsequent injury.

Seclusion and restraint are involuntary interventions, and as such their utilization is highly regulated. All efforts should be made to remove the patient from seclusion or restraint as soon as safely possible. The Joint Commission on Accreditation of Healthcare Standards has developed a set of standards to assist in regulating the usage of restraint and seclusion.[55] These standards include guidance on avoiding the use of restraints for the purposes of punishment, retaliation, or convenience; implementing a new order for each incident of seclusion or restraint; and evaluating a patient who is secluded or restrained within 1 hour of the initiation of the order. Documentation is required, including a description of the behavior leading to the seclusion or restraint and the patient's condition as a response to the intervention. Following the episode of seclusion or restraint, a debriefing discussion among staff is helpful to discuss what could have gone better, determine if safety is optimized, and plan for future management of the patient.

Early intervention with individuals who are exhibiting signs of agitation can in some cases prevent the ultimate need for seclusion and restraint. Recognition of risk factors is also helpful in this regard because studies have shown that restraints are more commonly utilized with patients who are younger, using substances, are psychotic, have limited insight, and arrive involuntarily.[2]

Conclusion

As the field of emergency psychiatry has developed, more nuanced approaches to the management of agitation have emerged. Verbal de-escalation is the desired initial intervention in many cases of agitation, with the goal of reducing the need for pharmacotherapy or physical management. Because each presentation is unique and multifactorial, including the presence or absence of substance intoxication, potential medical comorbidities, and different psychiatric diagnoses, it is important to understand the breadth of intervention options available. Keeping in mind the core principle of placing safety first, if one can stay organized from the pre-assessment through decision-making, then treatment can be optimized and adverse events can be minimized.

References

1. Miner JR, Klein LR, Cole JB, Driver BE, Moore JC, Ho JD. The characteristics and prevalence of agitation in an urban county emergency department. *Ann Emerg Med.* 2018;72(4):361–370. doi:10.1016/j.annemergmed.2018.06.001

2. Simpson SA, Joesch JM, West II, Pasic J. Risk for physical restraint or seclusion in the psychiatric emergency service (PES). *Gen Hosp Psychiatry.* 2014;36(1):113–118. doi:10.1016/j.genhosppsych.2013.09.009

3. Lindenmayer JP. The pathophysiology of agitation. *J Clin Psychiatry.* 2000;61(Suppl 14):5–10. http://www.ncbi.nlm.nih.gov/pubmed/11154018

4. Binder RL, McNiel DE. Contemporary practices in managing acutely violent patients in 20 psychiatric emergency rooms. *Psychiatr Serv.* 1999;50(12):1553–1554. doi:10.1176/ps.50.12.1553

5. Richmond JS, Berlin JS, Fishkind AB, et al. Verbal de-escalation of the agitated patient: Consensus statement of the American Association for Emergency Psychiatry Project BETA De-escalation Workgroup. *West J Emerg Med*. 2012;13(1):17–25. doi:10.5811/westjem.2011.9.6864

6. Swift RH, Harrigan EP, Cappelleri JC, Kramer D, Chandler LP. Validation of the Behavioural Activity Rating Scale (BARS): A novel measure of activity in agitated patients. *J Psychiatr Res*. 2002;36(2):87–95. doi:10.1016/S0022-3956(01)00052-8

7. Moore BJ, Stocks C, Owens PL. Trends in emergency department visits, 2006–2014. Statistical Brief 227. Healthcare Cost & Utilization Project. Published 2017. https://hcup-us.ahrq.gov/reports/statbriefs/sb227-Emergency-Department-Visit-Trends.jsp

8. Curran GM, Sullivan G, Williams K, Han X, Allee E, Kotrla KJ. The association of psychiatric comorbidity and use of the emergency department among persons with substance use disorders: An observational cohort study. *BMC Emerg Med*. 2008;8:1–6. doi:10.1186/1471-227X-8-17

9. Wilson MP, Pepper D, Currier GW, Holloman GH, Feifel D. The psychopharmacology of agitation: Consensus statement of the American Association for Emergency Psychiatry Project BETA Psychopharmacology Workgroup. *West J Emerg Med*. 2012;13(1):26–34. doi:10.5811/westjem.2011.9.6866

10. Cole JB, Klein LR, Martel ML. Parenteral antipsychotic choice and its association with emergency department length of stay for acute agitation secondary to alcohol intoxication. *Acad Emerg Med*. 2019;26(1):79–84. doi:10.1111/acem.13486

11. Moulin SRA, Mill JG, Rosa WCM, Hermisdorf SR, Caldeira LC, Zago-Gomes EMP. QT interval prolongation associated with low magnesium in chronic alcoholics. *Drug Alcohol Depend*. 2015;155:195–201. doi:10.1016/j.drugalcdep.2015.07.019

12. Bharadwaj B, Kattimani S. Clinical management of alcohol withdrawal: A systematic review. *Ind Psychiatry J*. 2013;22(2):100. doi:10.4103/0972-6748.132914

13. Mayo-Smith MF, Beecher LH, Fischer TL, et al. Management of alcohol withdrawal delirium: An evidence-based practice guideline. *Arch Intern Med*. 2004;164(13):1405–1412. doi:10.1001/archinte.164.13.1405

14. Scheuermeyer FX, Miles I, Lane DJ, et al. Lorazepam versus diazepam in the management of emergency department patients with alcohol withdrawal. *Ann Emerg Med*. 2020:76(6):774–781. doi:10.1016/j.annemergmed.2020.05.029

15. Soyka M. Treatment of benzodiazepine dependence. *N Engl J Med*. 2017;376(12):1147–1157. doi:10.1056/nejmra1611832

16. Pergolizzi J V., Raffa RB, Rosenblatt MH. Opioid withdrawal symptoms, a consequence of chronic opioid use and opioid use disorder: Current understanding and approaches to management. *J Clin Pharm Ther*. 2020;45(5):892–903. doi:10.1111/jcpt.13114

17. Herring AA, Perrone J, Nelson LS. Managing opioid withdrawal in the emergency department with buprenorphine. *Ann Emerg Med*. 2019;73(5):481–487. doi:10.1016/j.annemergmed.2018.11.032

18. D'Onofrio G, O'Connor PG, Pantalon MV, et al. Emergency department-initiated buprenorphine/naloxone treatment for opioid dependence: A randomized clinical trial. *JAMA*. 2015;313(16):1636–1644. doi:10.1001/jama.2015.3474

19. Mahoney JJ, Kalechstein AD, De La Garza R, Newton TF. Presence and persistence of psychotic symptoms in cocaine- versus methamphetamine-dependent participants. *Am J Addict*. 2008;17(2):83–98. doi:10.1080/10550490701861201

20. Jones R, Woods C, Usher K. Rates and features of methamphetamine-related presentations to emergency departments: An integrative literature review. *J Clin Nurs*. 2018;27(13–14):2569–2582. doi:10.1111/jocn.14493

21. Glasner-Edwards S, Mooney LJ. Methamphetamine psychosis: Epidemiology and management. *CNS Drugs*. 2014;28(12):1115–1126. doi:10.1007/s40263-014-0209-8

22. Dominici P, Kopec K, Manur R, Khalid A, Damiron K, Rowden A. Phencyclidine intoxication case series study. *J Med Toxicol*. 2015;11(3):321–325. doi:10.1007/s13181-014-0453-9

23. Journey JD, Bentley TP. Phencyclidine Toxicity. StatPearls; 2020. http://www.ncbi.nlm.nih.gov/pubmed/29939642

24. Giannini AJ, Nageotte C, Loiselle RH, Malone DA, Price WA. Comparison of chlorpromazine, haloperidol and pimozide in the treatment of phencyclidine psychosis: Da-2 receptor specificity. *Clin Toxicol*. 1984;22(6):573–579. doi:10.3109/15563658408992586

25. Macneal JJ, Cone DC, Sinha V, Tomassoni AJ. Use of haloperidol in PCP-intoxicated individuals. *Clin Toxicol*. 2012;50(9):851–853. doi:10.3109/15563650.2012.722222

26. Dines AM, Wood DM, Galicia M, et al. Presentations to the emergency department following cannabis use—A multi-centre case series from ten European countries. *J Med Toxicol*. 2015;11(4):415–421. doi:10.1007/s13181-014-0460-x

27. Bassir Nia A, Medrano B, Perkel C, Galynker I, Hurd YL. Psychiatric comorbidity associated with synthetic cannabinoid use compared to cannabis. *J Psychopharmacol*. 2016;30(12):1321–1330. doi:10.1177/0269881116658990

28. Mills B, Yepes A, Nugent K. Synthetic cannabinoids. *Am J Med Sci*. 2015;350(1):59–62. doi:10.1097/MAJ.0000000000000466

29. Allen MA, Debanné M, Lazignac C, Adam E, Dickinson LM, Damsa C. Effect of nicotine replacement therapy on agitation in smokers with schizophrenia. *Am J Psychiatry*. 2011;168(4):395–399. http://ajp.psychiatryonline.org/doi/pdf/10.1176/appi.ajp.2010.10040569

30. Goodwin RD, Hamilton SP. Lifetime comorbidity of antisocial personality disorder and anxiety disorders among adults in the community. *Psychiatry Res*. 2003;117(2):159–166. doi:10.1016/s0165-1781(02)00320-7

31. Hong V, Pirnie L, Shobassy A. Antisocial and borderline personality disorders in the emergency department: Conceptualizing and managing "malingered" or "exaggerated" symptoms. *Curr Behav Neurosci Rep*. 2019;6(4):127–132. doi:10.1007/s40473-019-00183-4

32. Pascual JC, Córcoles D, Castaño J, et al. Hospitalization and pharmacotherapy for borderline personality disorder in a psychiatric emergency service. *Psychiatr Serv*. 2007;58(9):1199–1204. doi:10.1176/ps.2007.58.9.1199

33. Hong V. Borderline personality disorder in the emergency department: Good psychiatric management. *Harv Rev Psychiatry*. 2016;24(5):357–366. doi:10.1097/HRP.0000000000000112

34. Rosenberg MS, Carpenter CR, Bromley M, et al. Geriatric emergency department guidelines. *Ann Emerg Med*. 2014;63(5):e7–e25. doi:10.1016/j.annemergmed.2014.02.008

35. Bessey LJ, Radue RM, Chapman EN, Boyle LL, Shah MN. Behavioral health needs of older adults in the emergency department. *Clin Geriatr Med*. 2018;34(3):469–489. doi:10.1016/j.cger.2018.05.002

36. Shenvi C, Wilson MP, Aldai A, Pepper D, Gerardi M. A research agenda for the assessment and management of acute behavioral changes in elderly emergency department patients. *West J Emerg Med*. 2019;20(2):393–402. doi:10.5811/westjem.2019.1.39262

37. Kales HC, Kim HM, Zivin K, et al. Risk of mortality among individual antipsychotics in patients with dementia. *Am J Psychiatry*. 2012;169(1):71–79. doi:10.1176/appi.ajp.2011.11030347

38. Reus VI, Fochtmann LJ, Eyler AE, et al. The American Psychiatric Association practice guideline on the use of antipsychotics to treat agitation or psychosis in patients with dementia. *Am J Psychiatry*. 2016;173(5):543–546. doi:10.1176/appi.ajp.2015.173501

39. Oh ES, Fong TG, Hshieh TT, Inouye SK. Delirium in older persons: Advances in diagnosis and treatment. *JAMA*. 2017;318(12):1161–1174. doi:10.1001/jama.2017.12067

40. Defrancesco M, Marksteiner J, Wolfgang Fleischhacker W, Blasko I. Use of benzodiazepines in Alzheimer's disease: A systematic review of literature. *Int J Neuropsychopharmacol*. 2015;18(10):1–11. doi:10.1093/ijnp/pyv055

41. Lonergan E, Luxenberg J, Areosa Sastre A. Benzodiazepines for delirium. *Cochrane Database Syst Rev*. 2009;2009(4):CD006379. doi:10.1002/14651858.CD006379.pub3

42. Marco CA, Vaughan J. Emergency management of agitation in schizophrenia. *Am J Emerg Med*. 2005;23(6):767–776. doi:10.1016/j.ajem.2005.02.050

43. Zeller SL, Citrome L. Managing agitation associated with schizophrenia and bipolar disorder in the emergency setting. *West J Emerg Med*. 2016;17(2):165–172. doi:10.5811/westjem.2015.12.28763

44. Niforatos JD, Wanta JW, Shapiro AP, Yax JA, Viguera AC. Q: How should I treat acute agitation in pregnancy? *Cleve Clin J Med*. 2019;86(4):243–247. doi:10.3949/ccjm.86a.18041

45. Aftab A, Shah AA. Behavioral emergencies: Special considerations in the pregnant patient. *Psychiatr Clin North Am*. 2017;40(3):435–448. doi:10.1016/j.psc.2017.05.017

46. Garriga M, Pacchiarotti I, Kasper S, et al. Assessment and management of agitation in psychiatry: Expert consensus. *World J Biol Psychiatry*. 2016;17(2):86–128. doi:10.3109/15622975.2015.1132007

47. Roppolo L, Morris D, Khan F, et al. Improving the management of acutely agitated patients in the emergency department through implementation of Project BETA (Best Practices in the Evaluation and Treatment of Agitation). *J Am Coll Emerg Physicians Open*. 2020;1(5):898–907. doi:10.1002/emp2.12138

48. Taylor DMD, Yap CYL, Knott JC, et al. Midazolam–droperidol, droperidol, or olanzapine for acute agitation: A randomized clinical trial. *Ann Emerg Med*. 2017;69(3):318–326.e1. doi:10.1016/j.annemergmed.2016.07.033

49. Patel MX, Sethi FN, Barnes TRE, et al. Joint BAP NAPICU evidence-based consensus guidelines for the clinical management of acute disturbance: De-escalation and rapid tranquillisation. *J Psychopharmacol*. 2018;32(6):601–640. doi:10.1177/0269881118776738

50. Klein LR, Driver BE, Miner JR, et al. Intramuscular midazolam, olanzapine, ziprasidone, or haloperidol for treating acute agitation in the emergency department. *Ann Emerg Med*. 2018;72(4):374–385. doi:10.1016/j.annemergmed.2018.04.027

51. Bak M, Weltens I, Bervoets C, et al. The pharmacological management of agitated and aggressive behaviour: A systematic review and meta-analysis. *Eur Psychiatry*. 2019;57(2019):78–100. doi:10.1016/j.eurpsy.2019.01.014

52. Meyer-Massetti C, Cheng CM, Sharpe BA, Meier CR, Guglielmo BJ. The FDA extended warning for intravenous haloperidol and torsades de pointes: How should institutions respond? *J Hosp Med*. 2010;5(4):E8–E16. doi:10.1002/jhm.691

53. Annas GJ. The last resort-The use of physical restraints in medical emergencies. *N Engl J Med*. 1999;341(18):1408–1412. doi:10.1056/NEJM199910283411182055.

54. Mohr WK, Petti TA, Mohr BD. Adverse effects associated with physical restraint. *Can J Psychiatry*. 2003;48(5):330–337. doi:10.1177/070674370304800509

55. Crisis Prevention Institute. Joint Commission Standards on Restraint and Seclusion/ Nonviolent Crisis Intervention training program. Published 2010. Accessed January 23, 2021. https://www.crisisprevention.com/CPI/media/Media/Resources/alignments/Joint-Commission-Restraint-Seclusion-Alignment-2011.pdf.

56. Chieze M, Hurst S, Kaiser S, Sentissi O. Effects of seclusion and restraint in adult psychiatry: A systematic review. *Front Psychiatry*. 2019;10:491. doi:10.3389/fpsyt.2019.00491

57. New A, Tucci VT, Rios J. A modern-day fight club? The stabilization and management of acutely agitated patients in the emergency department. *Psychiatr Clin North Am*. 2017;40(3):397–410. doi:10.1016/j.psc.2017.05.002

3

Medical Assessment of the Psychiatric Patient

Seth Thomas

Introduction

It is estimated that mental health-related complaints account for 1 in every 10 emergency department (ED) visits in the United States. Between 2009 and 2015, ED visits for mental health-related complaints increased by 40.8% for adults and by 56.4% for pediatric patients.[1] With such a significant percentage of ED visits attributed to these complaints, it is important for emergency physicians and psychiatrists to be familiar with the concept of the focused medical assessment and how to appropriately screen patients for underlying medical pathology that may contribute to their presentation.

From Medical Clearance to Focused Medical Assessment

In most jurisdictions within the United States, patients experiencing a behavioral health crisis must first present to their nearest ED to undergo what has been historically referred to as "medical clearance" before being transferred for care in an inpatient psychiatric facility. *Medical clearance* refers to a process by which a qualified medical provider, usually a physician, physician assistant, or nurse practitioner, performs an assessment of the patient to achieve two specific goals: (1) ensure patient stability; and (2) exclude organic conditions, such as delirium, as the primary etiology or contributing factor for the patient's symptoms.

The Emergency Medical Treatment and Labor Act (EMTALA), enacted in 1986, requires EDs associated with Medicare-participating hospitals to provide a Medical Screening Exam (MSE) to identify an Emergency Medical Condition (EMC) and provide stabilizing care for any patient requesting an examination regardless of their ability to pay.[2-4] At a minimum, the MSE must include a history and physical exam and may include diagnostic tests deemed necessary by the provider to adequately rule out an EMC. Providing an appropriate MSE for patients with a mental health chief complaint must mirror the process utilized for patients presenting with a medical chief complaint. In fact, according to EMTALA, a psychiatric emergency is considered an EMC and requires stabilizing care similar to that for other patients.[4,5] In essence, the medical clearance process for EDs includes an EMTALA-defined MSE but does not stop at the exclusion of an EMC: The process should also include a reasonable exclusion of organic etiologies of the patient's presentation. Unfortunately, the medical clearance process is ambiguous, lacks standardization, and expected elements are inconsistent from hospital to hospital and clinician to clinician.[6,7] Because there is no universally agreed upon definition of a "medically cleared" patient, psychiatric and non-psychiatric staff may be falsely assured and misled by the term, leading to poor patient care.[8]

Although the term medical clearance has been used for decades, it has begun to fall out of favor due to the lack of a clear definition, varying expectations, and the element of ambiguity described previously. Furthermore, medical clearance implies that a patient is ready for a follow-on action such as psychiatric evaluation, transfer to an acute psychiatric facility, or discharge, none of which is described by the term.[9] In 2006, the American College of Emergency Physicians (ACEP) published a clinical policy that addressed the issue of terminology. In its introductory remarks, the authors suggested that "focused medical assessment" be used as an alternative.[10] Other alternatives to the term medical clearance have been suggested; however, it is my opinion that "focused medical assessment" most accurately describes the process of the medical evaluation of the psychiatric patient.

History of the Medical Clearance Process

The concept of performing a focused medical assessment for patients suffering from psychiatric symptoms prior to, or in concurrence with, a psychiatric evaluation has been around for decades. Actual references to the term medical clearance in the literature date back as far as the late 1960s; however, some papers, such as that by Colodny et al.[11] in 1968, describe the process in the setting of performing medical examinations of children with learning disabilities and/or behavioral disturbances to clear them for entry into specific educational programs. Although this setting is not the same as providing a medical assessment for patients in the ED or other psychiatric settings, their paper did describe the process as one in which the physician performs "a thorough history and physical examination" prior to completing their assessment of the child.

Although the concept of medical clearance and the use of the term have been around for some time, the specific methodology and necessary elements have been the subject of considerable debate since the mid-20th century, particularly with regard to the need for routine comprehensive laboratory testing. Experts have repeatedly advocated for beginning the assessment with a thorough history and physical exam in order to identify potential medical etiologies or comorbid conditions that may be exacerbating the patient's psychiatric symptoms. Yet, over time, beginning in the 1960s, various publications and case reports advocated for structured and comprehensive screening protocols, including routine comprehensive laboratory testing and, in some instances, selective radiologic imaging. This conservative approach was motivated primarily out of fear of failure to identify a medical etiology of a patient's presentation given that several publications cited high prevalence of concomitant or causative medical conditions. However, subsequent review of these studies and expert consensus are in agreement that many of the earlier studies suffered from selection bias and also failed to examine the ability of a basic history and physical examination to identify medical conditions.

Few clinicians would argue the importance of performing a detailed history and physical exam on any patient presenting to an ED, regardless of a patient's complaint. However, as time progressed, newer studies called into question the practice of performing routine comprehensive testing based on what many believed to be more realistic estimates of the prevalence of medical illness in the psychiatric population. Authors then began trying to identify which medical conditions were most prevalent and how to best screen for them, representing a shift from routine comprehensive testing to the more contemporary approach of selective testing. Authors have since explored the possibility of utilizing standardized medical clearance protocols with a heavy emphasis on performing a thorough history and physical exam to help guide selective testing. Currently, more EDs utilize this approach—ensuring that a thorough history and physical exam are performed prior to the ordering of diagnostic tests. Although this is viewed by many to be best practice, some psychiatric facilities have been reluctant to accept this approach out of concern that patients may not have been adequately screened. Furthermore, psychiatric facilities often do not have access to rapid, in-house diagnostic testing.

Prevalence of Medical Illness in Psychiatric Patients

There is no doubt that patients with psychiatric emergencies have concurrent medical conditions that can exacerbate or complicate their presentations. In fact, studies have shown that psychiatric patients have a higher incidence of medical comorbidities and shorter life span compared with the general population.[12-18] Studies have cited the prevalence of organic etiologies in patients with an acute psychiatric condition to be between 0% and 63% and the frequency of major medical problems to range between 0% and 49%. Among these earlier studies, some authors suggested that the rate of medical problems that were suspected or confirmed to have caused the patient's psychiatric symptoms ranged from 0% to 42%.[19-30]

References to misdiagnosed or underdiagnosed medical conditions masquerading as psychiatric illness date back as far as the early 20th century. However, the most notable studies citing high rates of organic etiologies of their patients' presentations are those by Koranyi[27] and Hall et al.[28] Koranyi performed a retrospective analysis on clinic patients in an outpatient setting and cited that 43% of this population suffered from at least one physical illness and nearly half (46%) were undiagnosed by the referring source. He determined that these self and social agency–referred patients "almost always had undiagnosed physical illnesses," leading him to conclude that psychiatrists should be more familiar with screening patients for organic diseases. Hall et al. drew similar conclusions based on their study of 100 patients admitted to a state psychiatric research ward. This study found that 46% of these patients had medical illnesses that either caused or exacerbated their psychiatric condition. What was more surprising was that a staggering 80% of patients were noted to have a physical illness requiring treatment. As a result of these findings, the authors recommended routine, comprehensive screening for all hospitalized psychiatric patients consisting of a battery of tests including a 34-element metabolic panel (SMA-34), urinalysis, electrocardiogram, and post-sleep deprivation electroencephalogram. Their rationale was that this combination of tests identified more than 90% of the medical illnesses in their study population. Perhaps the most significant criticism of this study was the selection of the patient population. Compared to typical, community EDs or crisis stabilization units, the prevalence of organic disease in an inpatient research ward likely represents a much sicker population of patients. Furthermore, the authors did not expand upon the pre-admission screening or acceptance process or whether or not these medical illnesses would have been identified by thorough history and physical examination.

In 1982, Bunce et al.[31] published a retrospective analysis of 102 female patients admitted to the acute medical unit of a psychiatric hospital for "nonspecific changes in physical condition" or behavior. More than 70% of those patients were unable to adequately communicate with the physician, and unsurprisingly, 92% of them were diagnosed with at least one medical condition that was not predicted by their symptoms. Yet more than 50% of the patients had an initial presentation of "altered mental status," and 29% complained of weakness.

In 1994, Henneman et al.[32] prospectively studied the utility of a standardized medical evaluation of adult patients presenting to an academic emergency department with new psychiatric symptoms. The protocol consisted of a history and physical exam, comprehensive laboratory testing, and urine drug screen (UDS). Patients also received cranial computed tomography and a lumbar puncture if febrile. Of the 100 consecutive patients evaluated, 63% were found to have an organic etiology of their symptoms. Although this study cited a high prevalence of organic disease, this was because the study was designed to evaluate patients with *new psychiatric symptoms* and excluded those with psychiatric histories. Similar to Bunce et al.,[31] Henneman et al. also noted that 60% of the patients presented with disorientation and altered mental status, a complaint that is highly predictive of the presence of an organic etiology.

Other studies have revealed a lower prevalence of medical illness among patients with psychiatric presentations. Reeves et al.[33] performed a retrospective analysis of admissions to two separate inpatient psychiatric units over a 7-year period and found that 2.3% of patients had unrecognized delirium requiring rapid medical intervention. However, each of these patients presented with altered mentation identified on history and physical exam, indicating a high likelihood of organic disease.

These studies confirm that medical conditions are common among patients with psychiatric diagnoses and, in some circumstances, can cause or contribute to their psychiatric presentations. Based on these findings, some authors have recommended comprehensive laboratory testing to screen for and identify these conditions. However, the prevalence and relative effect of these conditions are highly variable and largely depend on study design and inclusion criteria. Furthermore, how any individual clinician defines medical clearance or considers a medical condition to be clinically relevant or contributory can significantly change the relative prevalence of medical conditions. It is also reassuring that in several of these studies, the medical conditions would have been identified or excluded during the history and physical exam.

Elements of the Focused Medical Assessment

It is clear that some patients presenting with psychiatric symptoms undoubtedly suffer from medical conditions, some of which may be minor and may not contribute directly to the patient's presentation, whereas others are significant and pose an immediate threat to the patient if not recognized. Yet it should also be apparent that there is no single, universal approach to the medical assessment to identify these conditions and, more important, to distinguish those that are important from those that are unimportant. However, there are elements of the focused medical assessment that are essential and should be applied to every patient, whereas there are others that should only be used selectively.

History and Physical Exam

The foundation of the focused medical assessment, psychiatric or otherwise, is performing a thorough history and physical exam. The history and physical exam should mirror the process for any patient without psychiatric complaints. Several studies highlighting the prevalence of medical conditions in psychiatric patients also either suggested or indirectly demonstrated that most medical conditions could be identified by history or physical exam.[31-35]

Unfortunately, it has been reported that patients do not always receive an adequate history and physical exam, which may cause clinicians to miss serious underlying medical conditions or inappropriately rely on diagnostic tests.[35,36-39] In 1981, Summers et al.[35] advocated for widespread adoption of a rapid, protocolized psychiatric physical examination after citing several reports that the majority of psychiatrists did not perform routine physical exams on their patients. Nearly a decade later, Riba and Hale[36] performed a retrospective chart review of 137 consecutive patients evaluated in an ED setting who were referred for psychiatric evaluation and found a high frequency of deficiencies. Their research revealed that 8% of patients did not receive a physical exam, 32% did not have vital signs obtained, and 67% had an incomplete history of present illness among other deficiencies. Another retrospective chart review published in 1994 measured the completeness of documentation and accuracy of the medical evaluation of 298 ED patients with psychiatric chief complaints.[37] This review found that 56% of patients did not have a documented mental status exam (the most common deficiency), and 4% of patients required medical treatment within 24 hours of admission to the psychiatric unit. Interestingly, the authors suggested that the ED history and physical alone should have identified the medical condition in 83% of these patients. In 2000, Reeves et al.[38] retrospectively reviewed 64 cases of medical emergencies inappropriately admitted to psychiatric units to determine the cause of the misdiagnosis. Patients with acute intoxication due to alcohol or other illicit substances (34.4%), drug or alcohol withdrawal, including delirium tremens (12.5%), and prescription drug overdoses (12.5%) were the most commonly missed medical diagnoses. Among these patients, none received appropriate mental status exams, and they often had inadequate physical exams (43.8%) and histories (34.4%) performed. According to the authors, the referring clinicians also failed to order indicated laboratory studies in 34.4% of these cases. The authors appropriately concluded that "a systematic approach is required for patients with altered mental status." This article reinforces the concept that a chief complaint of altered mental status is considered a red-flag presentation. Last, Szpakowicz and Herd[39] also performed a retrospective chart review of patients diagnosed with schizophrenia for the completeness of the medical clearance examination in the ED. The findings were consistent with those of previous studies which found that charts regularly lacked documentation of complete physical examinations. More alarmingly, complete vital signs were only recorded for 52% of patients, and in 6% of patients, no vital signs were recorded at all.

Despite the deficiencies that have been documented during the medical evaluation, at a minimum, patients presenting with psychiatric symptoms require a thorough history and physical exam. Performing an adequate history and physical exam should not be considered a formality and performed in a cursory fashion but, rather, viewed as an opportunity to get the assessment correct and to identify and address potentially unstable or causative conditions. It is an incredibly important part of a patient's evaluation and, depending on what is identified, will later direct which diagnostic tests, if any, should be ordered.

History

Obtaining a thorough history is perhaps the most important part of the medical evaluation. The value of a thorough history is seldom debated and has been confirmed by a 1997 study that calculated the history to be 94% sensitive for identifying medical conditions.[40] Intuitively this makes sense. Assuming the patient is cooperative and coherent enough, the history is where the patient will describe the onset and quality of symptoms and also confirm recent medication use and the presence of other medical conditions that may have precipitated their condition. The history should include a detailed assessment of a patient's presenting signs and symptoms and a review of their medical, psychiatric, medication, and social histories.[41] During the history, the clinician should pay special attention to a patient's quality, onset, and timing of symptoms, as well as any provoking and alleviating factors. It is also important to understand how the patient's symptoms or behaviors have changed from their baseline because this may hold valuable clues to identifying the precipitating etiology.[42]

Physical Exam

Performing a complete physical exam is an essential part of the focused medical assessment of the psychiatric patient and is also the next most sensitive element for identifying acute medical illness. Olshaker et al.[40] found that the physical exam had a sensitivity of 51% for identifying acute medical conditions in their retrospective analysis of 345 psychiatric patients. Every physical exam should begin with an assessment of the patient's vital signs, including temperature, heart rate, respiratory rate, blood pressure, and pulse oximetry without supplemental oxygenation.[43] Whereas some minor vital sign abnormalities, such as mild tachycardia, tachypnea, or hypertension, may not necessarily indicate an acute or unstable medical condition, others, such as fever, significant tachycardia, hypotension, or hypoxia, would be far more concerning and warrant further investigation.

The physical exam should include the elements outlined in Table 3.1 and, ideally, should be driven by the history of present illness, past medical history, and review of systems. Patients with physical complaints should have a complete and detailed exam of the affected organ system, and a brief exam of the remaining systems may suffice. Regardless of the complaint, special consideration should always be given to evaluating the patient's

Table 3.1 Physical Exam Elements

System	Critical Elements
General	Vital signs (temperature, heart rate, blood pressure, respiratory rate, pulse oximetry)
Cardiovascular	Respiratory effort/auscultation, cardiac auscultation, circulation
Musculoskeletal	Deformities, prosthetics
Integumentary	Rashes, lacerations, wounds
Neurologic	Mental status assessment

mental status. The mental status exam is an important element of the physical because it is used to evaluate patients for the presence of delirium, an important and potentially lethal condition.

The Mental Status Exam

Delirium is an acute, transient, and often reversible change in mental status marked by both a disturbance of consciousness/attention (drowsiness and reduced ability to focus, sustain, or shift attention) and a change in cognitive function affecting memory, orientation, visuospatial ability, or perception. In contrast to dementia and other permanent behavioral and cognitive diseases, delirium develops over hours to days and the symptoms typically fluctuate in intensity and often worsen at night.[44] Delirium is a syndrome, not a specific disease or etiology. As such, delirium may be caused by a wide range of medical conditions (Table 3.2), many of which are life-threatening and require urgent recognition and treatment.[45,46] In the ED setting, delirium is often caused by intoxication, medications, and infection; however, the incidence of each etiology is largely dependent on the patient's age group and specific risk factors.

Even for the experienced clinician, recognizing delirium presents a significant diagnostic challenge. Delirium is common, especially among elderly patients, yet is often missed. Some studies claim that clinicians recognize delirium in less than 20% of patients presenting with behavioral disturbances.[47] The high rate of under-recognition is alarming but understandable given that patients may present anywhere along the behavioral spectrum from hypoactivity to hyperactivity. Furthermore, the constellation of symptoms can mimic those of other neuropsychiatric conditions, leading to misdiagnosis. Therefore, any patient presenting with an acute change in behavior or altered mental status, especially among elderly patients or those with new onset of symptoms, should be screened for delirium before presuming that they are suffering from an acute psychiatric condition.

Table 3.2 Common Causes of Delirium

Category	Etiology
Cardiopulmonary	Hypoxia, hypercarbia, hypotension, acute coronary syndrome, heart failure, anemia
Endocrinopathies	Hypothyroidism, hyperthyroidism, hypopituitarism, hypoparathyroidism, hyperparathyroidism
Infection	Urinary tract infection, pneumonia, meningitis, encephalitis, intra-abdominal infections, sepsis
Medication	Anticholinergic agents, sedative hypnotics, antipsychotics, anticonvulsants, opioids, corticosteroids, polypharmacy
Metabolic	Hypo- or hyperglycemia, hypo- or hypernatremia, diabetic ketoacidosis, hepatic insufficiency, uremia, dehydration, thiamine deficiency (Wernicke's encephalopathy)
Neurologic	Stroke, transient ischemic attack, head injury, intracranial hemorrhage, intracranial mass, seizures, migraine
Toxicologic/withdrawal	Intoxication with alcohol or illicit drugs, alcohol or benzodiazepine withdrawal
Other	Environmental changes, insomnia, lack of hearing or vision aids, pain

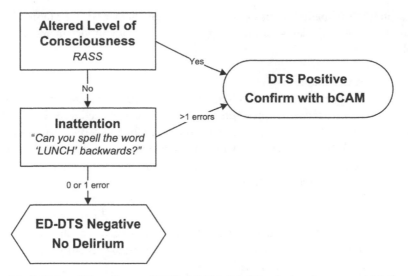

Figure 3.1 Delirium Triage Screen (DTS). bCAM, Brief Confusion Assessment Method; RASS, Richmond Agitation–Sedation Scale.

Several validated screening tools have been developed to assist the clinician in identifying delirium, including the Delirium Triage Screen (DTS), the Brief Confusion Assessment Method (bCAM), the 3D-Confusion Assessment Method, the Quick Confusion Scale, and the Confusion Assessment Method.[48–51] Screening tools should be quick to administer and must be highly sensitive in order to reliably exclude delirium from the differential. In consideration of these criteria, I recommend the DTS, which has proven to be 98% sensitive while only taking an average of 20 seconds to administer.[48] However, the DTS was designed as a screening tool and is only 55% specific when used alone. Therefore, patients who screen positive on the DTS must then undergo a more specific test, such as the bCAM, to confirm the presence of delirium. Both the DTS and the bCAM utilize the Richmond Agitation–Sedation Scale to screen for altered level of consciousness (Figure 3.1; Table 3.3).[52]

Table 3.3 Richmond Agitation–Sedation Scale

Points	Criteria	Definition
+4	Combative	Overtly combative, violent, immediate danger to staff
+3	Very agitated	Pulls or removes tube(s) or catheter(s), aggressive
+2	Agitated	Frequent nonpurposeful movement, fights ventilator
+1	Restless	Anxious but movements not aggressive vigorous
0	Alert and calm	
−1	Drowsy	Not fully alert, but has sustained awakening (eye opening/eye contact) to voice (>10 seconds)
−2	Light sedation	Briefly awakens with eye contact to voice (<10 seconds)
−3	Moderate sedation	Movement or eye opening to voice (but no eye contact)
−4	Deep sedation	No response to voice, but movement or eye movement to physical stimulation
−5	Unarousable	No response to voice or physical stimulation

Ancillary Testing

When completed appropriately, the history and physical examination will reliably identify the vast majority of medical conditions among patients presenting with psychiatric symptoms. Ancillary testing, such as laboratory tests, UDSs, and imaging, is not typically necessary for all patients and should be obtained as directed by the history and physical exam.

Utility of Laboratory Testing

Based on an unusually high prevalence of medical illnesses among patients with psychiatric presentations, many earlier studies advocated for the implementation of routine laboratory testing protocols to identify causative or comorbid medical conditions. However, most of these studies did not exclude patients with obvious organic etiologies, and they also suffered from significant selection bias, making their conclusions difficult to apply to typical modern EDs.

Several more recent studies have demonstrated that routine comprehensive testing is generally low yield and unnecessary, especially if patients are appropriately risk stratified. Dolan and Mushlin[53] studied the utility of routine laboratory testing among 250 psychiatric inpatients by searching for positive results that they termed "laboratory diagnoses." Patients underwent an average of 27.7 tests. They classified the results as either "true- or false-positive" and found a true-positive rate of only 1.8%, whereas false positives were eight times more frequent. Not surprisingly, their rate of laboratory diagnoses was only 0.08%. The authors concluded that extensive, routine testing is unnecessary, and they recommended that strategies for more accurate and efficient testing should be developed using clinical information. In 1997, Olshaker and colleagues[40] found in their analysis of 345 psychiatric patients that the vast majority of medical problems could be identified by history and physical alone. Three years later, Korn et al.[54] performed comprehensive laboratory testing on 212 consecutive patients with psychiatric complaints aged 16 years or older presenting to an ED during a 5-month period. Their protocol included a complete blood count, electrolyte analysis, toxicology screen, and a chest X-ray. Of the patients who presented with isolated psychiatric complaints and a documented past psychiatric history, none had positive screening laboratory or radiographic results. They concluded that patients with a psychiatric complaint, confirmed past psychiatric history, and who deny having medical problems can be referred directly to psychiatric services without ancillary testing, assuming they have stable vital signs and a normal physical exam.

Gregory et al.,[55] Janiak and Atteberry,[56] and Kagel et al.[57] all found similar results indicating that routine laboratory testing of patients presenting to the ED with psychiatric complaints is unnecessary and very low yield. According to their findings, patients with isolated psychiatric complaints, normal vital signs, and normal physical exams (with adequate mental status assessment) in the absence of high-risk medical conditions (elderly, new-onset psychiatric conditions, substance use, and preexisting medical conditions) should not undergo comprehensive testing but, rather, should receive selective testing.

Despite overwhelming evidence that routine laboratory testing is unnecessary among select patient groups, the debate among emergency physicians and psychiatrists has persisted. This is likely due to the fact that most EDs do not utilize a consistent and objective method for conducting the history and physical or risk stratifying patients in need of laboratory testing. In response, the professional societies ACEP and the American Association of Emergency Psychiatrists (AAEP) both issued clinical policies and consensus statements to guide the industry toward standard practice.

Box 3.1 AAEP's High-Risk Presentations

1. New-onset psychiatric symptoms after age 45 years
2. Advanced age (age 65 years or older)
3. Cognitive deficits or delirium
4. Positive review of systems indicative of a physical etiology, such as cough and fever
5. Focal neurologic findings or evidence of head injury
6. Substance intoxication, withdrawal, or exposure to toxins/drugs
7. Decreased level of awareness
8. Other indications, such as abnormal vital signs that direct further assessment

---

In 2006, ACEP published its clinical policy on the diagnosis and management of psychiatric patients in the ED.[10] In this review article, ACEP issued a "Level B recommendation" stating, "In adult patients with primary psychiatric complaints, diagnostic evaluation should be directed by the history and physical examination." ACEP added, "Routine laboratory testing of all patients is of very low yield and need not be performed as part of the ED assessment." Taking a less definitive yet more measured approach, an AAEP task force issued a consensus statement on the medical evaluation of psychiatric patients in 2017.[58] Among its eight recommendations, it suggested that psychiatric patients be universally screened, but it qualified this statement by recommending that, at a minimum, the screening should include vital signs, history and physical exam, and an assessment of mentation in the form of a brief cognitive exam. The task force also recommended a more rigorous evaluation for patients with high-risk presentations as outlined in Box 3.1, consistent with the recommendations of previous studies. In addition, the task force correctly noted that some psychiatric facilities have limited laboratory testing capabilities and that EDs should take this into consideration when labs are requested yet should not delay transfer.

After thorough review of the available literature from the past four decades, most clinicians would conclude that routine, comprehensive laboratory testing is unnecessary for most psychiatric patients and that emergency physicians should rely on the findings of their detailed history and physical exam to direct the need for further testing—in the words of Tolia and Wilson,[46] "examine thoroughly, test selectively." Gregory et al.[55] also summarized this approach well by stating, "Instead of routine laboratory screening testing in the ED, the data support more selective testing for patients at high risk of serious medical pathology."

Urine Drug Screen

Substance abuse and co-occurring mental health problems are a common presenting complaint in EDs. In fact, between 2010 and 2014, mental health issues, including substance abuse, were cited as the second most common reason for an ED visit (4.45%) after abdominal pain (11.75%).[59] More alarming was the rate of growth for mental health– and substance use–related complaints, estimated by a compound annual growth rate of 4.2%, second only to arthritis and joint problems.

The utility of the UDS in evaluating patients with psychiatric complaints has also been extensively deliberated. Classically speaking, psychiatrists believe the information provided by the UDS is of critical importance when identifying and differentiating the primary cause of a patient's change in behavior. In addition, positive findings on a UDS can help a psychiatrist identify a patient's triggers and reasons for decompensation. Alternatively, emergency physicians seldom rely on the results of a UDS to initiate resuscitative treatment or make disposition decisions. Emergency physicians not only view UDSs as providing low clinical value but also are reluctant to order UDSs because they have been known to increase cost and length of stay and, at their worst, may provide misleading information.

Studies have cited a relatively high sensitivity of the patient's self-reported social history in identifying recent substance use. Olshaker et al.[40] reported that the history is 91% sensitive in identifying illicit substance use and 96% sensitive in identifying alcohol use within the past 24 hours. A more recent study also confirmed high sensitivity of the social history, with 89.6% of UDS-positive patients reporting a history of drug use.[60] The authors concluded that the urine toxicology screen does not independently add diagnostic value when standard substance use histories have been implemented.

Although helping clinicians identify and document another 10% of substance use disorders in the ED setting may not seem overwhelmingly valuable, any diagnostic information that helps change a patient's management or disposition would be considered by many to add significant value. Naturally, then, the ability of the UDS to assist with management and disposition decisions has also been evaluated. Regardless of study type and design, several publications have confirmed what has been anecdotally known for years—that the results of a UDS for patients presenting to an ED or psychiatric emergency setting have little or no influence on the patient's acute management or ultimate disposition but can negatively impact cost and ED length of stay.[61-65] These findings and conclusions have also been confirmed among pediatric patients as well. Fortu et al.[66] retrospectively examined the charts of 652 ED pediatric patients aged 8–17 years who received a UDS for purposes of medical clearance. They categorized each UDS as "medically indicated" by the patient's presenting signs and symptoms or "routine-driven" when patients presented with uncomplicated symptoms. They evaluated the patients with routine-driven tests and determined how frequently the results of the UDS changed their management or disposition. Among the 385 patients with routine-driven tests, 95% of patients with negative screens and 97% of patients with positive screens were referred for psychiatric evaluation and treatment. The difference between the groups was determined to be statistically insignificant. In addition to concluding that the UDS did not influence the management of these patients, the authors also suggested that the UDS may increase evaluation cost ($154.00) and time.

Any cost–benefit analysis of a particular medical test would be incomplete without consideration of the test's accuracy and reliability. There is no such thing as the perfect diagnostic test (100% sensitive and 100% specific). Yet some tests clearly outperform others in their ability to rule in or rule out disease. The UDS, like any other test, is far from perfect, and depending on the particular technique and substance being screened for, its performance can vary significantly. Most hospital laboratories utilize an immunoassay technique for their UDS due to the fact that they are relatively low cost, simple to perform, and offer fast turnaround times. Unfortunately, some UDS immunoassay components lack specificity, are prone to false-positive results (especially amphetamines), and can be difficult or misleading for clinicians to interpret due to cross-reactivity with common therapeutic medications.[67-69]

Given the relatively high sensitivity of a thorough social history for the detection of drugs of abuse and in light of evidence suggesting that results of the UDS can be clinically misleading, unnecessarily increase diagnostic costs, and rarely change management in the ED setting, it is difficult to recommend the routine ordering of a UDS on all patients presenting to the ED for psychiatric symptoms. Rather, it is more logical for the evaluating clinician to selectively test patients with altered mental status or undifferentiated behavioral disturbances in the setting of a negative social history or among those with somatic complaints.

Blood Alcohol Levels

It is widely recognized that alcohol use and abuse are widespread among the U.S. population. It has been estimated that in 2017 and 2018, 69.5% of people aged 18 years or older consumed an alcoholic beverage within the last year and 25.8% reported heavy alcohol use or binge drinking within the last month. During the same time period, 14.1 million adults, or 5.6% of the population, aged 18 years or older suffered from alcohol use disorder.[70] Acute alcohol-related conditions increased rapidly during the past decade and in 2014 accounted for more than 2.7 million ED visits, a 51.5% increase over 2009.[71] With such high prevalence, it is understandable why emergency physicians and psychiatrists have become adept at evaluating patients impaired by alcohol. However, emergency physicians and psychiatrists often play different roles when assessing patients under the influence of alcohol. The emergency physician is expected to evaluate the patient through the lens of medical stability and, to a lesser extent, whether or not alcohol has played a significant role in the manifestation of their symptoms. On the other hand, alcohol can adversely influence the psychiatric assessment by preventing the exam altogether or by mimicking or exacerbating psychiatric symptoms.

The debate is not about whether or not alcohol can influence a patient's presentation but, rather, at what point during a patient's presentation is alcohol no longer considered an influential factor. As one might expect, this is not easy to determine, and there is no one single method that has been accepted to make this determination. Like many other things in medicine, it depends on the clinician's assessment and comfort level, the patient's level of impairment, and local customs and practice. But most psychiatric facilities refuse to accept patients who are impaired, and in some circumstances, they require objective evidence that a patient's blood alcohol level (BAL) is below a certain threshold before the patient is transferred. Ironically, most clinicians know through experience that a patient's BAL does not always predict their level of impairment. This phenomenon, thought to be due to physiologic differences in tolerance, has been studied and confirmed in the literature.[72,73] Despite widespread practice in EDs, there is no evidence to support that a patient is "cleared" for psychiatric assessment below a given BAL nor that a psychiatric assessment should be delayed until the patient achieves a specific BAL.

In 2006, ACEP published recommendations to address these inconsistencies.[10] In its evidence-based clinical policy, ACEP answered the question, "Does an elevated alcohol level preclude the initiation of a psychiatric evaluation in alert, cooperative patients with normal vital signs and a noncontributory history and physical examination?" ACEP's suggestions, classified as "Level C" recommendations, stated that a patient's level of cognition, rather than a specific BAL, should determine when the patient is ready to participate in the psychiatric evaluation. ACEP also recommended that clinicians consider observing patients to determine if their psychiatric symptoms resolve with their level of impairment.

Unfortunately, at the time of ACEP's publication, no standardized assessment had been developed to assist the clinician in objectively determining a patient's level of impairment. As a result, a patient's readiness for psychiatric assessments was, and to a large extent still is, being determined based on the emergency physician's subjective assessment of the patient or the patient's BAL. Since then, an objective bedside assessment tool called Hack's Impairment Index (HII) score has been developed and validated on an ED population. HII allows the clinician to reliably test and document levels of impairment.[74,75] The HII score was designed to be used by health care professionals (HCPs) in busy clinical environments and is composed of five simple tasks, each of which is scored objectively and may be repeated over time if necessary. The five tasks (speech and cognition, gross motor, nystagmus, finger-to-target, fine motor and coordination) were rooted in prior research and are scored by the HCP at the bedside on a 0–4 scale. Therefore, the lowest and highest possible HII scores are 0 and 20, respectively. In both the derivation study (Hack et al.[74]) and the validation study (Hack et al.[75]), the HII score demonstrated the ability to act as a quantitative, objective, and reliable assessment of alcohol impairment. The authors also noted how the HII score outperformed ethanol levels (BAL) as an objective measure of impairment.

Practicing clinicians evaluating patients with psychiatric complaints will commonly assess patients who are impaired by alcohol. As a result, they must be prepared to consider how they will assess patients' level of impairment and when they believe patients may participate in the psychiatric evaluation. Until 2014, clinicians had only two choices to evaluate impairment: subjective clinical assessment and BALs. However, now there are three with the introduction of the HII score. Given the unreliability, cost, and potential for delays in care, it may be time to transition away from ordering BALs, especially when patients do not appear to be impaired. Also, as an alternative to subjective clinical assessment, the HII score should be considered for ease of use, low cost, and ability to reliably assess level of impairment.

Pediatric Patients

In 2011, psychiatric chief complaints among children accounted for 7.2% of all ED visits, and between 2007 and 2016, despite stable pediatric ED volume, the rate of mental health-related disorders increased by 60%.[76,77] Even more alarmingly, during the same 9-year period, visits for deliberate self-harm increased by 329%. Yet the majority of research specifically addressing the medical evaluation of patients with psychiatric symptoms focuses on the adult population.

Recent studies have evaluated what is widely considered to be the most controversial topic regarding the assessment of pediatric patients: the need for comprehensive laboratory testing and UDS. Fortu et al.[64] and Shihabuddin et al.[66] both evaluated the utility of obtaining a routine UDS on pediatric patients and found that the results did not influence management or disposition. Similar to the adult population, Fortu et al. noted that the UDS had a negative impact on cost and ED length of stay. Routine, comprehensive laboratory testing has also been studied in the pediatric population. Donofrio et al.[78,79] performed a retrospective chart review of 1,082 pediatric patients presenting to the ED with psychiatric complaints. Of the 80.5% that received screening laboratory tests, only 7 resulted in disposition changes (0.8%), and only 1 of these patients had a non-contributory history and physical exam for a positive pregnancy test. Twenty-five patients (2.9%) with non-contributory history and physical exams had management-changing test results; however, all were considered non-urgent. The median charge for blood and urine testing among these patients was $1,235. The authors calculated the potential annual savings for provider-initiated selective testing to be up to $90 million without reducing the ability to diagnose emergency medical conditions.

Santillanes et al.[80] evaluated the possibility of developing pre-hospital criteria to divert pediatric patients with acute psychiatric symptoms away from the ED and directly to psychiatric facilities. They retrospectively reviewed the charts of 789 patients transported to the ED and determined that 90.9% did not require medical screening, potentially saving $1,241,295 by eliminating unnecessary laboratory tests and sitter wages. Based on their findings, they suggested developing high-risk criteria that would identify the need for medical screening, such as "altered mental status, ingestion, hanging, traumatic injury, unrelated medical complaints or rape."

Similar to adults, the literature available to date suggests that routine comprehensive testing of pediatric patients with psychiatric symptoms adds little value while increasing cost and delays in care. In 2016, the American Academy of Pediatrics in coordination with ACEP issued a summary and consensus statement on the medical clearance of pediatric patients that summarized current knowledge on the topic by stating that when patients are clinically stable, "routine diagnostic testing generally is low yield, costly, and unlikely to be of value or affect the disposition or management of ED psychiatric patients."[81] The logical conclusion that may be drawn from this statement and supporting literature is that routine comprehensive testing should not be performed indiscriminately on pediatric patients but, rather, that clinicians should test patients selectively based on findings revealed during the history and physical exam when compared to known, high-risk criteria.

Standardized Medical Clearance Protocols

Given the extent of literature suggesting that patients should undergo selective testing for medical clearance, it would be natural to assume that standardized protocols designed to guide the medical clearance process would be in wide use today. Unfortunately, this is not the case. However, standardized protocols have been discussed and evaluated in the literature, albeit with varying results. Zun and Downey[82] retrospectively reviewed the charts of 97 patients who underwent medical clearance before transfer to an inpatient psychiatric facility. Thirty-three charts were reviewed before and 64 charts after the implementation of a five-question protocol designed to identify patients who required further testing (Box 3.2). Although they found that the protocol did not influence length

---

Box 3.2 Zun and Downey's Screening Questions[82]

Does the patient have any new psychiatric condition?
Does the patient have any history of active illness needing evaluation?
Does the patient have any abnormal vital signs?
Does the patient have an abnormal physical exam (unclothed)?
Does the patient have any abnormal mental status?

of stay or rate of return to the ED, they did note a reduction of ancillary testing and cost ($352 before versus $269 after).

Shah et al.[83] evaluated the usefulness of a similar tool on a much larger cohort. The authors retrospectively reviewed the charts of 485 patients with primarily psychiatric complaints screened prior to transfer to a psychiatric crisis center. The tool consisted of a five-item questionnaire including the assessment for stable vital signs, prior psychiatric history, level of alertness and orientation, acute medical problems, and visual hallucinations. After screening with the tool, only 6 patients (1.2%) were sent back to the ED for further evaluation, and after laboratory and radiologic testing, none required more than an outpatient prescription.

Miller et al.[84] studied the performance of the triage algorithm for psychiatric screening (TAPS) on patients presenting to the ED with psychiatric chief complaints. TAPS assesses patients against seven potential exclusions: age younger than 65 years; normal vital signs; no medical complaints; no evidence of recent substance use; and no history of schizophrenia, mental retardation, or hallucinations. In a random sample of 100 TAPS-negative patients, none received a diagnosis of or treatment for acute medical illness. In a separate 2018 study, the TAPS protocol successfully identified low-risk patients without significant medical illness.[85]

More recently, the development of another screening tool, sponsored by the Sierra Sacramento Valley Medical Society (SSVMS), has received attention as a promising alternative to routine, comprehensive testing. In 2015, SSVMS published a white paper titled "Crisis in the Emergency Department: Removing Barriers to Timely and Appropriate Mental Health Treatment."[86] The second recommendation made in the white paper was to implement a regional, standardized medical clearance protocol that SSVMS refers to as SMART (Figure 3.2). SMART is an acronym reflecting each of five exclusionary categories designed to identify high-risk patients requiring selective laboratory testing (Box 3.3). In practice, the clinician evaluates each patient by reviewing the five SMART categories, and if the clinician scores the patients as "no" in all five, the patient is considered stable for psychiatric evaluation or transfer and does not require any additional testing. However, if the clinician answers "yes" to any element, further evaluation and consideration of testing are indicated. SMART was also designed to eliminate the reliance on BALs by incorporation of the HII score discussed previously.[74,75] Local and regional adoption of SMART medical clearance reflects the current industry appetite for effective protocol-based screening tools.[87,88]

With evidence that some local and regional protocols have been implemented successfully, one may wonder why there is no generally accepted industry standard. The reason likely has to do with local and regional variation in expectations among psychiatric receiving facilities. In general, emergency physicians would support the adoption of a protocol for assessing psychiatric patients, especially if it meant ordering fewer diagnostic tests and alleviating transfer delays. However, the accepting facilities must be willing to recognize that some patients can be adequately evaluated in the absence of ancillary testing. This would explain why local and regional coalitions have been successful in implementing these protocols. In order for change to occur, the literature must be recognized, consensus must be reached, and trust must be established.

We should also recognize that to date, the industry has not been pressured to change. In other words, payers and regulatory agencies have not yet expressed a desire to minimize the cost of the medical assessment. Now that it is evident that the medical assessment can be performed safely with a substantial reduction in laboratory testing, it may

SMART Medical Clearance Form

	No*	Yes	Time Resolved
Suspect <u>New Onset</u> Psychiatric Condition?	1		
Medical Conditions that Require Screening?	2		
Diabetes (FSBS less than 60 or greater than 250)			
Possibility of pregnancy (age 12-50)			
Other complaints that require screening			
Abnormal:	3		
Vital Signs?			
Temp: greater than 38.0°C (100.4°F)			
HR: less than 50 or greater than 110			
BP: less than 100 systolic or greater than 180/110 (2 consecutive readings 15 min apart)			
RR: less than 8 or greater than 22			
O_2 Sat: less than 95% on room air			
Mental Status?			
Cannot answer name, month/year and location (minimum A/O x 3)			
If clinically intoxicated, HII score 4 or more? (next page)			
Physical Exam (unclothed)?			
Risky Presentation?	4		
Age less than 12 or greater than 55			
Possibility of ingestion (screen all suicidal patients)			
Eating disorders			
Potential for alcohol withdrawal (daily use equal to or greater than 2 weeks) ...			
Ill-appearing, significant injury, prolonged struggle or "found down"			
Therapeutic Levels Needed?	5		
Phenytoin			
Valproic acid			
Lithium			
Digoxin			
Warfarin (INR)			

* If ALL five SMART categories are checked "NO" then the patient is considered medically cleared and no testing is indicated. If ANY category is checked "YES" then appropriate testing and/or documentation of rationale must be reflected in the medical record and time resolved must be documented above.

Date: _____ Time: _____ Completed by: _____ _____, MD/DO
                                                      Signature   Print

Figure 3.2 SMART Medical Clearance.

Box 3.3 SMART Medical Clearance Categories

Suspect new-onset psychiatric condition?
Medical conditions that require screening?
Abnormal: vital signs, mental status, physical exam (unclothed)?
Risky presentation?
Therapeutic levels needed?

just be a matter of time before expectations are placed upon evaluating clinicians to reduce the number of tests per patient.

Pitfalls of the Medical Assessment

Medically assessing patients with psychiatric symptoms in an ED setting can be a formi-
dable challenge. When performed as intended, patients are evaluated quickly, unstable
medical conditions are identified or excluded, and patients are transferred to the most
appropriate level of care. On the other hand, when performed inadequately, failure to
identify unstable medical conditions may go unrecognized and result in significant morbidity or mortality for the patient. To ensure patients receive a high-quality medical assessment, evaluating clinicians should avoid the following pitfalls:[42]

- Failure to perform an adequate history
- Failure to identify and address vital sign abnormalities
- Failure to perform an adequate physical exam
- Failure to assess mental status
- Ordering routine, comprehensive testing without clinical indication
- Relying on laboratory testing without performing an adequate history and phys-
  ical exam
- Anchoring on a psychiatric diagnosis

Assuming these common pitfalls are avoided, and clinicians embrace the evidence that
is currently available, patients will continue to receive high-quality medical assessments.

Conclusion

On the surface, the medical assessment of the psychiatric patient may seem simple,
yet in reality, emergency physicians are commonly faced with the complex task of
screening patients for unstable medical conditions and ruling out medical mimics of
psychiatric disease in a safe and resource-conscious fashion. Historically, the medical
assessment comprised a combination of the history and physical exam and routine
comprehensive testing in response to reports of surprisingly high rates of acute medical conditions among psychiatric patients. However, these studies were conducted
in atypical settings and included patients with high-risk complaints that would or-
dinarily be identified during the history and physical exam. Despite evidence that
routine comprehensive testing is unnecessary, costly, and can delay care, emergency
physicians are often expected to obtain them as part of their evaluation, regardless
of the patient's presentation.[89] Rationally, this makes little sense but is likely rooted
in the fact that emergency physicians have been shown to perform cursory exams on
psychiatric patients and even omit critical portions of the medical assessment, fueling
distrust among psychiatrists.

   Fortunately, the path forward is clear: It is time to move away from the compulsory
ordering of comprehensive testing and let the history and physical exam guide what is
necessary. However, to accomplish this and ensure consistency, the time has come to
advocate for widespread standardization and adoption of medical assessment guidelines

and protocols. The benefits to patients, clinicians, and the health care system as a whole are too great to ignore. It may be unreasonable to expect the medical community to adopt a single, specific protocol considering how widely individual practices and circumstances vary; however, one must believe it is possible to successfully implement them on regional or statewide levels.

References

1. Santillanes G, Axeen S, Lam CN, et al. National trends in mental health-related emergency department visits by children and adults. *Am J Emerg Med*. 2020;38(12):2536–2544.

2. Emergency Medical Treatment & Labor Act (EMTALA). Centers for Medicare & Medicaid Services. Updated March 26, 2012. Accessed December 30, 2020. https://www.cms.gov/Regulations-and-Guidance/Legislation/EMTALA

3. Compilation of the Social Security laws: Examination and treatment for emergency medical conditions and women in labor. Sec. 1867. Social Security Administration. Accessed December 30, 2020. https://www.ssa.gov/OP_Home/ssact/title18/1867.htm

4. State Operations Manual: Appendix V-Interpretive guidelines-Responsibilities of Medicare participating hospitals in emergency cases. Rev. 191. Centers for Medicare & Medicaid Services. Updated July 19, 2019. Accessed December 30, 2020. https://www.cms.gov/Regulations-and-Guidance/Guidance/Manuals/Downloads/som107ap_v_emerg.pdf

5. State Operations Manual (SOM) Emergency Medical Treatment and Labor Act (EMTALA) and death associated with restraint or seclusion complaint investigation timeline revisions. Centers for Medicare & Medicaid Services. Published June 4, 2019. Accessed December 30, 2020. https://www.cms.gov/Medicare/Provider-Enrollment-and-Certification/SurveyCertificationGenInfo/Policy-and-Memos-to-States-and-Regions-Items/QSO-19-14-Hospitals-CAHs

6. Zun LS, Hernandez R, Thompson R, et al. Comparison of EPs' and psychiatrists' laboratory assessment of psychiatric patients. *Am J Emerg Med*. 2004;22(3): 175–180.

7. Reeves RR, Perry CL, Burke RS. What does "medical clearance" for psychiatry really mean? *J Psychosoc Nurs Ment Health Serv*. 2010;48(8):2–4.

8. Weissberg MP. Emergency room medical clearance: An educational problem. *Am J Psychiatry*. 1979;136(6):787–790.

9. Anderson EL, Nordstrom K, Wilson MP, et al. American Association for Emergency Psychiatry Task Force on Medical Clearance of Adults Part I: Introduction, review and evidence-based guidelines. *West J Emerg Med*. 2017;18(2):235–242. doi:10.5811/westjem.2016.10.32258

10. Lukens TW, Wolf SJ, Edlow JA, et al. Clinical policy: Critical issues in the diagnosis and management of the adult psychiatric patient in the emergency department. *Ann Emerg Med*. 2006;47(1):79–99.

11. Colodny D, Kenny C, Kurlander LF. The educationally handicapped child: The physician's place in a program to overcome learning disability. *Calif Med*. 1968;109(1):15–18.

12. Goldman LS. Medical illness in patients with schizophrenia. *J Clin Psychiatry*. 1999;60(Suppl 21):10–15.

13. Felker B, Yazel JJ, Short D. Mortality and medical comorbidity among psychiatric patients: A review. *Psychiatr Serv*. 1996;47(12):1356–1363.

14. Young JQ, Kline-Simon AH, Mordecai DJ, Weisner C. Prevalence of behavioral health disorders and associated chronic disease burden in a commercially insured health system: findings of a case-control study. *Gen Hosp Psychiatry*. 2015;37(2):101–108.

15. Druss BG, von Esenwein SA, Compton MT, et al. Budget impact and sustainability of medical care management for persons with serious mental illness. *Am J Psychiatry*. 2011;168:1171–1178.

16. Kisely S, Sadek J, MacKenzie A, et al. Excess cancer mortality in psychiatric patients. *Can J Psychiatry*. 2008;53:753–761.

17. Kisely S, Preston N, Xiao J, et al. Reducing all-cause mortality among patients with psychiatric disorders: A population-based study. *CMAJ*. 2013;185:E50–E56.

18. Dickerson FB, Stallings C, Origoni A, et al. Predictors of occupational status six months after hospitalization in persons with a recent onset of psychosis. *Psychiatry Res*. 2008;160:278–284.

19. Marshall HES. Incidence of physical disorders among psychiatric in-patients. *Br Med J*. 1949;2(4625):468–470.

20. Herridge CF. Physical disorders in psychiatric illness. A study of 209 consecutive admissions. *Lancet*. 1960;2(7157):949–951.

21. Davies DW. Physical illness in psychiatric out-patients. *Br J Psychiatry*. 1965;111:27–33.

22. Johnson DA. The evaluation of routine physical examination in psychiatric cases. *Practitioner*. 1968;200(199):686–691.

23. Maguire GP, Granville-Grossman KL. Physical illness in psychiatric patients. *Br J Psychiatry*. 1968;114(516):1365–1369.

24. Koranyi EK. Physical health and illness in a psychiatric outpatient department population. *Can Psychiatr Assoc J*. 1972;17(2):SS109.

25. Willett AB, King T. Implementation of laboratory screening procedures on a short-term psychiatric inpatient unit. *Dis Nerv Syst*. 1977;38(11):867–870.

26. Hall RCW, Popkin MK, Devaul RA, et al. Physical illness presenting as a psychiatric disease. *Arch Gen Psychiatry*. 1978;35(11):1315–1320.

27. Koranyi EK. Morbidity and rate of undiagnosed physical illnesses in a psychiatric clinic population. *Arch Gen Psychiatry*. 1979;36(4):414–419.

28. Hall RC, Gardner ER, Popkin MK, Lecann AF, Stickney SK. Unrecognized physical illness prompting psychiatric admission: A prospective study. *Am J Psychiatry*. 1981;138(5):629–635.

29. Kolman PB. The value of laboratory investigations of elderly psychiatric patients. *J Clin Psychiatry*. 1984;45(3):112–116.

30. Ferguson B, Dudleston K. Detection of physical disorder in newly admitted psychiatric patients. *Acta Psychiatr Scand*. 1986;74(5):485–489.

31. Bunce DF, 2nd, Jones LR, Badger LW, Jones SE. Medical illness in psychiatric patients: Barriers to diagnosis and treatment. *South M J*. 1982;75(8):941–944.

32. Henneman PL, Mendoza R, Lewis RJ. Prospective evaluation of emergency department medical clearance. *Ann Emerg Med*. 1994;24(4):672–677.

33. Reeves RR, Parker JD, Burke RS, Hart RH. Inappropriate psychiatric admission of elderly patients with unrecognized delirium. *South Med J*. 2010;103(2):111–115.

34. Summers WK, Munoz RA, Read MR. The psychiatric physical exam-Part I: Methodology. *J Clin Psychiatry*. 1981;42(3):95–98.

35. Summers WK, Munoz RA, Read MR, Marsh GM. The psychiatric physical exam-Part II: Findings in 75 unselected psychiatric patients. *J Clin Psychiatry*. 1981;42(3):99–102.

36. Riba M, Hale M. Medical clearance: Fact or fiction in the hospital emergency room. *Psychosomatics*. 1990;31(4):400–404.

37. Tintinalli JE, Peacock FW 4th, Wright MA. Emergency medical evaluation of psychiatric patients. *Ann Emerg Med*. 1994;23(4):859–862.

38. Reeves RR, Pendarvis EJ, Kimble R. Unrecognized medical emergencies admitted to psychiatric units. *Am J Emerg Med*. 2000;18(4):390–393.

39. Szpakowicz M, Herd A. "Medically cleared": How well are patients with psychiatric presentations examined by emergency physicians? *J Emerg Med*. 2008;35(4):369–372.

40. Olshaker JS, Browne B, Jerrard DA, et al. Medical clearance and screening of psychiatric patients in the emergency department. *Acad Emerg Med*. 1997;4(2):124–128.

41. Zun LS. Emergency assessment and stabilization of behavioral disorders. In: Cydulka RK, Cline DM, Ma OJ, et al., eds. *Tintinalli's Emergency Medicine Manual*. 8th ed. McGraw-Hill; 2018:1007–1009.

42. Tucci VT, Moukaddam N, Alam A, Rachal J. Emergency department medical clearance of patients with psychiatric or behavioral emergencies, Part 1. *Psychiatr Clin North Am*. 2017;40(3):411–423.

43. Thomas S, Beckerman N. Medical evaluation of the agitated patient. In: Zeller SL, Nordstrom KD, Wilson MP, eds. The *Diagnosis* and *Management* of *Agitation*. Cambridge University Press; 2017:23–31.

44. Brown TM, Boyle MF. ABC of psychological medicine: Delirium. *BMJ*. 2002;325(7365): 644–647.

45. Shenvi C, Kennedy M, Austin CA, Wilson MP, Gerardi M, Schneider S. Managing delirium and agitation in the older emergency department patient: The ADEPT tool. *Ann Emerg Med*. 2020;75(2):136–145.

46. Tolia V, Wilson MP. The medical clearance process for psychiatric patients presenting acutely to the emergency department. In: Zun L, Chepenik L, Mallory MN, eds. *Behavioral Emergencies for the Emergency Physician*. Cambridge University Press; 2013:19–24.

47. LaMantia MA, Messina FC, Hobgood CD, Miller DK. Screening for delirium in the emergency department: A systematic review. *Ann Emerg Med*. 2014;63(5):551–560.

48. Han JH, Wilson A, Vasilevskis EE, et al. Diagnosing delirium in older emergency department patients: Validity and reliability of the Delirium Triage Screen and the Brief Confusion Assessment Method. *Ann Emerg Med*. 2013;62(5):457–465.

49. Marcantonio ER, Ngo LH, O'Connor M, et al. 3D-CAM: Derivation and validation of a 3-minute diagnostic interview for CAM-defined delirium: A cross-sectional diagnostic test study. *Ann Intern Med*. 2014;161(8):554–561. [Published correction appears in *Ann Intern Med*. 2014;161(10):764]

50. Bauer J, Roberts MR, Reisdorff EJ. Evaluation of behavioral and cognitive changes: The mental status examination. *Emerg Med Clin North Am*. 1991;9(1):1–12.

51. Wei LA, Fearing MA, Sternberg EJ, Inouye SK. The Confusion Assessment Method: A systematic review of current usage. *J Am Geriatr Soc*. 2008;56(5):823–830.

52. Sessler CN, Gosnell MS, Grap MJ, et al. The Richmond Agitation–Sedation Scale: Validity and reliability in adult intensive care unit patients. *Am J Respir Crit Care Med*. 2002;166(10):1338–1344.

53. Dolan JG, Mushlin AI. Routine laboratory testing for medical disorders in psychiatric inpatients. *Arch Intern Med*. 1985;145(11):2085–2088.

54. Korn CS, Currier GW, Henderson SO. "Medical clearance" of psychiatric patients without medical complaints in the emergency department. *J Emerg Med*. 2000;18(2):173–176.

55. Gregory RJ, Nihalani ND, Rodriguez E. Medical screening in the emergency department for psychiatric admissions: A procedural analysis. *Gen Hosp Psychiatry*. 2004;26(5):405–410.

56. Janiak BD, Atteberry S. Medical clearance of the psychiatric patient in the emergency department. *J Emerg Med*. 2012;43(5):866–870.

57. Kagel KE, Smith M, Latyshenko IV, Mitchell C, Kagel A. Effects of mandatory screening labs in directing the disposition of the apparently healthy psychiatric patient in the emergency department. *US Army Med Dep J*. 2017;(2-17):18–24.

58. Wilson MP, Nordstrom K, Anderson EL, et al. American Association for Emergency Psychiatry Task Force on Medical Clearance of Adult Psychiatric Patients. Part II: Controversies over medical assessment, and consensus recommendations. *West J Emerg Med*. 2017;18(4):640–646.

59. Hooker EA, Mallow PJ, Oglesby MM. Characteristics and trends of emergency department visits in the United States (2010–2014). *J Emerg Med*. 2019;56(3):344–351.

60. Kroll DS, Smallwood J, Chang G. Drug screens for psychiatric patients in the emergency department: Evaluation and recommendations. *Psychosomatics*. 2013;54(1):60–66.

61. Schiller MJ, Shumway M, Batki SL. Utility of routine drug screening in a psychiatric emergency setting. *Psychiatr Serv*. 2000;51(4):474–478.

62. Eisen JS, Sivilotti ML, Boyd KU, Barton DG, Fortier CJ, Collier CP. Screening urine for drugs of abuse in the emergency department: Do test results affect physicians' patient care decisions? *Can J Emerge Med*. 2004;6(2):104–111.

63. Tenenbein M. Do you really need that emergency drug screen? *Clin Toxicol*. 2009;47(4):286–291.

64. Shihabuddin BS, Hack CM, Sivitz AB. Role of urine drug screening in the medical clearance of pediatric psychiatric patients: Is there one? *Pediatr Emerg Care*. 2013;29(8):903–906.

65. Riccoboni ST, Darracq MA. Does the U stand for useless? The urine drug screen and emergency department psychiatric patients. *J Emerg Med*. 2018;54(4):500–506.

66. Fortu JM, Kim IK, Cooper A, Condra C, Lorenz DJ, Pierce MC. Psychiatric patients in the pediatric emergency department undergoing routine urine toxicology screens for medical clearance: Results and use. *Pediatr Emerg Care*. 2009;25(6):387–392.

67. Algren DA, Christian MR. Buyer beware: Pitfalls in toxicology laboratory testing. *Mo Med*. 2015;112(3):206–210.

68. Moeller KE, Lee KC, Kissack JC. Urine drug screening: Practical guide for clinicians. *Mayo Clin Proc*. 2008;83(1):66–76. [Published correction appears in *Mayo Clin Proc*. 2008;83(7):851]

69. Eskridge KD, Guthrie SK. Clinical issues associated with urine testing of substances of abuse. *Pharmacotherapy*. 1997;17(3):497–510.

70. Substance Abuse and Mental Health Services Administration. 2019 National Survey on Drug Use and Health (NSDUH). National Institute on Alcohol Abuse and Alcoholism. Published 2019. Accessed January 29, 2021. https://www.samhsa.gov/data/sites/defa ult/files/cbhsq-reports/NSDUHDetailedTabs2018R2/NSDUHDetTabsSect2pe2018. htm#tab2-1b

71. White AM, Slater ME, Ng G, Hingson R, Breslow R. Trends in alcohol-related emergency department visits in the United States: Results from the Nationwide Emergency Department Sample, 2006 to 2014. *Alcohol Clin Exp Res.* 2018;42(2):352–359.

72. Holt S, Stewart IC, Dixon JM, Elton RA, Taylor TV, Little K. Alcohol and the emergency service patient. *Br Med J.* 1980;281(6241):638–640.

73. Cherpitel C, Bond J, Ye Y, et al. Clinical assessment compared with breathalyser readings in the emergency room: Concordance of ICD-10 Y90 and Y91 codes. *Emerg Med J.* 2005;22(10):689–695.

74. Hack JB, Goldlust EJ, Gibbs F, Zink B. The H-Impairment Index (HII): A standardized assessment of alcohol-induced impairment in the emergency department. *Am J Drug Alcohol Abuse.* 2014;40(2):111–117.

75. Hack JB, Goldlust EJ, Ferrante D, Zink BJ. Performance of the Hack's Impairment Index Score: A novel tool to assess impairment from alcohol in emergency department patients. *Acad Emerg Med.* 2017;24(10):1193–1203.

76. Simon AE, Schoendorf KC. Emergency department visits for mental health conditions among US children, 2001–2011. *Clin Pediatr.* 2014;53(14):1359–1366.

77. Lo CB, Bridge JA, Shi J, Ludwig L, Stanley RM. Children's mental health emergency department visits: 2007–2016. *Pediatrics.* 2020;145(6):e20191536.

78. Donofrio JJ, Santillanes G, McCammack BD, et al. Clinical utility of screening laboratory tests in pediatric psychiatric patients presenting to the emergency department for medical clearance. *Ann Emerg Med.* 2014;63(6):666–75.e3.

79. Donofrio JJ, Horeczko T, Kaji A, Santillanes G, Claudius I. Most routine laboratory testing of pediatric psychiatric patients in the emergency department is not medically necessary. *Health Aff.* 2015;34(5):812–818.

80. Santillanes G, Donofrio JJ, Lam CN, Claudius I. Is medical clearance necessary for pediatric psychiatric patients? *J Emerg Med.* 2014;46(6):800–807.

81. Chun TH, Mace SE, Katz ER. American Academy of Pediatrics; Committee on Pediatric Emergency Medicine, and American College of Emergency Physicians; Pediatric Emergency Medicine Committee. Evaluation and management of children and adolescents with acute mental health or behavioral problems. Part I: Common clinical challenges of patients with mental health and/or behavioral emergencies. *Pediatrics.* 2016;138(3):e20161570.

82. Zun LS, Downey L. Application of a medical clearance protocol. *Prim Psychiatry.* 2007;14:47–51.

83. Shah SJ, Fiorito M, McNamara RM. A screening tool to medically clear psychiatric patients in the emergency department. *J Emerg Med.* 2012;43(5):871–875.

84. Miller AC, Frei SP, Rupp VA, Joho BS, Miller KM, Bond WF. Validation of a Triage Algorithm for Psychiatric Screening (TAPS) for patients with psychiatric chief complaints. *J Am Osteopath Assoc.* 2012;112(8):502–508.

85. Schieferle Uhlenbrock J, Hudson J, Prewitt J, Thompson JA, Pereira K. Retrospective chart review of the Triage Algorithm for Psychiatric Screening (TAPS) for patients who present to emergency departments with psychiatric chief complaints. *J Emerg Nurs.* 2018;44(5):459–465.

86. Wetzel AE, Thomas S, Balan Y, Hosein R, Noobakhsh A. Crisis in the emergency department: Removing barriers to timely and appropriate mental health treatment. Sierra Sacramento Valley Medical Society. Published 2015. Accessed January 30, 2021. http://smartmedicalclearance.org/wp-content/uploads/2017/09/ssvms-crisis_in_the_emergency_dept.pdf

87. MI-SMART psychiatric medical clearance. Michigan Psychiatric Care Improvement Project. Published 2019. Accessed January 30, 2021. https://www.mpcip.org/mpcip/mi-smart-psychiatric-medical-clearance

88. SMART medical clearance form. Tennessee Hospital Association. Published June 2020. Accessed January 30, 2021. https://tha.com/wp-content/uploads/2020/07/TN_SMART_form_July_1_2020.pdf

89. Broderick KB, Lerner EB, McCourt JD, Fraser E, Salerno K. Emergency physician practices and requirements regarding the medical screening examination of psychiatric patients. *Acad Emerg Med*. 2002;9(1):88–92.

4

Assessing for Suicidality and Overall Risk of Violence

Megan B. Schabbing

Epidemiology of Suicide

Suicide is defined as death caused by self-directed injurious behavior with intent to die as a result of the behavior.[1] According to the Centers for Disease Control and Prevention (CD), in 2018, suicide was the 10th leading cause of death in the United States, accounting for the deaths of more than 48,000 people. Suicide was the second leading cause of death among individuals aged 10–24 years and the fourth leading cause of death among individuals aged 35–54 years. Also in 2018, there were more than two and a half times as many suicides in the United States as there were homicides, and firearms were the most common method used in suicide deaths, accounting for approximately half of all suicide deaths.[1] Males are more likely to die by suicide than females.

Based on data from the 2019 National Survey on Drug Use and Health by the Substance Abuse and Mental Health Services Administration, 4.8% of adults aged 18 years or older in the United States had serious thoughts about suicide in 2019. Among adults across all age groups, the prevalence of serious suicidal thoughts was highest among young adults aged 18–25 years.[1] Regardless of chief complaint, 10% of people who present to the emergency department (ED) have been found to have suicidal thoughts or behaviors.[2,3]

What We Know About People Who Die by Suicide: Then and Now

To appreciate the importance of suicide risk assessment, it is imperative to consider trends regarding diagnosed mental illness in individuals who die by suicide. In 1959, Robins et al.[4] published a study in which all suicides occurring in metropolitan St. Louis, Missouri, in a 1-year period were studied by means of interviews with relatives, friends, job associates, physicians, and others soon after each suicide. Of 134 individuals who died by suicide, 94% of them were found to have had psychiatric illness. This high percentage is consistent with early suicide research, which suggested that approximately 90% of people who died by suicide carried a mental illness diagnosis.[5,6] However, in 2018, the CDC released a report showing that from 1999 to 2018, the total age-adjusted suicide rate in the United States increased by 35%.[1] Perhaps the most notable finding in the CDC report was that more than 50% of people who died by suicide did not have a known mental health condition, which starkly contrasted with previous studies showing a relatively high percentage of diagnosed mental illness in completed suicides.[1]

Despite the shift in the prevalence of diagnosed mental illness in people who die by suicide, one factor that has remained constant is the significance of a recent stressful life event as a risk factor for suicide. Dorpat and Ripley[7] found that in Seattle, Washington, 27% of individuals who completed suicide had suffered loss of a family member by death, separation, or divorce within 1 year of the suicide. Similarly, Robins et al.[4] found that 26.4% of suicides involved recent loss.[8]

Many factors can contribute to suicide among those with and without known mental health conditions, including problems related to relationships, finances, employment, housing, and substance use disorders.[9] When a patient expresses feelings of hopelessness or being "stuck," particular attention should be paid to this condition. Often, if a patient is supported in moving past the feeling of hopelessness, a subsequent crisis can be avoided. A study of more than 500 people who attempted suicide by jumping off the Golden Gate Bridge from 1937 to 1971 showed that 26 years later, 94% of the attempters were still alive; only 5–7% went on to complete suicide.[10] Interviews of Golden Gate Bridge suicide survivors revealed that they often regretted their decision mid-air.[11] Survivor Ken Baldwin stated, "I instantly realized that everything in my life that I'd thought was unfixable was totally fixable—except for having just jumped."[11]

The Etiology of Suicide

Shea[12] describes three different etiologies of suicide: situational, psychological, and biological. Whereas situational factors may include stressful events or other external factors, psychological factors often entail cognitive distortions. Significant evidence supports dysregulation in stress response systems, particularly the hypothalamic–pituitary–adrenal axis, as a diathesis for suicide.[13] In Mann's stress-diathesis model of suicide, it is postulated that suicide may be triggered by a life event or psychiatric episode in an individual with genetic risk, combined with traumatic events and mental and physical illness, leading to neurobiological changes.[14] Unlike Beck's similar model,[15] Mann's model suggests that life stressors lead to suicide only when combined with vulnerability. Neuroimaging studies have identified a variety of neuroanatomical abnormalities, such as volume changes, associated with suicide in numerous psychiatric disorders, therefore providing valuable information on the neural circuitry associated with suicide risk.[16] Evidence indicates that a family history of suicide and a history of a suicide attempt by violent means may be associated with particular volume changes that could be considered "neural phenotypes."[17]

Fawcett[18] noted that before a serious suicide attempt, individuals often experience increased anxiety and agitation, or "psychic pain."[19] Galyenker[20] hypothesized that prior to attempting suicide, individuals enter a state of cognitive and affective dysregulation, or the acute suicide crisis syndrome (SCS). Galyenker found that SCS includes three factors: frantic hopelessness, an affective state of entrapment, dread, and hopelessness; ruminative flooding, a cognitive state of incessant rumination and a sense of one's head bursting with uncontrollable thoughts; and near-psychotic somatization, a state of strange somatic experiences in the context of severe anxiety and panic.[20] It is possible that SCS has contributed to the higher number of completed suicides in individuals without a mental health diagnosis because this transient state can occur in people with or without mental illness, particularly following a stressful life event.

Screening for Suicide

Prevention of suicide depends on the recognition of patients who should be the clinical focus of special concern and further evaluation.[21] Approximately 80% of people who died by suicide had contact with a primary care provider in the year before their death,[22] although fewer than 20% of people who died by suicide had contact with a mental health provider in the month prior to their death.[23] These data underscore the importance of screening for suicide in primary care settings, including EDs. Validated instruments can be used in primary care settings to identify patients who are at risk for suicide. However, it is important to remember that these instruments do not predict suicide but, rather, serve as a way to determine which patients require further assessment for suicide risk. The Patient Health Questionnaire (PHQ-9) is used to screen for depression in the outpatient setting.[24] Although early studies suggested that suicidal ideation reported on the PHQ-9 was a predictor of suicide attempts and deaths,[25] subsequent research published by Na et al.[26] showed that the PHQ-9 is an insufficient assessment tool for suicide risk and suicidal ideation. Validated screening tools frequently used in the emergency department setting include the Columbia Suicide Severity Rating Scale, the Suicide Assessment Five-Step Evaluation and Triage, and the Ask Suicide-Screening Questions–4.[27-29] Of course, once an individual is identified as at risk for suicide, it is imperative that the individual undergoes a thorough risk assessment so that a treatment plan is determined based on optimal modification of that individual's risk factors for suicide.

Risk Factors for Suicide

Previous Suicide Attempt

Numerous biological and environmental factors contribute to an individual's risk for suicide. Although many individuals who attempt suicide do not ultimately die by suicide, as shown in studies of Golden Gate Bridge survivors, a prior history of attempted suicide is the strongest single factor predictive of suicide.[30] Studies of individuals who have attempted suicide multiple times show that multiple attempters are more likely to have diagnosed psychiatric disorders, family history of suicide, and interpersonal conflict or limited social support.[31] Following a suicide attempt, the risk of suicide is particularly higher in the first year among patients with unipolar or bipolar depression and schizophrenia.[32]

Psychiatric Disorders

Numerous psychiatric disorders are associated with an increased risk for suicide. Approximately 75% of ED visits for suicidal ideation had an associated diagnosis of mood disorders, and 43% had a substance-related disorder.[33] The lifetime risk of suicide in individuals with bipolar disorder is estimated to be at least 15 times that of the general population, and bipolar disorder may account for 25% of completed suicides. Approximately 5% or 6% of individuals with schizophrenia die by suicide, and approximately 20% attempt suicide.[34] In individuals with major depressive disorder, a history of suicide attempts correlated with feelings of worthlessness and concurrent personality disorder.[35] Although borderline personality disorder is often recognized for its association with chronic suicidal thoughts and gestures, approximately 8–10% of individuals with borderline personality disorder were found to have died by suicide in retrospective studies.[36,37] Anxiety disorders more than double the risk of suicide attempts.[38] For all patients, the risk of suicide attempt or death by suicide is highest within 30 days of discharge from an ED or inpatient psychiatric unit.[39]

Recent Stressful Event

According to the CDC's National Violent Death Reporting System, numerous factors contribute to suicide among those with and without mental health conditions. These factors include a relationship problem, crisis in the past or upcoming 2 weeks, problematic substance use, physical health problems, job-related or financial problems, legal problems, and loss of housing.[9] For many individuals, such stressful life events drive a feeling of hopelessness or being stuck in a situation from which escape seems impossible. It is important to pay careful attention anytime you identify a patient who is in this state of mind, which is suggestive of an ongoing high risk of suicide. In fact, hopelessness is associated with suicidal ideation and behavior across psychiatric disorders.[40]

Family History of Suicide

Family history of suicide increases the risk for suicide in both individuals with and without a history of psychiatric illness.[41,42] An individual with a family history of completed suicide is twice as likely to die by suicide as an individual with no family history of suicide.[42] Adoption, twin, and family studies suggest that this increased risk has both genetic and environmental components.[41,43] There is evidence that a genetic component of this increased risk may be mediated by the transmission of intermediate phenotypes, such as impulsive aggression.[44] Jollant et al.[17] showed that in suicide attempters, a family history of suicide was associated with reduced volumes in bilateral temporal regions, right dorsolateral prefrontal cortex, and left putamen.

Access to Firearms

More than half of suicides in the United States occur by firearms.[45,46] Firearms in the home are associated with a fivefold greater risk of suicide.[47] Firearms are a particularly lethal method for attempting suicide, with a mortality rate of 92%, compared with 67% for drowning, 78% for hanging, and 2% for intentional overdoses.[48,49]

Substance Use Disorders

Many substance use disorders are associated with a higher risk of suicide. A meta-analysis of 31 studies pooling data from more than 400,000 participants found an association between alcohol use disorder and suicidal ideation, suicide attempt, and completed suicide.[50] Studies have shown that completed suicides rise by a factor of 14 in heroin users, and cocaine and methamphetamine have been shown to be related to suicide attempts in 20% of users and to suicidality in approximately two-thirds of users.[51]

Other Risk Factors

Other risk factors for suicide include childhood adversity, single marital status, being in a sexual minority, military service, medical illnesses, chronic pain, neurologic disorders, occupations, anti-depressant medication, and rural residence.

Protective Factors for Suicide

To date, protective factors for suicide have not been studied as extensively as risk factors for suicide, and therefore evidence for protective factors for suicide is equivocal. There is evidence indicating that family and community support, or connectedness, is a protective factor. Suicidal patients often report that they did not act on suicidal thoughts due to not wanting to leave behind a friend or a pet, and therefore a significant protective factor can be a family member, friend, or pet. Cultural, religious, and spiritual beliefs that discourage suicide and support self-preservation are also protective factors. Other protective factors for suicide include an alliance with an outpatient treatment provider, access to treatment, skills in problem-solving, conflict resolution, and nonviolent ways of handling disputes.[52,53]

Assessing Risk for Suicide

Talking to a Patient About Suicide

Performing a comprehensive risk assessment is one of the most challenging skills to develop and hone as a psychiatrist. Iannuzzi et al.[54] describe a five-step suicide assessment, loosely based on the Columbia-Suicide Severity Rating Scale,[27] which can be integrated into a clinician's routine evaluation: (1) explore the chief complaint; (2) identify suicidal behavior; (3) evaluate risk and protective factors; (4) obtain collateral information; and (5) document your decision.

Prior to exploring the chief complaint, a clinician must make an effort to develop rapport with the patient. Developing rapport with a patient is particularly important when addressing suicidality. If a patient trusts a provider, it is more likely that the patient will be honest when discussing suicidal thoughts and other related issues. It is important to meet the patient where the patient is and find a way to connect with them. Connecting may or may not involve some degree of small talk, but it must entail creation of an atmosphere in which the patient feels safe and supported by the clinician. It is also important to remember that many patients feel embarrassed when talking about suicidality. It can help to remind the patient why you are asking such personal questions. You might say, "I understand that it can be hard to talk about these thoughts and feelings, but it's important that you be honest with me so that I can understand how to best help you." Presenting yourself in a confident and calm manner can also be reassuring to the patient and help the patient feel more comfortable talking about suicide.

Box 4.1 How to Ask About Suicide: The Spectrum of Suicidal Thinking

---

"Have you ever thought 'I wish I wasn't here?' or 'I wish I didn't wake up in the morning?'"

"Have you ever wished you were dead?"

"Have you ever thought about doing something to make it so that you were no longer living?"

"Have you ever taken any steps toward enacting a plan for suicide?"

"Have you ever actually tried to kill yourself?"

"Have you thought about killing yourself here in the emergency department?"

Suicidality can be considered a spectrum, starting with passive death wishes and ending with intent for suicide with a specific plan. When a patient presents with suicidal thoughts, it can be helpful to start with questions about passive death wishes, moving your way up the spectrum of suicidal thoughts. A starting point to evaluate for passive death wishes may be, "Have you ever thought 'I wish I wasn't here?' or 'I wish I didn't wake up in the morning?'" The next step involves a stronger version of a passive death wish: "Have you ever wished you were dead?" To inquire about a plan for suicide, it can be asked, "Have you ever thought about doing something to make it so that you were no longer living?" or "Have you ever taken any steps toward enacting a plan for suicide?" Finally, it should be asked whether the patient has ever attempted suicide: "Have you ever actually tried to kill yourself?" Ongoing active suicidality in the ED should also be assessed by asking, "Have you thought about killing yourself here in the emergency department?" See Box 4.1.

To optimally assess ongoing risk for suicide in someone who recently attempted suicide, it is important to understand the patient's thought process at the time of the suicide attempt. This process can be evaluated with various questions, such as "What was going through your head when you took the pills?" or "What were you hoping would happen when you tied the rope around your neck?" It is also important to explore the patient's thoughts and feelings after the attempt by asking how the patient felt upon waking up and realizing that they were still alive. Many patients with psychiatric illness are too guarded or too embarrassed to discuss their suicidal thoughts, particularly after attempting suicide. Fear of psychiatric hospitalization and desire to follow through with suicide may also prevent a patient from answering honestly.

Suicidality may also be explored within the context of a patient's particular complaint. For instance, in a patient who endorses feelings of anxiety, one might ask, "I can imagine that those worries could be pretty disturbing. Do they ever get so bad that they make you wish you weren't here?" In a patient who presents with paranoia or delusional thinking, probing for suicidality may entail a question such as "Do you ever feel scared or threatened to the extent that you wish you were dead?" Or, for a patient who is hallucinating, it could be asked, "Do the voices ever make you want to kill yourself?" If a patient endorses depressed mood, a clinician may say, "Sometimes when people feel down, they think about ending their life. Do you ever feel like that?" See Table 4.1.

Table 4.1 Exploring Suicidal Thoughts Based on the Presenting Symptom

Presenting Symptom	Sample Question or Comment
Anxiety	"I can imagine that these worries could be pretty disturbing. Do they ever get so bad that they make you wish you weren't here?"
Depressed mood	"I'm sorry to hear you're having a rough time. Do you ever feel so down that you want to die?"
Paranoid ideation or delusional thinking	"Do you ever feel scared or threatened to the extent that you wish you were dead?"
Auditory hallucinations	"Do the voices ever make you want to kill yourself?"

Medical Record Review and Collateral Information

Doing a suicide risk assessment based solely on patient interview is comparable to attempting to assemble a puzzle with a myriad of missing puzzle pieces. Studies of patients who complete suicide on an inpatient unit or within 72 hours of discharge show that up to 78% of people deny suicidal thoughts in the last contact prior to completing suicide[55] A thorough review of the patient's current and past medical record, when available, is an important part of a suicide risk assessment. Suicidal comments made by the patient throughout the encounter should be addressed, particularly if they involve mention of a specific suicide plan. For instance, on arrival to the ED, a patient may tell a triage nurse that he wanted to take a bottle of pills but may deny thoughts of suicide to subsequent hospital staff. In order to optimally assess the patient's suicide risk, the suicide plan to overdose must be addressed with the patient and further explored. Previous medical records can also be helpful in revealing valuable details about the patient's history of suicidal behaviors, psychiatric disorders, family history, and other key risk factors. For a patient who refuses to provide collateral contact information, this information can often be obtained from records of the patient's past visits.

The patient's family members, friends, coworkers, and others often provide valuable collateral information necessary to understand the patient's recent and longitudinal history, and therefore accurately assess the patient's risk for suicide. Most important, collateral information can help you, as the provider, determine whether the patient is minimizing symptoms, which could lead to an underestimation of the patient's suicide risk. Of course, some patients are resistant to providing permission to contact others for such information. In this case, it can be helpful to explain to the patient why this information is being requested. You may tell the patient, "In order for me to figure out how to best help you, I need to better understand your life. Talking to someone who knows you can really help me to better understand how to help you." It can also be helpful to explain to the patient that your primary goal is to ask questions of the collateral contact person, as opposed to dispense information about the patient. If collateral information obtained from a family member or other person strongly contradicts the patient's reports, it may be necessary to obtain another source of collateral information; if no further collateral sources are available, consideration of previous medical records and the patient's current mental status examination may help inform a final disposition decision.

Making an Accurate Diagnosis

A step often overlooked in performing a thorough suicide risk assessment is making an accurate diagnosis. As Charles Zorumski[56] wrote in the Foreword to the sixth edition of *Goodwin & Guze's Psychiatric Diagnosis*, "Diagnosis is the cornerstone of medicine. . . . In the absence of accurate diagnosis, medicine largely becomes a 'Tower of Babel' where no one understands what is going on."[p.xxv] An optimal and comprehensive risk assessment cannot be completed in the absence of an accurate diagnosis. The way to best modify a patient's risk for suicide is different for a patient who meets criteria for a substance use disorder but has no primary mood, anxiety, or psychotic disorder compared to a patient whose sole diagnosis is a primary mood disorder. Therefore, making an accurate diagnosis helps not only identify the appropriate risk factors for suicide but also determine how to best modify the patient's risk for suicide at a particular point in time.

Formulating and Documenting a Suicide Risk Assessment

The purpose of suicide risk assessment is not to predict suicide but, rather, to identify treatable and modifiable risks and protective factors that inform the patient's treatment and safety management requirements.[57] Formulating a suicide risk assessment involves more than simply a weighing of risk factors versus protective factors. Rather, it should involve putting together the pieces of the patient's puzzle, including past history, subjective patient report, collateral information, and mental status examination, to determine which factors are driving the patient's risk for suicide at that point in time so that the disposition and treatment plan are tailored to modify these risk factors. Although there is no universally accepted standardized and validated tool for suicide risk assessment, it is standard of care to consider and document both risk factors for suicide and protective factors for suicide with a clinical determination of how to best modify the patient's risk for suicide. Shea[58] describes the following three elements of a sound suicide assessment approach: (1) gathering information related to risk factors, protective factors, and warning signs of suicide; (2) collecting information related to the patient's suicidal ideation, planning, behaviors, desire, and intent; and (3) making a clinical formulation of risk based on these two databases.

Information involving the patient's risk factors, protective factors, warning signs, and suicidal thoughts and behaviors should be obtained from multiple sources. In addition to patient interview, information should be gathered from past medical and legal records, when available, as well as from people who known the patient, such as family, friends, or coworkers. Considering input from ED staff can also be helpful because social workers, nurses, psych techs, and protective services officers who have observed and interacted with the patient during the patient's stay in the ED are often able to provide insight regarding the patient's behavior and current mental state. Contacting the patient's outpatient provider can also be instrumental in determining contributing factors to the patient's suicidality, particularly in patients with frequent ED visits and patients who may be deceptive on interview. The following case illustrates this approach to suicide risk assessment.

Case Example

Jessica, 32 years old, presented to the ED stating that she took "a bunch of pills" in a suicide attempt. Her medical evaluation revealed no evidence of overdose. ED staff reported that Jessica was preoccupied with eating and joked frequently with various staff members. She had presented to the ED last week, voicing suicidal thoughts due to being dissatisfied with her housing situation. On exam, she continued to voice suicidal thoughts and stated that she would walk into traffic if discharged, although her affect was noted to be bright and full range. An extensive review of her medical record revealed a history of presenting to the ED with suicidal gesturing in the context of social stressors, with more than 30 psychiatric hospitalizations, and a diagnosis of borderline personality disorder and intellectual disability. Her outpatient treatment team was contacted and shared the details of her outpatient treatment plan, which involved avoidance of repeated hospitalization when possible. Both her therapist and her mother, who was her legal guardian, supported discharge back to group home. She voiced dissatisfaction with this decision but was ultimately cooperative with discharge after receiving a dose of lorazepam.

In this case example, although the patient is endorsing active suicidal thoughts and plan, numerous aspects of her presentation necessitate acquisition of further information prior to determining whether inpatient psychiatric admission is appropriate. Her recent ED visit in the setting of dissatisfaction with her housing situation and discrepancy between her subjective report and objective exam are concerning for malingering. In the absence of a comorbid mood or psychotic or anxiety disorder, her diagnoses of borderline personality disorder and intellectual disability make it less likely that she would benefit from acute psychiatric hospitalization.

The case example illustrates the challenge in following through with discharge in a patient who is resistant to it. Although borderline personality disorder and intellectual disability alone are not disorders for which psychiatric admission is typically shown to be the most effective treatment strategy, it is important to rule out other comorbidities that may necessitate inpatient admission and involve the patient's family and outpatient treatment team in safety and disposition planning. Finally, for a patient who is resistant to discharge, it may be helpful to consider medication for agitation prior to discharge to reduce the risk of impulsive aggression or other behavior that may prevent a successful discharge.

Because many patients have multiple risk factors for suicide, it is important to remember that a patient's risk factors may change from one ED presentation to the next. In addition to having a primary psychiatric disorder, such as schizophrenia, major depressive disorder, or bipolar disorder, many patients have comorbid substance abuse, maladaptive personality traits, and psychosocial stressors that complicate their diagnostic picture and create a challenge in the determination of disposition. It is imperative to appreciate the fact that such a complex patient may present to the ED one day with complaints centered around unstable housing; in the absence of acute psychiatric decompensation, it may be determined that the patient's risk for suicide at that time is most strongly tied to unstable housing and not likely to be modified by acute psychiatric hospitalization. However, the same patient may present days or weeks later acutely psychotic in the context of acute amphetamine intoxication, at which time it may be determined that the patient's risk for suicide is best modified by chemical dependency treatment. Finally, the same patient may present another time with severe depressive symptoms and hopelessness with nihilistic thinking, which may be determined to be tied to underlying psychiatric illness. In this instance, the patient's risk for suicide would likely be best modified by acute psychiatric hospitalization for the purpose of adjustment of psychotropic medication to stabilize the acute decompensation. It is important to look at every patient with a fresh set of eyes at each encounter and avoid labeling a patient or assuming that the patient's risk for suicide is always modified with the same disposition plan.

Safety and Disposition Planning

The transition from inpatient to outpatient psychiatric treatment is a critical time for patients at risk for suicide. In the month following discharge from inpatient psychiatric treatment, an individual's suicide death rate is 200 times higher than that of the general population.[59] Subsequently, suicide prevention efforts involve significant focus on careful management of patients during this transition period. The National Action Alliance for Suicide Prevention has made several recommendations for providers to close potential gaps surrounding transition of care.[60] Use of a standardized safety plan individualized for each patient is considered best practice in the care of patients with suicide-related complaints. Interventions involving development of a safety plan in the ED have been shown to decrease suicide attempts and increase treatment engagement.[61] An optimal safety plan should be individualized for each patient, engage the patient, include lethal means counseling, and involve the patient's friends or family when possible. Elimination of access to firearms is an effective way to reduce suicide risk, particularly given the combination of the often transient and impulsive nature of suicidal thoughts and behaviors and the high lethality potential of firearms. It is important to remember that lethal means counseling is not exclusive to discussion of firearms. In a patient who has attempted suicide by overdose, it is important to consider ways to limit the patient's access to pills, which may involve storage of medications in a lockbox controlled by a patient's friend or family member or administration of medications by a home health service associate. Timely follow-up is also an important component of this transition period, and it is recommended that a follow-up appointment be scheduled within no more than 7 days of discharge. There is also evidence to support the use of Caring Contacts, in which a patient at risk for suicide is contacted within 24 hours of discharge, as means of reducing subsequent suicidal thoughts and attempts, as well as recurrent hospitalization.[62]

Assessing Risk for Violence

Violence and Psychiatric Illness

Although most violence in society is not committed by psychiatric patients, certain psychiatric disorders, including substance use disorders, can elevate a patient's risk for violence. Stimulant intoxication can drive violent behavior through agitation, irritability, paranoia, and even delirium,[63,64] whereas alcohol intoxication can lead to violence through disinhibition, emotional lability, and impaired judgment.[65–67] Violence occurs in the context of intoxication with hallucinogens, particularly phencyclidine, which can also lead to suicide and bizarre behavior.[68] With a clinical picture similar to that of stimulant intoxication, ingestion of synthetic cathinones or "bath salts" has also been associated with violent behavior.[69]

In individuals with schizophrenia, violence may be associated with a perceived threat related to hallucinations and delusional thinking, although the most common external factor associated with violence in schizophrenia is substance abuse. Particular attention should be paid early on in the course of psychotic illness because 40% of homicides committed by schizophrenics occur during the first psychotic episode.[70] Individuals with bipolar spectrum disorders can experience agitation and impulsive aggression during mixed and manic episodes, as well as irritability during depressive episodes, both of which have the potential to drive violent behavior. Borderline personality disorder and antisocial personality disorder are also associated with violence toward others.[71] Intermittent explosive disorder is characterized by violent behavioral outbursts and aggression out of proportion to the provocation or precipitating factors. In children and adolescents, violence can be related to behavioral disorders or intellectual disability.[72]

Rozel[73] describes six maxims involving the relationship between violence and psychiatric illness First, most violence is not due to mental illness. In fact, it is estimated that less than 10% of the violence that occurs in our society is attributable to psychiatric illness.[74–76] Second, most people with mental illness are not violent. Third, people with mental illness are more likely to be a victim of violence than a perpetrator of violence.[74,77] Fourth, there is an intersection between psychiatric illness and violence, and it is critical for clinicians to effectively identify and manage this risk. Fifth, even when risk for violence is not driven by psychiatric illness, clinicians should optimize opportunities to mitigate risk. Finally, the most robust risk factors for violence are similar for individuals with and without mental illness. These maxims are particularly important to remember when faced with societal misconceptions involving a categorical perceived dangerousness in individuals with mental health disorders.

Models of Violence

Violence can be approached as a medical syndrome with psychotic, impulsive, and predatory subtypes because growing evidence supports these discrete phenotypes for violence.[78] This model is useful in determining how to best modify a patient's risk for violence based on etiology. For instance, if a patient's homicidal thoughts are rooted in antisocial traits driving a pattern of predatory violence, acute psychiatric hospitalization is less likely to modify this patient's risk. Conversely, if a patient's homicidal thoughts are driven by persecutory delusions, acute psychiatric hospitalization, for the purpose of optimization of antipsychotic medication, is more likely to modify the patient's risk for violence. Another model of violence is the quadripartite model of violence, also known as the four R's—rage, revenge, reward, and recreation.[79] This model considers the four categories as being either high or low impulsivity and either high or low affect. These models may help improve understanding of the different driving forces behind an individual's violent behavior, which is important to determine in order to develop a disposition and treatment plan focused on modification of the individual's risk factors.

Risk Factors and Protective Factors for Violence

Violence is studied and characterized in categories, such as intimate partner violence, sexual violence, and youth violence. It is beyond the scope of this chapter to discuss in detail the difference in risk factors among these groups. Collective risk factors for violence include history of violent victimization, heavy alcohol and drug use, lack of empathy, poor behavioral control, suicidal behavior, access to firearms or other weapons, and previous violent or aggressive behavior. Risk factors for violence in the context of psychosis include dynamic factors such as hostile behavior, poor impulse control, lack of insight, recent alcohol or drug misuse, and non-adherence with psychological therapies and medication.[80] Protective factors for violence include social support, emotional health and connectedness, religious or spiritual beliefs, and intolerance to deviance.[81]

Evaluation of the Violent Patient

Evaluation of a patient who presents with violent behavior should include an assessment of the chief complaint, history of the present illness, family history, personal and developmental history, medical history, mental status, physical examination, and laboratory tests and imaging, when indicated.[71] It is important to remember that patients will often attempt to minimize their violence, and therefore it is imperative to make all attempts possible to obtain collateral information about the patient's recent and remote history.

First, the nature of the threat is explored, particularly in terms of any degree of planning that done by the patient. For instance, if the patient voices thoughts of killing his neighbor, it is important to ask whether the patient has taken any steps toward doing so, such as formulating a specific plan or obtaining weapons. It is important to ascertain through patient interview, collateral information from friends and family, and review of medical and criminal records, when possible, whether the patient has a history of violence. Many patients, particularly those with antisocial and narcissistic traits, become defensive when questioned about legal history. It can be helpful to explain to the patient why you are asking these questions and why this information is relevant to a psychiatric evaluation. A nonjudgmental approach may help develop rapport with a patient when asking about such sensitive topics.

A thorough history of present illness should include pertinent positives and negatives, including consideration of previously mentioned risk factors, such as substance abuse and access to firearms. Family history should be obtained because it may help clarify the likelihood of a primary psychiatric disorder in the patient, which can help determine how best to modify the patient's risk for violence. Similarly, personal and developmental history, including childhood abuse or neglect, helps shed light on potential risk factors for violence. Medical history, laboratory testing, and imaging may uncover underlying medical problems and neurologic disorders, such as traumatic brain injury or temporal lobe epilepsy, that may elevate a patient's risk for violence.[71]

Formulating and Documenting a Violence Risk Assessment

Three approaches to violence risk assessment are clinical, structured clinical judgment, and actuarial. In a clinical assessment, which is most commonly used in the ED, the clinician formulates a risk assessment based on patient interview, collateral information, and review of the medical record. In an actuarial approach, more commonly done in a forensic setting, standardized clinical tools are used to perform a more extensive and systematic review. A structured clinical judgment approach combines the former two approaches.

The ability to predict violence is limited to the short term, using a process analogous to that of predicting suicide potential.[71,82] Once the nature of the threat is explored, similar to suicide risk assessment, risk factors and protective factors must be considered and weighed so as to determine the best way by which to modify the patient's risk for violence. Similar to suicide risk assessment, it is important to consider the nature of the risk factors for violence, as opposed to simply the quantity of risk factors versus protective factors. A psychotic patient may have a myriad of protective factors, with the only risk factor being psychosis, but if the violence is being driven by psychosis, psychiatric hospitalization may be the best course of action for the purpose of initiating antipsychotic treatment. Again, a previous history of violence must be particularly carefully considered when determining disposition. This history can be ascertained not only from interviewing the patient but also from collateral information from family or friends, the medical record, and any accessible legal records, such as public court records. The importance of obtaining collateral information, and other elements of violence risk assessment, is illustrated in two clinical scenarios.

Case Example

Matt, age 19 years, presented to the ED by police on an involuntary psychiatric hold after he reportedly called the suicide hotline and made suicidal statements about suicide by cop, claiming to have an AR-15 and a Glock. In the ED, he denied suicidal thoughts or access to a gun, reporting that he had only been "venting" due to anger toward his parents and inability to contact his friends. His history is notable for one previous psychiatric hospitalization following an "aborted suicide attempt" 2 years ago, after he had disclosed a history of sexual abuse as a teenager. He voiced a desire for outpatient treatment, including counseling, to deal with previous trauma. He was noted to be very insightful but refused to provide permission to contact his parents. Following discussion of the patient on multidisciplinary rounds, the patient was told that for discharge to be a possibility, further information must be obtained from the patient's parents. With the patient's permission, the ED social worker contacted the patient's mother, who reported that the patient was visiting crime scenes and tracking crime scenes and had recently sent her a picture of a handgun and suicidal texts. She also reported that the patient often became "scary and volatile" with suicidal threats when his parents refused to give him money. She stated that the patient's father did have a gun and agreed to have it removed from the home. The information obtained from the patient's mother was addressed with the patient in a subsequent interview by the attending psychiatrist. Upon further evaluation, the patient admitted that he occasionally experienced vague suicidal thoughts, particularly during times of stress, and stated that he often made suicidal and homicidal threats to his parents during arguments as means of manipulating them. He did not endorse any symptoms consistent with a primary mood, anxiety, or psychotic disorder. He agreed to meet with a therapist to work on improving his coping strategies, as it was determined that his suicide risk was tied most strongly to his maladaptive personality traits and limited coping strategies. His family was involved in safety planning and supported the plan for therapy and firearm removal.

In this case example, multiple aspects of the patient's presentation should trigger concern on the part of the clinician. First, he expressed anger toward his parents. Second, there was a gun mentioned in the involuntary paperwork completed by police, although the patient later denied having a gun. His history of an aborted suicide attempt and subsequent psychiatric hospitalization should also raise concern. Finally, of particular concern is his refusal to provide permission to talk to his parents. This case highlights a number of teaching points. First and most important, it illustrates the value of obtaining collateral information, particularly when concern exists for access to firearms. Although inpatient admission was not indicated for this patient, his risk for both violence and suicide was modified by not only therapy but also removal of firearms from the home. It also shows how a patient is often more likely to open up about details surrounding suicidal thoughts and behavior if the right questions are posed.

Case Example

Gary, aged 55 years, presented to the ED with complaints of rectal pain. He expressed concern that he might have been sexually assaulted by his roommate and requested a sexual assault evaluation. He stated that he snored loudly and believed that his snoring indicated to his roommate that he was asleep and could be assaulted. He also expressed the belief that his roommate was drugging him and admitted that he had stopped eating at home for this reason and subsequently lost 20 pounds. He denied feelings of anger and denied suicidal or homicidal thoughts, although he was noted to have been guarded and paranoid on exam. His medical evaluation showed no evidence of sexual assault. He refused to provide consent to contact his roommate or others and declined psychiatric hospitalization or treatment. A review of his medical record showed more than 15 visits to other local hospitals during the previous 3 months with similar complaints. He was diagnosed with delusional disorder versus paranoid personality disorder, and he was discharged due to not meeting criteria for involuntary admission. The attending psychiatrist evaluated the patient, who initially remained resistant to contacting his roommate. It was suggested to the patient that if he disclosed further details about his experience, it would be more likely that he could be helped to better manage his stressful living situation. Gary ultimately admitted that he heard voices telling him to shoot his roommate and had been taking steps toward buying a gun. He was psychiatrically admitted and prescribed antipsychotic medication.

In this case example, the patient's initial evaluation was particularly notable for delusions of reference and a perceived threat by his roommate. Although it was initially thought that the patient did not meet criteria for involuntary psychiatric admission, it could be argued that his psychosis was limiting his ability to care for himself, particularly given that paranoid delusions were the cause of his decreased eating and subsequent weight loss. Ultimately, Gary opened up about his thoughts once it was framed to him that his stressful situation could possibly be improved. In Gary's case, his risk for violence was clearly tied to his psychosis and best modified by acute psychiatric hospitalization for the purpose of initiating antipsychotic medication. With a guarded patient such as Gary, it is particularly important not to rush through an interview because psychotic patients often take more time to open up about their thoughts, particularly those involving violence or suicide.

Documentation of Suicide and Violence Risk Assessment

Documentation is addressed in Chapter 21. It is worth repeating, however, that thorough and accurate documentation is an essential component of an optimal suicide or violence risk assessment. A general format should include consideration of key risk factors and protective factors and explanation of how modification of these risk factors dictates the treatment plan and disposition. The risk assessment should not include personal opinions but, rather, objective notation of how the formulated treatment plan and disposition address the patient's risk for suicide or violence.

Conclusion

Assessing for suicidality and risk of violence is a complex and multifaceted process. Although there is no single validated tool for suicide or violence risk assessment, it is considered standard of care to perform a thorough exploration of risk factors and protective factors using a combination of resources, including patient interview, medical record review, and collateral information obtained from family, friends, and outpatient providers. Collateral information is particularly important in establishing a clear and comprehensive understanding of all factors contributing to a patient's risk. These factors are used to formulate a risk assessment that helps determine how to best modify the patient's risk at that point in time and drives the development of a disposition and treatment plan. Because most patients have multiple risk factors, it is important to consider risk assessment a fluid process that may differ from one encounter to the next.

References

1. Suicide is a leading cause of death in the United States. National Institute of Mental Health. Published 2021. Accessed January 20, 2021. https://www.nimh.nih.gov/health/statistics/suicide.shtml

2. Classen CA, Larkin, GL. Occult suicidality in an emergency department population. *Br J Psychiatry*. 2005;186:352–353.

3. Ilgen MA, Walton MA, Cunningham RM, et al. Recent suicidal ideation among patients in an inner city emergency department. *Suicide Life Threat Behav*. 2009;39(5):508–517.

4. Robins E, Murphy GE, Wilkinson RH Jr, Gassner S, Kayes J. Some clinical considerations in the prevention of suicide based on a study of 134 successful suicides. *Am J Public Health*. 1959;49:888–899.

5. Hirschfeld RM, Russell JM. Assessment and treatment of suicidal patients. *N Engl J Med*. 1997; 337:910–915.

6. Moscicki E. Epidemiology of suicide. In: Goldsmith S, ed. Suicide Prevention and Intervention. National Academies Press, 2001.

7. Dorpat TL, Ripley HS. A study of suicide in the Seattle area. *Compr Psychiat*. 1960;1: 349–359.

8. Murphy GE, Robins E. Social factors in suicide. *JAMA*. 1967;199(5):303–308.

9. Suicide rates increased in every state. Centers for Disease Control and Prevention. Published June 7, 2018. Accessed December 20, 2021. https://www.cdc.gov/vitalsigns/suicide/index.html

10. Seiden RH: Where are they now? A follow-up study of suicide attempters from the Golden Gate Bridge. *Suicide Life Threat Behav*. 1978:8(4):203–216.

11. Friend T. Jumpers: The fatal grandeur of the Golden Gate Bridge. *The New Yorker*. October 13, 2003.

12. Shea SC. *The Practical Art of Suicide Assessment: A Guide for Mental Health Professionals and Substance Abuse Counselors*. Wiley; 1999.

13. Oquendo MA, Sullivan GM, Sudol K, et al. Toward a biosignature for suicide. *Am J Psychiatry*. 2014; 171 (12): 1259–1277.

14. Mann JJ, Wateraux C, Hass GL, Maloe KM. Toward a clinical model of suicidal behavior in psychiatric patients. *Am J Psychiatry*. 1999;156:181–189.

15. Wenzel A, Beck A. A cognitive model of suicidal behavior: Theory and treatment. *Appl Prev Psychol*. 2008;12:189–201.

16. Balcioglu YH, Kose S. Neural substrates of suicide and suicidal behavior: From a neuroimaging perspective. *Psychiatry Clin Psychopharmacol*. 2018;28(3):314–328.

17. Jollant F, Wagner G, Richard-Devantoy S, et al. Neuroimaging-informed phenotypes of suicidal behavior: A family history of suicide and the use of a violent suicidal means. *Transl Psychiatry*. 2018;8(1):120.

18. Fawcett J. Depressive disorders. In: Simon RI, Hales RE, eds. *Textbook of Suicide Assessment and Management*. American Psychiatric Publishing; 2006:1–24.

19. Fawcett J, Scheftner WA, Fogg L, et al. Time-related predictors of suicide in major affective disorder. *Am J Psychiatry*. 1990;147(9):1189–1194.

20. Galyenker I. The Suicidal Crisis. Oxford University Press; 2017.

21. Wetzel RD, Murphy GE. Suicide. In: Rubin E, Zorumski C, eds. Adult Psychiatry. 2nd ed. Blackwell; 2005:409–419.

22. Stene-Larsen K, Reneflot A. Contact with primary care and mental health care prior to suicide: A systematic review of the literature from 2000 to 2017. *Scand J Public Health*. 2019;47(1):9–17.

23. Luoma JB, Martin CE, Pearson JL. Contact with mental health and primary care providers before suicide: A review of the evidence. *Am J Psychiatry*. 2002;159(6):909–916.

24. Kroenke K, Spitzer RL, Williams JG. The PHQ-9: Validity of a brief depression severity measure. *J Gen Intern Med*. 2001;16(9):606–613.

25. Rossum RC, Coleman KJ, Ahmedani BK, et al. Suicidal ideation reported on the PHQ9 and risk of suicidal behavior across age groups. *J Affect Disord*. 2017;215:77–84.

26. Na PJ, Yaramala S, Kim J. The PHQ-9 Item 9 based screening for suicide risk: A validation study of the Patient Health Questionnaire (PHQ)-9 Item 9 with the Columbia Suicide Severity Rating Scale (C-SSRS). *J Affect Disord*. 2018;232:34–40.

27. Columbia Lighthouse Project. Columbia-Suicide Severity Rating Scale. Published 2016. Accessed January 10, 2021. https://cssrs.columbia.edu

28. Suicide Assessment Five-Step Evaluation and Triage SAFE-T pocket card. Suicide Prevention Resource Center. Published 2009. Accessed January 3, 2021. https://sprc.org/resources-programs/suicide-assessment-five-step-evaluation-and-triage-safe-t-pocket-card

29. Horowitz LM, Bridge JA, Teach SJ, et al. Ask Suicide-Screening Questions (ASQ): A brief instrument for the pediatric emergency department. *Arch Pediatr Adolesc Med*. 2012;166(12):1170–1176.

30. World Health Organization. *Preventing Suicide: A Global Imperative*. World Health Organization; 2014.

31. Choi KH, Wang S, Yeon B, et al. Risk and protective factors predicting multiple suicide attempts. *Psychiatry Res.* 2013;10(3):957–961.

32. Tidemalm D, Långström N, Lichtenstein P, Runeson B. Risk of suicide after suicide attempt according to coexisting psychiatric disorder: Swedish cohort study with long-term follow-up. *BMJ.* 2008;337:a2205.

33. Owens PL, Fingar KR, Heslin KC, Mutter R, Booth CL. Emergency department visits related to suicidal ideation, 2006–2013. HCUP Statistical Brief no. 220. Agency for Healthcare Research and Quality; January 2017.

34. American Psychiatric Association. *Diagnostic and Statistical Manual of Mental Disorders.* 5th ed. American Psychiatric Publishing; 2013:104–131.

35. Bolton JM, Belik SL, Enns MW, et al. Exploring the correlates of suicide attempts among individuals with major depressive disorder: Findings from the National Epidemiologic Survey on Alcohol and Related Conditions. *J Clin Psychiatry.* 2008;69:1139–1149.

36. Paris J. Implications of long-term outcome research for the management of patients with borderline personality disorder. *Harv Rev Psychiatry.* 2002;10:315–323.

37. Pompili M, Girardi P, Ruberto A, Tatarelli R. Suicide in borderline personality disorder: A meta-analysis. *Nord J Psychiatry.* 2005; 59:319–324.

38. Bolton JM, Belik SL, Enns MW, et al. Exploring the correlates of suicide attempts among individuals with major depressive disorder: Findings from the National Epidemiologic Survey on Alcohol and Related Conditions. *J Clin Psychiatry.* 2008;69:1139–1149.

39. Knesper DJ, American Association of Suicidology, Suicide Prevention Resource Center. *Continuity of Care for Suicide Prevention and Research: Suicide Attempts and Suicide Deaths Subsequent to Discharge from the Emergency Department or Psychiatric Inpatient Unit.* Education Development Center; 2010.

40. Ribeiro JD, Huang X, Fox KR, Franklin JC. Depression and hopelessness as risk factors for suicide ideation, attempts and death: Meta-analysis of longitudinal studies. *Br J Psychiatr.* 2018;212:279–286.

41. Egeland JA, Sussex JN. Suicide and family loading for affective disorders. *JAMA.* 1985;254:915–918.

42. Qin P, Agerbo E, Mortensen PB. Suicide risk in relation to family history of completed suicide and psychiatric disorders: A nested case–control study based on longitudinal registers. *Lancet.* 2002;360:1126–1130.

43. Roy A, Segal NL, Centerwall BS, Robinette CD. Suicide in twins. *Arch Gen Psychiatry.* 1991;48:29–32.

44. Brent DA, Melhem N. Familial transmission of suicidal behavior. *Psychiatr Clin North Am.* 2008;31(2):157–177.

45. Ivey-Stephenson AZ, Crosby AE, Jack SPD, et al. Suicide trends among and within urbanization levels by sex, race/ethnicity, age group, and mechanism of death—United States, 2001–2015. *MMWR Surveill Summ.* 2017;66:1–16.

46. Kaufman EJ, Morrison CN, Branas CC, Wiebe DJ. State firearm laws and interstate firearm deaths from homicide and suicide in the United States: A cross-sectional analysis of data by county. *JAMA Intern Med.* 2018;178:692–700.

47. Kellermann AL, Rivara FP, Somes G, et al. Suicide in the home in relation to gun ownership. *N Engl J Med.* 1992;327:467–472.

48. Mann JJ, Michel CA. Prevention of firearm suicide in the United States: What works and what is possible. *Am J Psychiatry.* 2006;173(10):969–979.

49. Chapdelaine A, Samson E, Kimberley MD, Viau L. Firearm-related injuries in Canada: Issues for prevention. *CMAJ*. 1991;145:1217–1223.

50. Spicer RS, Miller TR: Suicide acts in 8 states: Incidence and case fatality rates by demographics and method. *Am J Public Health*. 2000;90:1885–1189.

51. Darvishi N, Farhadi M, Haghtalab T, Poorolajal J. Alcohol-related risk of suicidal ideation, suicide attempt, and completed suicide: A meta-analysis. *PLoS One*. 2015;10(5):e0126870.

52. Bachman S. Epidemiology of suicide and the psychiatric perspective. *Int J Environ Res Public Health*. 2018;15:1425.

53. Risk and protective factors. Centers for Disease Control and Prevention. Published 2018. Accessed January 18, 2021. https://www.cdc.gov/suicide/factors

54. Iannuzzi GL, Ruth LJ, Wagoner RC, Currier GW. Suicide. In: Glick RL, Zeller SL, Berlin JS, eds. Emergency Psychiatry: Principles and Practice. 2nd ed. Wolters Kluwer; 2021:323–331.

55. Busch KA, Fawcett J, Jacobs DG. Clinical correlates of inpatient suicide. *J Clin Psychiatry*. 2003;64:14–19.

56. Zorumski CF. Looking forward. In: North CS, Yutzy SH, eds. *Goodwin & Guze's Psychiatric Diagnosis*. 6th ed. Oxford University Press; 2010.

57. Simon RI. Improving suicide risk assessment. *Psychiatric Times*. 2011;28(11).

58. Shea SC. Suicide assessment. *Psychiatric Times*. 2009;26(12).

59. Chung DT, Hadzi-Pavlovic D, Wang M, et al. Meta-analysis of suicide rates in the first week and the first month after psychiatric hospitalisation. *BMJ Open*. 2018;9(3).

60. Closing a deadly gap in health care. National Action Alliance for Suicide Prevention. Accessed December 1, 2021. https://theactionalliance.org/sites/default/files/handout_-_best_practices_in_care_transitions_final.pdf

61. Stanley B, Brown GK, Brenner LA, et al. Comparison of the safety planning intervention with follow-up vs usual care of suicidal patients treated in the emergency department. *JAMA Psychiatry*. 2018;75(9):894–900.

62. Motto JA, Bostrom AG. A randomized controlled trial of postcrisis suicide prevention. *Psychiatr Serv*. 2001;52(6):828–833.

63. Lowenstein DH, Massa SM, Rowbotham MC, et al. Acute neurologic and psychiatric complications associated with cocaine abuse. *Am J Med*. 1987;83:841–846.

64. Zweben JE, Cohen JB, Christian D, et al. Psychiatric symptoms in methamphetamine users. *Am J Addict*. 2004;13(2):181–190.

65. Holcomb WR, Anderson WP. Alcohol and multiple drug use in accused murderers. *Psychol. Rep*. 1983;52:159–264.

66. Swanson JW, Holzer CE, Ganu VK, et al. Violence and psychiatric disorder in the community: Evidence from the Epidemiologic Catchment Area surveys. *Hospital and Community Psychiatry*; 1990;41:761–770.

67. Eronen M, Hakila P, Tiihonen J. Mental disorders and homicidal behavior in Finland. *Archives of General Psychiatry*. 1996;53:497–501.

68. Budd RD, Lindstrom DM. Characteristics of victims of PCP-related deaths in Los Angeles County. *J Toxicol Clin Toxicol*. 1982;19:997–1004.

69. Schifano F, Napoletano F, Arillotta D, et al. The clinical challenges of synthetic cathinones. *Br J Clin Pharmacol*. 2020;86(3):410–419.

70. Rund BR. The association between schizophrenia and violence. *Schiz Res*. 2018;199:39–40.

71. Tardiff K. Violence: Causes and non-psychopharmacological treatment. In: Rosner R, ed. *Principles & Practice in Forensic Psychiatry*. 2nd ed. Oxford University Press, 2003:572–578.

72. Pfeffer C, Plutchnik R, Miziuchi M. Predictors of assaultiveness in latency age children. *Am J Psychiat*. 193;150:1368–1373.

73. Rozel JS. Violence: Violence risk as a psychiatric emergency. In: Glick RP, Zeller SL, Berlin JS, eds. Emergency Psychiatry Principles and Practice. 2nd ed. Wolters Kluwer; 2021;332–344.

74. Choe JY, Teplin LA, Abram K, et al. Perpetration of violence, violent victimization, and severe mental illness: Balancing public health concerns. *Psychiatric Services*. 2008;59(2):153–164.

75. Beeber LS. Disentangling mental illness and violence. *J Am Psychiatr Nurses Assoc*. 2018;24(4):360–362.

76. Ahonen L, Loeber R, Brent DA. The association between serious mental health problems and violence. Some common assumptions and misconceptions. *Trauma Violence Abuse*. 2017;20(5):613–625.

77. Bhavsar V, Bhugra D. Violence toward people with mental illness: Assessment, risk factors, and management. *Psychiatry Clin Neurosci*. 2018;72:811–820.

78. Stahl SM. Deconstructing violence as a medical syndrome: Mapping psychotic, impulsive, and predatory subtypes to malfunctioning brain circuits. *CNS Spectr*. 2014;19(5):357–365.

79. Runions KC, Salmivalli C, Shaw T, et al. Toward a conceptual model of motive and self-control in cyberaggression: Rage, revenge, reward, and recreation. *J Youth Adolesc*. 2013:42(5):751–777.

80. Witt K, Van dorn R, Fazel S. Risk factors for violence in psychosis: Systematic review and meta-regression analysis of 110 studies. *PLoS One*. 2013;8(2):e55942.

81. Violence prevention. Centers for Disease Control and Prevention. Published 2020. Accessed January 5, 2020. https://www.cdc.gov/violenceprevention/youthviolence/riskprotectivefact ors.html

82. Tardiff, K. The past as prologue: The assessment of future violence in individuals with a history of past violence. In Simon R., Shuman D, eds. *Predicting the Past: The Retrospective Assessment of Mental States in Civil and Criminal Litigation*. American Psychiatric Press; 2001.

5

Telepsychiatry and Beyond

Future Directions in Emergency Psychiatry

Katherine Maloy

The Changing Landscape of Telemedicine

During the past decade, psychiatric presentations to emergency departments have continued to increase. A shortage of inpatient beds, crisis resources, and urgent outpatient follow-up has continued to be a problem, despite the Affordable Care Act's impact on increasing the number of insured individuals overall and despite efforts to expand primary care–based treatment of anxiety and depression. In the emergency setting, providing thorough and skilled evaluations to patients in crisis is only part of the puzzle. Provision of aftercare, wraparound services, and mobile outreach all factor into an emergency service's ability to triage effectively and move patients on to the most appropriate setting. As inpatient bed availability continues to be a challenge, providing treatment and re-evaluation while patients "board" is also essential.[1]

In 2020, the entire medical community faced the unprecedented challenge of a lethal global pandemic. In an already highly stressed health care system, hospitals have been left scrambling for adequate supplies of personal protective equipment (PPE) for providers; forced to cancel elective procedures that typically offset funding challenges for other hospital services, including mental health; and are dealing with the mental health ramifications of economic uncertainty, unemployment, and trauma that the massive death toll has taken on patients and providers. Demand for intensive care unit and medical beds has led to closure of mental health beds throughout the United States, further limiting access to this already scarce resource, and COVID-related precautions on existing units have altered the milieu of inpatient treatment.[2] Patients stayed away from emergency departments during the initial first wave of the epidemic in the spring of 2020,[3] presumably due to fear of contracting the illness in the emergency room, among other factors, and one can imagine people who clearly needed help not believing that it was safe to access it. Given PPE shortages and other concerns about exposure, many providers began to use telemedicine as a primary treatment option, at the same time that many medical services also did so. In some areas, home-based or mobile crisis teams using telephone screening are used to triage cases or provide follow-up, providing in-person services only when absolutely necessary.

Thus, the COVID epidemic has pushed telemedicine forward with an unprecedented swiftness.[4] Faced with having to re-evaluate the safety of even basic clinical encounters and rationing of PPE, as well as the impact of travel to and from appointments, exposure from waiting rooms, and all the other associated potential avenues of transmission, telemedicine has exploded, particularly for services such as psychiatric evaluation that rely most heavily on narrative history-taking. The crisis has thrust all aspects of telemedicine forward with an immediacy that has pushed aside years of individual and systemic resistance, including funding barriers. For example, a review of Massachusetts General Hospital's utilization of telepsychiatry comparing March 2019 to March 2020 showed a near complete reversal of rates of in-person and virtual care, from less than 5% utilization of virtual visits to 97%.[5] The same article also notes a shift in the risk:benefit analysis regarding sending patients for hospitalization or emergency care, given the risks of exposure in the hospital setting. This rapid change has occurred in departments of psychiatry and private practices throughout the country and forced providers who previously would not have considered telepsychiatry to become more familiar with the technology's advantages and disadvantages. During the pandemic, it has become more apparent than ever before that adaptation and modification are necessary skills to meet the demand for services.

Although telepsychiatry studies prior to the pandemic have shown overall that telepsychiatry is largely accepted by a wide range of patients, concerns have been raised that the most vulnerable—homeless patients, those without access to the internet, those without phones, paranoid or reclusive patients, the elderly or otherwise homebound, and those in abusive relationships—may be the least able to access mobile technologies or to have a private, safe space to see their provider.[6] For example, how does a homeless patient living in a congregate shelter setting access a private place to talk to their psychiatrist? How does a patient in an abusive relationship find a way to convey what is going on in their home if they cannot visit a provider's office for privacy? If patients are less able or willing to contact their outpatient provider via telemedicine, and simultaneously avoiding the emergency department for fear of contracting COVID, these vulnerable populations may become even more isolated or wait to present until they are more severely symptomatic, thus further increasing the burden on emergency services once they do arrive needing treatment.

It is also not possible at this stage to gauge the impact that the trauma of the pandemic may have on mental health overall. Frontline medical providers, including those who work in emergency psychiatric services—some of whom have been pressed into service on medical units due to staffing shortages or work in medical settings in which the impact of COVID is intense and immediate—will likely be dealing with the aftermath of the pandemic long after it subsides. The mental health burden on these providers and everyone in the general population who has been affected by the pandemic is not possible to estimate but likely to be profound. What the health care system will look like, and how it will be able to handle the trauma implications, is an open question.

This chapter discusses the use of telemedicine in an emergency psychiatric setting and explores possible avenues for innovation in provision of services. The landscape of mental health services has changed rapidly due to the COVID-19 pandemic and will likely continue to evolve. Telemedicine can incorporate a wide variety of modalities, from video visits to phone-based consultation and chart review. For the purposes of this chapter, *telepsychiatry* refers to the provision of mental health services by a psychiatric provider through use of video telemedicine technology. Other options, such as phone follow-up, phone consultation, and providing supervision remotely, are also discussed. In the world of emergency psychiatry, the most common clinical scenario is a patient who presents needing an evaluation and disposition, be that admission, discharge, or a short-term hold in a crisis center. This kind of evaluation, whether it is accomplished by a psychiatrist, nurse practitioner, social worker, or other provider, and how to perform it through video technology are primarily the focus of this chapter.

This chapter discusses the evidence for telepsychiatry as a viable model of care; explores different models of providing telepsychiatry services; discusses regulatory and legal requirements; and considers issues of technique, technology, and therapeutic approaches during the evaluation.

Models of Care

In approaching the initiation of any new program or model of care, an essential first step is conducting a needs assessment to match the goals of the program to the patient population and existing system. The needs assessment phase of planning should include review of current patient volume, reasons for presentation, identified existing providers, funding streams, and other available resources. A small hospital that averages, for example, a few visits a month will have very different needs than a tertiary care center with onsite psychiatric beds.[7] An ideal system will endeavor to match the needs of the patient population and regulatory requirements of a given community with the most appropriate level of care. Here, the different models that have been used in a variety of systems are briefly reviewed.

Hub-and-Spoke/Comprehensive Psychiatric Emergency Program

One model that addresses the scarcity of psychiatric resources involves the creation of a network of referring hospitals and crisis centers that access a common tertiary-care psychiatric facility to provide comprehensive evaluations and care.[8] Patients present referred from medical emergency departments, as walk-ins, or by direct ambulance, with a specific medical triage system designating patients as sufficiently medically stable to bypass evaluation at a medical emergency department. Many systems throughout the country have adopted this model. In a setting in which volume of psychiatric presentations at community hospitals is low, and thus the cost of having comprehensive onsite services, or even a dedicated consulting provider, is high, it makes sense to centralize resources to provide the highest level of care possible to a wider geographic area.

The Comprehensive Psychiatric Emergency Program (CPEP), originally implemented in New York City to deal with the high volume of presentations in a dense, urban setting, could be viewed as a model of what services can be provided onsite by a "hub" hospital. The New York State Office of Mental Health requires that all licensed CPEPs provide a specialized unit for 72-hour monitoring (extended observation units), interim crisis aftercare services including mobile crisis, and availability of crisis respite beds for patients not requiring admission but who would benefit from a short-term more supportive setting.

A major disadvantage of a centralized model is the necessity for transport, sometimes across long distances. CPEPs originated in New York City, where there is sufficient patient population to support multiple facilities in each borough, thus decreasing transport times. There is also a robust public transportation system, reducing difficulty of traveling to follow-up. In rural areas, however, the designated hub may be very far away from the patient's home, outpatient providers, and support system. If a decision is made to discharge the patient, accessing follow-up care onsite at the hub may not be a feasible option. In addition, if the hub is full, patients can be stuck waiting for transport. If transport is reliant on law enforcement, further delays related to availability of staffing and prioritization of the transport by a busy police service may be a problem as well.

Telepsychiatry can address some of these concerns if the tertiary care hospital can provide evaluations remotely. Evaluation via video consultation can eliminate the need for patients to travel to a hub facility and can potentially decrease the need for admission or transport to the tertiary care hospital. Telepsychiatry could also be utilized to provide follow-up at home for discharged patients who cannot return for a clinic appointment or who do not have resources available where they live. One could also imagine a system in which a client in crisis could potentially access video telepsychiatry services from their clinic appointment or from their home. If the tertiary care center is already staffing providers on-site, those providers could be enlisted to provide this consultation or screening evaluation to remote facilities, with one incentive being that they can prevent unnecessary admissions or transfers.

Some systems provide all the services of a tertiary care center but with the psychiatrist available via telepsychiatry. For example, one program in east Texas combines the full services of a comprehensive psychiatric emergency program with psychiatric coverage provided by telepsychiatry videoconference. In this system, mental health calls are triaged by phone with a standardized protocol to determine medical stability and appropriateness. In cases in which there is a question about whether the patient needs to come to the center, mobile crisis services can be sent out to do an on-site evaluation. Once the patient arrives at the center, the psychiatric evaluation is completed by videoconferencing. This model reportedly has decreased waiting times by eliminating the need for all psychiatric patients to pass through a medical emergency room, and it has decreased law enforcement involvement by eliminating the need for law enforcement supervision of patients being medically cleared or awaiting transport.[9]

An existing hub facility may already have trained staff with a high level of experience who could be trained to extend their services via telemedicine or offer supervision and consultation to providers at a remote facility. Utilization of telepsychiatry technology to provide attending-level supervision of trainees could also provide a better educational experience and increased support to trainees working in high-acuity settings, without requiring that attending to be on-site overnight, which can be a staffing challenge.

Consultant Model

Probably the most commonly used model in psychiatric emergency evaluation, consultation is the most easily adapted to telemedicine technology. In this model, a primary on-site team provides care, including medical stabilization, optimization for psychiatric admission if needed, and referral to aftercare, while the psychiatric practitioner evaluates the patient and provides recommendations.

There are many advantages of a consultant telepsychiatry model. First, in terms of staffing and service design, the psychiatric practitioner can provide consultation to multiple lower volume locations at the same time, allowing, for example, a network of hospitals to cover a variety of locations. The consultant does not even need to be based in the emergency department and could be part of a consult-liaison service or even an outpatient setting. Staffing costs can be distributed across a network of consortium of emergency departments, with utilization driving the portion of funding contributed by each individual system. Lower volume hospitals could thus potentially have access to a higher level of care than they could otherwise afford.

For the provider, the focus of the consultant is on evaluating the patient and providing recommendations, as opposed to having to follow up more immediate moment-to-moment management. This can allow the provider to provide consultation as an adjunct to other clinical tasks because they are not bound to a specific location or workflow.

Finally, there is potential for faster turnover of patients and decreased boarding time if patients can be evaluated in real time instead of waiting for regular business hours. If a hospital that provides in-person psychiatric evaluations during regular business hours can supplement those services with a telepsychiatry consultation on weekends, nights, and holidays, it can avoid a backlog of patients taking up valuable medical emergency department resources.

The consultant model can be challenging, however, because of the potential loss of the "liaison" function of an on-site consultant. The consultant who is based in the hospital and can be easily contacted while they are seeing another patient or paged for a question while they are already in-house may be able to provide support to the emergency department and improve teamwork more easily than a consultant who is not located on-site and has to be summoned through video technology for a full visit. Developing an alliance and partnership with the primary team takes time. If a provider is only interacting with the patient during video evaluation, developing a relationship with other staff can be more complicated and requires concerted effort on both sides. The consultant is also more dependent on the primary team to implement its recommendations, and the primary team may not have sufficient training in behavioral emergencies or sufficient resources or motivation to provide a therapeutic milieu. If the consultant is also providing care at a primary site, juggling responsibilities and triaging between in-person and remote consultation can be difficult.

One example of a consultant service is the South Carolina Department of Mental Health's 2009 initiative. Previous research had shown that only 32% of South Carolina's emergency departments had a psychiatric emergency service. Follow-up research compared a matched control group of patients who did not receive telepsychiatry services with those who did and found that admission rates decreased and follow-up improve at 30 and 90 days.[10] Another system in Washington state implemented a telepsychiatry consultation service primarily to manage involuntarily detained patients awaiting beds. However, the service was found to have additional benefits in terms of providing support to the community hospitals. In particular, it was noted that

> it changes the hospitalist–psychiatrist dynamic, often for the better, when the subtext of the consult does not include the expectation that the psychiatrist will be able to personally find an acute psychiatric bed for the patient. . . .They were pleased to have a psychiatrist to help with agitated patients, to evaluate suicidality, and to initiate psychiatric treatment.[11]

This highlights the importance of clearly establishing the role of the consultant, defining the scope of their work carefully, and appropriately assessing the needs that the service is trying to address.

In the New York area, one major health system has utilized telepsychiatry consultation to evaluate patients presenting at its network facilities that do not have on-site psychiatric services. If patients need admission, they can be transferred within the health system to an available bed at one of the affiliated hospitals. If discharged, follow-up planning can also be facilitated by telehealth social work services and case management.

Follow-Up, Supervision, and Other Uses of Telepsychiatry

The collaborative care model for integrating behavioral health into primary care settings has been used for several years, and telepsychiatry has been adapted to fill the role of the consulting psychiatrist in the primary care model.[12] The emergency department could potentially use similar models, utilizing a tiered system in which the psychiatrist only sees the most acute or emergent cases and provides periodic supervision and chart-based case tracking of other less severe cases, with utilization of nurses, social workers, Credentialed Alcohol and Substance Abuse Counselors, or peers to provide the in-the-moment care for more "routine" or "non-emergent" emergency department presentations.

For example, if a patient presents to an emergency department with acute psychosis and behavioral disturbance, the psychiatric consultant might be called on to evaluate the patient and offer recommendations immediately via a video visit. The several other patients who present during the week with anxiety, depression, or mild substance abuse might be primarily seen by a social worker, referred to aftercare with peer support follow-up before the appointment, and the case reviewed at a weekly conference call after the doctor has had a chance to review the week's charts. The psychiatrist could also consult with emergency department physicians regarding starting medications such as antidepressants or for substance use disorders. This consultation may be easier to provide remotely, through videoconferencing or conference calls, rather than requiring the psychiatrist to be on-site. A study from Norway described the positive impact that availability of a video evaluation by a psychiatrist had on consultation by local psychiatric nurses who provided on-site in-person evaluation, increasing confidence of the nurse provider.[13]

An example of a hybrid program based out of the University of Rochester Medical Center utilized a psychiatric assessment officer (PAO) model in which telepsychiatry was provided as a resource to support the on-site PAO, who was a social worker, nurse, or licensed mental health counselor. Notably, prior to this program, there were no psychiatric services at the participating rural hospitals. The PAO performed primary evaluations, interventions, and coordination of care, with support from the telepsychiatrist, who could also see the patient directly if needed through a mobile tablet-based telemedicine platform. The PAO intervention group was associated with a statistically significant reduction in the emergency department revisit rate.[14]

For follow-up care, some systems have utilized a crisis clinic model. When combined with mobile crisis services and respite housing, immediately available high-acuity aftercare can potentially divert patients from requiring psychiatric admission. Instead of referring to outside providers, the facility refers the patient back to a follow-up clinic on-site or at an affiliated facility, where they meet with a non-MD provider for additional stabilization, with psychiatrist backup to provide prescriptions if indicated. Peers can be enlisted as well to provide support between the initial visit and follow-up or to act as an advocate in navigating aftercare systems. In some systems, walk-in non-emergent evaluations are also available, where patients can be triaged to the emergency department if needed but can avoid it altogether if the issue is not life-threatening. The non-MD provider can triage the patient, present the case to the psychiatric provider, and then the psychiatric provider can see the patient via video if needed—for example, if medication is being prescribed or if there is a question about diagnosis or need for hospitalization. Again, in this scenario, the telepsychiatry model could potentially alleviate the need to have a dedicated prescriber on-site, with the psychiatrist or psychiatric nurse practitioner being able to provide consultation remotely.

Mobile crisis is more challenging for telepsychiatry simply because the purpose of the team is to go to the patient instead of expecting the patient to cooperate, call in, or make an appointment. Mobile crisis calls are generally high-acuity and frequently not self-referred; thus, initial phone contact may unfortunately give the patient more of a chance to avoid treatment or intervention. However, during the initial spring surge of COVID-19 in New York City, some teams did utilize telephone visits, particularly for follow-up, to minimize the need for in-person visits and the associated exposure risk. One could also imagine a model in which a psychiatric provider could video-call into a mobile visit when needed to provide supervision or could offer case conferencing via videoconferencing or conference call. Given the prevalence of smartphones with video-call capability, and the availability of phone or tablet-based telemedicine software, it is now more possible than ever to bring the consultant clinician directly into the patient's home, possibly preventing the need for hospital transfer in some cases.

Child psychiatrists or psychiatric providers with child and adolescent expertise or training are in even shorter supply than adult psychiatric services, so the need for access to alternate forms of evaluations and services has led programs to experiment with a variety of options. One service implemented a Web-based evaluation to assess adolescents for depression, suicidal ideation, post-traumatic stress disorder, substance use, and exposure to violence which could be self-administered. This intervention led to small but significant increases in identification of patients who otherwise would not have been recognized.[15] A 12-month prospective study in Toronto, Canada, found that telepsychiatry was an acceptable option to child and adolescent patients and their parents, reducing unnecessary travel to urban centers.[16] In general, children and adolescents have spent their entire lives in a world in which video-call technology exists and is readily available on most smartphones, and thus they may be less reluctant to utilize the technology than older patients.

Regulatory Issues

Federal Regulations

In the United States, telemedicine is federally regulated via the Drug Enforcement Administration (DEA), with regard to prescribing, and through the Centers for Medicare & Medicaid Services (CMS), with regard to Medicare and Medicaid billing. The aim of the DEA regulations around telemedicine has been primarily focused on prevention of drug trafficking through internet-based or phone-based distribution. Unfortunately, due to some high-profile criminal cases, the definition of "telemedicine" became tied up in extremely minimal clinical interactions (e.g., filling out an online questionnaire or completing a brief phone call) rather than a full psychiatric visit with videoconferencing as part of a licensed health care facility. Prior to COVID, Medicare reimbursement for telepsychiatry was also limited, focusing only on high-need areas. Medicare has also required that the provider be located within the United States. The state of emergency under COVID has led to significant relaxing of some of these regulations, albeit temporarily.[17] Given the current state of flux of the health care system, it makes the most sense to consult with an expert on CMS, federal regulations, DEA regulations, and Joint Commission expectations when designing a telepsychiatry service.

Privacy Regulations

In addition to the privacy of the medical record, two aspects of privacy to consider in telepsychiatry are that of the clinical interaction and that of the technology used. Each side of the clinical interaction should be conducted in a space that provides privacy. Providers working from home need to be particularly mindful of these issues, and busy emergency departments may struggle with finding adequate space. In terms of data transmission, adequate encryption and secure medical record systems are essential, as is adequate internet bandwidth to support the level of encryption required.

State/Local Regulations

Every state has a different set of regulations regarding psychiatric holds and admissions; therefore, it is important to take into account any state or local regulations around these issues when setting up an emergency telepsychiatry service. In addition, state or county offices of mental health may have regulations or guidelines around telepsychiatry in facilities that they license. Some states require admission decisions to be made by non-physician practitioners, some counties allow nurse practitioners or psychologists to place a patient on or remove them from a hold, and some states specifically require a board-certified or board-eligible psychiatrist. When considering staffing remotely, the licensure and credentials of the consultant should match the requirements of the system. In addition, telepsychiatry services should follow locally established guidelines. If there are no existing guidelines, consultation with the local regulatory agencies is recommended.[18]

In addition, the location of the provider must be considered. If the patient is in one state and the provider is in another, the provider will likely be required to be licensed in both states in order to provide care. However, this varies by state, and it has been further diffused by emergency waivers related to COVID. The practitioner should ensure they are following all local licensure guidelines and consult with the state medical boards before taking on a position that involves crossing state lines because physicians have been held liable for taking the word of staffing agencies and not consulting medical boards.[19]

Prescribing of controlled substances via telemedicine is another issue where guidelines need to be closely consulted. Although COVID emergency provisions temporarily waived the in-person visit requirement for prescribing controlled substances in certain circumstances,[20] this will likely not continue indefinitely. The issue of prescribing, including specific concerns for controlled substances, should be clearly specified in any telepsychiatry plan. If the clinician is serving primarily as a consultant providing recommendations to a primary team, the prescribing issue may be avoided altogether.

Finally, states may have their own regulations regarding privacy of electronic transfer of protected health information, and typically if those regulations are more stringent than what is specified in HIPAA, the state regulations take precedence.

Billing

During COVID-19, Medicare billing for telemedicine services was broadly expanded to permit providers to continue care without requiring in-person visits, which were being minimized so as to avoid shortages of PPE, unnecessary travel, crowding of waiting rooms, and unnecessary emergency room visits.[17] Many states also passed regulations or executive orders mandating that insurance companies waive copays for telemedicine visits and that reimbursement for telemedicine be equivalent to that for in-person visits for the duration of the epidemic. Prior to the epidemic, insurance companies varied widely with regard to their reimbursement and understanding of telemedicine. It remains to be seen what changes pushed forward by COVID remain permanent. In summary, before making any assumptions about profitability, it is important for hospital systems to get an informed opinion as to the revenue they may expect from a telepsychiatry emergency service and weigh that against savings related to unnecessary admissions, boarding, or transfers.

Technical and Design Issues

A safe, quiet, and private location for the patient to be evaluated is essential. In a busy emergency department, rooms can be scarce. To improve the flexibility of the assessment, use of a mobile cart with a moveable camera can facilitate evaluation in a variety of spaces in the emergency department and allow an on-site provider to show close-ups of relevant physical findings.

In addition to conducting the interview, clinicians will require a means of documenting in the record. Accessing the medical record remotely if not working from another site in the same health system would be ideal but can be complicated and slow depending on the system. The clinician also will need a means of communicating with the on-site staff that can accommodate addressing an emergent clinical change. Backup procedures should also be considered for periods of electronic medical record downtime, power failures, or internet disruption.

Interpretation services for both spoken and sign language will need to be adapted to the telemedicine setting. Planning ahead for how to incorporate telephone interpreters or video relay of sign language can avoid delays of care for individuals needing those services. Many hospitals rely on phone-based language interpretation and video relay–based sign language services, both of which may be complicated to adapt to the video visit.

Technique and Clinical Approach

In general, efficacy of care and satisfaction of patients has been shown to be equivalent to in-person care for telemental health modalities. An extensive review of available evidence in 2013 showed telemental health to overall be comparable to in-person care and to increase access.[21] However, despite the best technology available, there will always be a difference between evaluating a patient in person and remotely, and technique needs to be adapted accordingly. The loss of the utilization of all of the doctor's senses is not something to take for granted. Most emergency psychiatrists can recall when an odor has helped inform their decision-making or when being able to observe the patient covertly in the milieu has broadened their understanding of the clinical situation. To be even more concrete, how much of the patient's body is visible on the video? The condition of a patient's feet or personal hygiene or the way they are sitting or lying down can give important clues as to their overall functioning. Placing a patient in front of a camera with an escort nearby may create an artificial sense of order and calm that lowers the psychiatrist's ability to detect instability. Conversely, the psychiatrist unaccustomed to remote evaluations or concerned about liability may be reluctant to discharge or release a patient from a hold if they are not able to see the patient in person. The remote provider is also more reliant on the primary team to determine medical stability. It is therefore important that the consultant take into account as many sources of information as possible to correct for the change in perspective and lack of immediacy that telemedicine may cause. Careful review of the chart and discussion with the on-site providers help set the stage for a focused and informed assessment.

In some cases, the patient may be too paranoid, agitated, or somnolent to participate in a video interview. Cultural factors should also be considered, with patients who have less familiarity or comfort with technology being more reluctant to engage by video.[22] Discussion and cooperation with the on-site providers are therefore key in getting additional information if the patient is uncooperative or unable to participate and providing support to the remote clinician by explaining the process to the patient in advance. Encouraging patients to voice their concerns and ask questions can go a long way toward providing reassurance that the interaction will be private and in the patient's interest in terms of facilitating care.

There may be some advantages to distance, however. In emergency settings, with a high degree of acuity, the remote consultant does not need to be physically afraid for their safety and thus may be freed up from any conscious or unconscious fears that would interfere with their ability to engage. More clinicians may be willing to work from home or from a location close to their residence than they would be to travel to a distant location where they are required to remain for an entire shift. Depending on volume, the consultant can intersperse emergency evaluations with other forms of psychiatric care, allowing for a more varied practice, which may be more appealing to some clinicians than full-time emergency work. In the time of COVID-19, in which hospitals have struggled with having sufficient PPE and clinicians and patients are routinely wearing masks for all clinical interactions, telepsychiatry allows the patient and clinician to see each other's faces safely.

Practice is essential to mastering the video patient encounter. Clinicians should arrange for a trial run of the technology platform with someone who can provide feedback about how they are presenting on camera and what is visible to the patient in the clinician's consulting office. If the telepsychiatry setup has additional features, such as being able to zoom the remote camera or zoom the clinician's own camera, the clinician should have practice in using them. Clinicians should get feedback about whether they appear to be making eye contact and whether they are speaking clearly and in a normal manner. It may not be apparent where to look when facing a telepsychiatry screen, and most people have a tendency to look at themselves instead of the patient. For some clinicians, minimizing or hiding the view of their own face can limit this distraction. It may also be easier to be distracted by phones, pagers, or any other items out of immediate camera range; clearing the workspace and closing other browser windows can be helpful if this is an issue. Use of a headset or earbuds can reduce ambient noise interference and improve privacy in a setting in which the clinician may be overheard. Whatever system is used, practice and planning ahead are crucial.

Clinicians should address any privacy concerns the patient may have up front, explain the parameters of the assessment, and ask the patient to notify them immediately if there are any technical issues. Acknowledging the reality of the artificiality of the telemedicine situation goes a long way toward establishing rapport. Clinicians may find themselves needing to be more explicit than they are accustomed to—for example, asking the patient to sit up so they are more visible or asking the patient to show their hands to assess for tremor. Similarly, the clinician should solicit feedback from the patient about whether they can hear and see the clinician adequately and ask them to let the clinician know if something disrupts the connection.

In some settings, depending on local or facility regulations, a staff member may be required to be in the room with the patient during the video encounter. Clinicians should ascertain who is in the room with the patient and document the name of that person in the record. It is also helpful to let that person know they can relay any acute concerns that develop during the interview (e.g., if they observe some indicator of agitation or the patient's vital signs change). In addition to whoever is in the room, it is helpful to understand the circumstances of where the patient is located: Is the patient in a private room with the door closed by themselves? Is the sitter or escort in the room or outside the door? Or, does the patient have any privacy at all? Asking if there is anyone else present off-camera (e.g., an escorting police officer, a hospital security guard, or a family member) can help contextualize the interview and establish whether the patient has adequate privacy to respond honestly.

Risk Management Issues

Emergency psychiatry focuses largely on decisions around risk, in that most patients present in crisis and a decision is typically being made as to whether hospitalization is indicated. The standard of care for determining risk does not change because the evaluation is done by video telemedicine. Some clinicians, accustomed to primarily in-person evaluations, may find themselves more reluctant to discharge or release a patient from a hold via a telepsychiatry evaluation only. If there is something missing from the video evaluation, then a plan for how to correct for that should be documented and pursued.

For example, one can easily imagine a patient who is so intoxicated and uncooperative that they cannot answer any questions and will not sit in front of the camera. The issue at hand is an inability to evaluate the patient's safety due to their intoxication, and a plan should be documented as to how the patient should be monitored and re-evaluated, just as in any other clinical setting. However, given that the clinician evaluating remotely cannot smell the patient's breath or may not see whether the patient can walk with a steady gait, confirmation from the on-site team verifying that they, too, think intoxication is the issue and that there is not some other medical problem would be important to verify as well. In summary, it is not sufficient to attribute gaps in information needed to make a decision either to retain or discharge a patient to the video visit. A plan should be documented to resolve the discrepancy or get more information.

Documentation that the patient consented to the video evaluation is also important, as is the reason for the evaluation being conducted by video instead of in person.[19] It is also important to document the type of evaluation taking place because telemedicine with video is different from a phone conversation or reviewing a chart electronically. Make sure to report all the different ways that you obtained information—reviewing the chart, speaking with on-site providers, speaking with collateral contacts by phone, interviewing the patient by video, etc.—and also to document what information you were not able to obtain, such as aspects of a physical exam that cannot be done remotely. Finally, documentation should include a plan for relaying the conclusions and recommendations to the primary team. Because the telepsychiatry provider is inherently less accessible than if they were located on-site, documentation should be as clear and direct as possible, with encouragement to contact the provider if clarification is needed.

Support and Supervision

A doctor or other psychiatric clinician working in a hospital system, emergency department, or crisis center is always subject to—and, it is hoped, supported by—a health care cultural system. Anyone who has worked in a variety of settings can attest to the various esoteric differences of "the way things are done" that develop over time and in reaction to various experiences or outcomes. Psychiatric providers working remotely may not have the firsthand experience of everyday interactions with other staff that contribute to a hospital's culture, and as a result they may struggle to fit in with the team. Training and ongoing feedback are essential to integrating the remote provider into the primary team. Training should ideally include feedback and guidelines specific and unique to telepsychiatry. Hospital systems should anticipate providing regular supervision, support, and mentoring for remote providers, whether through regular case conferences, individual meetings, or more informal check-ins.

On the provider side, it is important to anticipate and be conscious of the difference between working directly with a team on-site and working remotely and also to take steps to ensure a productive relationship is being cultivated. The liaison function of a consultant—responding to "curbside" questions, being responsive to questions, and providing support around managing complex and difficult patients—can be lost if the clinical interaction is confined solely to the video visit.

Future Directions

The state of U.S. health care is changing so rapidly that it is not possible to predict where we will land. COVID-19 continues to surge, putting unimaginable strain on hospitals, providers, and patients. There continues to be a shortage of psychiatric care overall; the opioid epidemic has arguably worsened under COVID-19; and health coverage continues to be primarily tied to employment, despite the Affordable Care Act. One thing seems clear: Efforts to contain costs and provide care in innovative ways will continue to be needed. Vast numbers of psychiatric providers—from outpatient counselors to inpatient psychiatrists—have now had experience with utilizing videoconferencing technology to see patients; many of these providers had no interest in doing so prior to the COVID-19 pandemic. Although there will always be a role for in-person evaluation and treatment, it seems likely that the convenience afforded to both providers and patients will set a precedent for incorporation of telepsychiatry even after the COVID-19 pandemic.

References

1. Nordstrom K, Berlin JS, Nash SS, Shah SB, Schmelzer NA, Worley L. Boarding of mentally ill patients in emergency departments: American Psychiatric Association resource document. *West J Emerg Med*. 2019;20(5):690–695. https://doi.org/10.5811/westjem.2019.6.42422

2. Bojdani E, Rajagopalan A, Chen A, et al. COVID-19 pandemic: Impact on psychiatric care in the United States. *Psychiatry Res*. 2020;289:113069. https://doi.org/10.1016/j.psych res.2020.113069

3. Hartnett KP, Kite-Powell A, DeVies J, et al. Impact of the COVID-19 pandemic on emergency department visits—United States, January1, 2019–May 30, 2020. *MMWR Morb Mortal Wkly Rep*. 2020;69:699–704. http://dx.doi.org/10.15585/mmwr.mm6923e1

4. Koonin LM, Hoots B, Tsang CA, et al. Trends in the use of telehealth during the emergence of the COVID-19 pandemic—United States, January–March 2020. *MMWR Morb Mortal Wkly Rep*. 2020;69:1595–1599. http://dx.doi.org/10.15585/mmwr.mm6943a3

5. Chen J, Cheung W, Young S, et al. COVID-19 and telepsychiatry: Early outpatient experiences and implications for the future. *Gen Hosp Psychiatry*. 2020;66:89–95. https://doi.org/10.1016/j.genhosppsych.2020.07.002

6. Ojha R, Syed S. Challenges faced by mental health providers and patients during the coronavirus 2019 pandemic due to technological barriers. *Internet Interv*. 2020;21:100330. https://doi.org/10.1016/j.invent.2020.100330

7. Butterfield A. Telepsychiatric evaluation and consultation in emergency care settings. *Child Adolesc Psychiatr Clin North Am*. 2018;27:467–478.

8. Zeller S. Hospital-level psychiatric emergency department models. *Psychiatric Times* 2019;36(12). https://www.psychiatrictimes.com/psychiatric-emergencies/hospital-level-psychiatric-emergency-department-models

9. American Psychiatric Association. 2011 APA Gold Award: A telepsychiatry solution for rural eastern Texas. *Psychiatr Serv*. 2011;62(11):1384–1386.

10. Narasimhan M, Druss B, Hockenberry J, et al. Impact of a statewide telepsychiatry program at emergency departments statewide on the quality, utilization and costs of mental health services. *Psychiatr Serv*. 2015;66(11):1167–1172.

11. Kimmel R, Toor R. Telepsychiatry by a public, academic medical center for inpatient consults at an unaffiliated, community hospital. *Psychosomatics*. 2019;60(5):468–473.

12. Al Achkar M, Bennett I, Chwastiak L, et al.. Telepsychiatric consultation as a training and workforce development strategy for rural primary care. *Ann Fam Med*. 2020;18(5):438–445. doi:10/1370/afm.2561

13. Trondsen M, Tjora A, Broom A, Scambler G. The symbolic affordances of a video-mediated gaze in emergency psychiatry. *Soc Sci Med*. 2018;197:87–94. https://doi.org/10.1016/j.socsci med.2017.11.056

14. Maeng D, Richman J, Lee B, Hasselberg M. Impact of integrating psychiatric assessment officers via telepsychiatry on rural hospitals' emergency revisit rates. *J Psychosom Res*. 2020;133:109997. https://doi.org/10.1016/j.jpsychores.2020.109997

15. Fein J, Pailler M, Barg F, et al. Feasibility and effects of a Web-based adolescent psychiatric assessment administered by clinical staff in the pediatric emergency department. *Arch Pediatr Adolesc Med.* 2010;164(12):1112–1117.

16. Roberts N, Hu T, Axas N, Repetti L. Child and adolescent emergency and urgent mental health delivery through telepsychiatry: 12-Month prospective study. *Telemed J E Health.* 2017;23(10):842–846. doi:10.1089/tmj/2016/0269

17. Physicians and other clinicians: CMS flexibilities to fight COVID-19. Centers for Medicare and Medicaid Services. Published 2020. https://www.cms.gov/files/document/physicians-and-other-clinicians-cms-flexibilities-fight-covid-19.pdf

18. Shore J, Savin D, Novins D, Manson S. Cultural aspects of telepsychiatry. *J Telemed Telecare.* 2006;12:116–121.

19. Vanderpool D. Top 10 myths about telepsychiatry. *Innov Clin Neurosci.* 2017;14(9–10):13–15.

20. How to prescribe controlled substances to patients during the COVID-19 emergency. Drug Enforcement Administration. Published 2020. Accessed November 21, 2020. https://www.deadiversion.usdoj.gov/GDP/(DEA-DC-023)(DEA075)Decision_Tree_(Final)_33120_2007.pdf

21. Hilty D, Ferrer D, Parish M, Johnston B, Callahan E, Yellowlees P. The effectiveness of telemental health: A 2013 review. *Telemed J E Health.* 2013;19(6):444–454. doi:10.1089/tmj.2013.0075

22. Shore J, Savin D, Novins D, Manson S. Cultural aspects of telepsychiatry. *J Telemed Telecare.* 2006;12:116–121.

6

Cultural Competence in Emergency Psychiatry

Arpit Aggarwal and Oluwole Popoola

Introduction

The use of psychiatry emergency services is strongly influenced by cultural attitudes and beliefs of patients. The clinicians' cultural attitudes and beliefs also affect the quality of patients' experience and thus indirectly influence their utilization of psychiatric emergency services. Because patients of various cultural and ethnic background visit the emergency department, it is important for clinicians to be culturally competent. The process of evaluating and managing culturally diverse patient populations in the emergency setting requires special expertise and unique approaches while working under time constraints.

Definitions

Culture: Integrated pattern of human behaviors including thoughts, communication, actions, customs, beliefs, values, and institutions of a racial, ethnic, religious, or social nature[1]

Cultural competence: Set of congruent behaviors, attitudes, and policies found in a system, agency, or professionals that enables them to work effectively in a context of cultural difference[2]

Acculturation: Process of change in the cultures of two or more groups of individuals from different cultures, resulting from their continuous firsthand contact[3]

Culture and Psychiatry

Psychiatric presentations are strongly influenced by cultural contexts. To properly understand the cultural dimensions, culture can be divided into the culture of the patient, the culture of the clinician, and the medical culture of the place where the clinical work is being performed.

The Role of the Patient's Culture

Individual factors such as personal life experiences, medical knowledge, socioeconomic status, and personal beliefs contribute to the patient's understanding of illness and reaction to the illness. Culture directly affects patients in how they describe their symptoms to clinicians. There are different cultural views of subjective experiences and distress and how much stigma surrounds an illness.[4]

Psychiatric disorders are considered to result from a complex interaction between biological, psychological, social, and cultural factors, and the role of one or more of these factors can be stronger or weaker depending on the kind of disorder.[5]

Culture also relates to the patient's coping strategies, likelihood of treatment seeking, expectations from the clinician, motivation for treatment, and compliance with treatment recommendations.[5]

The Role of the Clinician's Culture

Clinicians, as individuals, have their own cultural identity based on race, ethnicity, gender identification, religion, immigration status, and other sociodemographic characteristics. Another significant contributor to the clinician's culture is the professional culture of the clinician, which is largely informed by the culture of mental health treatment—usually the cultural context of the clinician's training. These can have a significant impact on patient care.[5] The culture of mental health treatment exerts its effect on patient assessment and care directly and indirectly (through its impact on the clinician's cultural identity). It is important for clinicians to be aware of the various ways that conflicts between their cultures and those of their patients could impact on assessment, diagnosis, and treatment. They can then work to reduce the negative effects and maximize outcomes from the clinical encounter.

Issues that could arise from cultural conflicts between clinicians and their patients include conflicting explanatory models of the patient's illness; the clinician's biases, attitudes, and stereotypes; and mistrust and hostility between the patient and the clinician due to a history of sociopolitical tension between their cultural groups.[5]

Although matching a patient with an ethnoculturally similar clinician certainly has benefits, there are some potential disadvantages. Negative transference and countertransference can occur, resulting in ambivalence, mistrust, and anger. For example, a patient may perceive the ethnoculturally similar clinician as a betrayer because they sold out their shared culture, or the clinician may overidentify with the patient and wrongly assume comprehension of the cultural context of the patient's illness.[6]

The Role of the Medical Culture

Medical culture includes customs, regulations, and attitudes that have developed in the medical service setting beyond medical knowledge.[7] Clinicians become accustomed to living within this cultural system and may be unaware of its influence on their practice.

Cultural Challenges in Emergency Psychiatry

Patients from diverse cultural and ethnic backgrounds present to emergency psychiatry services, which raises potential problems that are unique to this setting. The emergency department is the most accessible part of the health care system for patients who do not have an adequate crisis resolution network. Because emergency psychiatric evaluations are usually time limited, treatment of patients can be very challenging for clinicians who are not culturally competent. Timely diagnosis and immediate care can be difficult if the clinician is not familiar with the patient's cultural and social background. Language barriers can also pose a serious challenge in an emergency setting.

Assessment of suicide risk is commonly performed in emergency settings and can be challenging because in many cultures suicide is associated with shame and patients from these cultures might not easily share their suicidal ideation with others. There is also a potential for bias in deciding patient disposition and diagnosis; race and ethnicity play an important role in the severity of diagnosis given and rates of hospitalization.[8]

Role of Culture in Emergency Psychiatric Assessment and Diagnosis

A preliminary diagnostic formulation is essential for the patient presenting in a psychiatric emergency to be properly triaged and for treatment planning. It is important to consider cultural influences on the patient's presentation during psychiatric emergency encounters because a culturally sensitive assessment is crucial to meaningfully formulate a preliminary diagnosis. One of the significant adverse consequences of ignoring this is that the clinician may misinterpret a patient's behavior or misconstrue the severity of the presenting problem, leading to misdiagnosis and mismanagement of the patient. For example, a study by Adeponle et al.[9] found that psychotic disorders were misdiagnosed in patients from all ethnocultural backgrounds. Among immigrants and refugees from South Asia, post-traumatic stress disorder and adjustment disorders were often misdiagnosed as psychotic disorders.[9] On the other hand, a culturally sensitive assessment has been noted to improve clinical rapport, patient engagement, and therapeutic efficacy.[10]

The Culturally Sensitive Emergency Psychiatric Assessment

It is helpful for the clinician to have a broad knowledge of cultural groups to which patients may belong. The clinician should also be aware of their own culture and strive to recognize how their culture and the mental health treatment culture might impact on their conceptualization of the patient's symptoms.[5] However, due to the complex relationship between culture and mental illness, it is useful to have a framework that helps elicit, organize, and analyze information that reflects the impact of the patient's culture on their illness. The Cultural Formulation Interview (CFI) in the fifth edition of the *Diagnostic and Statistical Manual of Mental Disorders* (DSM-5) is an internationally validated tool jointly produced and disseminated by the American Psychiatric Association and the DSM-5 Cross-Cultural Issues Subgroup. It offers a good framework for a culturally sensitive psychiatric assessment and treatment planning, and it can be applied in various settings, including the emergency psychiatric setting.[11] It contains questions that elicit the patient and their social network's narrative and views about the patient's illness and how they seek help. It provides an opportunity for the clinician to identify subtle sociocultural factors that meaningfully impact diagnoses and patient care.[12] The CFI is widely used in operationalizing cultural assessment of psychiatric patients. It is feasible, widely accepted, improves clinician–patient communication, and is publicly available.[13,14]

The Cultural Formulation Interview

The CFI is a brief semistructured interview with three components: the core, informant, and supplementary modules. The core and informant version CFIs are aimed at eliciting information from the patient and people closest to the patient, respectively. The informant version is particularly useful when patients are unable to provide meaningful or coherent information due to significant cognitive impairment, psychosis, or agitation or when patients are young children. The supplementary modules contain additional questions used to obtain more information than was elicited by the core and informant components.[15]

It is highly encouraged to be flexible in the use of the CFI. It is intended to guide a culturally sensitive assessment and should not get in the way of the natural flow of the interview and maintenance of rapport with the patient. Based on the clinical setting, the entire CFI could be used, or as in the case of psychiatric emergencies, certain aspects of it could be incorporated into the clinical evaluation as necessary. The following four domains of cultural impact on illness are addressed by the CFI:[15]

- Cultural definition of the problem—aims to elicit and facilitate the patient's description of their view of their illness.
- Cultural perceptions of cause, context, and support—aims to enunciate the patient's perception and their social network's perception or explanation of the cause(s) of the illness, social problems that worsen the illness, and social supports that make it better.
- Cultural factors that affect self-coping and past help seeking—aims to explore what methods the patient has employed to cope with the illness, what ways the patient has sought help (within and outside the biomedical system) for their illness, and what barriers they have encountered in the process of seeking help.
- Cultural factors that affect current help seeking—aims to explore the patient's treatment preferences and those of the patient's close associates. It also gives the patient an opportunity to express how perceived differences with the clinician could affect their care.

Although operationalizing the full complement of questions in the CFI may not be feasible for every patient presenting in a psychiatric emergency, bearing in mind the concepts of these four domains and incorporating relevant elements in them into the assessment and overall evaluation of the patient afford a culturally sensitive assessment.

Using Language Interpreters and Cultural Informants

Language interpreters or translators are indispensable to effective communication and therapeutic alliance when there are significant differences in language ability and proficiency between the patient and the clinician. Basic English proficiency may not suffice for an adequate psychiatric assessment because in contrast to general medical interviews, the expression of social and emotional distress usually requires more proficiency. Important considerations in the use of translators include the following:

- Awareness of the nonverbal component of communication: Individuals (patient, clinician, and interpreter) should be positioned in a triangular formation, such that each person has a clear view of the others. When appropriate, the clinician can ask the interpreter to help contextualize nonverbal communication by the patient.
- Training in competencies that include the necessary technical medical and psychiatric vocabulary, knowledge of the patient's cultural background, and ethical and interpersonal issues.
- When feasible and appropriate, it is helpful for the clinician to prepare the translator by reviewing the patient's sociodemographic details and presenting complaint with the translator prior to the patient encounter and also to review the session together after the encounter to clarify possible areas of misunderstandings.[16]

One common pitfall to avoid is the use of family members or friends as translators. Although they may be English proficient, family dynamics and personal interpretation of the content of the patient's response could inadvertently mislead the clinician.[17]

Cultural informants are also known as cultural brokers or cultural consultants. They have knowledge of a cultural group by experience gained from belonging to such a group and usually have other key roles within the group. Sometimes, language interpreters can double as cultural informants. Mental health providers, community leaders, and religious leaders can also serve as cultural informants. Their knowledge as participants and leaders in the cultural group makes them a resource for clarification and information about attitudes, perspectives, and other cultural underpinnings of patients' illnesses.[17] In the emergency psychiatric setting, consulting with a cultural informant could take the form of obtaining collateral information from the pastor of a patient whose religion strongly underlies their explanatory model of their illness. Also, if a language interpreter was used during the assessment, the clinician could gauge their appropriateness to serve as a cultural informant by inquiring about their level of participation in the cultural group.

The Culturally Sensitive Emergency Psychiatric Diagnostic Formulation

Once a psychiatric diagnosis is made, deductions about the impact of the patient's culture on their presentation should be included in the diagnostic formulation to clarify the patient's symptoms and etiological attributions. If the presentation does not meet criteria for a specified or unspecified mental disorder, the DSM-5 has V and Z codes that may be relevant, such as acculturation difficulty, social exclusion or rejection, parent–child relational problems, or religious or spiritual problems.[15] Also, the DSM-5 contains a glossary of cultural concepts of distress (a more acceptable term than culture-bound syndromes), some of which are discussed in the next section, especially those likely to be encountered in the emergency psychiatric setting.

Cultural Concepts of Distress (Culture-Bound Syndromes)

Cultural concepts of distress refer to ways that cultural groups experience, understand, and communicate suffering, behavioral problems, or troubling thoughts and emotions.

There are three main types of cultural concepts of distress: cultural syndromes, cultural idioms of distress, and cultural explanations or perceived causes. The term "cultural concepts of distress" acknowledges that distress in all forms is shaped by cultural contexts and that the individual's experience and explanations of distress account for the clinically relevant cultural differences in presentation. *Culture-bound syndrome*, on the other hand, suggests that certain types of distress and symptom configurations are peculiar to and localized in specific cultures.[15] Some cultural concepts of distress that may be encountered in the emergency psychiatric setting are presented next.

Amok

This syndrome is usually described in males and is often associated with mass homicide. It occurs as a dissociative episode characterized by an initial period of depressed mood and brooding followed by aggressive, violent, or homicidal behavior until the individual becomes exhausted, is restrained, or sometimes killed. When not killed, the individual has complete or partial amnesia of the episode.[18] The episode is often associated with persecutory ideas or feelings of prejudice and automatism. It was initially described in Malay tribesmen and is derived from the Malay word *mengamok*, which means to make a furious and desperate charge. The Malay culture tolerates this syndrome based on the belief that it is an involuntary behavior caused by possession by an evil tiger. It has also been observed in primitive tribes in the Philippines, Laos, Puerto Rico, and Papua New Guinea. Notably, whereas the modern occurrence of amok in primitive tribes decreased to the point that it was almost unheard of by the mid-20th century, similar occurrences of violence in industrial societies have been increasing.[19]

Ataque de Nervios (Attack of Nerves)

Also known as Puerto Rican syndrome, *ataque de nervios* refers to an idiom of distress characterized by a general sense of being out of control that is prominent among Puerto Rican females and other Latino groups.[20] Although more common among people of Latino descent, this syndrome has been reported among non-Latinos as well.[21,22] Commonly reported symptoms include uncontrollable screaming or shouting, crying fits, trembling, sensation of heat in the chest rising into the head, verbal or physical aggression, dissociative experiences, seizure-like or fainting episodes, and suicidal gestures.[20] A prominent feature of ataque de nervios is a sense of being out of control. Events causing acute anxiety, grief, or anger, such as the death of a loved one or intense interpersonal conflicts, may trigger an attack. Among individuals with an underlying history of trauma, attacks may occur without a triggering event. Although symptoms of ataque de nervios may appear similar to panic attacks, a main distinguishing feature between these two is the absence of intense fear or sense of impending doom in ataque de nervios, whereas these are prominent in panic attacks.[23-25]

Khyal Cap or Wind Attacks

This is a culturally shaped experience of anxiety and trauma-related disorder commonly found among Cambodians and other Southeast Asians. Common symptoms of khyal attacks include those of panic attacks (dizziness, palpitations, shortness of breath, and cold extremities) and other symptoms of anxiety and autonomic arousal, such as tinnitus and muscle tension. These symptoms are usually interpreted as arising from "kyal," a windlike substance that is thought to rise in the body and blood, wreaking havoc such as entering the ears to cause tinnitus, compressing the lungs to cause shortness of breath, clogging up the vessels to cause heart attack, and potentially leading to death. Common triggers for this attack include worry, orthostasis, going into crowded spaces or riding in a car, and specific odors with negative associations. In some cases, it may be unprovoked.[26,27]

Koro

Although originally described and common among Asian cultures, koro has been reported among individuals of various cultures.[28,29] Depending on the patient's culture, it is known by a variety of names—shuk yang, suo yang (Chinese), jinjinia bemar (Assam), or rok-joo (Thailand). It refers to sudden intense fear or perception that the penis (or vulva and nipples in females) is receding into the body and will cause death despite the lack of obvious changes to the sexual organs. Victims and their relatives try several remedies to prevent the penis from shrinking, including tying the penis or asking several family members to grasp and prevent the penis from retracting.[29,30] It is reported in connection with different mental and physical disorders, and medications aimed at treatment of underlying disorders have shown promise.[30,31]

Boufee Delirante

This is a French term referring to an acute and brief psychotic episode not due to an underlying mental disorder or substances, observed in various francophone countries.[32] Usually seen in young people (aged 20–40 years), typical symptoms include delusions, hallucinations, psychomotor excitement, agitated and aggressive behavior, and dissociative experiences or marked confusion.[33]

Qi-Gong Psychotic Reaction

This is an acute and transient dissociative or psychotic episode that may occur after participation in *qi-gong*, a Chinese health-enhancing practice. Individuals who become overly invested in the practice are vulnerable to developing qi-gong psychotic reaction. Symptoms may include hallucinations, delusions, extreme anxiety, discomfort, and uncontrolled spontaneous movement.[34]

Role of Culture in Emergency Psychiatric Treatment

Just as with emergency psychiatric assessment and diagnosis, the impact of culture on the patient's response to psychiatric treatment is complex. The patient's culture as well as that of the clinician can affect the patient's response to treatment.[5,10] Aspects of the patient's culture can be protective. For example, the significant cross-cultural variance in schizophrenia prognosis can be largely accounted for by culturally unique personal dynamics within the family. These can be capitalized upon for culturally sensitive treatment planning.[35] Also, more relevant to the emergency setting are known ethnic-related biological variations in psychiatric medication metabolism that exert influence on medication response, knowledge of which is indispensable to efficient and appropriate selection of psychotropic medications.[36]

CFI and Treatment Planning

The last two domains in the CFI capture cultural factors that affect the patient's self-coping and current and past attempts to seek help for their illness. Information from these aspects of the assessment should be factored into the intervention and treatment plan. The patient's culturally acceptable self-coping and previous help-seeking patterns that are beneficial should be incorporated into the treatment plan. For example, a religious patient whose explanatory model of their illness is significantly influenced by their religion and who has benefited previously from religious-based counseling should be encouraged to re-engage in such. For cultural influences on current help seeking, the patient's treatment preferences and those of their close associates should shape management.[12] As in the assessment, the clinician should continue to be aware of the potential for clashes between their culture and that of their patient and how this could impact on the treatment. Cultural variations in prescription patterns may be partially accounted for by the clinician's stereotypes and biases about the patient. For example, stereotypes of "the angry Black male" and misunderstanding of the expressive, vocal demeanor of the African American male have been found to be associated with overdiagnosis, overtreatment, and misjudgment of treatment response.[17] This may be one reason why African American patients are prescribed higher doses of antipsychotics and have higher rates of being on long-acting injectable antipsychotics and first-generation antipsychotics.[36]

Ethnic Variations in the Metabolism of Psychotropic Medications

There is a sizable amount of literature on variation in medication metabolism and clinical response. Ethnically specific polymorphic variability accounts for a large part of this variation.[37] Some of the variability has been found to be associated with variations in genetic as well as nongenetic mechanisms that drive psychotropic medication metabolism, although other ethnic-specific factors, such as diet and societal attitudes, likely have a significant impact.[36] One of the known genetic variations that account for the ethnic-related variations in antidepressant, antipsychotic, and benzodiazepine response and side effect profiles is in the cytochrome P450 drug-metabolizing enzymes.[36–38] One example of this is in different polymorphisms of CYP2D6, which is one of the most important CYP enzymes in psychiatry because it is the major pathway for the metabolism of many antipsychotics, some tricyclic antidepressants, and selective serotonin reuptake inhibitors.[37] Many of the mutations in CYP2D6 are ethnic-specific, resulting in polymorphisms that are more common in certain cultural groups. The finding that Asians require lower therapeutic doses of antidepressants and antipsychotics may be related to the unique presence of two alleles of the CYP2D6 gene, which is associated with slower enzyme activity and medication metabolism.[37] Conversely, Mexican Americans have remarkably faster 2D6 activity because they have low rates of these mutations.[39] In treating ethnic minority patients, it is recommended to start psychotropic medications at a low dose and increase the dose slowly; ask about diet, smoking, and use of herbal medications to evaluate for potential drug–drug interactions; check plasma levels when appropriate; and involve the patient's family or close associates.

References

1. Pumariega AJ, Rothe E, Mian A, et al. Practice parameter for cultural competence in child and adolescent psychiatric practice. *J Am Acad Child Adolesc Psychiatry*. 2013;52(10):1101–1115.

2. Cross T, Bazron B, Dennis K, Isaacs M. *Towards a culturally competent system of care*. Vol. 1. CASSP Technical Assistance Center; 1989.

3. Rothe EM, Tzuang D, Pumariega AJ. Acculturation, development, and adaptation. *Child Adolesc Psychiatr Clin N Am*. 2010;19(4):681–696.

4. Kleinman A. *Rethinking Psychiatry*. Simon & Schuster; 2008.

5. Office of the Surgeon General, Center for Mental Health Services, National Institute of Mental Health. Mental health: Culture, race, and ethnicity: A supplement to mental health: A report of the Surgeon General. Substance Abuse and Mental Health Services Administration; 2001.

6. Comas-Diaz L, Jacobsen FM. Ethnocultural transference and countertransference in the therapeutic dyad. *Am J Orthopsychiatry*. 1991;61(3):392–402.

7. Tseng W-S, Streltzer J. *Cultural Competence in Clinical Psychiatry*. American Psychiatric Publishing; 2008.

8. Strakowski SM, Lonczak HS, Sax KW, et al. The effects of race on diagnosis and disposition from a psychiatric emergency service. *J Clin Psychiatry*. 1995;56(3):101–107.

9. Adeponle AB, Thombs BD, Groleau D, Jarvis E, Kirmayer LJ. Using the cultural formulation to resolve uncertainty in diagnoses of psychosis among ethnoculturally diverse patients. *Psychiatr Serv*. 2012;63(2):147–153.

10. Alarcon RD, Westermeyer J, Foulks EF, Ruiz P. Clinical relevance of contemporary cultural psychiatry. *J Nerv Ment Dis*. 1999;187(8):465–471.

11. Aggarwal NK, Glass A, Tirado A, et al. The development of the DSM-5 Cultural Formulation Interview–Fidelity Instrument (CFI-FI): A pilot study. *J Health Care Poor Underserved*. 2014;25(3):1397–1417.

12. DeSilva R, Aggarwal NK, Lewis-Fernandez R. The DSM-5 cultural formulation interview and the evolution of cultural assessment in psychiatry. *Psychiatric Times*. 2015;32(6).

13. Lewis-Fernandez R, Aggarwal NK, Baarnhielm S, et al. Culture and psychiatric evaluation: Operationalizing cultural formulation for DSM-5. *Psychiatry*. 2014;77(2):130–154.

14. Lewis-Fernandez R, Aggarwal NK, Lam PC, et al. Feasibility, acceptability and clinical utility of the Cultural Formulation Interview: Mixed-methods results from the DSM-5 International Field Trial. *Br J Psychiatry*. 2017;210(4):290–297.

15. American Psychiatric Association. *Diagnostic and Statistical Manual of Mental Disorders*. 5th ed. American Psychiatric Publishing; 2013.

16. Lee E. Cross-cultural communication: Therapeutic use of interpreters. 1997:477–489.

17. Lim RF. *Clinical Manual of Cultural Psychiatry*. American Psychiatric Publishing; 2015.

18. Schmidt K, Hill L, Guthrie G. Running amok. *Int J Soc Psychiatry*. 1977;23(4):264–274.

19. Saint Martin ML. Running amok: A modern perspective on a culture-bound syndrome. *Prim Care Companion J Clin Psychiatry*. 1999;1(3):66–70.

20. Guarnaccia PJ, Rivera M, Franco F, Neighbors C. The experiences of ataques de nervios: Towards an anthropology of emotions in Puerto Rico. *Cult Med Psychiatry.* 1996;20(3):343–367.

21. Interian A, Guarnaccia PJ, Vega WA, et al. The relationship between ataque de nervios and unexplained neurological symptoms: A preliminary analysis. *J Nerv Ment Dis.* 2005;193(1):32–39.

22. Keough ME, Timpano KR, Schmidt NB. Ataques de nervios: Culturally bound and distinct from panic attacks? *Depress Anxiety.* 2009;26(1):16–21.

23. Lewis-Fernandez R, Garrido-Castillo P, Bennasar MC, et al. Dissociation, childhood trauma, and ataque de nervios among Puerto Rican psychiatric outpatients. *Am J Psychiatry.* 2002;159(9):1603–1605.

24. Lewis-Fernandez R, Guarnaccia PJ, Martinez IE, Salman E, Schmidt A, Liebowitz M. Comparative phenomenology of ataques de nervios, panic attacks, and panic disorder. *Cult Med Psychiatry.* 2002;26(2):199–223.

25. Lewis-Fernandez R, Gorritz M, Raggio GA, Pelaez C, Chen H, Guarnaccia PJ. Association of trauma-related disorders and dissociation with four idioms of distress among Latino psychiatric outpatients. *Cult Med Psychiatry.* 2010;34(2):219–243.

26. Hinton DE, Hinton AL, Eng KT, Choung S. PTSD and key somatic complaints and cultural syndromes among rural Cambodians: The results of a needs assessment survey. *Med Anthropol Q.* 2012;26(3):383–407.

27. Hinton DE, Pich V, Marques L, Nickerson A, Pollack MH. Khyal attacks: A key idiom of distress among traumatized Cambodia refugees. *Cult Med Psychiatry.* 2010;34(2):244–278.

28. Adeniran RA, Jones JR. Koro: Culture-bound disorder or universal symptom? *Br J Psychiatry.* 1994;164(4):559–561.

29. Chowdhury AN. The definition and classification of Koro. *Cult Med Psychiatry.* 1996;20(1):41–65.

30. Garlipp P. Koro–A culture-bound phenomenon intercultural psychiatric implications. *German J Psychiatry* 2008;11(1):21–28.

31. Roy D, Hazarika S, Bhattacharya A, Das S, Nath K, Saddichha S. Koro: Culture bound or mass hysteria? *Aust N Z J Psychiatry.* 2011;45(8):683.

32. Chabrol H. Chronic hallucinatory psychosis, bouffee delirante, and the classification of psychosis in French psychiatry. *Curr Psychiatry Rep.* 2003;5(3):187–191.

33. Pillmann F, Haring A, Balzuweit S, Bloink R, Marneros A. Bouffee delirante and ICD-10 acute and transient psychoses: A comparative study. *Aust N Z J Psychiatry.* 2003;37(3):327–333.

34. Hwang WC. Qi-gong psychotic reaction in a Chinese American woman. *Cult Med Psychiatry.* 2007;31(4):547–560.

35. Marcolin MA. The prognosis of schizophrenia across cultures. *Ethn Dis.* 1991;1(1):99–104.

36. Chaudhry I, Neelam K, Duddu V, Husain N. Ethnicity and psychopharmacology. *J Psychopharmacol.* 2008;22(6):673–680.

37. Lin KM, Smith MW, Ortiz V. Culture and psychopharmacology. *Psychiatr Clin North Am.* 2001;24(3):523–38.

38. Sramek JJ, Pi EH. Ethnicity and antidepressant response. *Mt Sinai J Med.* 1996;63(5–6):320–325.

39. Mendoza R, Wan YJ, Poland RE, et al. CYP2D6 polymorphism in a Mexican American population. *Clin Pharmacol Ther.* 2001;70(6):552–560.

SECTION II

SPECIFIC DISORDERS, DIAGNOSES, AND SYMPTOMS FREQUENTLY ENCOUNTERED AS PSYCHIATRIC EMERGENCIES

7

Altered Mental Status and Neurologic Syndromes

Thomas W. Heinrich, Ian Steele, and Sara Brady

Introduction

A patient presenting to the emergency department often represents a diagnostic enigma. The patient may present with a single pathognomonic symptom or sign or a myriad of vague, inconclusive signs and symptoms. When a patient presents to the emergency department with a neuropsychiatric complaint, the diligent clinician should include various medical, surgical, and neurologic conditions in their differential diagnosis. This chapter discusses medical conditions that should be considered in the differential diagnosis of patients presenting to the emergency department with neuropsychiatric signs and symptoms.

Delirium

Clinical Presentation

Delirium is an acute confusional state resulting from an underlying physiologic disturbance commonly observed among medically ill patients. According to the fifth edition of the *Diagnostic and Statistical Manual of Mental Disorders* (DSM-5),[1] delirium is characterized by a disturbance in attention (i.e., reduced ability to direct, focus, sustain, and shift attention) and awareness (reduced orientation to the environment) that develops over a short period of time (usually hours to a few days) and often fluctuates in severity during the course of a day. This disturbance is accompanied by at least one other cognitive deficit (e.g., memory, orientation, language, visuospatial ability, or perception). Finally, this disturbance in consciousness and cognition cannot be better attributed to a preexisting neurocognitive disorder.

Perceptual disturbances and transient psychotic symptoms, such as hallucinations or delusions, occur in 50% of delirious patients.[2] Hallucinations are often visual, whereas delusional content involves misidentifications, themes of imminent danger, or bizarre events in the immediate environment.[3] Patients often experience disruptions in the sleep–wake cycle, with marked periods of drowsiness, sleep during the day, and insomnia at night.[4]

There are three motor subtypes of delirium: hyperactive, hypoactive, and mixed. The hyperactive subtype presents with an increased quantity of motor activity, loss of control of activity, restlessness, and/or wandering. The hypoactive subtype manifests with decreased activity, psychomotor slowing, withdrawal, diminished speech, listlessness, and/or reduced awareness of surroundings.[5] In mixed delirium, features of both hyperactive and hypoactive delirium are observed in the patient. Although hyperactive delirium is most readily recognized, it accounts for only 25% of delirium cases. Often, hypoactive or mixed delirium is associated with poorer outcomes.[6]

Prevalence and Risk Factors

Delirium is a common psychiatric syndrome observed in medically ill patients. Delirium is estimated to occur in 11% of elderly emergency department patients,[7] 37% of postoperative patients,[8] and as many as 80% of critically ill patients receiving mechanical ventilation.[9] Delirium affects up to 85% of terminally ill patients during their last weeks of life.[10]

Significant risk factors for delirium include age and cognitive impairment, including both mild cognitive disorder and dementia.[11] A preexisting diagnosis of dementia increases the risk for delirium fivefold.[12] Additional risk factors include severity of acute illness, length of hospital stay, visual impairment, urinary catheterization, and nutritional deficiency.[13] Common deliriogenic medication classes include anticholinergics, narcotics, and hypnotics (e.g., benzodiazepines).[14]

Pathogenesis

Symptoms of delirium arise from an underlying etiology that is often multifactorial and may vary over time (e.g., acute trauma, metabolic derangements, and infection). The underlying etiologies often induce inflammation, oxidative stress, hypoxia, and various toxic–metabolic insults that manifest as the syndrome of delirium.[15]

Symptom Course

DSM-5 delineates between acute delirium (i.e., symptoms lasting a few hours or days) and persistent delirium (i.e., symptoms lasting weeks or months). Although delirium was previously thought to be a temporary cognitive disruption, evidence now suggests that delirium is associated with long-term sequelae. These include prolonged hospital length of stay,[16] as well as increased risk of institutionalization, sustained cognitive impairment, and death.[17] It is not uncommon for symptoms of delirium to continue for weeks to months beyond the time of initial diagnosis.[18]

Diagnosis

Although delirium is common, the diagnosis relies on a high index of suspicion, as it often goes undetected or misdiagnosed. Up to 40% of hospitalized patients referred for psychiatric consultation for depression were diagnosed with delirium.[19]

Unfortunately, there is no clinical study or biomarker with robust accuracy for the diagnosis of delirium. Although electroencephalography (EEG) studies typically show generalized slowing in delirium, the false-negative and false-positive rates approach 20%, limiting the utility of this tool.[20] Several validated delirium screening tools with high sensitivity and specificity have been developed, including the Confusion Assessment Method (CAM), that improve the detection of delirium by multidisciplinary health care providers.[21] Nevertheless, the gold standard for diagnosing delirium remains a thorough clinical evaluation.

The clinical assessment for delirium focuses on reviewing information regarding acuity of mental status changes, previous history of delirium or cognitive impairment, and potential precipitating factors. A delirious patient may or may not be able to participate in the interview, depending on the severity of disturbance in their awareness and attention. Therefore, it is critical to obtain collateral information through record review, collaboration with other treatment providers (e.g., nursing staff and personal care attendants), and conversation with family. Assessment of the patient's appearance, psychomotor activity, level of consciousness, and ability to sustain attention during the interview provides essential diagnostic information. However, as previously noted, the diagnosis of delirium relies on a high index of suspicion because cases frequently go undiagnosed.

Nonpharmacologic Interventions

The definitive treatment of delirium includes identification and treatment of the underlying medical illness. However, a single underlying etiology is not often readily apparent; rather, multiple insults coalesce to create the neuropsychiatric syndrome of delirium. Several factors may contribute to the propagation of delirium, including use of physical restraints for behavioral control, polypharmacy (initiating three or more medications during the period 24–48 hours before the onset of delirium), use of a bladder catheter, and any iatrogenic event.[22]

Behavioral interventions, such as providing a calm environment, frequent reorientation, availability of sensory aids (glasses and hearing aids), and preservation of the sleep–wake cycle, should be implemented to reduce confusion and agitation. Catheters and lines should be removed or replaced as soon as medically appropriate. Supportive measures, including addressing nutritional and volume status, should also be incorporated. Nutritional deficiencies, particularly thiamine (vitamin B_1), can lead to delirium.[23] Early mobilization and deep vein thrombosis prophylaxis are important to reduce iatrogenic risks, including deep vein thrombosis, pressure ulcers, and aspiration pneumonia. Finally, a thorough medication reconciliation should be performed, with attention to deliriogenic medication classes and potential drug–drug interactions.

Pharmacologic Intervention: Antipsychotics

Although there is no U.S. Food and Drug Administration (FDA)-approved medication for the treatment of delirium, antipsychotics are the most used class of medication to manage symptoms of delirium while one addresses the underlying medical etiologies. Recent high-quality systematic reviews and meta-analyses indicate that antipsychotics do not significantly impact delirium incidence, duration, severity, or hospital length of stay,[24,25] but there are no systematic reviews or meta-analyses that evaluate the effect of antipsychotics on patient-centered measures of delirium, including their impact on psychotic symptoms, emotional distress, and long-term functional outcomes. Clinical experience and multiple consensus statements, including those by the American Psychiatric Association[26] and the National Institute for Health and Care Excellence,[27] suggest using antipsychotics to target specific symptoms of delirium when the symptoms create patient distress, pose an immediate physical safety risk, or impede the delivery of medical care.

In these cases, it is reasonable to embark on a judicious, time-limited trial of antipsychotics to target specific symptoms such as insomnia, hallucinations, paranoia, delusions, or psychomotor agitation. Because no single antipsychotic has been demonstrated as superior to others in treating delirium, the selection of an antipsychotic agent should be based on optimization of the medication's pharmacodynamics, side effect profile, and available route of administration to the clinical situation. Haloperidol may be administered orally, intramuscularly, or intravenously, although the intravenous (IV) route is not approved by the FDA. In addition, haloperidol minimally affects vital signs, possesses negligible anticholinergic activity, and has few medication interactions; thus, it may be most appropriate for medically unstable or critically ill patients.[28] For patients who have difficulty swallowing tablets, both risperidone and olanzapine are available in dissolvable tablet preparations. Patients experiencing a disrupted sleep–wake cycle may benefit from more sedating antipsychotics dosed at bedtime, such as olanzapine or quetiapine. In terms of disease-specific considerations, patients with Parkinson's disease or degenerative dopaminergic neuron disease should be treated with antipsychotics such as quetiapine, which are less likely to worsen the motor symptoms of Parkinson's disease.[29] Patients receiving chemotherapy often benefit from the antiemetic properties of olanzapine.[30]

Three of the most serious medical risks of antipsychotic use are prolonged QTc interval, extrapyramidal side effects (EPS), and neuroleptic malignant syndrome (NMS). QTc prolongation, particularly in patients with medical illness, has been associated with lethal ventricular arrhythmias, such as torsades de pointes. Although all antipsychotics can increase the QTc interval, absolute increases tend to be modest, ranging from 5 to 20 msec depending on which formula is used to calculate the QTc (e.g., Bazett, Fridericia, Framingham, or Hodges).[31] It is important to obtain a baseline electrocardiogram, address modifiable risk factors for prolonged QTc (e.g., replete electrolytes and minimize other medications that prolong QTc), and reassess the QTc interval after initiating an antipsychotic to ensure it has not significantly increased. Patients must also be monitored for EPS, including acute dystonia and akathisia, which can exacerbate symptoms of restlessness in delirium. IV haloperidol has been observed to be associated with little of the EPS that often complicate the use of oral or intramuscular haloperidol.[32] Finally, all patients who are newly initiated on antipsychotic treatment must be routinely assessed for NMS, a rare but life-threatening condition characterized by lead-pipe rigidity, hyperthermia, mental status changes, and autonomic instability.[33] If NMS is suspected, the antipsychotic medication should be immediately discontinued and aggressive supportive care should be initiated. Finally, antipsychotics should be initiated at low doses. Doses may be gradually titrated to efficacy while monitoring for side effects to maximize tolerability. Antipsychotics should be used for the shortest duration necessary and with a clear plan to taper or discontinue before discharge.

Alternative Pharmacotherapy: Benzodiazepines, Alpha Agonists, and Antiepileptics

Although antipsychotic medications are most used to manage delirium symptoms, other classes of medications may be helpful in specific clinical situations. Benzodiazepines are typically discontinued during acute delirium due to their propensity to perpetuate delirium; however, benzodiazepines are often the preferred agent in the treatment of delirium resulting from alcohol or benzodiazepine withdrawal. When benzodiazepines are administered, patients must be carefully monitored for signs of benzodiazepine intoxication, including nystagmus, ataxia, slurred speech, and oversedation (leading to respiratory depression). Dexmedetomidine, a parenterally administered selective α_2 agonist, may be used as an alternative or augmentation sedation strategy in intensive care settings. Dexmedetomidine's use is limited to the intensive care setting due to the risk of bradycardia and hypotension. Clonidine, an oral α_2 agonist, has less central nervous system selectivity than dexmedetomidine but can be safely administered in non-intensive care unit settings.

Among patients for whom antipsychotics are poorly tolerated or relatively contraindicated (e.g., history of NMS or prolonged QTc in an unstable cardiac patient), antiepileptic drugs may be considered for the management of agitation associated with delirium. A retrospective study demonstrated that valproic acid is effective in reducing agitation and duration of delirium.[34] Baseline liver enzymes and complete blood counts (CBCs) should be obtained before initiating valproic acid.

Serotonin Syndrome

Introduction

A syndrome that is becoming increasingly important for a psychiatrist working in the emergency department to detect is serotonin syndrome. The recent increase in serotonin syndrome is most likely due to the increasing number of antidepressant prescriptions prescribed each year and the increased use of synthetically created illicit substances (methamphetamine, MDMA, LSD, etc.).[35,36]

Epidemiology

The true yearly incidence of serotonin syndrome is difficult to determine because the syndrome ranges from mild to severe, and mild cases may have the symptoms attributed to other causes.[37] In 2018, there were 125,358 incidents of exposure to an antidepressant (tricyclic antidepressant [TCA], selective serotonin reuptake inhibitor [SSRI], serotonin–norepinephrine uptake inhibitor [SNRI], monoamine oxidase inhibitor [MAOI], etc.), according to the Toxic Exposure Surveillance System.[36] Of those exposed only to a single antidepressant, 10,091 had moderate to severe symptoms of serotonin toxicity.[36] This is a 24% increase in exposures from 2002 to 2018.[38]

A significant number of medications and substances can lead to the development of serotonin syndrome, including antidepressants (MAOIs, TCAs, SSRIs, and SNRIs), opiate analgesics, over-the-counter cough medicines (dextromethorphan), antibiotics (linezolid), antivirals (ritonavir), weight-reduction agents, antiemetics, antimigraine agents, drugs of abuse, and herbal products.[37,39]

Risk factors that may predispose an individual to develop serotonin syndrome include serum iron deficiency, taking a serotonergic agent with a prolonged half-life, co-ingestion of a shorter acting serotonergic agent, and end-stage renal disease on hemodialysis.[39,40] Medications that slow or inhibit the hepatic metabolism of serotonergic agents (specifically cytochrome P-450 enzymes 3A4, 2D6, 2C9, 2C19, and 1A2) also increase the risk of developing serotonin syndrome due to higher levels of the agent in the bloodstream.

Clinical Presentation

The presentation of serotonin syndrome has a wide range from mild to severe. It is essential to know what symptoms are present in each stage.

In mild cases of serotonin syndrome, the neurological symptoms that one may see include tremor, myoclonus, and hyperreflexia. The mental status may include dizziness, insomnia, incoordination, and restlessness, whereas autonomic symptoms include shivering, diaphoresis, or mydriasis. Patients will often be afebrile but can have tachycardia, and they may have physical complaints of nausea and diarrhea.[41]

In moderate cases of serotonin syndrome, the physical symptoms include hyperactive bowel sounds. Neurological symptoms include hyperreflexia and clonus, which may be more pronounced in the lower extremities than the upper extremities.[37] Patients may exhibit horizontal ocular clonus, and mental status changes may often be present in this stage. As the severity of serotonin toxicity escalates, the patient's autonomic symptoms will also be more pronounced and include tachycardia, hypertension, diaphoresis, dyspnea, and hyperthermia. A core temperature as high as 40°C is common in moderate intoxication.

The presentation of severe serotonin syndrome is quite pronounced with neurologic signs including seizures, extreme clonus, and muscle rigidity. The individual's mental status would also be significantly altered and often agitated. Individuals' autonomic symptoms would demonstrate extreme labile blood pressures, extreme tachycardia, and hyperthermia greater than 41.1°C. Individuals with severe cases are also at risk for developing metabolic acidosis, rhabdomyolysis, elevated liver function tests, renal failure, acute respiratory distress, disseminated intravascular coagulopathy, and even coma or death.

Some studies have examined which symptoms are more significantly associated with serotonin syndrome, and being aware of these will help clinicians more readily diagnose potential serotonin syndrome. The most significant ones were neuromuscular and included hyperreflexia, inducible clonus, myoclonus, and ocular clonus. Autonomic symptoms included tachycardia and shivering, whereas clonus (inducible, spontaneous, and ocular) was the most crucial finding in establishing the diagnosis of the serotonin syndrome because it is seen in even mild cases.[35,37,40]

The diagnosis of serotonin syndrome cannot be established solely with laboratory or imaging studies. When performing the history, one should pay particular attention to any medication changes (new additions or dose adjustments), if the patient has taken any over-the-counter supplements, and if any illicit substances have been used.[37,39] Symptoms of serotonin syndrome can start within 1 or 2 hours of ingestion of a serotonergic agent, especially if the medication has a short half-life.[39] Most cases present within 6–24 hours of initiation, change in dosing, or overdose of the serotonergic agent.[35,37,41,42]

In addition, mild cases may present with subacute or chronic-appearing symptoms, whereas severe cases often present with rapid onset and changes of symptoms.[37]

Treatment

The first step in the treatment of serotonin syndrome is to discontinue any serotonergic agents. In mild to moderate cases, symptoms usually resolve on their own approximately 1–3 days after cessation of offending agents.[37,39]

Much of the treatment for serotonin syndrome is supportive care, which includes aggressive hydration and correction of vital sign abnormalities (hypertension and tachycardia). Most mild cases can be treated with supportive measures along with discontinuation of the offending agent(s).[35,37,39] In cases of moderate to severe serotonin syndrome, a 5-HT 2A antagonist (cyproheptadine) should be administered in addition to the IV fluids and management of autonomic symptoms. Dosing of cyproheptadine is usually an initial dose of 12 mg and then 2 mg every 2 hours if symptoms continue, up to 32 mg during a 24-hour period (a dose binds 85–95% of serotonin receptors).[35,37,39] Other agents that have been used successfully but not rigorously studied include olanzapine and chlorpromazine. Chlorpromazine may be utilized in the rare case in which the patient requires acute parenteral therapy. In this case, the patient is often hypertensive and is not ambulatory; therefore, the associated risk of orthostatic hypotension is minimized. Chlorpromazine should not be administered to a patient with hypotension or neuroleptic malignant syndrome because the drug could potentially exacerbate these conditions.[35,37,39,40]

Agitation associated with serotonin toxicity should be managed primarily with benzodiazepines (i.e., lorazepam and diazepam). They have been shown to blunt the hyperadrenergic component of the syndrome.[35,37,39] If the individual requires physical restraint, it should be of short duration. Restraints may increase the risk of mortality due to escalating agitation as the individual struggles against the restraints, potentially contributing to the development of lactic acidosis and exacerbating hyperthermia. If you are unable to manage agitation with benzodiazepines and release the physical restraints safely, then transfer to the intensive care unit and chemical sedation should be considered.

Therapies that should be avoided include propranolol, bromocriptine, and dantrolene. Propranolol can blunt the tachycardia associated with serotonin syndrome, but this reduction in heart rate may mask the efficacy of cyproheptadine. It may also lead to hypotension and shock in those with severe autonomic instability.[35,37,40] Bromocriptine, a dopamine agonist, has been implicated in the development of serotonin syndrome.[37,40] Dantrolene has not been shown to be helpful in the treatment of serotonin syndrome, may worsen the patient's symptoms, and has not been shown to have a positive effect on survival in animal models.[37,40]

Neuroleptic Malignant Syndrome

Introduction

A relatively rare but significant side effect from antipsychotic medication is NMS. It is an important syndrome to diagnose in the emergency department because misdiagnosis can lead to significant morbidity and mortality.

Epidemiology

The overall prevalence of NMS has been decreasing during the past few decades, likely due to the use of newer antipsychotics with improved side effect profiles in terms of extra-pyramidal effects.[43] The most recent data show an overall incidence range of 0.01–0.02% of individuals treated with antipsychotics, which is improved from earlier data that had a range of 0.02–3.23%.[44,45] Although this occurs rarely, the mortality of NMS can be quite high, up to 30%.[43] However, mortality rates have also been decreasing during the past decades, likely due to higher awareness of the syndrome with quicker identification and rapid discontinuation of antipsychotics.[44] Neuroleptic malignant syndrome is most often due to antipsychotic medications; however, other medications have also been associated with the development of NMS, including antiemetics (prochlorperazine, meto-clopramide, and droperidol), antidepressants (amoxapine, phenelzine, desipramine, trimipramine, and dosulepin), tetrabenazine, promethazine, and diatrizoate.[45,46] Abrupt withdrawal of medications, primarily dopamine agonists (i.e., carbidopa-levodopa and amantadine), has also been associated with the emergence of NMS.[45,47]

Pharmacological risk factors for NMS include the initiation, high doses, rapid titration, and parental routes of dopamine antagonists.[45,46] Polypharmacy with more than one dopamine antagonist along with coadministration of lithium or carbamazepine may also increase an individual's risk of developing NMS.[45,46,48] Environmental risk factors include the individual being in physical restraints, high external temperatures, and agitation.[45,46,48] Non-modifiable risk factors include older age, having medical comorbidities, and previous episodes of NMS or catatonia.[45,46,48] The medical comorbidities that increase an individual's risk include dehydration, hyponatremia, iron deficiency, thyrotoxicosis, substance abuse, and the presence of a structural or functional brain disorder (delirium, encephalitis, tumor, or dementia).[45,46,48]

Clinical Presentation

When gathering the history, it is vital to determine what medications patients are taking and any recent medication additions or dosing changes within the previous days to weeks. Most patients who develop NMS had a medication change (most commonly an addition or dose increase of a medication) within the past 1 or 2 weeks, although it can be seen after 1 month.[44,45,47,49] The first symptoms commonly seen are tremor and rigidity (often referred to as "lead-pipe rigidity"), followed by hyperthermia within several hours. The hyperthermia does not fluctuate, is not accompanied by chills, and is not responsive to normal antipyretics. Patients will also have altered mental status ranging from mild confusion to severe delirium and agitation. The overall progression of these is relatively rapid and can peak over 2 or 3 days.[45,48] As the syndrome progresses, autonomic dysfunction may be seen, with symptoms including labile blood pressures, tachycardia, tachypnea, sialorrhea, diaphoresis, incontinence, pallor, and flushing.[45–47] Other symptoms associated with NMS include dysphagia, dyspnea, abnormal reflexes, and mutism.[45–47] The clinical course usually resolves within 3–14 days of medication cessation unless complications occur or the NMS is prolonged by the use of a long-acting injectable antipsychotic.[46,47]

Although neuroleptic malignant syndrome is primarily diagnosed with a history and physical exam, laboratory studies may be helpful in the diagnosis but are most often used to monitor the severity of the syndrome. Laboratory studies include CBC for leukocytosis, creatinine kinase (CK), lactate dehydrogenase, aspartate transaminase, alanine transaminase, C-reactive protein, fibrinogen, and erythrocyte sedimentation rate.[46,48,49] Imaging will not help with diagnosis, but it may rule out other etiologies if the diagnosis of NMS remains uncertain. An EEG will often show generalized slowing.[48]

Some literature describes "atypical neuroleptic malignant syndrome," which attempts to capture individuals presenting with subthreshold NMS symptoms. It is recommended that for the diagnosis of atypical NMS, four of the following symptoms must be present: hyperthermia, rigidity, Altered Mental Status (AMS), autonomic dysfunction, elevated CK.[50] Compared to typical NMS cases, atypical NMS cases most often had an absence of rigidity (65%) or hyperthermia (30%).[48,50] Individuals who developed atypical NMS were often challenged with a second-generation antipsychotics, most commonly olanzapine and clozapine, but otherwise had a similar patient profile and onset of symptoms after medication change.[50]

Complications in NMS include rhabdomyolysis, renal failure, electrolyte imbalances, thrombosis, pulmonary artery embolism, pneumonia, seizures, reversible dilated myocardiopathy, multiorgan failure, and even death.[45-47,49] A study examining risk factors for mortality in NMS found that sepsis, acute kidney injury, comorbid congestive heart failure, and acute respiratory failure were predictors of mortality, with acute respiratory failure having the highest mortality.[43]

Treatment

After successfully diagnosing an individual with NMS, the first step in management is to discontinue the offending dopamine antagonist or restart the recently discontinued dopamine agonist.[45,47] Treatments include aggressive IV fluids, treatment of autonomic dysfunction (for blood pressure, calcium channel blockers are the first choice), nutritional supplementation if unable to take orally, mechanical cooling (because elevated temperatures do not respond to antipyretics), and prophylactic anticoagulation.[45-47] Use of physical restraints in individuals with NMS should be avoided because it can increase CK levels and contribute to the development of rhabdomyolysis.[46] If an individual is agitated, it is recommended to use benzodiazepines.[45,51]

The literature is heterogeneous regarding specific targeted medication management of NMS. Guidelines differ between countries about when to start, how to dose, and when to discontinue these medications.[52] Commonly utilized treatments include the medications dantrolene and bromocriptine, as well as electroconvulsive therapy (ECT). When using dantrolene, the recommended starting dose is 1–2.5 mg/kg IV followed by 1 mg/kg every 6 hours up to a maximum dose of 10 mg/kg/day.[45,46,51,52] When using bromocriptine, start with 2.5 mg TID PO and increase 2.5–7.5mg per day (maximum of 45 mg per day) while monitoring for nausea, vomiting, and declining mental status.[45,46,51,52] These medications have been used in combination, most commonly in severe cases, but determining which one to start first has not been consistently established.[46,51] Some studies have recommended starting with bromocriptine in moderate to severe cases and adding dantrolene only in the most severe cases.[51,52] Most studies suggest a slow taper over several days of whichever medication is utilized once symptoms resolve to avoid rebound NMS.[45,51] Other studies recommend continuing these medications for 10 days after the resolution of NMS and only then initiating a gradual wean over several days.[44,45,51] If patients do not respond to these medications, it is appropriate to consider a trial of ECT.[45,46,51] Some case studies have used other dopamine agonists to treat NMS, including amantadine, levodopa, and apomorphine.[45,51] Anticholinergic medications should be avoided in NMS because they may exacerbate temperature dysregulation and contribute to hyperthermia.[46,51]

Catatonia

Introduction

Another important condition that providers working in the emergency department should be aware of is catatonia. Catatonia is a neuropsychiatric syndrome composed of symptoms and signs of motor dysregulation; correspondingly, it is caused by a wide variety of medical, neurologic, and psychiatric illnesses.

Epidemiology

The overall prevalence of catatonia is challenging to determine because it varies based on the setting in which catatonia is studied (inpatient psychiatry units, medical units, outpatient, etc.). The prevalence of catatonia in inpatient psychiatry units is approximately 10%, although it ranges from 4.8%–20%.[53-58] When considering patients admitted to a general medical hospital, the prevalence appears to be approximately 4% or 5%, with a range from 1.6% to 6.3%.[59-61]

The most common etiologies on inpatient psychiatric units appear to be affective disorders followed by primary psychotic disorders, but medical/neurological etiologies are also found in these settings. The predominate psychiatric illness responsible for catatonia is bipolar disorder (20.1–46%),[58,62] followed by schizophrenia (20–33%),[58,63,64] schizoaffective disorder (2–6%),[58,63] and major depressive disorder (2.9–18%).[63]

Catatonia on medical/surgical floors is three times more likely to be from neurological or medical problems than psychiatric illness.[53,65,66] The most common etiologies appear to be encephalitis (25–38.2%),[53,66-68] central nervous system structural abnormalities (up to 30%),[61] psychiatric disorder (17%),[53] epilepsy (8–15%),[53,61,67] and drug-/medication-related conditions such as abrupt dopamine agonist withdrawal (10–29%).[53,69]

Risk factors for catatonia include exposure to infections during the perinatal period, previous episodes of catatonia, a history of experiencing EPS from antipsychotics, and a recent substantial weight loss (>5% loss of body weight in 3 weeks or >20% loss of body weight in 6 months).[69] Among the neurological and medical patient population, females may be at higher risk for catatonia due to anti-NMDA receptor encephalitis because this entity is far more common in women.[70]

Clinical Presentation

Catatonia is composed of the following 23 psychomotor symptoms: excitement, immobility/stupor, mutism, staring, grimacing, stereotypy, mannerisms, rigidity, negativism (automatic resistance to instructions or attempts to examine the patient/does the exact opposite of instruction), withdrawal, posturing/catalepsy, echopraxia/echolalia, verbigeration (i.e., repetition of phrases or sentences like a scratched record), waxy flexibility, impulsivity, automatic obedience, mitgehen ("Anglepoise lamp" arm raising in response to light pressure of a finger, despite the instruction to the contrary), gegenhalten (resistance to passive movement, which is proportional to the strength of stimulus and appears automatic rather than willful), ambitendency (the patient appears motorically "stuck" in indecisive, hesitant movements), grasp reflex, perseveration, combativeness, and autonomic.[71] The most common symptoms present in individuals with catatonia are staring (87%), immobility/stupor (90.6%), mutism (84.4%), and withdrawal (90%).[53,54,72] There are three different subtypes of catatonia: stuporous, excited, or mixed (showing both stuporous and excited symptoms).[70] In addition to the physical symptoms, patients will often have concurrent psychotic symptoms (present in approximately 77% of patients with catatonia), which often go unnoticed given the mutism and stupor.[54,73]

The most used rating scale is the Bush Francis Catatonia Rating Scale (BFCRS),[74] a 23-item scale that assesses the symptoms and signs of catatonia. In the screening portion of the scale, which comprises the first 14 items, each item is scored as either "absent" or "present." If two or more of these symptoms are present for 24 hours or longer, catatonia is considered a possibility. All items on the BFCRS are also rated on a scale from 0 to 3 points, with higher scores correlating with a higher severity of catatonia.[74,75] The diagnosis also requires a careful physical exam and a diligent review of medications and laboratory data. The DSM-5 diagnostic criteria require the patient to have three symptoms (instead of the two required by the BFCRS) to diagnose catatonia. Concerns have been raised that the diagnostic criteria for catatonic disorder due to another medical condition states that the disturbance does not occur exclusively during delirium, which has been proposed to be incorrect.[61,72]

The workup for catatonia should involve several laboratory tests, including CBC, electrolytes, blood urea nitrogen, creatinine, hepatic enzymes, CK, serum iron levels, thyroid function tests, toxic panels, and a urinalysis.[54,61] Other tests included in the workup are neuroimaging (magnetic resonance imaging [MRI] or computed tomography [CT]), EEG, and lumbar puncture. In cases of a psychiatric etiology, the EEG is normal early, but over time it may start to demonstrate a pattern of generalized slowing.[76] Catatonia due to medical causes (encephalitis, seizures, etc.) is more likely to have an abnormal EEG early in the disease course, most commonly consisting of diffuse slowing.[61,71] When performing a lumbar puncture, the sample should be tested for antibodies associated with autoimmune encepahalitis.[71]

One must be vigilant regarding the comorbidities and complications associated with catatonia. Patients with stuporous catatonia are at high risk for developing dehydration, metabolic derangements, constipation, severe weight loss, malnutrition, and vitamin deficiencies due to lack of eating and drinking for a prolonged period. Complications such as pressure wounds, contractures, and deep vein thrombosis/pulmonary emboli may occur for those who have been immobile for long periods. On the opposite end, patients with excited catatonia are at risk for hyperthermia, seizures, or death due to complications of excessive motor activity.[59,70,71] Malignant catatonia, a particularly severe form of catatonia, is characterized by hyperthermia and dramatic autonomic instability. It is associated with mortality rates as high as 75–100% in some studies.[64,69] Given that untreated catatonia can last for weeks, months, or even years, timely diagnosis and effective treatments have contributed to a shortening of its course.[69,77]

Treatment

The first step should be to discontinue any neuroleptics and other dopamine depleters or restart any recently stopped dopamine agonists.[71,78] Next, one should proceed with supportive care consisting of hydration, nutrition, mobilization, anticoagulation, and aspiration precautions.[71,78,79]

The first-line treatment for catatonia, regardless of the underlying etiology, is with benzodiazepines. The most commonly utilized and evidence-based agent is lorazepam; subsequently, approximately 60–90% of patients with catatonia will respond to lorazepam.[54,73] A "lorazepam challenge" is often used to determine if a patient will respond to benzodiazepines. The challenge is to start with lorazepam 1 or 2 mg IV and monitor for effect, which usually appears within 5–10 minutes. If there is no effect after 20 minutes, another dose is given. A positive response is at least a 50% reduction in symptoms on the BFCRS.[54,69,71] Typical dosages of lorazepam in the treatment of catatonia range from 8 to 24 mg per day (via any route IV/intramuscular [IM]/PO) and are often tolerated without excess sedation.[78,79] The recommendation for the initial regimen is to start with lorazepam 1 or 2 mg Q4-12H and adjust the dose based on the alleviation of symptoms without sedating the patient.[78,79] Starting with lower doses in elderly, young, or medically compromised patients, especially patients with obstructive sleep apnea, is recommended.[55] When treated with benzodiazepines, complete resolution of symptoms occurs on average 3–7 days after treatment initiation.[71,78,80] It is important to avoid discontinuing the benzodiazepine too quickly because catatonia may reemerge.[78]

The second-line treatment of catatonia is ECT. The response rates for ECT in catatonic patients range from 60% to 100%.[78,81] This treatment is often initiated when there is an insufficient response to benzodiazepines or in life-threatening conditions such as malignant catatonia.

There is limited evidence regarding the use of non-benzodiazepine hypnotics in the treatment of catatonia. Dose ranges were typically 7.5–40 mg per day.[78] Like the lorazepam challenge test, there is a zolpidem challenge test that involves administering 10 mg of zolpidem orally (no current IV/IM route) and examining the patient after 30 minutes. A positive response is a reduction of at least 50% of the BFCRS score.

Transcranial magnetic stimulation has also been employed in the treatment of catatonia. It has been used in patients with catatonia due to various etiologies (psychosis, mood, autism, and neurological) as a monotherapy agent. However, these were only single case reports.[57,82]

The use of antipsychotics in catatonia is reserved for patients with a primary diagnosis of schizophrenia,[57] given that usage here may worsen catatonia or contribute to the development of NMS.[55] Once the symptoms of catatonia start to improve, there may be a role for an antipsychotic to help treat the underlying psychotic illness.[78] If an antipsychotic is to be initiated, a second-generation antipsychotic with relatively lower D_2 receptor blockade (quetiapine, olanzapine, or clozapine) or with D_2 partial agonism (aripiprazole) is preferable.[78]

Case reports have demonstrated successful use of NMDA receptor antagonists (e.g., amantadine and memantine) to treat catatonia after failed trials of a benzodiazepine. Amantadine has been successfully used as monotherapy for the treatment of catatonia in both psychiatric and medical etiologies.[57,59,78,81,83,84] Dosages have been 100–600 mg daily, averaging 200 mg daily. Memantine has also been successfully used in the treatment of catatonia. Dosages were 5–20 mg per day.[57,84] The evidence for using these medications is currently based on case reports, and no extensive studies have been completed comparing them to other treatments.

Mood stabilizers have also been used to treat catatonia, with valproic acid being shown to be helpful.[57,78] Topiramate, in conjunction with benzodiazepines, has also been found to help treat catatonia. In addition, monotherapy with carbamazepine was found to be successful in resolving several cases of catatonia in patients with mood disorders.[57,81] Lithium has also been reported to be helpful in the treatment of catatonia.[78]

Epilepsy and Seizures

Introduction

Epilepsy is a complex and often chronic condition that results from recurrent epileptic seizures. Epilepsy is a common disorder, with a point prevalence of 6.38 per 1,000 persons and a lifetime prevalence of 7.60 per 1,000 persons.[85] Episodes of isolated seizure activity are an even more common occurrence, affecting an estimated 4% of individuals over a lifetime.[86] In fact, it is estimated that seizure activity may be responsible for approximately 1% of emergency department visits.[87] It is important to recognize that seizures are a heterogeneous condition with multiple potential causes and numerous clinical presentations.

Classification of Seizures

Generalized tonic–clonic seizures often present dramatically with motor activity and loss of consciousness. The seizure starts with a sudden loss of consciousness and sustained muscle contractions of all limbs (tonic phase), followed by a period of sustained rhythmic muscle contractions (clonic phase). It is often during the tonic phase of the seizure that the patient bites their tongue, and various autonomic changes and urinary incontinence may also accompany generalized tonic–clonic seizures. Immediately after the seizure (i.e., the postictal period), the patient is drowsy and often confused. Absence seizures are brief generalized seizures that often present with a behavioral arrest consisting of staring, unresponsiveness, and automatisms. Absence seizures are not associated with an aura or postictal confusion.

Partial or focal seizures are differentiated by how they impact the patient's level of consciousness or arousal. Partial seizures are classified as simple, complex, or secondarily generalized. Simple partial seizures do not impair consciousness. They often involve impact-limited neuronal networks in the brain. Their clinical presentation is dependent on the anatomic location of the seizure activity so that autonomic, cognitive (déjà vu or jamais vu), emotional, sensory, or motor activity may occur. The patient may also experience an aura at the onset of a complex partial seizure, with the aura itself representing a brief, simple partial seizure, and the content of the aura will depend on the area of the brain experiencing the abnormal electrical discharges. Symptoms of an aura include hallucinations, intense emotional experiences, cognitive distortions such as déjà vu or jamais vu, and depersonalization. Complex partial seizures are also commonly associated with postictal confusion and amnesia for the seizure event.

The temporal lobe is the focus of a majority of focal seizure activity, with ictal symptoms of temporal lobe epilepsy including olfactory hallucinations, usually involving unpleasant odors such as burning rubber. Gustatory sensations, such as nausea or a sense of "gastric rising," have also been reported, as have behavioral manifestations such as intense emotional outbursts unrelated to events happening at the time. Complex focal seizures that impact the frontal lobes often represent a diagnostic challenge because they may not be associated with postictal confusion, and the seizure activity often occurs in clusters with bizarre motor symptoms such as bicycling of the legs.

Convulsive status epilepticus is defined as at least 5 minutes of continuous seizure activity or an incomplete recovery between seizures.[88] It represents a neurological emergency and is associated with a time-dependent relationship to morbidity and mortality.[89] Treatment is most commonly accomplished in the emergency department through the parental use of benzodiazepines (IM midazolam 10 mg if >40 kg or IV lorazepam 0.1 mg/kg/dose, maximum 4 mg/dose).[89]

Nonconvulsive status epilepticus has multiple definitions but is most defined by more than 30 minutes of electrographic seizure activity resulting in nonconvulsive clinical symptoms.[90] In all cases of status epilepticus, it is imperative to perform a thorough evaluation for potential etiologies and address any identified etiology or etiologies to terminate the seizure activity.

The Evaluation of Epilepsy

Once the patient's presentation is determined to be secondary to underlying seizure activity, a diagnostic workup must be undertaken to determine an underlying cause(s) of the seizure. If a structural abnormality is identified on neuroimaging that correlates EEG findings and the seizure's phenotype, then the etiology is most likely structural. Infectious etiologies for seizures are common in the developing world, whereas a metabolic etiology may occur in patients with significant metabolic derangements. Seizures secondary to autoimmune processes are becoming recognized as potential causes of epilepsy; however, the etiology of seizure activity is unclear in up to one-third of patients.[91]

The episodic nature of seizure disorders limits the usefulness of routine time-limited "spot" EEGs; however, continuous EEG monitoring, capturing the paroxysmal event that constitutes the proposed seizure activity, may help further clarify the presence of seizure activity. The absence of active ictal findings or interictal epileptiform discharges does not rule out the possibility of a seizure disorder. Epilepsy is a clinical diagnosis in which the EEG provides supporting evidence.[92]

A cranial MRI with contrast is the structural neuroimaging modality of choice in patients presenting with seizure activity, although CT may have to suffice in an emergency.[93] Neuroimaging may help identify potential anatomic pathologies associated with the onset of seizures, including mesial temporal sclerosis, tumor, vascular malformation, or pathology associated with a traumatic brain injury.

Differential Diagnosis

The differential diagnosis of epilepsy is broad because numerous neurologic and non-neurologic conditions may present to the emergency department with paroxysms of

---

Box 7.1 Differential Diagnosis of Epilepsy

Neurologic
    Migraine headaches
    Movement disorders
    Transient ischemic events
    Transient global amnesia
Medical
    Syncope
    Hypoglycemia
    Cardiac arrhythmias
Psychiatric
    Panic attacks
    Dissociative disorder
    PNES/conversion disorder
    • Factitious disorder
    • Malingering

PNES, psychogenic nonepileptic seizures.

---

behavior that may mimic seizure activity (Box 7.1). Syncope is the most common non-neurologic paroxysmal disorder that may be confused with seizure activity.[94] Neurologic conditions that may mimic epilepsy include transient ischemic attacks, migraine headaches, and movement disorders. In addition, various behavioral conditions may also imitate seizure activity, including psychogenic nonepileptic seizures (PNES). PNES are paroxysmal behavioral episodes that lack ictal epileptiform discharges on EEG and are thought to be secondary to psychological distress.

Psychiatric Comorbidity of Epilepsy

The comorbidity of epilepsy and psychiatric illnesses is common and multifaceted.[95] There appears to be a bidirectional relationship between psychiatric conditions and epilepsy, with studies suggesting that patients with a primary psychiatric disorder may be at greater risk of developing seizures. In contrast, some patients with epilepsy are at greater risk of developing psychiatric disorders.[96] Population-based studies have identified up to a 35% lifetime prevalence of psychiatric comorbidities in patients with epilepsy, most commonly mood and anxiety disorders.[97] It is crucial to identify and address co-occurring psychiatric conditions in patients with epilepsy because failure to treat psychiatric comorbidity is associated with various adverse outcomes, such as the increased risk of suicide, impaired quality of life, and intolerance to antiepileptic medications (AEDs).[95]

Classification of Psychiatric Comorbidity

In patients with epilepsy, the classification of the clinical psychiatric symptoms and signs depends on when they occur in relation to seizure activity (Figure 7.1). They may appear

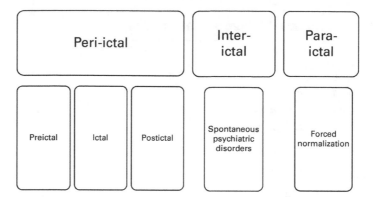

Figure 7.1 Classification of neuropsychiatric presentations in epilepsy.

directly as a result of the seizure activity, such as those occurring during the seizure (ictal manifestations); before the onset of the seizure (preictal); or following the termination of the seizure (postictal manifestations). Alternatively, psychiatric symptoms and signs may occur in the context of epilepsy but between seizure episodes and are not directly related to the seizure activity (interictal presentations). Serious consideration must also be given to iatrogenic neuropsychiatric signs and symptoms in patients with epilepsy due to the adverse effects of pharmacotherapy or surgical interventions.

Preictal neuropsychiatric manifestations, which most commonly manifest as a dysphoric mood or irritability, typically occur in the days or hours before the onset of the seizure. Postictal psychiatric symptoms generally are observed after a symptom-free period following the cessation of seizure activity. This asymptomatic period may last between several hours and 1 week and is often a source of diagnostic confusion because the ictal event itself may manifest with psychiatric symptoms. Most commonly, this takes the form of ictal panic or fear, but it may also present as dysphoria. Para-ictal neuropsychiatric presentations are related to a decrease or total remission of seizure activity, and these rare presentations are often caused by forced normalization, a rare but important phenomenon discussed later in this chapter.[98]

The treatment of epilepsy may also be associated with various neuropsychiatric adverse effects, more likely occurring in patients with a personal or family history of psychiatric disorders.[99] These adverse effects may be secondary to the pharmacokinetic impact of specific AEDs, such as carbamazepine, which may induce psychotropic medications' metabolism, reducing serum levels and limiting their efficacy. Other AEDs, such as phenobarbital, topiramate, zonisamide, and levetiracetam, have exhibited various idiopathic adverse neuropsychiatric events.[100]

Depression

Depression is a common psychiatric comorbidity in people with epilepsy. Many factors contribute to this significant comorbidity, including seizure-specific considerations such as duration, focus, and perceived stigma of seizures, along with general risks such as a family history of mood disorders, lack of social support, and personality structure.[101] Coexisting anxiety also often complicates depression in patients with epilepsy.[102] A meta-analysis of population-based studies examining depression in epilepsy yielded an estimated overall incidence of active depression of almost 25%.[103] In the case of depression, is the mood disorder directly related to the occurrence of seizures (peri-ictal depression), or does it occur in the context of an underlying seizure disorder (interictal depression)? A preictal prodrome of dysphoria and irritability may occur in the hours or days before a seizure in approximately 10% of patients with focal epilepsy.[104] These preictal affective symptoms tend to escalate in the hours immediately prior to the seizure and often remit entirely following the ictal event. The dysphoric effect experienced by the patient with ictal depression is often incongruent with their state of mind immediately before the onset of the seizure. Ictal dysphoria is often very acute and intense, and it may be associated with the sudden onset of suicidality.[105] Postictal depression occurs within 1 week following the occurrence of the latest seizure activity. If the depressed mood represents a postictal phenomenon, it rarely persists beyond 7 days.[106]

Anxiety

Anxiety is also common in patients, with population-based studies estimating lifetime prevalence rates of approximately 25% for anxiety disorders in patients with epilepsy.[97] Interictal anxiety may manifest as all typical anxiety disorders, including generalized anxiety disorder, panic disorder, and social anxiety disorder. However, epilepsy patients may also exhibit specific seizure-related concerns, such as anticipatory anxiety surrounding the occurrence of a seizure or an excessive fear of being seen by others during a seizure.[107]

Preictal anxiety symptoms can occur in the hours or days leading up to the seizure. It is often challenging to distinguish preictal anxiety from the psychological distress that may precipitate a seizure. Focal seizures might present with isolated ictal psychological symptoms such as panic or fear, whereas ictal anxiety leads to intense symptoms, often lasting only for seconds to minutes. These psychological symptoms represent a frequent presentation of a type of simple partial seizures estimated to account for 60% of all psychiatric auras.[108] In the case of temporal lobe focus, there may also be the associated symptoms of déjà vu, olfactory hallucinations, or a sensation of epigastric rising. In addition, when present, postictal anxiety symptoms are often confounded by co-occurring symptoms of depression. Postictal anxiety or fear may persist for up to 1 week following the last seizure.[109]

Psychosis

Psychosis in epilepsy is an important diagnostic consideration for the clinician practicing in the emergency medical setting. Like other psychological presentations related to epilepsy, it is essential to determine its relationship to ongoing seizure activity. This determination allows the clinician to identify if the psychosis represents an interictal phenomenon or a peri-ictal psychotic presentation. Evidence suggests that the prevalence of interictal psychosis may be as high as 3–9% in patients with epilepsy, with the higher rates occurring in patients with a temporal lobe focus.[110] Although interictal psychosis is often chronic, it usually has a later age of onset than schizophrenia.[111] In addition, interictal psychosis is often less severe with better insight and a relative lack of significant negative symptoms compared to schizophrenia.[112] This may present as an acute episode, lasting days to weeks, or a more chronic condition that may last for years.

Ictal psychosis is uncommon, and when it does occur, the psychotic symptoms appear suddenly and are of short duration, terminating with the conclusion of the seizure. In addition to the psychotic symptoms inherent in ictal psychosis, there are often other manifestations of ongoing seizure activity, such as automatisms.

Postictal psychosis is a fairly common occurrence, with a prevalence of approximately 2%.[110] The psychotic symptoms tend to occur within a couple of days of the seizure activity's cessation, following an initial lucid period.[113] The lucid period between the termination of the seizure and the onset of the psychosis is often key to differentiating postictal psychosis from other types of psychosis in this patient population. The duration of the psychosis may be brief, lasting less than 1 day, or more prolonged, persisting for months.[114] Postictal psychosis is often best characterized by affectively laden positive symptoms and may be complicated by significant agitation. Fortunately, these episodes of postictal psychosis tend to resolve spontaneously, but if the symptoms persist, low-dose antipsychotics are often helpful.[113] Regardless of when the antipsychotic is initiated, the goal should be to attempt to taper the medication off within 2 or 3 months of symptoms remission.[115] There is currently little evidence to guide providers on which antipsychotic medication to utilize in patients with epilepsy, other than to avoid medications known to lower the seizure threshold (i.e., clozapine). Most patients experiencing postictal psychosis respond well to treatment (AED and antipsychotics); however, if symptoms fail to remit, then consideration should be given to the presence of an interictal psychotic disorder and longer term maintenance therapy with antipsychotic medication.

Suicide

Suicide occurring in the context of epilepsy is an important consideration, especially for clinicians practicing in the field of emergency psychiatry. Suicide occurs at a higher rate in people with epilepsy than in the general population.[115] For example, when contrasted to the general population, the suicide-specific standardized mortality ratio has been estimated to be 3.3 (95% confidence interval = 2.8–3.7).[116] Among individuals with epilepsy, the risk may be higher in those with temporal lobe epilepsy (6.6) and new-onset epilepsy (2.1). However, comorbid mood disorders are the most common condition independently associated with suicide in individuals with epilepsy.[117]

Treatment of Epilepsy

Antiepileptic drugs have demonstrated diverse neuropsychiatric effects. Some AEDs have shown positive effects on mood, whereas others can be associated with adverse neuropsychiatric side effects. Valproic acid, carbamazepine, and lamotrigine are mood stabilizers but may negatively affect cognition at higher doses.[118] Most of the newer AEDs appear to be well-tolerated, except for levetiracetam and topiramate. As many as 31% of individuals taking levetiracetam may experience adverse neuropsychiatric effects including irritability (29%), aggression (10%), and psychosis (5%).[119] Topiramate has also been linked to mood lability (17%) and depression (11%) at higher doses.[120] As a result, clinicians may wish to avoid levetiracetam and topiramate in patients with a personal or family history of psychiatric illness.

Psychiatric Medications in Patients with Epilepsy

The primary pharmacological intervention in depressive and anxiety disorders should be SSRIs and SNRIs. These agents are preferred over TCAs and bupropion, which may lower the seizure threshold. Certain antiepileptic drugs, such as pregabalin, may exhibit anxiolytic properties and may be considered when anxiety disorders co-occur with epilepsy. Lamotrigine, valproate, and carbamazepine may be useful AEDs in the setting of depression and comorbid epilepsy.

The use of antipsychotics in patients with epilepsy represents more of a challenge than that of antidepressants. For example, there is a clear dose–response relationship between escalating doses of clozapine and the onset of seizures. When dosed at greater than 600 mg/day, clozapine has been reported to cause seizures in 4.4% of patients, whereas when used at doses less than 300 mg/day, the incidence of seizures is less than 1%.[121] However, clozapine can lower the seizure threshold at any dose and should be used with caution in patients with risk factors for seizures. Although structurally similar to clozapine, olanzapine's association with lowering the seizure threshold is less consistent.[122] Among the typical antipsychotics, chlorpromazine, loxapine, and perphenazine have been noted to have the highest risk of seizures, whereas haloperidol appears to be associated with a lower risk.

A potential association between the use of AEDs, suicidal ideation, and suicidal behavior has been recorded in the literature. These reports led the FDA to issue a warning linking AED use to suicidality in 2008.[123] However, these initial studies may have methodological flaws that limited their clinical relevance. When studies controlled for conditions related to suicidal behavior in patients with epilepsy, there was no association between AED use and suicidal behavior.[124] Although close adverse event monitoring is warranted following an AED prescription, most clinicians and researchers think current evidence is lacking to support a direct link between AEDs and increased suicidal behavior.[112]

Forced Normalization

Forced normalization is characterized by the emergence of psychiatric symptoms following either a significant reduction or outright cessation of seizure activity. The psychiatric presentation most commonly associated with forced normalization is psychosis, but mood disturbances and dissociation have also been reported in the literature.[98] Forced normalization is most common in patients with a history of long-standing and previously refractory temporal lobe epilepsy. This was first noted in 1954 by Landolt, who observed that the resolution of electrographic evidence of seizure activity in certain patients with refractory seizures was associated with behavioral symptoms.[125] Precipitants of forced normalization may include the initiation of specific AEDs or epilepsy surgery. Treatment of the psychological sequelae of forced normalization is usually successful and most commonly involves tapering or discontinuing the offending AED. Antipsychotic medications are less effective than AED withdrawal but may be necessary to manage psychotic symptoms following epilepsy surgery or when it is not feasible to withdraw the AED. When the trigger of forced normalization is epilepsy surgery, the prognosis is poorer than that for an AED trigger, with a high risk of persistent psychotic symptoms despite ongoing antipsychotic treatment.[98]

Psychogenic Nonepileptic Seizures

Psychogenic nonepileptic seizures are an essential consideration in the differential diagnoses of patients presenting to the emergency department with possible seizure activity.

PNES include alterations in arousal, behavior, and/or movement that resemble epileptic seizures. These paroxysmal behaviors, however, lack an associated electrophysiological epileptic discharge on EEG. PNES may be differentiated from epilepsy through various symptoms and signs, but none of these differences are pathognomonic for PNES (Box 7.2). Complicating the presentation of PNES is the fact that approximately 10% of patients with PNES also experience co-occurring epileptic seizures.[126]

Video EEG supports the presence of PNES by documenting that the patient's typical behavioral paroxysm is not associated with epileptiform activity immediately before, during, or after the event. A serum prolactin level within 20 minutes of the paroxysmal event that is less than twice the individual's normal level also suggests the occurrence of PNES rather than epileptic seizures.[127]

Individuals presenting to the emergency department with PNES represent a heterogeneous patient population with a wide variety of predisposing, precipitating, and perpetuating factors. A history of trauma may increase a patient's predisposition to PNES, whereas acute stressors or trauma may precipitate an acute episode and the resulting presentation to the emergency department. Studies suggest that up to three-fourths of adults with PNES report prior traumatic experiences.[128] A history of sexual abuse has been associated with an earlier onset, significant diagnostic delay, and more severe paroxysmal PNES events.[128] Misdiagnosis coupled with concurrent medical, neurologic, and/or psychiatric conditions may contribute to the perpetuation of PNES.[129]

Treatment

The treatment of PNES begins at the time of diagnosis, with the communication of the diagnosis to the patient and the patient's support system being critical. A straightforward, empathetic, nonjudgmental, and educational approach to delivering the diagnosis is an essential first therapeutic step in treating PNES. The establishment of a therapeutic alliance with a health care provider who can provide long-term care is essential given the chronic nature of PNES. If a patient exhibits an appreciation that psychological factors may contribute or even precipitate their paroxysmal episodes, a formal psychiatric or psychological consultation should be requested to assess and treat any identified psychiatric conditions. Unfortunately, even after PNES is appropriately diagnosed, studies suggest that many patients continue to experience paroxysmal episodes consistent with PNES.[130]

Box 7.2 Characteristics of Psychogenic Non-Epileptic Seizures

Asynchronous limb movements
Shaking movements intermittent with episodes of inactivity
Side-to-side head movements
Dystonic body posturing
Eyes closed during event
Preserved awareness during the event
Ability of bystanders to modulation the event
Recall of information presented during the event
Non-stereotypical seizure pattern
Prolonged event followed by a rapid recovery without drowsiness

References

1. American Psychiatric Association. *Diagnostic and Statistical Manual of Mental Disorders*. 5th ed. American Psychiatric Publishing; 2013.

2. Gupta N, de Jonghe J, Schieveld J, Leonard M, Meagher D. Delirium phenomenology: What can we learn from the symptoms of delirium? *J Psychosom Res*. 2008;65(3):215–222.

3. Cutting J. The phenomenology of acute organic psychosis: Comparison with acute schizophrenia. *Br J Psychiatry*. 1987;151:324–332.

4. Watson PL, Ceriana P, Fanfulla F. Delirium: Is sleep important? *Best Pract Res Clin Anaesthesiol*. 2012;26(3):355–366.

5. Meagher D, Moran M, Raju B, et al. A new data-based motor subtype schema for delirium. *J Neuropsychiatry Clin Neurosci*. 2008;20(2):185–193.

6. Meagher DJ, Leonard M, Donnelly S, Conroy M, Adamis D, Trzepacz PT. A longitudinal study of motor subtypes in delirium: Relationship with other phenomenology, etiology, medication exposure and prognosis. *J Psychosom Res*. 2011;71(6):395–403.

7. Han JH, Morandi A, Ely EW, et al. Delirium in the nursing home patients seen in the emergency department. *J Am Geriatr Soc*. 2009;57(5):889–894.

8. Dyer CB, Ashton CM, Teasdale TA. Postoperative delirium: A review of 80 primary data-collection studies. *Arch Intern Med*. 1995;155:461–465.

9. Girard TD, Pandharipande PP, Ely EW. Delirium in the intensive care unit. *Crit Care*. 2008;12(Suppl 3):S3.

10. Breitbart W, Strout D. Delirium in the terminally ill. *Clin Geriatr Med*. 2000;16:357–372.

11. Racine AM, Fong TG, Gou Y, et al. Clinical outcomes in older surgical patients with mild cognitive impairment. *Alzheimers Dement*. 2018;14(5):590–600.

12. Elie M, Cole MG, Primeau FJ, Bellavance F. Delirium risk factors in elderly hospitalized patients. *J Gen Intern Med*. 1998;13(3):204–212.

13. Ahmed S, Leurent B, Sampson EL. Risk factors for incident delirium among older people in acute hospital medical units: A systematic review and meta-analysis. *Age Ageing*. 2014;43:326–333.

14. Gaudreau JD, Gagnon P, Roy MA, Harel F, Tremblay A. Association between psychoactive medications and delirium in hospitalized patients: A critical review. *Psychosomatics*. 2005;46(4):302–216.

15. Maldonado JR. Neuropathogenesis of delirium: Review of current etiologic theories and common pathways. *Am J Geriatr Psychiatry*. 2013;21(12):1190–1222.

16. McCusker J, Cole M, Dendukuri N, Han L, Belzile E. The course of delirium in older medical inpatients: A prospective study. *J Gen Intern Med*. 2003;18(9):696–704.

17. Leslie DL, Marcantonio ER, Zhang Y, Leo-Summers L, Inouye SK. One-year health care costs associated with delirium in the elderly population. *Arch Intern Med*. 2008;168(1):27–32.

18. Cole MG, Ciampi A, Belzile E, Zhong L. Persistent delirium in older hospital patients: A systematic review of frequency and prognosis. *Age Ageing*. 2009;38(1):19–26.

19. Farrell KR, Ganzini L. Misdiagnosing delirium as depression in medically ill elderly patients. *Arch Intern Med*. 1995;155(22):2459–2464.

20. Trzepacz PT, Brenner RP, Coffman G, van Thiel DH. Delirium in liver transplantation candidates: Discriminant analysis of multiple test variables. *Biol Psychiatry*. 1988;24(1):3–14.

21. Ely EW, Margolin R, Francis J, et al. Evaluation of delirium in critically ill patients: Validation of the Confusion Assessment Method for the Intensive Care Unit (CAM-ICU). *Crit Care Med*. 2001;29(7):1370–1379.

22. Kim MY, Park UJ, Kim HT, Cho WH. DELirium Prediction based on Hospital Information (Delphi) in general surgery patients. *Medicine*. 2016;95(12):e3072.

23. El-Gabalawy R, Patel R, Kilborn K, et al. A novel stress-diathesis model to predict risk of post-operative delirium: Implications for intra-operative management. *Front Aging Neurosci*. 2017;9:274.

24. Neufeld KJ, Yue J, Robinson TN, Inouye SK, Needham DM. Antipsychotic medication for prevention and treatment of delirium in hospitalized adults: A systematic review and meta-analysis. *J Am Geriatr Soc*. 2016;64(4):705–714.

25. Siddiqi N, Harrison JK, Clegg A, et al. Interventions for preventing delirium in hospitalised non-ICU patients. *Cochrane Database Syst Rev*. 2016;3:CD005563.

26. American Psychiatric Association. Practice guideline for the treatment of patients with delirium. *Am J Psychiatry*. 1999;156(5 Suppl):1–20.

27. Young J, Murthy L, Westby M, Akunne A, O'Mahony R; Guideline Development Group. Diagnosis, prevention, and management of delirium: Summary of NICE guidance. *BMJ*. 2010;341:c3704.

28. Zayed Y, Barbarawi M, Kheiri B, et al. Haloperidol for the management of delirium in adult intensive care unit patients: A systematic review and meta-analysis of randomized controlled trials. *J Crit Care*. 2019;50:280–286.

29. Desmarais P, Massoud F, Filion J, Nguyen QD, Bajsarowicz P. Quetiapine for psychosis in Parkinson disease and neurodegenerative Parkinsonian disorders: A systematic review. *J Geriatr Psychiatry Neurol*. 2016;29(4):227–236.

30. Navari RM, Gray SE, Kerr AC. Olanzapine versus aprepitant for the prevention of chemotherapy-induced nausea and vomiting: A randomized phase III trial. *J Support Oncol*. 2011;9(5):188–195.

31. Beach SR, Celano CM, Noseworthy PA, Januzzi JL, Huffman JC. QTc prolongation, torsades de pointes, and psychotropic medications. *Psychosomatics*. 2013;54(1):1–13.

32. Menza MA, Murray GB, Holmes VF, Rafuls WA. Decreased extrapyramidal symptoms with intravenous haloperidol. *J Clin Psychiatry*. 1987;48:278–280.

33. Seitz DP, Gill SS. Neuroleptic malignant syndrome complicating antipsychotic treatment of delirium or agitation in medical and surgical patients: Case reports and a review of the literature. *Psychosomatics*. 2009;50(1):8–15.

34. Gagnon DJ, Fontaine GV, Smith KE, et al. Valproate for agitation in critically ill patients: A retrospective study. *J Crit Care*. 2017;37:119–125.

35. Scotton W, Hill L, Williams A, Barnes N. Serotonin syndrome: Pathophysiology, clinical features, management, and potential future directions. *Int J Tryptophan Res*. 2019;12:1–14.

36. Gummin DD, Mowry JB, Spyker DA, et al. Annual report of the American Association of Poison Control Centers' National Poison Data System (NPDS): 36th annual report. *Clin Toxicol*. 2019;57(12):1220–1413.

37. Boyer E, Shannon M. The serotonin syndrome. *N Engl J Med*. 2005;352:1112–1120.

38. Watson WA, Litovitz TL, Rodgers GC Jr, et al. 2002 annual report of the American Association of Poison Control Centers Toxic Exposure Surveillance System. *Am J Emerg Med*. 2003;21:353–421.

39. Talton CW. Serotonin syndrome/serotonin toxicity. *Fed Pract*. 2020;37(10):452–459.

40. Volpi-Abadie J, Kaye AM, Kaye AD. Serotonin syndrome. *The Ochsner J*. 2013;13:533–540.

41. Werneke U, Jamshidi F, Taylor D, Ott M. Conundrums in neurology: Diagnosing serotonin syndrome—A meta-analysis of cases. *BMC Neurol*. 2016;16:97.

42. Iqbal M, Basil M, Kaplan J, Iqbal T. Overview of serotonin syndrome. *Ann Clin Psychiatry*. 2012;24(4):310–318.

43. Modi S, Dharaiya D, Schultz L, Varelas P. Neuroleptic malignant syndrome: Complications, outcomes, and mortality. *Neurocrit Care*. 2016;24:97–103.

44. Ware M, Feller D, Hall K. Neuroleptic malignant syndrome: Diagnosis and management. *Prim Care Companion CNS Disord*. 2018;20(1):17r02185.

45. Berman B. Neuroleptic malignant syndrome: A review for neurohospitalists. *Neurohospitalist*. 2011;1(1):41–47.

46. Tse L, Barr AM, Scarapicchia V, Vila-Rodriguez F. Neuroleptic malignant syndrome: A review from a clinically oriented perspective. *Curr Neuropharmacol*. 2015;13:395–406.

47. Kuhlwilm L, Schonfeldt-Lucuona C, Gahr M, Connemann BJ, Keller F, Sartoris A. The neuroleptic malignant syndrome—A systematic case series analysis focusing on therapy regimes and outcome. *Acta Psychiatr Scand*. 2020;142:233–241.

48. Oruch R, Pryme I, Engelsen B, Lund A. Neuroleptic malignant syndrome: An easily overlooked neurologic emergency. *Neuropsychiatr Dis Treat*. 2017;13:161–175.

49. Perry P, Wilborn C. Serotonin syndrome vs neuroleptic malignant syndrome: A contrast of causes, diagnoses, and management. *Ann Clin Psychiatry*. 2012;24(2):155–162.

50. Signhai K, Kuppili P, Nebhinani N. Atypical neuroleptic malignant syndrome: A systematic review of case reports. *Gen Hosp Psychiatry*. 2019;60:12–19.

51. Pileggi D, Cook A. Neuroleptic malignant syndrome. *Ann Pharmacother*. 2016;50(11):973–981.

52. Schonfeldt-Lucuona C, Kuhlwilm L, Cronemeyer M, et al. Treatment of the neuroleptic malignant syndrome in international therapy guidelines: A comparative analysis. *Pharmacopsychiatry*. 2020;53:51–59.

53. Espinola-Nadurille M, Ramirez-Bermudez J, Fricchione GL, et al. Catatonia in neurologic and psychiatric patients at a tertiary neurological center. *J Neuropsychiatry Clin Neurosci*. 2016;28(2):124–130.

54. Rasmussen SA, Mazurek MF, Rosebush PI. Catatonia: Our current understanding of its diagnosis, treatment and pathophysiology. *World J Psychiatr*. 2016;6(4):391–398.

55. Brar K, Kaushik SS, Lippmann S. Catatonia update. *Prim Care Companion CNS Disord*. 2017;19(5):16br02023.

56. Walther S, Strik W. Catatonia. *CNS Spectr*. 2016;21:341–348.

57. Beach SR, Gomez-Bernal F, Huffman JC, Fricchione GL. Alternative treatment strategies for catatonia: A systematic review. *Gen Hosp Psychiatry*. 2017;48:1–19.

58. Rosenbush PI, Mazurek MF. Catatonia and its treatment. *Schizophr Bull*. 2010;36(2):239–242.

59. Saddawi-Konefka D, Berg SM, Nejad SH, Bittner EA. Catatonia in the ICU: An important and underdiagnosed cause of altered mental status. A case series and review of the literature. *Online Case Rep*. 2013;42(3):e234–e241.

60. Jaimes-Albornoz W, Serra-Mestres J. Catatonia in a liaison psychiatry service of a general hospital: Prevalence and clinical features. *Eur Psychiatry*. 2015;30(Suppl 1):28–31.

61. Oldham M, Lee HB. Catatonia vis-à-vis delirium: The significance of recognizing catatonia in altered mental status. *Gen Hosp Psychiatry*. 2015;37:554–559.

62. Solmi M, Pigato GG, Roiter B, et al. Prevalence of catatonia and its moderators in clinical samples: Results from a meta-analysis and meta-regression analysis. *Schizophr Bull*. 2018;44(5):1133–1150.

63. Grover S, Chakrabarti S, Ghormode D, et al. Catatonia in inpatients with psychiatric disorders: A comparison of schizophrenia and mood disorders. *Psychiatry Res*. 2015;229:919–925.

64. Ungvari S, Caroff N, Gerevich J. The catatonia conundrum: Evidence of psychomotor phenomena as a symptom dimension in psychotic disorders. *Schizophr Bull*. 2010;36(2):231–238.

65. Rizos D, Peritogiannis V, Gkogkos C. Catatonia in the intensive care unit. *Gen Hosp Psychiatry*. 2011;33(1):500–505.

66. Carroll BT, Anfinson TJ, Kennedy JC, Yendreck R, Boutros M, Bilon A. Catatonic disorder due to general medical conditions. *J Neuropsychiatry Clin Neurosci*. 1994;6:122–133.

67. De Figueiredo NS, Angst DB, Neto AM, et al. Catatonia, beyond a psychiatric syndrome. *Dement Neuropsychol*. 2017;11(2):209–212.

68. Smith JH, Smith VD, Philbrick KL, Kumar N. Catatonia disorder due to a general medical or psychiatric condition. *J Neuropsychiatry Clin Neurosci*. 2012;24:198–207.

69. Fink M, Taylor MA. *Catatonia: A Clinician's Guide to Diagnosis and Treatment*. Cambridge University Press; 2003.

70. Brar K, Kaushik SS, Lippmann S. Catatonia Update. *Prim Care Companion CNS Disord*. 2017;19(5):16br02023.

71. Rustad JK, Landsman HS, Ivkovic A, Finn CT, Stern TA. Catatonia: An approach to diagnosis and treatment. *Prim Care Companion CNS Disord*. 2018;20(1):17f02202.

72. Wilson JE, Niu K, Nicolson SE, Levine SZ, Heckers S. The diagnostic criteria and structure of catatonia. *Schizophr Res*. 2015;164:256–262.

73. Northoff G. What catatonia can tell us about "top-down modulation": A neuropsychiatric hypothesis. *Behav Brain Sci*. 2002;25:555–604.

74. Bush G, Fink M, Petride G, Dowling F, Francis A. Catatonia I. Rating scale and standardizing examination. *Acta Psychiatr Scand*. 1996;93:129–136.

75. Sienaert P, Rooseleer J, De Fruyt J. Measuring catatonia: A systematic review of rating scales. *J Affect Disord*. 2011;135:1–9.

76. Carroll BT, Boutros NN. Clinical electroencephalograms in patients with catatonic disorders. *Clin Electroencephalogr*. 1995;26(1):60–64.

77. Wilcox JA, Duffy PR. The syndrome of catatonia. *Behav Sci*. 2015:5:576–588.

78. Sienaert P, Dhossche DM, Vancampfort D, De Hert M, Gazdag G. A clinical review of the treatment of catatonia. *Front Psychiatry*. 2014;5:181.

79. Clinebell K, Azzam PN, Gopalan P, Haskett R. Guidelines for preventing common medical complications of catatonia: Case report and literature review. *J Clin Psychiatry*. 2014;75(6):644–651.

80. Narayanaswamy JC, Tibrewal P, Zutshi A, Srinivasaraju R, Math SB. Clinical predictors of response to treatment in catatonia. *Gen Hosp Psychiatry*. 2012;34:312–316.

81. Pelzer A, van der Heijden F, den Boer E. Systematic review of catatonia treatment. *Neuropsychiatr Dis Treat*. 2018;14:317–326.

82. Costanzo F, Menghini D, Casula L, et al. Transcranial direct current stimulation treatment in an adolescent with autism and drug-resistant catatonia. *Brain Stimul*. 2015;8(6):1223–1240.

83. Gregory D, Brown G, Muzyk A, Preud'Homme X. Prolonged delirium with catatonia following orthotopic liver transplant responsive to memantine. *J Psychiatr Pract.*
2016;22(2):128–132.

84. Carroll BT, Goforth HW, Thomas C, et al. Review of adjunctive glutamate antagonist therapy
in the treatment of catatonic syndromes. *J Neuropsychiatry Clin Neurosci.* 2007;19:406–412.

85. Fiest KM, Sauro KM, Wiebe S, et al. Prevalence and incidence of epilepsy: A systematic review and meta-analysis of international studies. *Neurology.* 2017;88(3):296–303.

86. Annegers JF, Hauser WA, Lee JR, Rocca WA. Incidence of acute symptomatic seizures in
Rochester, Minnesota, 1935–1984. *Epilepsia.* 1995;36(4):327–333.

87. Huff JS, Morris DL, Kothari RU, Gibbs MA; Emergency Medicine Seizure Study Group.
Emergency department management of patients with seizures: A multicenter study. *Acad
Emerg Med.* 2001;8(6):622–628.

88. Lowenstein DH, Bleck T, Macdonald RL. It's time to revise the definition of status epilepticus. *Epilepsia.* 1999;40(1):120–122.

89. VanHaerents S, Gerard EE. Epilepsy emergencies: Status epilepticus, acute repetitive seizures, and autoimmune encephalitis. *Continuum.* 2019;25(2):454–476.

90. Walker M, Cross H, Smith S, et al. Nonconvulsive status epilepticus: Epilepsy Research
Foundation workshop reports. *Epileptic Disord.* 2005;7(3):253–296.

91. Thomas RH, Berkovic SF. The hidden genetics of epilepsy—A clinically important new paradigm. *Nat Rev Neurol.* 2014;10(5):283–292.

92. St. Louis EK, Cascino GD. Diagnosis of epilepsy and related episodic disorders. *Continuum.*
2016;22(1):15–37.

93. Ho K, Lawn N, Bynevelt M, Lee J, Dunne J. Neuroimaging of first-ever seizure: Contribution
of MRI if CT is normal. *Neurol Clin Pract.* 2013;3(5):398–403.

94. Saklani P, Krahn A, Klein G. Syncope. *Circulation.* 2013;127(12):1330–1339.

95. Kanner AM. Management of psychiatric and neurological comorbidities in epilepsy. *Nat
Rev Neurol.* 2016;12(2):106–116.

96. Hesdorffer DC, Ishihara L, Mynepalli L, Webb DJ, Weil J, Hauser WA. Epilepsy, suicidality,
and psychiatric disorders: A bidirectional association. *Ann Neurol.* 2012;72(2):184–191.

97. Tellez-Zenteno JF, Patten SB, Jetté N, Williams J, Wiebe S. Psychiatric comorbidity in epilepsy: A population-based analysis. *Epilepsia.* 2007;48(12):2336–2344.

98. Calle-López Y, Ladino LD, Benjumea-Cuartas V, Castrillón-Velilla DM, Téllez-Zenteno JF,
Wolf P. Forced normalization: A systematic review. *Epilepsia.* 2019;60(8):1610–1618.

99. Mula M, Trimble MR, Yuen A, Liu RS, Sander JW. Psychiatric adverse events during levetiracetam therapy. *Neurology.* 2003;61(5):704–706.

100. Kanner AM, Rivas-Grajales AM. Psychosis of epilepsy: A multifaceted neuropsychiatric
disorder. *CNS Spectr.* 2016;21(3):247–257.

101. Hermann BP, Seidenberg M, Bell B. Psychiatric comorbidity in chronic epilepsy: Identification,
consequences, and treatment of major depression. *Epilepsia.* 2000;41(Suppl 2):S31–S41.

102. Kanner AM, Cole AJ. Comorbid depressive disorders in epilepsy. *CNS Spectr.* 2010;15(2
Suppl 4):3–6.

103. Fiest KM, Dykeman J, Patten SB, et al. Depression in epilepsy: A systematic review and
meta-analysis. *Neurology.* 2013;80(6):590–599.

104. Mula M, Jauch R, Cavanna A, et al. Interictal dysphoric disorder and periictal dysphoric
symptoms in patients with epilepsy. *Epilepsia.* 2010;51(7):1139–1145.

105. Gaitatzis A, Trimble MR, Sander JW. The psychiatric comorbidity of epilepsy. *Acta Neurol Scand*. 2004;110(4):207–220.

106. Kanner AM, Soto A, Gross-Kanner H. Prevalence and clinical characteristics of postictal psychiatric symptoms in partial epilepsy. *Neurology*. 2004;62(5):708–713.

107. Hingray C, McGonigal A, Kotwas I, Micoulaud-Franchi JA. The relationship between epilepsy and anxiety disorders. *Curr Psychiatry Rep*. 2019;21(6):40.

108. Kanner AM. Ictal panic and interictal panic attacks: Diagnostic and therapeutic principles. *Neurol Clin*. 2011;29(1):163–175.

109. Torta R, Keller R. Behavioral, psychotic, and anxiety disorders in epilepsy: Etiology, clinical features, and therapeutic implications. *Epilepsia*. 1999;40(Suppl 10):S2–S20.

110. Clancy MJ, Clarke MC, Connor DJ, Cannon M, Cotter DR. The prevalence of psychosis in epilepsy: A systematic review and meta-analysis. *BMC Psychiatry*. 2014;14:75.

111. Slater E, Beard AW, Glithero E. The schizophrenia-like psychoses of epilepsy. *Br J Psychiatry*. 1963;109:95–150.

112. Josephson CB, Jetté N. Psychiatric comorbidities in epilepsy. *Int Rev Psychiatry*. 2017;29(5):409–424.

113. Kanner AM, Stagno S, Kotagal P, Morris HH. Postictal psychiatric events during prolonged video-electroencephalographic monitoring studies. *Arch Neurol*. 1996;53(3):258–263.

114. Logsdail SJ, Toone BK. Post-ictal psychoses. A clinical and phenomenological description. *Br J Psychiatry*. 1988;152:246–252.

115. Pompili M, Girardi P, Ruberto A, Tatarelli R. Suicide in the epilepsies: A meta-analytic investigation of 29 cohorts. *Epilepsy Behav*. 2005;7(2):305–310.

116. Bell GS, Gaitatzis A, Bell CL, Johnson AL, Sander JW. Suicide in people with epilepsy: How great is the risk? *Epilepsia*. 2009;50(8):1933–1942.

117. Altura KC, Patten SB, Fiest KM, Atta C, Bulloch AG, Jetté N. Suicidal ideation in persons with neurological conditions: Prevalence, associations and validation of the PHQ-9 for suicidal ideation. *Gen Hosp Psychiatry*. 2016;42:22–26.

118. Kwan P, Brodie MJ. Neuropsychological effects of epilepsy and antiepileptic drugs. *Lancet*. 2001;357(9251):216–222.

119. Penovich PE. Much ado about something or nothing: Behavioral problems with levetiracetam use in epilepsy patients. *Epilepsy Curr*. 2004;4(4):145–146.

120. Mula M, Trimble MR, Lhatoo SD, Sander JW. Topiramate and psychiatric adverse events in patients with epilepsy. *Epilepsia*. 2003;44(5):659–663.

121. Devinsky O, Honigfeld G, Patin J. Clozapine-related seizures. *Neurology*. 1991;41(3):369–371.

122. Alper K, Schwartz KA, Kolts RL, Khan A. Seizure incidence in psychopharmacological clinical trials: An analysis of Food and Drug Administration (FDA) summary basis of approval reports. *Biol Psychiatry*. 2007;62(4):345–354.

123. Patorno E, Bohn RL, Wahl PM, et al. Anticonvulsant medications and the risk of suicide, attempted suicide, or violent death. *JAMA*. 2010;303(14):1401–1409.

124. Arana A, Wentworth CE, Ayuso-Mateos JL, Arellano FM. Suicide-related events in patients treated with antiepileptic drugs. *N Engl J Med*. 2010;363(6):542–551.

125. Landolt H. Some clinical EEG correlations in epileptic psychosis (twilight states). *EEG Clin Neurophysiol*. 1953;5:121.

126. Duncan R, Oto M. Predictors of antecedent factors in psychogenic nonepileptic attacks: Multivariate analysis. *Neurology.* 2008;71(13):1000–1005.

127. Chen DK, So YT, Fisher RS. Use of serum prolactin in diagnosing epileptic seizures: Report of the Therapeutics and Technology Assessment Subcommittee of the American Academy of Neurology. *Neurology.* 2005;65:668–675.

128. Selkirk M, Duncan R, Oto M, Pelosi A. Clinical differences between patients with nonepileptic seizures who report antecedent sexual abuse and those who do not. *Epilepsia.* 2008;49(8):1446–1450.

129. Perez DL, LaFrance WC Jr. Nonepileptic seizures: An updated review. *CNS Spectr.* 2016;21(3):239–246.

130. Durrant J, Rickards H, Cavanna AE. Prognosis and outcome predictors in psychogenic nonepileptic seizures. *Epilepsy Res Treat.* 2011;2011:274736.

8

Intoxication, Withdrawal, and Symptoms of Substance Use Disorders

Annaliese Koller Shumate

Substance use disorders (SUDs) are quite common and lead to significant morbidity and mortality. In 2019, in the United States alone, more than 19.3 million people aged 18 years or older had an SUD.[1] Substance use and psychiatric illness are commonly comorbid. The etiology of SUDs is a multifactorial interplay between nature and nurture drawing on genetics, neuronal circuitry reinforcement, and environmental factors. Substance use of any kind triggers the brain's mesolimbic dopaminergic reward pathway, and reinforcement occurs as a result of acute intoxication and also becomes hardwired into the brain by activating the amygdala.[2] Unfortunately, those with SUDs continue to be a highly stigmatized patient population and deserve nonjudgmental treatment and access to pharmacologic treatment and therapy. Substance use, although prevalent, is treatable, and early intervention and action in places such as a psychiatric emergency service (PES) can lead to improved long-term sequelae in patients with SUDs. Table 8.1 lists the fifth edition of the *Diagnostic and Statistical Manual of Mental Disorders* (DSM-5) criteria for SUDs.[3]

The PES is often the first access point to psychiatric services for those with SADs. The interaction can occur when a patient is acutely intoxicated, withdrawing from certain substances, or in the midst of another crisis in which a SUD can be revealed. PESs can be a vital interaction, allowing a clinician to intercede both pharmacologically and by introducing the therapeutic framework to help treat those with SUDs longitudinally.

What kind of situations are seen in the PES? Frequently, patients present with acute intoxication leading to alterations in their mental status, agitation, worsened suicidal ideations, gestures, or attempts, and exacerbations in the dynamics of their interpersonal relationships resulting in a an acute crisis requiring evaluation in the psychiatric emergency room (ER). Patients also can present in times of withdrawal or increased cravings. At times, patients present with alterations in mental status and behavioral disturbances, and a skilled clinician might not be able to elicit a cogent history or obtain a urine drug screen but will presume based on clinical presentation that substances could be contributing to the patient's symptomatology. As such, an understanding of the symptoms associated with various SUDs and the stages of acute intoxication and withdrawal is vital to practicing emergency psychiatry.

Initial Assessment

Psychiatric emergency services are similar to other emergency services in that patients present with acute concerns, and staff and physicians triage patients

Table 8.1 Substance Use Disorders Criteria and Severity

Criteria	Severity
Using larger amounts than intended	0–1 criteria = no SUD
Persistent desire to cut down or quit	2–3 criteria = mild SUD
	4–5 criteria = moderate SUD
Significant time spent taking or obtaining substance	>5 criteria = severe SUD
Craving or urge to use substance	
Failure to fulfill obligations	
Continued use despite negative interpersonal consequences	
Reduced social or recreational activities	
Use in physically hazardous situations	
Use despite knowledge of harms	
Tolerance (excludes prescription medication)	
Withdrawal (excludes prescription medication)	

SUD, substance use disorder.

according to the level of care the patients require. Full assessments are often unable to be completed in the ER. Patients may be uncooperative, on psychiatric holds, altered, agitated, or collateral history may be unattainable. Security should have first contact with the patient and should have removed any personal property, which can often be telling, as can nursing assessments in which vitals should be obtained, including a blood alcohol concentration (BAC) and urine drug screen. Legal status should be confirmed. Is the patient seeking care voluntarily or is the encounter involuntary? This is another important point of collateral offering how, why, and by whom the patient came to the PES. Flow of information in the PES is vitally important because one member of the team often possesses additional knowledge from the patient and outside sources to aid in the full assessment of the patient. Initial physician assessment should include these important pieces of information and help clarify the clinical picture. On first interaction with a patient, one can immediately assess consciousness in the patient and determine whether a higher level of medical care is imminently needed.

Depressants

Alcohol

Alcohol is a major contributing factor to both presentations to the ER and to hospitals worldwide. It is frequently seen in the PES, and acute intoxication is often comorbid with either other substance use or other co-occurring mental illness. Both acute alcohol poisoning and alcohol withdrawal can be life-threatening. Identification and treatment are essential to reduce morbidity and mortality.

The following are symptoms of an alcohol use disorder according to DSM-5 criteria, with severity based on number of criteria present—mild, two or three criteria; moderate, four or five criteria; and severe, six or more criteria:

- Recurrent drinking resulting in failure to fulfill role obligations
- Recurrent drinking in hazardous situations
- Continued drinking despite alcohol-related social or interpersonal problems
- Evidence of tolerance
- Evidence of alcohol withdrawal or use of alcohol for relief or avoidance of withdrawal
- Drinking in larger amounts or over longer periods than intended
- Persistent desire or unsuccessful attempts to stop or reduce drinking
- Great deal of time spent obtaining, using, or recovering from alcohol
- Important activities given up or reduced because of drinking
- Continued drinking despite knowledge of physical or psychological problems caused by alcohol
- Alcohol craving

Alcohol's effect on the central nervous system (CNS) is that of a depressant working to stimulate γ-aminobutyric acid (GABA), which is an inhibitory neurotransmitter in the CNS, and then to inhibit glutamate, an excitatory neurotransmitter, resulting in sedation, disinhibition, and relaxation.[4] Alcohol also works on other neurotransmitters. It potentiates dopamine release and stimulates the μ-opioid receptors positively. It also affects serotonin neurotransmitters by increasing serotonin with acute alcohol ingestion and reducing its transmission during alcohol withdrawal.[5] Alcohol also has associations with endocannabinoids, calcium channels, G proteins, and neurosteroids, leading to further motor instability, memory loss, gait instability, and disturbances in sleep.[4]

Acute Intoxication

Alcohol absorption and resulting intoxication depend on numerous factors, including body weight of the individual, period of time over which the alcohol was consumed, percentage of alcohol consumed, and the tolerance of the individual. Obtaining a BAC is the gold standard. Although one can certainly see symptoms suggestive of a certain BAC, those with chronic use will often demonstrate the same symptoms but at higher BAC (Table 8.2).

Table 8.2 Blood Alcohol Level and Corresponding Clinical Effect

Blood Alcohol Concentration	Clinical Effects
20–50 mg/dL (4.4–11 mmol/L)	Diminished fine motor coordination
50–100 mg/dL (11–22 mmol/L)	Impaired judgment, impaired coordination, euphoria or dysphoria, sexual disinhibition
100–150 mg/dL (22–33 mmol/L)	Difficulty with gait and balance
150–250 mg/dL (33–55 mmol/L)	Slurred speech, ataxia, diplopia, nausea, tachycardia, lethargy, difficulty sitting upright without assistance, mood lability
300 mg/dL (66 mmol/L)	Stupor to coma in the nonhabituated drinker
≥400 mg/dL (88 mmol/L)	Coma in the nonhabituated drinker to respiratory paralysis

Adapted from Marx.[6]

Treatment of Acute Alcohol Intoxication

Most patients presenting with acute intoxication will require supportive care and observation to ensure return to sobriety. Again, careful observation of vital signs, blood sugar, and serial observation for signs of withdrawal is called for. Alcohol generally clears from the bloodstream at approximately 20 mg/dL per hour and slightly faster in the habituated drinker. When clinically sober, the patient can likely be discharged should they no longer be an acute danger to themself or others. At this time, assessing further detoxification needs should be accomplished with motivational interviewing allowing the clinician to identify further needs to best aid the patient in their treatment options.

Intravenous fluids may be needed if a patient demonstrates signs of volume depletion, hypotension, or malnutrition. Severe intoxication or alcohol poisoning requires a higher level of supervision and medical care than most PESs can provide. Patients with severe intoxication in which stupor or coma is present must have aggressive supportive care, including possible mechanical ventilation and hemodynamic support. Intravenous thiamine should be administered to prevent Wernicke's encephalopathy. Intensive care unit (ICU) admission may be necessary (Table 8.3).

Treating acute withdrawal should employ clinically useful tools such as the Clinical Institute Withdrawal Assessment for Alcohol–Revised (CIWA-R; Figure 8.1) along with benzodiazepines or gabapentin as indicated in Box 8.1.

Table 8.3 Alcohol Withdrawal Timeline and Clinical Findings

Syndrome	Onset After Last Drink	Clinical Findings
Minor withdrawal	6–36 hours	Insomnia Tremulousness Mild anxiety Gastrointestinal upset, anorexia Headache Diaphoresis Palpitations
Seizures	6–48 hours	Single generalized tonic–clonic seizure or brief burst of seizure activity Short postictal period Status epilepticus rare
Alcoholic hallucinosis	12–48 hours	Usually visual hallucinations (auditory and/or tactile hallucinations can occur), intact orientation and normal vital signs Resolve by 48 hours
Delirium tremens	48–96 hours	Delirium Agitation Tachycardia Hypertension Fever Diaphoresis

Adapted from Hoffman and Weinhouse.[7]

Clinical Institute Withdrawal Assessment of Alcohol Scale, Revised (CIWA-Ar)

Patient:_____ Date: _____ Time: _____ (24 hour clock, midnight = 00:00)

Pulse or heart rate, taken for one minute:_____ Blood pressure:_____

NAUSEA AND VOMITING -- Ask "Do you feel sick to your stomach? Have you vomited?" Observation.
0 no nausea and no vomiting
1 mild nausea with no vomiting
2
3
4 intermittent nausea with dry heaves
5
6
7 constant nausea, frequent dry heaves and vomiting

TACTILE DISTURBANCES -- Ask "Have you any itching, pins and needles sensations, any burning, any numbness, or do you feel bugs crawling on or under your skin?" Observation.
0 none
1 very mild itching, pins and needles, burning or numbness
2 mild itching, pins and needles, burning or numbness
3 moderate itching, pins and needles, burning or numbness
4 moderately severe hallucinations
5 severe hallucinations
6 extremely severe hallucinations
7 continuous hallucinations

TREMOR -- Arms extended and fingers spread apart. Observation.
0 no tremor
1 not visible, but can be felt fingertip to fingertip
2
3
4 moderate, with patient's arms extended
5
6
7 severe, even with arms not extended

AUDITORY DISTURBANCES -- Ask "Are you more aware of sounds around you? Are they harsh? Do they frighten you? Are you hearing anything that is disturbing to you? Are you hearing things you know are not there?" Observation.
0 not present
1 very mild harshness or ability to frighten
2 mild harshness or ability to frighten
3 moderate harshness or ability to frighten
4 moderately severe hallucinations
5 severe hallucinations
6 extremely severe hallucinations
7 continuous hallucinations

PAROXYSMAL SWEATS -- Observation.
0 no sweat visible
1 barely perceptible sweating, palms moist
2
3
4 beads of sweat obvious on forehead
5
6
7 drenching sweats

VISUAL DISTURBANCES -- Ask "Does the light appear to be too bright? Is its color different? Does it hurt your eyes? Are you seeing anything that is disturbing to you? Are you seeing things you know are not there?" Observation.
0 not present
1 very mild sensitivity
2 mild sensitivity
3 moderate sensitivity
4 moderately severe hallucinations
5 severe hallucinations
6 extremely severe hallucinations
7 continuous hallucinations

ANXIETY -- Ask "Do you feel nervous?" Observation.
0 no anxiety, at ease
1 mild anxious
2
3
4 moderately anxious, or guarded, so anxiety is inferred
5
6
7 equivalent to acute panic states as seen in severe delirium or acute schizophrenic reactions

HEADACHE, FULLNESS IN HEAD -- Ask "Does your head feel different? Does it feel like there is a band around your head?" Do not rate for dizziness or lightheadedness. Otherwise, rate severity.
0 not present
1 very mild
2 mild
3 moderate
4 moderately severe
5 severe
6 very severe
7 extremely severe

AGITATION -- Observation.
0 normal activity
1 somewhat more than normal activity
2
3
4 moderately fidgety and restless
5
6
7 paces back and forth during most of the interview, or constantly thrashes about

ORIENTATION AND CLOUDING OF SENSORIUM -- Ask "What day is this? Where are you? Who am I?"
0 oriented and can do serial additions
1 cannot do serial additions or is uncertain about date
2 disoriented for date by no more than 2 calendar days
3 disoriented for date by more than 2 calendar days
4 disoriented for place/or person

Total **CIWA-Ar** Score _____
Rater's Initials _____
Maximum Possible Score 67

Figure 8.1 The Clinical Institute Withdrawal Assessment for Alcohol Scale–Revised.

Maintenance Treatment

Naltrexone is a U.S. Food and Drug Administration (FDA)-approved medication for alcohol use disorders that works by blocking μ-opioid receptors, thus disrupting the reinforcement pathway, leading to reduced cravings and reduced heavy drinking.[9] A daily oral formulation of 50 mg and an intramuscular monthly formulation of 380

Box 8.1 Treatment of Acute Withdrawal

Benzodiazepine (CIWA-Ar score <10)—symptom-triggered
  Chlordiazepoxide (long acting)
    Day 1: 50 mg every 6–12 hours as needed
    Days 2–5: 25 mg every 6 hours as needed
  Diazepam (long acting)
    Day 1: 20 mg every 6–12 hours as needed
    Days 2–5: 10 mg every 6–12 hours as needed
  Lorazepam (shorter acting)
    Day 1: 2–4 mg every 6 hours as needed
    Days 2–5: 2 mg every 6 hours as needed

Benzodiazepines (CIWA-Ar score 10–15)—fixed dose
  Chlordiazepoxide (long acting)
    Day 1: 50 mg every 6–12 hours
    Day 2: 25 mg every 6 hours
    Day 3: 25 mg twice a day
    Day 4: 25 mg at night
  Diazepam (long acting)
    Day 1: 20 mg every 6–12 hours
    Day 2: 10 mg every 6 hours
    Day 3: 10 mg twice a day
    Day 4: 10 mg at night
  Lorazepam (shorter acting)
    Day 1: 2–4 mg every 6 hours
    Day 2: 2 mg every 8 hours
    Day 3: 2 mg every 12 hours
    Day 4: 2 mg at night

Gabapentin (CIWA-Ar score 0–15)—fixed dosing
  Gabapentin
    Day 1: 300 mg every 6 hours
    Day 2: 300 mg every 8 hours
    Day 3: 300 mg every 12 hours
    Day 4: 300 mg one dose

Nutritional support
  Thiamine 100 mg for 3 days, multivitamins maintenance

CIWA-Ar, Clinical Institute Withdrawal Assessment for Alcohol Scale–Revised.
Adapted from Holt and Tetrault.[8]

---

mg every 4 weeks are available. Liver function should be monitored regularly, and unless the patient has decompensated cirrhosis or acute hepatitis, naltrexone can likely be safely used.[10]

Acamprosate is thought to moderate glutamate and works to reduce cravings. Dosing is 666 mg three times daily. It is an FDA-approved medication to help "sustain abstinence in patients with AUD [alcohol use disorder] who are abstinent at treatment initiation."[11]

Disulfiram works by blocking the metabolism of alcohol, leading to the accumulation of acetaldehyde and resulting in unpleasant effects such as flushing, headache, palpitations, and diaphoresis. Although FDA approved for alcohol use disorder, disulfiram requires a very motivated patient and is not considered first-line treatment. This medication should be started following a period of abstinence, with dosing of 500 mg once daily for 1 or 2 weeks and then reduced dosing of 125–250 mg once daily.

Opioids

Opioid misuse and abuse is a worldwide problem with significant morbidity and mortality. In the United States, drug overdose is the leading cause of accidental death, and opioids are the most commonly implicated drug, with the Centers for Disease Control and Prevention estimating that ERs see more than 1,000 emergency department visits daily related to the misuse of opioids and approximately 91 opioid overdose deaths every day.[12]

Opioids (substances that work on the opioid receptors) are both natural and synthetic and work via the endogenous opioid system. Throughout the CNS, peripheral nervous system, and the gut, there are μ-, κ-, and δ-opioid receptors. Opioids mediate these receptors as agonists, partial agonists, or agonist–antagonists of opioid receptors, leading to lower perceptions of pain, dopamine release, euphoria, sedation, dysmotility, dependence, and respiratory depression.[12] Opiates have various means of administration, including intravenously (IV), intramuscularly (IM), topically, inhaled, sublingual, or oral. Peak effect of the drug depends on when and how it is administered, with IV and intranasal administration resulting in peak effect sometimes in minutes.

Symptoms of an Opioid Use Disorder

The DSM-5 carefully distinguishes opioid use that is therapeutic under the direction of a physician and misuse or illicit use. Two or more of the following DSM-5 criteria present in a 12-month period indicate opioid use disorder:

- Opioids are often taken in larger amounts or over a longer period than was intended.
- There is a persistent desire or unsuccessful efforts to cut down or control opioid use.
- A great deal of time is spent in activities necessary to obtain the opioid, use the opioid, or recover from its effects.
- Craving, or a strong desire or urge to use opioids.
- Recurrent opioid use resulting in failure to fulfill major role obligations at work, school, or home.
- Continued opioid use despite having persistent or recurrent social or interpersonal problems caused or exacerbated by the effects of opioids.
- Important social, occupational, or recreational activities given up or reduced because of opioid use.
- Recurrent opioid use in situations in which it is physically hazardous.
- Continued opioid use despite knowledge of having a persistent or recurrent physical or psychological problem that is likely to have been caused or exacerbated by the substance.
- Tolerance
- Withdrawal

Table 8.4 Opioid Use and Its Effects on the Body

Organ System	Mechanism	Side Effects
Skin	Administration of opioid Release of histamine	Check skin for patch marks related to inhalation Track marks Cellulitis around injection site Itching, flushing, urticaria
Pulmonary	Respiratory suppression in the pons	Decreased respirations Decreased tidal volume
Cardiovascular	Peripheral vasodilation	Hypotension (which responds to change in positioning or fluid administration) Decreased heart rate Decreased blood pressure
Gastrointestinal	Gastric aperistalsis Slowed motility	Nausea Vomiting
Neurologic	Paradoxical excitation	Lowered seizure threshold Hearing loss Loss of consciousness Coma Hypothermia
Psychiatric		Anxiety Agitation Depression Dysphoria Hallucinations Nightmares Paranoia

Adapted from Stolbach and Hoffman.[13]

Acute Intoxication

The symptoms of acute opioid intoxication range from euphoria to sedation (Table 8.4). Acute overdose can result in respiratory depression, which can lead to coma and death. Vital signs need to be obtained, and careful assessment of level of consciousness must occur. The triad of respiratory depression, depressed levels of consciousness, and pinpoint pupils points to acute intoxication. Vitals can include reduced heart rate, reduced respirations, hypotension, and hypothermia.

Management

Always obtain vital signs and monitor levels of consciousness. Remember your ABCs: airway, breathing, circulation. If an airway cannot be maintained, the patient requires an elevated level of medical care that can often not be provided in a PES. If this is the case, escalating care to a medical ER is necessary and appropriate because cardiopulmonary support may be needed. If you suspect that a patient has had an opiate overdose, naloxone should be administered to reverse respiratory depression. Naloxone administered via IV is preferred, but intranasal, subcutaneous, IM, and interosseous routes can be used if IV is unavailable. Naloxone is a short-acting opioid antagonist. Be prepared, as naloxone works quickly to reverse the opiate binding, which can lead to aggression and agitation.

Keep in mind that specific toxicities can be associated with specific substances. For instance, buprenorphine, a partial agonist, can induce withdrawal in those with full agonists on board. Dextromethorphan and meperidine can provoke seizures. Loperamide and methadone can prolong QTc, and hydrocodone is often one part of a combination drug with acetaminophen and can cause acetaminophen toxicity. One should always obtain a blood sugar, serum drug screen to assess for acetaminophen toxicity, a serum creatinine kinase, and an electrocardiogram.

Withdrawal

Early withdrawal from short-acting opioids such as heroin occurs within several hours. Signs and symptoms of early withdrawal, which can occur 8–24 hours after last use, include mydriasis, piloerection, muscle twitching, lacrimation, rhinorrhea, diaphoresis, yawning, tremor, restlessness, myalgia, arthralgia, abdominal pain, nausea, and vomiting. Fully developed withdrawal can occur 24 hours out from discontinuing short-acting opioids or 3 or 4 days after long-acting opioids. There you will see tachycardia, tachypnea, hypertension or hypotension, dehydration, hypoglycemia, fever, anorexia, and nausea, vomiting, and diarrhea.

Treatment of Opioid Withdrawal

Methadone, a long-acting full μ-agonist, blocks other opiates from binding to the receptor and suppresses cravings. Typically, a patient can be started on methadone during withdrawal via induction and either started on maintenance dosing or tapered while in the inpatient setting with typical daily dosing ranging from 80 to 120 mg. This is accomplished by observation and treatment based on Clinical Opiate Withdrawal Scale symptomatology (Table 8.5). Methadone can be fatal in overdose; thus, risk is mitigated by a strict regulatory process of distribution in which patients present daily for observed ingestion.

Outcomes of methadone maintenance include the following:[15]

- Increased retention in treatment
- Decreased illicit opioid use
- Decreased transmission of hepatitis C virus and HIV
- Reduced rates of incarceration
- Increased employment
- Increased survival

Buprenorphine, a partial opioid agonist at the μ-receptor, must be initiated after a period of withdrawal because it is often co-formulated with naloxone under the brand name Suboxone. Dosing is typically once daily and generally ranges from 16 to 24 mg daily. It also can be prescribed as an outpatient, which allows for additional treatment options for patients (Table 8.6).

In general, pregnant patients with opioid use disorder should be maintained on medication-assisted therapy with either methadone or buprenorphine as opposed to medically assisted withdrawal.[17] Both of these maintenance medications are preferred over continued substance use (Box 8.2).

Table 8.5 Clinical Opioid Withdrawal Scale (COWS)

Patient's name: _____   Date and time: ___/___/___: _____

Reason for this assessment: _____

Resting pulse rate: beats/minute
Measured after patient is sitting or lying for
  one minute
0 pulse rate 80 or below
1 pulse rate 81 to 100
2 pulse rate 101 to 120
4 pulse rate greater than 120

GI upset: Over last half-hour
0 no GI symptoms
1 stomach cramps
2 nausea or loose stool
3 vomiting or diarrhea
5 multiple episodes of diarrhea or vomiting

Sweating: Over past half-hour not accounted
  for by room temperature or patient
  activity
0 no report of chills or flushing
1 subjective report of chills or flushing
2 flushed or observable moistness on face
3 beads of sweat on brow or face
4 sweat streaming off face

Tremor: Observation of outstretched hands
0 no tremor
1 tremor can be felt, but not observed
2 slight tremor observable
4 gross tremor or muscle twitching

Restlessness: Observation during assessment
0 able to sit still
1 reports difficulty sitting still, but is able
  to do so
3 frequent shifting or extraneous movements
  of legs/arms
5 unable to sit still for more than a few seconds

Yawning: Observation during assessment
0 no yawning
1 yawning once or twice during assessment
2 yawning three or more times during
  assessment
4 yawning several times/minute

Pupil size
0 pupils pinned or normal size for room light
1 pupils possibly larger than normal for
  room light
2 pupils moderately dilated
5 pupils so dilated that only the rim of the iris
  is visible

Anxiety or irritability
0 none
1 patient reports increasing irritability or
  anxiousness
2 patient obviously irritable or anxious
4 patient so irritable or anxious that
  participation in the assessment is difficult

Bone or joint aches: If patient was having
  pain previously, only the additional
  component attributed to opiates
  withdrawal is scored
0 not present
1 mild diffuse discomfort
2 patient reports severe diffuse aching of
  joints/muscles
4 patient is rubbing joints or muscles and is
  unable to sit still because of discomfort

Gooseflesh skin
0 skin is smooth
3 piloerection of skin can be felt or hairs
  standing up on arms
5 prominent piloerection

Runny nose or tearing: Not accounted for by
  cold symptoms or allergies
0 not present
1 nasal stuffiness or unusually moist eyes
2 nose running or tearing
4 nose constantly running or tears streaming
  down cheeks

Total score:_____

The total score is the sum of all 11 items
Score: 5 to 12 = mild
13 to 24 = moderate
25 to 36 = moderately severe;
More than 36 = severe withdrawal

Reproduced from Wesson and Ling.[14]

Table 8.6 Pharmacologic Treatment for Opioid Withdrawal

Symptoms	Medication	Usual Effective Dose Range (Adult)	Notes
Anxiety Irritability	Diphenhydramine	50–100 mg orally every 4–6 hours as needed (maximum 300 mg daily)	May also treat nausea Use reduced dose in hepatic impairment
	Hydroxyzine	25–100 mg orally every 6–8 hours as needed (maximum 400 mg daily)	May also treat lacrimation and rhinorrhea Reduced dose (50%) in renal or hepatic impairment
	Clonazepam Lorazepam Oxazepam	0.5–1.5 mg 3–4 times daily (maximum 6 mg) 1 mg 4–6 hours as needed (maximum 6 mg) 15–30 mg every 6–8 hours (maximum 120 mg)	Clonazepam use with caution in mild hepatic and renal impairment Avoid in moderate to severe hepatic impairment or hepatic encephalopathy Lorazepam and oxazepam safer in mild hepatic and renal impairment
Abdominal cramping	Dicyclomine	10–20 mg orally every 6–8 hours as needed (maximum 160 mg daily)	IM administration available (lower doses are used) Caution/reduce dose in renal/hepatic impairment
Diarrhea	Bismuth	~524 mg orally every 30–60 minutes as needed (up to 4,200 mg daily)	Monitor for dehydration and maintain fluid levels with oral and/or IV hydration
	Loperamide	4 mg orally followed by 2 mg after each loose stool (maximum 16 mg)	
Nausea/ vomiting	Ondansetron	4–8 mg orally or IV every 12 hours as needed (maximum 16 mg/day)	Monitor for dehydration Dose-dependent QT interval prolongation Caution/reduced dose (50%) in severe hepatic impairment
	Prochlorperazine	5–10 mg orally 3 times daily before meals or every 6 hours as needed (maximum 40 mg/day)	Monitor for dehydration and maintain fluid levels with oral and/or IV hydration Use with caution in mild to moderate hepatic impairment; avoid in severe hepatic impairment IM and rectal administration available
	Promethazine	25 mg orally every 4–6 hours as needed (maximum 50 mg/day)	Monitor for dehydration and maintain fluid levels with oral and/or IV hydration Use with caution in mild to moderate hepatic impairment; avoid in severe hepatic impairment IM and rectal administration available (IV use not recommended)

Table 8.6 Continued

Symptoms	Medication	Usual Effective Dose Range (Adult)	Notes
Insomnia	Trazodone	25–100 mg orally at bedtime	May titrate nightly up to 300 mg at bedtime if needed
	Doxepin	6–50 mg orally at bedtime	Use with caution and reduce dose in severe hepatic impairment
	Mirtazapine	7.5–15 mg orally at bedtime	Consider reduced dose in moderate to severe hepatic or renal impairment
	Quetiapine	50–100 mg orally at bedtime	Use lower initial dose (25 mg) in hepatic impairment and adjust
	Zolpidem	5–10 mg orally at bedtime	Avoid in severe hepatic impairment or hepatic encephalopathy
Aches	Ibuprofen	400 mg orally every 4–6 hours as needed (maximum 2,400 mg daily)	Caution in mild to moderate hepatic or renal impairment and avoid in severe
	Acetaminophen	650–1,000 mg orally every 4–6 hours as needed (maximum 4,000 mg daily)	Appropriate analgesic for most patients Use reduced dose (i.e., 2000 mg daily) or avoid in hepatic impairment or if malnourished
	Naproxen	500 mg orally twice daily with meals	Patient should be well hydrated and without significant kidney disease Use with caution in mild to moderate hepatic or renal impairment Avoid all NSAIDs in severe renal or hepatic impairment or cirrhosis
Muscle spasm, restless legs	Cyclobenzaprine	5–10 mg orally every 8 hours as needed (maximum 30 mg daily)	Use reduced dose in mild hepatic impairment Avoid in moderate to severe haptic impairment
	Baclofen	5–10 mg orally every 8 hours as needed (max 60 mg daily)	Use reduced dose in renal impairment
	Diazepam	5–10 mg orally every 6–12 hours as needed (maximum 40 mg daily)	Use with caution in hepatic or renal impairment. Avoid in severe hepatic impairment or hepatic encephalopathy.
	Methocarbamol	750–1,500 mg orally every 8 hours as needed (maximum 6 g/day)	Use with caution in hepatic or renal impairment

IM, intramuscular; IV, intravenous; NSAIDs, nonsteroidal anti-inflammatory drugs.

Adapted from Severino.[16]

Box 8.2 Maintenance for People with Opioid Use Disorder

Screen for HIV, hepatitis B virus, hepatitis C virus, sexually transmitted infections, and tuberculosis (at least annually for most patients).

Vaccinate against hepatitis A, hepatitis B, tetanus, diphtheria–pertussis, influenza, and pneumococcus.

Aggressively manage cardiac risk factors, including hypertension, lipid control, and smoking, particularly for people who also use stimulants or tobacco.

Treat other comorbid substance use disorders, including tobacco and alcohol use disorders.

Treat comorbid psychiatric disorders.

Educate patients about safer injection practices and provide clean injection equipment.

Offer preexposure HIV prophylaxis for patients who inject drugs or have other risk factors.

Prescribe naloxone and discuss precautions such as test shots and using with friends.

Offer methadone, buprenorphine, or naltrexone (Vivitrol) to all patients.

Adapted from San Francisco Department of Public Health.[18]

Benzodiazepines

Benzodiazepines are drugs with which you will become very familiar while working in the PES. They are frequently used in various stages of acute intoxication of multiple substances and management of resulting agitation. They are prescribed in stages of withdrawal and are used to treat seizures. They can be very clinically helpful in the PES, but they can also be abused and are one of the most frequently misused prescription medications. Often, they will be co-ingested with other substances and fail to screen positively on some urine drug screens, so clinical suspicion must be high.

Acute Intoxication

Overdose of benzodiazepines is rarely lethal.[19] However, overdose of benzodiazepines with other substances co-ingested, especially alcohol and opioids, can be a very lethal combination. Acute intoxication leads to CNS depression, with patients becoming lethargic, ataxic, and slurring speech. They are generally arousable, and vital signs are normal.

Most benzodiazepine overdose is treated with supportive care. Assess airway and circulation. Assess for co-ingestion and escalate medical needs for the patient if needed.

Flumazenil is rarely used because in individuals who have tolerance to benzodiazepines, it can precipitate seizures and is less clinically useful in a PES as opposed to being used to reverse sedation under anesthesia.

Withdrawal

Withdrawal from benzodiazepines can be life-threatening. Benzodiazepines work by modulating and downregulating GABA. Less GABA means less disinhibition and a more excitatory state. Severity of withdrawal depends of many factors, including half-life of the drug, how long a patient has been using the drug, and how rapidly the drug was discontinued. In general, withdrawal can produce the following symptoms:[20]

- Tremors
- Anxiety
- Perceptual disturbances
- Dysphoria
- Psychosis
- Seizures
- Autonomic instability

Treatment Options

Treatment options for those with benzodiazepine use disorder can focus on either abstinence or maintenance. In general, shorter acting benzodiazepines such as alprazolam have a higher likelihood of misuse. The safest option for patients is to convert the type of benzodiazepine to its longer acting equivalent, such as diazepam, and then either taper as an inpatient using scales such as the CIWA or taper slowly over several weeks to months to maintenance dosing of long-acting benzodiazepines, which have less abuse potential (Table 8.7).

Table 8.7 Benzodiazepine and Z-Drugs Half-Life and Conversion Table

Drug	Approximate Half-Life (Hours)	Dose of Oral Benzodiazepine Approximately Equivalent to Diazepam 5 mg (mg)
Short- to intermediate-acting		
Triazolam	1–3	0.25
Oxazepam	4–15	15
Temazepam	5–15	10
Lorazepam	12–16	1
Bromazepam	20	3
Alprazolam	6–25	0.5
Flunitrazepam	20–30	0.5
Nitrazepam	16–48	5
Clobazam	17–49	10
Long-acting		
Clonazepam	22–54	0.5
Diazepam	20–80	5
Z-drugs		
Zolpidem	2.4	10
Zopiclone	5.2	7.5

From Sareen et al.[21]

Barbiturates

In the past, barbiturates were heavily abused and misused as co-ingestants, leading to fatal overdose. They are much less common now, but a skilled clinician should still be alert to signs of misuse in a patient's history or aware of signs of respiratory depression similar to alcohol or benzodiazepine intoxication. Barbiturates withdrawal can be fatal.

Inhalants

Inhalants are also classified as a CNS depressant. These substances are volatile hydrocarbons or nitrous oxide. They are typically found in compounds that have a variety of uses, such as in glue, shoe polish, paint thinner, keyboard cleaner, or nitrous oxide whippets. In short, their intoxication is similar to that of alcohol or marijuana but only lasts for 15–30 minutes, thus requiring continued abuse to sustain a high (Table 8.8).[22]

Lethality arises from risk of asphyxia or other trauma, such as burns or aspiration when attempting to abuse inhalants. Sudden sniffing death can occur, as can methemoglobinemia resulting from nitrous oxide ingestion. Inhalant abuse can cause significant long-term multiorgan system morbidity, including severe neurotoxic effects such as parkinsonism, encephalopathy, neuropathies, dementia, cardiomyopathy, leukemia, hepatocellular carcinoma, and renal toxicities.[24]

Again, acute treatment focuses on supportive care. Check your ABCs. Check for co-ingestion. Treat agitation. If there is concern for methemoglobinemia, administering intravenous methylene blue will be necessary. Avoid pressors or bronchodilators.[24]

There is no formal withdrawal; however, some case reports discuss withdrawal-like phenomena that include cravings, increased irritability, or anxiety. Also, some have

Table 8.8 Stages of Acute Inhalant Intoxication

Phase	Symptoms
First phase Within minutes Usually resolves within 2 hours	Euphoria, excitation Sneezing, coughing, salivating Rhinitis, increased sputum, conjunctival injection, epistaxis Nausea and vomiting Dyspnea, heart palpitations
Second phase CNS depression worsens	Slurred speech, visual changes Delusions and disorientation Confusion, tremor, weakness Headache Visual hallucinations
Third phase Further CNS depression	Obtunded Ataxia Decreased reflexes and nystagmus
Fourth phase	Stupor including coma, seizures Sudden death

CNS, central nervous system.
Adapted from Kurtzman et al.[23]

noted headaches, nausea or vomiting, hallucinations, runny eyes or nose, craving, tachycardia, depressed mood, and anxiety during withdrawal from inhalants.[25]

Stimulants

Stimulant abuse is a significant problem throughout the United States. According to the 2018 National Survey on Drug Use and Health, more than 5 million individuals misused stimulants, 1.9 million used methamphetamines, and more than 5.5 million used cocaine.[26] From caffeine to cocaine use to methamphetamine use, stimulant abuse contributes to significant disease burden, with little or no treatment options readily available in the form of pharmacologic management. The mainstay of treatment for stimulant use disorders are psychosocial interventions and various forms of psychotherapy. Identifying stimulant use disorders, reducing burden of acute intoxication, working toward sustainable psychosocial interventions, and working to treat comorbid mental illness can all be accomplished in a PES.

Cocaine

Cocaine is an indirect sympathomimetic agent that affects serotonin, dopamine, norepinephrine, and epinephrine by blocking their reuptake. Cocaine affects adrenergic activity on cardiac and peripheral vasculature, resulting in vasoconstriction. Its effects on serotonin and dopamine lead to a euphoric feeling when acutely intoxicated and cause reinforcement with addiction. Cocaine increases the excitatory neurotransmitters in the brain, glutamate and aspartate. It also has a significant effect on sodium channels, causing blockade that locally causes anesthesia and on cardiac muscle prolongs QRS.

Acute Intoxication
Cocaine affects multiple organ systems (Table 8.9). It is rapidly absorbed into the body through multiple routes of administration. It works on the cardiovascular system through vasoconstriction, which causes tachycardia and hypertension. It can cause agitation, seizure, or coma. It can cause hyperthermia as a result of peripheral vasoconstriction, and mortality can occur in up to one-third of individuals when cocaine-induced hyperthermia occurs.[27]

Managing acute cocaine intoxication in the PES is often aimed at treating associated agitation and providing supportive care. Vitals need to be obtained, as does a careful history because cocaine can affect virtually every organ system and result in end organ damage. If hypertensive urgency occurs, transfer to a medical emergency room where further medical workup is indicated. Benzodiazepines are the treatment of choice in acute agitation resulting from cocaine ingestion. Avoid β-blockers because of β blockade.

Withdrawal
Symptoms of acute withdrawal from cocaine are generally mild and not life-threatening. They include depression, anxiety, anhedonia, mental fog, and fatigue. They also can be associated with cravings, increased appetite, and increased sleep. The cocaine crash can be observed and generally includes a "crash" of psychomotor retardation, increased sleep, and severe depression with suicidal ideation.

Table 8.9 Cocaine Effects on Multiple Organ Systems

Organ System	Causes	Acute Effects	Chronic Effects

Cardiovascular	Vasoconstriction
	↑ Cardiac
	  oxygen demand
	Negative inotropy
		Tachycardia
		Hypertension
		Cardiac ischemia
		Dysrhythmia
		Heart failure
		Aortic dissection and
		  rupture
			Atherogenesis
			Left ventricular
			  hypertrophy
			All increase risk
			  of ischemia and
			  cardiomyopathy

CNS	↑ Glutamate ↑ Aspartate ↑ Serotonin ↑ Dopamine	Agitation Seizures Coma Headache	
Neurologic	Vasoconstriction	TIA or stroke Intracerebral hemorrhage	

Pulmonary	Method of ingestion
	Vasoconstriction/
	  vasospasm
	↑ Thrombus
		Angioedema and burns of
		  airways
		Pneumothorax
		Pneumomediastinum
		Pneumopericardium
		Pulmonary infarction
		Pulmonary embolism	

Gastrointestinal		Ulcers Ischemia and infarction throughout the gut Renal/splenic infarction	
Musculoskeletal	Electrolyte abnormality	Rhabdomyolysis Muscle pain Compartment syndrome	

CNS, central nervous system; TIA, transient ischemic attack.
Adapted from Nelson and Odujebe.[28]

Amphetamine-Type Substances

Stimulants, methamphetamine, ephedrine, pseudoephedrine, MDMA ("ecstasy" or "molly"), and catathiones ("bath salts") all fall under the class of phenylethylamines because of their structural similarities in addition to their pharmacodynamic properties.[29] They all cause the neurotransmitters norepinephrine, epinephrine, and serotonin to be released postsynaptically while also blocking its reuptake, causing a huge surge in these neurotransmitters. Dopamine is also increased, activating the drug reward pathway in the brain and thus increasing cravings and drug-seeking. As such, they are discussed as a group because they generally present similar symptoms of acute intoxication and withdrawal.

The following are the DSM-5 criteria for an amphetamine-type substance use disorder, with two or more symptoms in a 12-month period signifying a disorder:

- Methamphetamine is often taken in larger amounts or over a longer period than was intended.
- There is a persistent desire or unsuccessful efforts to cut down or control methamphetamine use.

- A great deal of time is spent in activities necessary to obtain methamphetamine, use methamphetamine, or recover from its effects.
- Craving, or a strong desire or urge to use methamphetamine.
- Recurrent methamphetamine use resulting in a failure to fulfill major role obligations at work, school, or home.
- Continued methamphetamine use despite having persistent or recurrent social or interpersonal problems caused or exacerbated by the effects of methamphetamine.
- Important social, occupational, or recreational activities are given up or reduced because of methamphetamine use.
- Recurrent methamphetamine use in situations in which it is physically hazardous.
- Continued methamphetamine use despite knowledge of having a persistent or recurrent physical or psychological problem that is likely to have been caused or exacerbated by methamphetamine.
- Tolerance
- Withdrawal

Acute Intoxication

Amphetamine intoxication can occur within seconds of ingestion. Amphetamines are frequently ingested via inhalation or intranasally but can be ingested orally or injected intravenously. Acute ingestion can lead to agitation related to the serotonin and dopamine surge. Psychomotor agitation can be severe and requires aggressive benzodiazepine treatment. Psychosis and tachycardia are frequently present. Amphetamine ingestion can be fatal. Watch for the following symptoms: hypertension, tachycardia, severely agitated delirium, hyperthermia, metabolic acidosis, and seizures.[30] Of note, hallucinations may persist beyond acute ingestion and often do not respond to antipsychotics (Table 8.10).

Treatment Options

Again, the majority of the time, treatment requires supportive care. Think reduced environmental stimuli such as a dark room, a less active milieu, and not a complete psychiatric history and evaluation. A patient takes cues from the environment, and agitation may be increased with bright lights, a loud milieu, and lengthy questioning. Ensure stable vitals, blood sugar, nutritional status, and hydration. Aggressive treatment including benzodiazepines for agitation, antipsychotics for psychosis, and β-blockers for the treatment of hypertension and tachycardia is supported in the literature.[32] Should agitation be present, and it often is, the first-line treatment is aggressive benzodiazepine treatment. Intravenous benzodiazepines are preferred but often unable to be accomplished in the PES. Oral benzodiazepines should be offered, but IM may be needed. Should psychosis or paranoia be present, antipsychotics including haloperidol, olanzapine, risperidone, and ziprasidone are often used in oral, IV, or IM formulations. Psychosis including profound paranoia and auditory, visual, or tactile hallucinations has been demonstrated in up to 42% of patients with methamphetamine intoxication.[33]

Withdrawal

DSM-5's diagnostic criteria for stimulant withdrawal include cessation of use of amphetamine-type substances, cocaine, and other stimulants and dysphoric mood and also at least two additional symptoms: fatigue, vivid or unpleasant dreams, insomnia or hypersomnia, increased appetite, and psychomotor agitation or retardation. These can

Table 8.10 Acute and Chronic Effects of Methamphetamine Abuse

Organ System	Acute Effects	Chronic Effects
Cardiovascular	Tachycardia Hypertension Cardiac ischemia Cardiomyopathy MI Cardiovascular collapse Cardiac arrest	Cardiomyopathy Coronary heart disease Left ventricular hypertrophy
HEENT	Mydriasis Mucosal injury Oropharyngeal burns Bruxism	"Meth mouth" Extensive tooth decay
Pulmonary	↑ Respirations ↑ Tidal volume Pulmonary edema Pulmonary hypertension	
Gastrointestinal	Vomiting/diarrhea Bowel ischemia	
Skin	Cellulitis Burns	Formication "crank bugs" Excoriations Jaundice
Neurologic	Choreiform movements Ischemia Seizures	
Psychiatric	Delirium Paranoia Psychosis Suicidality/homicidality	Psychosis may persist and may not respond to treatment

HEENT, head, eyes, ears, nose, and throat, MI, myocardial infarction.
Adapted from Arnold and Ryan.[31]

be seen within hours to several days following last use. Anhedonia and drug cravings are also seen clinically. A crash can occur during withdrawal associated with binge use of any stimulant type, despite being most associated with cocaine. Again, no pharmacologic treatment has demonstrated sufficient data to prove effective in the withdrawal phases of stimulant use.[34] Treatment in the acute phase is supportive, and long-term maintenance is focused on psychosocial support and therapy.

Caffeine

Caffeine is the most commonly used stimulant in the world. It is not discussed in detail here but, rather, mentioned as a reminder that it is frequently co-consumed with other substances. Similar to other stimulants, caffeine can lead to dependence and cause withdrawal. Symptoms of acute intoxication include palpitations, agitation, tremor, and gastrointestinal upset. Hallucinations, seizures, arrhythmias, or cardiac ischemia may also be seen.[35] It is important to screen for caffeine usage, especially because caffeine is formulated in energy drinks and supplements.

Caffeine withdrawal is common—so common, in fact, that you have likely experienced it yourself in the form of a headache. The following are common symptoms of caffeine withdrawal, which typically occurs within 12–24 hours after last use and can last for up to 9 days:[36]

- Headache
- Tiredness/fatigue
- Decreased energy
- Decreased alertness
- Drowsiness
- Decreased contentedness
- Depressed mood
- Difficulty concentrating
- Irritability
- Fuzzy/not as mentally sharp

Tobacco

Tobacco derives its psychoactive properties from nicotine, which is a CNS stimulant. Nicotine binds to nicotinic acetylcholine receptors and causes the release of dopamine, serotonin, and norepinephrine, as well as adrenaline. Nicotine exerts two effects—a stimulant effect exerted at the locus coeruleus and a reward effect in the limbic system.[37] Acute intoxication with nicotine can affect the heart, causing either tachycardia or bradycardia; it can also cause respiratory difficulty, nausea, vomiting, diarrhea, and hallucinations. It can also cause more severe side effects such as seizures, hypotension, respiratory depression, and death.[38]

The DSM-5 reports seven primary symptoms associated with nicotine withdrawal: irritability/anger/frustration, anxiety, depressed mood, difficulty concentrating, increased appetite, insomnia, and restlessness. These symptoms will peak within the first 3 days after cessation and take up to 1 month to clear. Clinically, the following may also be seen:[39]

- Anxiety
- Anhedonia
- Dysphoria
- Hyperalgesia
- Irritability
- Tremors
- Bradycardia
- Gastrointestinal discomfort
- Increased appetite
- Nightmares
- Sore throat
- Difficulty concentrating
- Impaired memory

Although it is unlikely that a patient would present to the PES solely for tobacco abuse or acute nicotine intoxication or withdrawal, tobacco use disorder is a frequent comorbidity not only in the PES but also in most every other clinical setting in medicine. The ability to identify this disorder will help the patient acutely and in the long term given the heavy toll of continued tobacco use. First-line treatment for tobacco use includes nicotine replacement, varenicline, and bupropion. Nicotine patches are applied daily with strength of the patch corresponding to how many cigarettes are consumed daily, with 21-mg dosing corresponding to >10 cigarettes and 14-mg dosing corresponding with <10 cigarettes. Nicotine gum, which is available in dosages of 2 or 4 mg, can be chewed hourly. Lozenges work in a similar manner as the gum. These two are interesting in that they also provide an oral habit substitute. Nicotine replacement is also available in an inhaler and an intranasal spray, which are used every 1 or 2 hours as needed. Varenicline, a partial nicotine agonist, works by relieving nicotine withdrawal and blocking the reward from smoking. Bupropion is another consideration in treatment.

Hallucinogens

Hallucinogenic drugs are considered as a group with some selective hallucinogens singled out below (Table 8.11). As discussed above, some hallucinogens are also stimulants of the phenylethylamine group. Also included are phencyclidine (PCP) and lysergic acid diethylamide (LSD), and although not as much abuse of these drugs is being seen as in previous decades, they still exist (and may be laced in other drugs of abuse). Ingestion of dextromethorphan, salvia, or psilocybin is common. It is important to be concerned about co-ingestions, especially in cases of dextromethorphan in which the over-the-counter preparations often include acetaminophen or anticholinergics.

On the whole, hallucinogens work by modulating serotonin, dopamine, and glutamate. Others also have some effect on opioid receptors in the brain. As noted previously with other drugs that work on these same receptors, sympathomimetic effects are seen, including tachycardia, hypertension, hyperthermia, and mydriasis, along with increased plasma cortisol and increases in prolactin, oxytocin, and epinephrine.[41] This modulation will also result in psychosis and can lead to serotonin syndrome. Although the intended effect may have been to have an altered state of consciousness, the PES frequently sees patients who have taken a "bad trip" or a psychosis that leads to dysphoria or severe agitation.

Acute intoxication often does not have severe vital sign derangement; however, you will likely see clinical features that may have been desired effects of drug usage versus the "bad trip": euphoria or dysphoria, heightened senses, perceptual disturbances, depersonalization, synesthesia (the blending of senses), the classic LSD associated symptom of "hearing colors," fear, panic, paranoia, psychosis, and dread.

Watch out for serotonin syndrome (altered mental status, neuromuscular abnormalities, and autonomic hyperactivity) and hyperthermia and cardiovascular collapse, which has been seen in massive overdose[42] and can be life-threatening. Hyperthermia, if observed, is a medical emergency and will likely need to be treated in a critical care setting. Most patients do well with only supportive care and treatment with benzodiazepines and antipsychotics. Most of the time, morbidity is associated with poor decision-making while intoxicated as opposed to the direct effects of the drugs on the body.

Table 8.11 Common Names and Classification of Select Hallucinogens

Common Name	Active Ingredient	Drug Class
2CB, "Bromo," "Nexus"	25B-NBOMe	Phenylethylamine
2CT-7, "Blue Mystic"	25C-NBOMe	Phenylethylamine
25I, "N-bomb," "Smiles"	25I-NBOMe	Phenylethylamine
AMT	α-Methyltryptamine	Indolealkylamine (tryptamine)
DMT, *Ayahuasca*	Dimethyltryptamine	Indolealkylamine (tryptamine)
Dextromethorphan, DXM	Dextromethorphan	Arylcyclohexylamine (piperidine)
"Foxy methoxy"	5-MeO-DIPT (5-methoxydimethyl tryptamine)	Indolealkylamine (tryptamine)
Hawaiian baby woodrose (*Argyreia nervosa*)	Ergine	Lysergamide
Ibogaine	12-Methoxybogamine	Indolealkylamine (tryptamine)
Ketamine, "Special K"	Ketamine	Arylcyclohexylamine (piperidine)
LSD	D-Lysergic acid diethylamide	Lysergamide
Mescaline, peyote	3,4,5-Trimethoxy-phenethylamine	Phenylethylamine
Morning glory (*Ipomoea violacea*)	Lysergic acid hydroxyethylamide	Lysergamide
PCP, "angel dust"	Phencyclidine	Arylcyclohexylamine (piperidine)
Psilocybin, "magic mushroom"	Psilocin (*N,N*-dimethyl-4-phosphoryloxytryptamine)	Indolealkylamine (tryptamine)
Salvia divinorum	Salvinorin A	Diterpene alkaloid

From Delgado.[40]

Phencyclidine

Phencyclidine affects the brain via three sites of action. First, it antagonizes NMDA receptors in the brain, causing a release of glutamate, glycine, and aspartate leading to psychosis, agitation, and seizures.[43] It also works on inhibiting the reuptake for dopamine, norepinephrine, and serotonin.[44] Third, it binds to the sigma receptor complex, also leading to psychosis, anticholinergic effects, and movement abnormalities.[45]

Clinically, one will see alterations in vital signs with ingestion of PCP, which is frequently co-ingested with other drugs of abuse. Hypertension and tachycardia are seen. One can also see violent or bizarre behavior, nystagmus, and motor incoordination. Motor signs include grand mal seizures, generalized rigidity, localized dystonias, catalepsy, and athetosis.[46]

The hallmark of treatment for acute intoxication with PCP is good management of agitation, which often involves higher doses of benzodiazepines. If psychomotor agitation is severe, consider ICU admission and propofol for sedation.

Dextromethorphan

Dextromethorphan is another hallucinogen that is commonly abused, especially in teens and young adults due to its relative ease of availability as a component in most over-the-counter cough and cold preparations. Using dextromethorphan is frequently called "robo-tripping" due to the fact that it is being a component of Robitussin. It has several street names, including purple drank, triple C's, DXM, Skittles, and poor man's PCP. In general, side effects of use are dose dependent (Table 8.12).

Marijuana

Cannabis is the most commonly used illicit drug in the world.[48] Cannabis works by its psychoactive component δ-9-tetrahydrocannabinol (THC) on cannabinoid CB1 and CB2 receptors throughout the brain and body, including vascular endothelium, liver, adipose, immune cells, and neurons.[49] By activating CB1 receptors, dopamine is released, leading to the dopamine reward pathway associated with substance abuse. Regular use is associated with downregulation of CB1 cannabinoid receptors.

Frequently, cannabis is smoked. However, new formulations in addition to synthetic derivations have introduced higher potency THC cannabinoids in multiple different forms, ranging from traditional form to oils, wax, and edibles. Table 8.13 highlights both states of intoxication and withdrawal informed from DSM-5 criteria.

Synthetic Cannabinoids

Synthetic cannabinoids are recreational drugs that are synthetically produced to mimic the effect of acute intoxication with cannabis as above; however, clinically they produce much more severe neuropsychiatric effects and contain much more THC in addition to other chemical derivatives that can also be neurotoxic. They are generally available under different names, such as K2, Kush, or Spice, and sold as incense or herbal products. In fact, those with synthetic cannabinoid exposure versus those with only cannabinoid exposure had higher odds of coma, respiratory depression, and seizures.[50] Synthetic

Table 8.12 Dextromethorphan Plateaus of Abuse

Plateau 1 (1.5–2.5 mg/kg)	Plateau 2 (2.5–7.5 mg/kg)	Plateau 3 (7.5–15 mg/kg)	Plateau 4 (>15 mg/kg)
Total intake 100–200 mg (4–6 capsules or 35–60 mL of syrup)	Total dose 200–500 mg (7–18 capsules or 60–185 mL of syrup)	Total dose 500–1000 mg (18–33 capsules or 185–375 mL of syrup)	Total dose >1000 mg (>33 capsules or >375 mL of syrup)
Restlessness, euphoria	Exaggerated auditory and visual sensations, closed-eye hallucinations, imbalance	Visual and auditory disturbances, altered consciousness, delayed reaction times, mania, panic, partial dissociation	Hallucinations, delusions, ataxia, complete dissociation

From Antoniou and Juurlink.[47]

Table 8.13 DSM-5 Cannabis Intoxication and Withdrawal

Intoxication	Withdrawal
Impaired motor coordination	Irritability, anger, or depression
Euphoria	Nervousness or anxiety
Anxiety	Sleep difficulty (i.e., insomnia, disturbing dreams)
Sensation of slowed time	Decreased appetite or weight loss
Paranoia	Restlessness
Conjunctival injection	Depressed mood
Increased appetite	At least one physical symptom causing discomfort
Dry mouth	(i.e., abdominal pain, shakiness/tremors,
Tachycardia	sweating, fever, chills, headache)
Perceptual disturbances	

cannabinoid intoxication can affect multiple organ systems. Neuropsychiatric, cardiac, and renal sequelae have all been identified, including reports of death. Based on an examination of the data on acute intoxication with synthetic cannabis from 2010 to 2015, toxicologists reported the effects shown in Table 8.14.

Treatment

Acute intoxication with both cannabis and synthetic cannabis is treated by supportive care and managing agitation with benzodiazepines, treating psychosis with antipsychotics, and escalating medical needs when severe agitation is present or there is concern for end organ damage.

Treatment for cannabis use disorder is aimed at psychosocial treatment, with cognitive–behavioral therapy and motivational interviewing the best modalities of therapy, similar to treatment for stimulant use disorder. N-acetylcysteine and gabapentin have shown some reduction of use in limited studies.[52,53] Again, treat any co-occurring mood disorder.

Table 8.14 Effects of Synthetic Cannabis

System/Syndrome	Effects	%
Nervous	Agitation, coma, toxic psychosis, other	66.1
Cardiovascular	Bradycardia, tachycardia, other	17.0
Pulmonary	Respiratory depression	5.4
	Other	2.2
Renal/muscle	Acute kidney injury	4.0
	Rhabdomyolysis	6.1
Other	Metabolic	8.7
	Gastrointestinal/hepatic	1.4
	Significant leukocytosis	2.9
Toxidrome	Sedative–hypnotic	6.9
	Sympathomimetic syndrome	5.4
	Other	2.2

From Riederer et al.[51]

Steroids

Androgenic steroids are another potential drug of abuse you could encounter while working in the PES. Although likely ingested for performance0enhancing qualities, these are illicit drugs and can be toxic, resulting in both acute and long-term consequences for the user other than just bulking up (Box 8.3). There is not a complete clinical picture of what acute intoxication or toxicity looks like; rather, "synthetic androgen intoxication can be defined by a pattern of poor self-regulation characterized by increased

---

Box 8.3 Adverse Effects and Complications of Androgenic Steroids

Cardiovascular
   Coronary heart disease
   Cardiomyopathy
   Erythrocytosis
   Hemostasis/coagulation abnormalities
   Dyslipidemia
   Hypertension
Infection
   HIV, hepatitis B and C, MRSA
   Unsafe needle practices
   Contaminated products
Musculoskeletal
   Tendon rupture
Neuropsychiatric
   Major mood disorders
   Aggression, violence
   Dependence
Men (reproductive)
   Hypogonadism (following withdrawal)
   Gynecomastia
   Acne
   Premature epiphyseal closure (when taken before completion of puberty)
   Prostate (potential increased risk for cancer)
Women (reproductive)
   Acne
   Virilization (hirsutism, deepening of voice, clitoromegaly)
   Irregular menses
Hepatic (only with oral 17-α-alkylated androgens)
   Cholestasis
   Peliosis hepatis
   Hepatic neoplasms

MRSA, methicillin-resistant *Staphylococcus aureus*.
From Snyder.[55]

propensity for a range of behaviors (e.g., aggression, sex, drug seeking, exercise, etc.) via androgen mediated effects on general brain arousal."[54]

Conclusion

Assess your patient early. Early intervention is key. Listen to your collateral sources, including your nurses, to get a more thorough clinical picture. Offer oral medications should you have a patient who is agitated or psychotic as a result of their substance use. Early intervention and medication can reduce increased agitation, episodes of violence, and worsened morbidity and mortality, which is safest for both the patient and staff. Always attempt oral medications and verbal de-escalation first-line. A consensus statement from the American Association for Emergency Psychiatry De-escalation Workgroup describes the following 10 key elements for verbal de-escalation:[56]

- Respect personal space: Maintain a distance of two arm's length and provide space for easy exit for either party.
- Do not be provocative: Keep your hands relaxed, maintain a non-confrontational body posture, and do not stare at the patient.
- Establish verbal contact: The first person to contact the patient should be the leader.
- Use concise, simple language: Elaborate and technical terms are difficult for an impaired person to understand.
- Identify feelings and desires: "What are you hoping for?"
- Listen closely to what the patient is saying: After listening, restate what the patient said to improve mutual understanding (e.g., "Tell me if I have this right . . .").
- Agree or agree to disagree: (1) Agree with clear specific truths; (2) agree in general—"Yes, everyone should be treated respectfully"; (3) agree with minority situations—"There are others who would feel like you."
- Lay down the law and set clear limits: Inform the patient that violence or abuse cannot be tolerated.
- Offer choices and optimism: Patients feel empowered if they have some choice in matters.
- Debrief the patient and staff.

If a patient is not willing to take oral medications but is acutely dangerous either to themself or others (think posturing, restless pacing, harming themself, and targeting other peers), than IM medications or restraints may be needed. Restraints should be used as a means of allowing one to chemically sedate a patient so that restraints may be rapidly removed. Restrain to medicate. Remember that with special populations such as pregnant patients, risk of untreated SUD and the acute effects of intoxication or withdrawal are more harmful to the fetus that most interventions you could create by medicating your patient.

In the PES, best medication management for acute intoxication and related agitation follows guidelines set forth by Project BETA (Best Practices in the Evaluation and Treatment of Agitation) by the American Association of Emergency Psychiatry (Figure 8.2).[57]

Remember, being able to identify and treat SUDs, both in stages of acute intoxication and withdrawal, will benefit you and your patients. Working toward next steps after

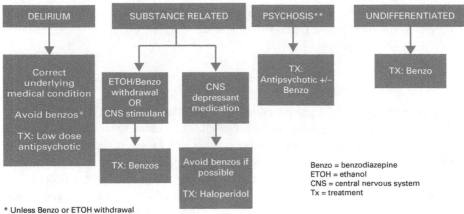

Figure 8.2 Project BETA guidelines for medication management of acute intoxication and related agitation.
Reproduced from Roppolo et al.[57]

stabilizing your patient will help guide them toward recovery. Use motivational interviewing and help them identify goals toward recovery. Manage your own countertransference while also using subject matter expertise if needed (e.g., U.S. Poison Control Network at 1-800-222-1222). Substance use is a relapsing illness with a large genetic component, several different mechanisms of neuronal feedback reinforcing use, and strong psychosocial factors affecting continued use. Working in the PES will give you ample opportunities to treat patients who have SUDs.

References

1. McCance-Katz E. The National Survey on Drug Use and Health: 2019. Substance Abuse and Mental Health Services Administration. Published 2019. Accessed September 2020. https://www.samhsa.gov/data/sites/default/files/reports/rpt29392/Assistant-Secretary-nsduh2019_presentation/Assistant-Secretary-nsduh2019_presentation.pdf

2. Adinoff B. Neurobiologic processes in drug reward and addiction. *Harv Rev Psychiatry.* 2004;12(6):305–320. doi:10.1080/10673220490910844

3. American Psychiatric Association. *Diagnostic and Statistical Manual of Mental Disorders.* 5th ed. American Psychiatric Publishing; 2013.

4. Costardi JV, Nampo RA, Silva GL, et al. A review on alcohol: From the central action mechanism to chemical dependency. *Rev Assoc Med Bras (1992).* 2015;61(4):381–387. doi:10.1590/1806-9282.61.04.381

5. Vengeliene V, Bilbao A, Molander A, Spanagel R. Neuropharmacology of alcohol addiction. *Br J Pharmacol.* 2008;154(2):299–315. doi:10.1038/bjp.2008.30

6. Marx JA. *Rosen's Emergency Medicine: Concepts and Clinical Practice.* 5th ed. Mosby; 2002.

7. Hoffman RS, Weinhouse GL. Management of moderate and severe alcohol withdrawal syndromes. UpToDate. Accessed January 18, 2021. https://www.uptodate.com/contents/management-of-moderate-and-severe-alcohol-withdrawal-syndromes#!

8. Holt SR, Tetrault JM. Ambulatory management of alcohol withdrawal. UpToDate. Accessed January 18, 2021. https://www.uptodate.com/contents/ambulatory-management-of-alcohol-withdrawal#!

9. Maisel NC, Blodgett JC, Wilbourne PL, Humphreys K, Finney JW. Meta-analysis of naltrexone and acamprosate for treating alcohol use disorders: When are these medications most helpful? *Addiction.* 2013;108(2):275–93. doi:10.1111/j.1360-0443.2012.04054.x

10. Klein JW. Pharmacotherapy for substance use disorders. *Med Clin North Am.* 2016;100(4):891–910. doi:10.1016/j.mcna.2016.03.011

11. Kranzler HR, Soyka M. Diagnosis and pharmacotherapy of alcohol use disorder: A review. *JAMA.* 2018;320(8):815–824. doi:10.1001/jama.2018.11406

12. Schiller EY, Goyal A, Mechanic OJ. Opioid overdose. In: *StatPearls.* StatPearls Publishing; 2020.

13. Stolbach A, Hoffman RS. Acute opioid intoxication in adults. UpToDate. Accessed January 24, 2021. https://www.uptodate.com/contents/acute-opioid-intoxication-in-adults?search=Acute%20opioid%20intoxication%20in%20adults&source=search_result&selectedTitle=1~150&usage_type=default&display_rank=1

14. Wesson DR, Ling W. The Clinical Opiate Withdrawal Scale (COWS). *J Psychoactive Drugs.* 2003;35:253.

15. Mattick RP, Breen C, Kimber J, et al. Methadone maintenance therapy versus no opioid replacement therapy for opioid dependence. *Cochrane Database Syst Rev.* 2009;2009(3):CD002209.

16. Severino KW. Medically supervised opioid withdrawal during treatment of addiction. UpToDate. Accessed January 22, 2021. https://www.uptodate.com/contents/medically-supervised-opioid-withdrawal-during-treatment-for-addiction#!

17. Committee Opinion No. 711: Opioid use and opioid use disorder in pregnancy. *Obstet Gynecol.* 2017;130(2):e81–e94. doi:10.1097/AOG.0000000000002235

18. San Francisco Department of Public Health. Opioid stewardship and chronic pain: A guide for primary care providers. March 2018.

19. Höjer J, Baehrendtz S, Gustafsson L. Benzodiazepine poisoning: Experience of 702 admissions to an intensive care unit during a 14-year period. *J Intern Med.* 1989;226(2):117–122. doi:10.1111/j.1365-2796.1989.tb01365.x

20. Marriott S, Tyrer P. Benzodiazepine dependence. Avoidance and withdrawal. *Drug Saf.* 1993;9(2):93–103. doi:10.2165/00002018-199309020-00003

21. Sareen J, Katz C, Stein MB. Treatment of benzodiazepine dependence. *N Engl J Med.* 2017;376(24):2398. doi:10.1056/NEJMc1705239

22. Brust JC. Other agents: Phencyclidine, marijuana, hallucinogens, inhalants, and anticholinergics. *Neurol Clin.* 1993;11(3):555–561.

23. Kurtzman TL, Otsuka KN, Wahl RA. Inhalant abuse by adolescents. *J Adolesc Health.* 2001;28(3):170–180. doi:10.1016/s1054-139x(00)00159-2

24. Williams JF, Storck M; American Academy of Pediatrics Committee on Substance Abuse; American Academy of Pediatrics Committee on Native American Child Health. Inhalant abuse. *Pediatrics.* 2007;119(5):1009–1017. doi:10.1542/peds.2007-0470

25. Perron BE, Howard MO, Vaughn MG, Jarman CN. Inhalant withdrawal as a clinically significant feature of inhalant dependence disorder. *Med Hypotheses.* 2009;73(6):935–937. doi:10.1016/j.mehy.2009.06.036

26. Substance Abuse and Mental Health Services Administration. Key substance use and mental health indicators in the United States: Results from the 2018 National Survey on Drug Use and Health. HHS Publication No. PEP19-5068, NSDUH Series H-54. Center for Behavioral Health Statistics and Quality, Substance Abuse and Mental Health Services Administration; 2019.

27. Marzuk PM, Tardiff K, Leon AC, et al. Ambient temperature and mortality from unintentional cocaine overdose. *JAMA*. 1998;279(22):1795–1800. doi:10.1001/jama.279.22.1795

28. Nelson L, Odujebe O. Cocaine, acute intoxication. UpToDate. Accessed January 22, 2021. https://www.uptodate.com/contents/cocaine-acute-intoxication#!

29. Hill SL, Thomas SH. Clinical toxicology of newer recreational drugs. *Clin Toxicol*. 2011;49(8):705–719. doi:10.3109/15563650.2011.615318. Erratum in: *Clin Toxicol*. 2011;49(9):880.

30. Chan P, Chen JH, Lee MH, Deng JF. Fatal and nonfatal methamphetamine intoxication in the intensive care unit. *J Toxicol Clin Toxicol*. 1994;32(2):147–155. doi:10.3109/15563659409000444

31. Arnold TC, Ryan ML. Acute amphetamine and synthetic cathinone ("bath salt") intoxication. UpToDate. Accessed January 25, 2021. https://www.uptodate.com/contents/acute-amphetamine-and-synthetic-cathinone-bath-salt-intoxication#!

32. Richards JR, Albertson TE, Derlet RW, Lange RA, Olson KR, Horowitz BZ. Treatment of toxicity from amphetamines, related derivatives, and analogues: A systematic clinical review. *Drug Alcohol Depend*. 2015;150:1–13.

33. Lecomte T, Dumais A, Dugré JR, Potvin S. The prevalence of substance-induced psychotic disorder in methamphetamine misusers: A meta-analysis. *Psychiatry Res*. 2018;268:189–192. doi:10.1016/j.psychres.2018.05.033

34. Shoptaw SJ, Kao U, Heinzerling K, Ling W. Treatment for amphetamine withdrawal. *Cochrane Database Syst Rev*. 2009;2009(2):CD003021. doi:10.1002/14651858.CD003021.pub2

35. Gunja N, Brown JA. Energy drinks: Health risks and toxicity. *Med J Aust*. 2012;196(1):46–49. doi:10.5694/mja11.10838

36. Juliano LM, Griffiths RR. A critical review of caffeine withdrawal: Empirical validation of symptoms and signs, incidence, severity, and associated features. *Psychopharmacology*. 2004;176(1):1–29. doi:10.1007/s00213-004-2000-x

37. Nicotine. PubChem. https://pubchem.ncbi.nlm.nih.gov/compound/Nicotine#section=Pharmacology-and-Biochemistry

38. Alkam T, Nabeshima T. Molecular mechanisms for nicotine intoxication. *Neurochem Int*. 2019;125:117–126. doi:10.1016/j.neuint.2019.02.006

39. Heishman SJ, Kleykamp BA, Singleton EG. Meta-analysis of the acute effects of nicotine and smoking on human performance. *Psychopharmacology*. 2010;210:453–469.

40. Delgado J. Intoxication from LSD and other common hallucinogens. UpToDate. Accessed January 25, 2021. https://www.uptodate.com/contents/intoxication-from-lsd-and-other-common-hallucinogens#!

41. Schmid Y, Liechti ME. Long-lasting subjective effects of LSD in normal subjects. *Psychopharmacology*. 2018;235(2):535–545. doi:10.1007/s00213-017-4733-3

42. Klock JC, Boerner U, Becker CE. Coma, hyperthermia and bleeding associated with massive LSD overdose: A report of eight cases. *West J Med*. 1974;120(3):183–188.

43. Javitt DC, Zukin SR. Recent advances in the phencyclidine model of schizophrenia. *Am J Psychiatry*. 1991;148:1301.

44. Akunne HC, Reid AA, Thurkauf A, et al. [3H]1-[2-(2-thienyl)cyclohexyl]piperidine labels two high-affinity binding sites in human cortex: Further evidence for phencyclidine binding sites associated with the biogenic amine reuptake complex. *Synapse*. 1991;8:289.

45. Wolfe SA Jr, De Souza EB. Sigma and phencyclidine receptors in the brain–endocrine–immune axis. *NIDA Res Monogr*. 1993;133:95.

46. McCarron MM, Schulze BW, Thompson GA, Conder MC, Goetz WA. Acute phencyclidine intoxication: Incidence of clinical findings in 1,000 cases. *Ann Emerg Med*. 1981;10(5):237–242. doi:10.1016/s0196-0644(81)80047-9

47. Antoniou T, Juurlink DN. Dextromethorphan abuse. *Can Med Assoc J*. 2014;186(16):E631. https://doi.org/10.1503/cmaj.131676

48. United Nations Office on Drugs and Crime. World drug report 2016. Published 2016. https://www.unodc.org/doc/wdr2016/WORLD_DRUG_REPORT_2016_web.pdf

49. Mechoulam R, Parker LA. The endocannabinoid system and the brain. *Annu Rev Psychol*. 2013;64:21–47. doi:10.1146/annurev-psych-113011-143739

50. Anderson SAR, Oprescu AM, Calello DP, et al.; ToxIC Investigators. Neuropsychiatric sequelae in adolescents with acute synthetic cannabinoid toxicity. *Pediatrics*. 2019;144(2):e20182690. doi:10.1542/peds.2018-2690

51. Riederer AM, Campleman SL, Carlson RG, et al.; Toxicology Investigators Consortium (ToxIC). Acute poisonings from synthetic cannabinoids: 50 U.S. Toxicology Investigators Consortium registry sites, 2010–2015. *MMWR Morb Mortal Wkly Rep*. 2016;65(27):692–695. doi:10.15585/mmwr.mm6527a2

52. Gray KM, Carpenter MJ, Baker NL, et al. A double-blind randomized controlled trial of *N*-acetylcysteine in cannabis-dependent adolescents. *Am J Psychiatry*. 2012;169(8):805–812. doi:10.1176/appi.ajp.2012.12010055. Erratum in *Am J Psychiatry*. 2012;169(8):869.

53. Mason BJ, Crean R, Goodell V, et al. A proof-of-concept randomized controlled study of gabapentin: Effects on cannabis use, withdrawal and executive function deficits in cannabis-dependent adults. *Neuropsychopharmacology*. 2012;37(7):1689–1698. doi:10.1038/npp.2012.14

54. Hildebrandt T, Heywood A, Wesley D, Schulz K. Defining the construct of synthetic androgen intoxication: An application of general brain arousal. *Front Psychol*. 2018;9:390. doi:10.3389/fpsyg.2018.00390

55. Snyder PJ. Use of androgens and other hormones by athletes. UpToDate. Accessed January 27, 2021. https://www.uptodate.com/contents/use-of-androgens-and-other-hormones-by-athletes#!

56. Richmond JS, Berlin JS, Fishkind AB, et al. Verbal de-escalation of the agitated patient: Consensus statement of the American Association for Emergency Psychiatry Project BETA De-escalation Workgroup. *West J Emerg Med*. 2012;13(1):17–25. doi:10.5811/westjem.2011.9.6864

57. Roppolo LP, Morris DW, Khan F, et al. Improving the management of acutely agitated patients in the emergency department through implementation of Project BETA (Best Practices in the Evaluation and Treatment of Agitation). *J Am Coll Emerg Physicians Open*. 2020;1(5):898–907. doi:10.1002/emp2.12138.

9

Psychosis, Psychotic Disorders, and the Schizophrenia Spectrum

Chelsea Wolf and Helena Winston

Introduction

Individuals experiencing psychotic symptoms may present to an emergency setting at any age, with new-onset psychosis, a relapse of a known psychiatric disorder, or psychosis due to substance intoxication or withdrawal. These patients may present with behavioral agitation or social withdrawal, in the presence or absence of other medical conditions. Regardless of the presentation, the emergency department (ED) is frequently the first point of contact between a patient with psychosis and the medical professional.

Encountering a patient experiencing psychosis in an emergency setting can be stressful for all who are involved. The situation may feel unpredictable and unsettling for staff, particularly when patients are agitated or aggressive. The undifferentiated nature of psychotic symptoms may seem daunting to the providers, who recognize the gravity of the presenting features and the need for rapid management. And, for the patients, an unfamiliar ED may feel terrifying, particularly if they are not there of their own volition but, rather, at the directive of the police or a concerned party.

Nevertheless, for all parties the encounter may be emotionally charged, fraught with tension and uncertainty. Given this, a systematic process is imperative to effectively manage the emergent situation and to evaluate and treat the patient. This chapter provides background information and a structured approach that can be used in the evaluation and management of psychotic patients in an emergency setting. Specifically, this approach includes the following:

- Initial assessment and management
- Diagnostic workup and differential diagnosis
- Treatment of psychotic symptoms
- Appropriate disposition

Epidemiology

In the United States, more than 20% of adults (51.5 million) and 16% of youth aged 6–17 years (7.7 million) experience a mental illness, which is defined by the National Institute of Mental Health as "a mental, behavioral, or emotional disorder."[1,2] Furthermore, for more than 5% of U.S. adults, their mental illness contributes to a severe functional impairment.[1] The lifetime prevalence of schizoaffective disorder is approximately 0.3%, and that of schizophrenia is estimated between 0.3% and 0.7%.[3] In addition, between 5% and 8% of all U.S. adults report having had psychotic experiences, defined as psychotic symptoms in which some degree of insight is maintained.[4]

Despite this high prevalence of mental health disorders in the general population, many have difficulty accessing, or choose not to access, outpatient services, leaving them to seek psychiatric care in the ED. In 2014, the second most common reason for an ED visit was for mental health or substance abuse complaints.[5] And, the number of patients presenting to the ED with psychiatric issues continues to rise. In 2007, mental health diagnoses constituted 6.6% of all ED visits. By 2016, nearly 11% of all ED visits were for mental health concerns, an increase of 44%.[6]

Psychosis is common among patients presenting to the ED with mental health concerns and is considered a medical emergency.[7] Indeed, EDs are frequently the initial point of contact for individuals experiencing a first psychotic break, and many with a severe mental illness turn to this acute hospital setting for much of their mental health care. Although certainly not all individuals experiencing psychosis require an ED visit, psychosis is a common presentation and, as such, it is vital that providers in an emergency setting are able to appropriately evaluate and manage patients who demonstrate these symptoms.

Definition of Terms

Because acute psychosis exists at the intersection of emergency medicine and psychiatry, it is important to ensure a common vocabulary. Terms such as positive symptoms and negative symptoms tend to be more specialty specific. These phrases and descriptors are frequently used in the field of psychiatry but may be less familiar to ED providers. Having a common language when discussing symptoms can be valuable in order to convey concise and accurate information about a patient to staff, colleagues, and consulting providers. Below, we briefly define some of the more common psychiatric terminology regarding psychosis and psychotic symptoms.

Psychosis
Psychosis is not a specific disease or disorder. Instead, the term encompasses a group of symptoms, or a syndrome, and is ultimately a clinical diagnosis. In general, individuals with psychotic symptoms experience an alternative reality and may have *impaired reality testing*, or an impaired ability to distinguish that which is real from that which is not. Psychosis may impair one's cognition; ability to relate to others; and emotional responses to people, objects, or events.[8] There are multiple ways in which psychosis can manifest, and within the field of psychiatry, one common means of describing psychosis is by delineation into positive and negative symptoms.

Positive Symptoms
Positive symptoms can be thought of as the presence of atypical behaviors or perceptions. These are often the most dramatic symptoms and, as such, may be the precipitant of the patient being brought to the attention of emergency services. Positive symptoms include the following:

- *Hallucinations* are sensory perceptions in the absence of an existent external stimulus. Hallucinations can take an auditory, visual, tactile, olfactory, or gustatory form, and they seem completely real to the individual who is experiencing them. Auditory hallucinations are the most common type of hallucinations in those with primary psychotic disorders and can manifest in a wide spectrum of ways to the individual—from barely audible mumbling to loud derogatory commentary and commands to harm oneself or others. Individuals experiencing hallucinations may talk or gesture to themselves, commonly referred to as responding to internal stimuli.

- *Delusions* are fixed false beliefs that are not consistent with common cultural beliefs and do not shift despite reason or evidence to the contrary. Delusions may include persecutory, somatic, religious, and grandiose themes. Ideas of reference are a specific type of delusion in which the individual believes that an innocuous event has a direct and special personal significance. For example, the individual may believe that an internet news story was written specifically about them or is sending them a special message.

- *Disorganized thought process* can present as illogical thoughts or as thoughts coming too fast or too slow. It can also manifest as a loosening of associations, in which there are unclear connections between thoughts or ideas. This also includes a tangential thought process (thoughts that digress from the original topic and do not return) as well as a circumstantial thought process (circuitous thoughts that digress from the original subject but do eventually return to the original topic). Disorganized thought process can lead to disordered speech in which there is a breakdown of grammatical structure ranging from perseveration on a single word or phrase to word salad, a kind of jumbled nonsense.

- *Disorganized behavior* encompasses a wide spectrum of behavior. It can include unpredictable motor agitation, disinhibition, or difficulty maintaining goal-directed behavior. It also includes behavior that appears unusual or bizarre to onlookers and is not consistent with one's cultural norms. Examples include wearing clothing not appropriate to the weather (e.g., multiple layers of sweaters in the summer or going barefoot in freezing temperatures) or socially inappropriate outbursts.

Negative Symptoms

Negative symptoms can be thought of as the absence of, or reduction in, behaviors or perceptions that are commonly present in others. Negative symptoms may not be as dramatic as positive symptoms of psychosis, and thus they may be less likely to immediately draw the attention of others. Nonetheless, negative symptoms can be equally, if not more, debilitating to the individual and distressing to family members because they frequently lead to social and functional decline. As such, they are an important, although often overlooked, component of psychotic illnesses, particularly schizophrenia. They can manifest in the prodromal period of a primary psychotic disorder and can persist over the course of a lifetime, even as positive symptoms may decrease in intensity.[9] Negative symptoms include the following, often referred to as the "5 A's":

- *Alogia* is poverty of speech, or decreased speech output. It also refers to a lack of spontaneous elaboration in speech, often reflected as single-word responses to questions.
- *Affective blunting* refers to a decreased intensity in emotional expression or reactions, through language, gestures, or facial expression. Although an individual may

indeed endorse a particular mood state such as a depression or happiness, with affective blunting, there is a significantly decreased outward expression of this emotion. In the most extreme, affective flattening refers to a near absence of emotional expression.

- *Anhedonia* is a decreased capacity to experience pleasure or pleasant emotions.
- *Asociality* is defined as a diminished desire to form close relationships with others. This also includes a decreased initiative to engage in social interactions. This can manifest as withdrawal from family, friends, and engagements and even complete social isolation. Individuals may have a decreased ability to read social cues—for example, staring intensely at others, unaware of the discomfort this may cause.
- *Avolition* is decreased motivation and diminished initiation of goal-oriented behavior, including taking medications, procuring food, or maintaining hygiene. This can make maintaining employment or participation in school difficult and can also impact an individual's capacity to attend outpatient case management or mental health care appointments.

What Constitutes a Psychotic Psychiatric Emergency?

There is a wide spectrum in the acuity and severity of psychotic symptoms. Some individuals may experience auditory hallucinations chronically, despite adherence to antipsychotic medications. These individuals may talk or gesture to themselves, responding visibly to the internal stimuli of hallucinations. Other individuals may have paranoia at baseline, voicing persistent concern that their phone has been hacked or that they are being pursued by others. Still others may dress eccentrically and struggle to communicate in a linear or organized fashion.

In each of these examples, the individuals are experiencing symptoms of psychosis. However, simply because an individual is experiencing psychosis—hallucinations, delusions, disorganized thoughts or behavior, or negative symptoms—does not automatically mean that the individual requires acute medical or psychiatric attention. Many people experience psychosis chronically yet are able to care adequately for themselves and function adequately in the community. Although their behavior may be perceived as odd or atypical, this does not necessarily necessitate a visit to the ED or admission to a hospital.

There are certainly instances, however, when psychosis does constitute an emergency. Psychosis is an emergency if the individual is an imminent danger to themself or others or if the individual is unable to care for themself or provide for their basic needs. Furthermore, because psychosis can arise due to multiple organic etiologies, a new onset of psychosis typically requires emergent evaluation and workup. These situations are described in more detail below.

Danger to Self

Individuals with psychotic symptoms have an increased risk of suicidal ideation, suicide attempts, and suicide. Individuals experiencing a major depressive episode with active psychotic features have a twofold risk for suicide attempts compared to those without psychotic features and a 1.21-fold lifetime risk of suicide.[10]

In individuals with schizophrenia, the lifetime risk of dying due to suicide is 5%.[11] Specific risk factors include young age, male gender, and having a higher level of education. Prior suicide attempts, depressed mood, active hallucinations and delusions, and insight into the illness also confer a higher risk. Strikingly, following a hospitalization for first-episode schizophrenia, individuals who do not take a regular antipsychotic medication have a 37-fold increase in dying by suicide.[12]

Even among individuals who may not meet the criteria for a full psychotic disorder but have had psychotic experiences in the past, there are increased odds of suicidal ideation, suicide attempts, and dying by suicide.[13]

Particularly given the statistics presented above, it is imperative that a thorough risk assessment be performed when someone presents to an emergency setting with psychotic symptoms. In general, it is important to directly ask the patient whether they are experiencing thoughts of suicide—including the frequency and intensity of these thoughts—and whether they have a plan or intent to kill themselves currently or have attempted suicide in the past.[14] It is also important to inquire as to whether an individual is having command hallucinations to kill or harm themselves, because they may not "want" to but are being "told" to do so. However, given that individuals with psychosis may be unwilling or unable to provide reliable responses or an accurate history, it is also important to gather collateral information from family, friends, as well as prehospital responders and the patient's outpatient care team when possible to determine safety risk.

If a there is a concern that the patient is an imminent risk to themself—based on the patient's self-reported suicidal ideation, a recent suicide attempt, or collateral information—the patient should not be allowed to leave the ED until the risk evaluation is complete. While in the ED, it is important to prevent the patient from immediate self-harm or a suicide attempt. Steps to do so may include placing the patient in a private room with constant observation by a trained staff member. In addition, it is important to ensure that the immediate environment is safe for the patient. This includes searching the patient, their belongings, and the room for weapons, illicit substances, or bottles of medications that could be used for self-harm. Similarly, ligature risks such as belts, gowns with strings, shoelaces, oxygen tubing, and room-dividing curtains, as well as sharp objects such as scalpels or scissors, should be identified and secured, or removed from the vicinity of the patient.

Danger to Others

Violence in the emergency setting is a common occurrence. Eighty percent of emergency medical services (EMS) personnel report being the victim of physical assault while working in the prehospital setting.[15] More than 50% of ED physicians report having experienced one or more incidents of violence in the workplace,[16] and more than 80% of ED nurses report a physical assault in the workplace during the previous year.[17]

Among those perpetrating assaults in ED, mental illness or substance intoxication was found to be a frequent characteristic.[18] Agitation is a common manifestation in those experiencing psychosis, and it is imperative that it is managed appropriately in an emergency setting in order to reduce the risk to the patient and staff. Agitation is often characterized by restlessness, excessive psychomotor activity, increased verbal activity, and irritability. Individuals can quickly and unpredictably escalate, and although not every patient experiencing agitation is a danger to themself or others, agitation can lead to aggression, placing the patient and others at risk of harm.

In addition to acute agitation, patients, both those experiencing psychosis and those who are not, may experience homicidal thoughts or homicidal ideation. As when assessing for a patient's risk to self, it is important to ask the patient whether they are experiencing thoughts of wanting to harm or kill others and, if so, to further inquire about the intensity and nature of those thoughts, as well as about a plan, intent, and means to do so. Ask about whether the patient is experiencing any command hallucinations to harm others. This differentiates between the "ideation" or desire to harm others and feeling compelled to do so due to psychosis. If a patient says that they are hearing voices telling them to harm others, ask them if they believe they can resist these commands. Some people can and some cannot. Again, it is important to ensure that the physical environment is kept safe as well by placing the agitated patient in a private room under constant observation and by ensuring that the room and the patient's belongings are cleared of items that can be used to inflict harm. The presence of lethal weapons increases the likelihood for violence, and as such it is vital that these are removed from the possession of the patient both in the ED and at their home.

It is important to note, however, that most patients with psychotic symptoms pose little threat to others. Unfortunately, high-profile cases contribute to the stigma that individuals with psychosis are inherently violent. Although this is certainly not true, some studies have found that patients with psychosis are more likely than those in the general population to engage in violent behavior, particularly if there are comorbid substance use disorders, medication nonadherence, or if the individual has been a target of violence themself.[19] Still other studies, however, have found that psychosis is not related to violence.[20] Much of the violence perpetrated by those with psychosis is impulsive and unplanned, often due to the individual feeling threatened in some way, and is not premediated.

Regardless, because agitation can so quickly and abruptly escalate to aggression, it is imperative that agitation be addressed and managed quickly and appropriately in order to not only maintain the safety of others but also reduce the emotional and potentially physical harm to the patient. Indeed, given the importance of rapid and appropriate assessment and management of agitation, several medical societies have developed guidelines and consensus statements for the management of acute agitation.[16,21,22]

These guidelines include the use of verbal de-escalation and nonpharmacologic interventions; medications such as benzodiazepines and antipsychotics; and, when necessary, physical restraints. Some patients with acute agitation can recover rapidly with verbal de-escalation, metabolization of alcohol or substances, or with the administration of a medication. However, others will remain agitated without full resolution for a longer period and will need to either remain under observation in the emergency setting or be admitted to a medical or psychiatric unit following a medical evaluation.

Gravely Disabled

Yet another type of emergency for the patient experiencing psychotic symptoms is grave disability or an inability to care for oneself. This can include an inability to provide oneself with food, clothing, or shelter or to care for one's own medical needs. Grave disability can take many forms. Perhaps the patient is unable to distinguish food items from nonedible items because of significant thought disorganization. Perhaps the patient is not taking their insulin because they hear voices telling them that the medication has been poisoned. Or perhaps the patient has been wandering outside in freezing temperatures, inadequately clothed or without shoes, due to a delusion that they are being followed by a drug cartel or the Federal Bureau of Investigation.

In each of these instances, the patient's psychosis is directly interfering with their capacity to care for their basic needs; as a result, their health, and indeed their life, is at significant risk. Careful medical workup is imperative to reduce morbidity and mortality for these individuals.

New-Onset Psychosis

New acute onset of psychosis constitutes an emergency as well. As discussed in detail later, there are many causes of acute psychosis, ranging from high-risk medical conditions such as infection, metabolic disarray, or trauma to primary psychotic disorders such as schizophrenia. Many of the medical causes of psychosis can lead to significant morbidity and mortality if left undiagnosed and untreated.

The presentation of psychosis in a patient outside of the typical age of onset for a psychotic disorder, as detailed later, or without a prodromal period, previous mood episode, or a family history of a mental disorder should raise particular concern for a medical cause to the psychosis. The American Association for Emergency Psychiatry recommends further medical evaluation (beyond vital signs and a mental status exam) for the following:[23]

- Patients aged 45 years or older with new psychiatric symptoms
- Patients aged 65 years or older
- Evidence of delirium or cognitive deficits
- Patients with physical signs or symptoms that may be consistent with a medical cause of the psychiatric symptoms
- Neurological deficits or head trauma
- Alcohol or substance intoxication or withdrawal
- Decreased level of consciousness
- Other, including abnormal vital signs

However, it is also important to be cognizant that individuals with a preexisting psychiatric disorder can develop a new physical illness (e.g., infection, metabolic disarray, and endocrine abnormalities) that contributes to a worsening or a change in the nature of the psychotic symptoms. Providers should use caution to not anchor to a previous psychiatric diagnosis as a way of explaining all symptoms of psychosis.[24]

Medical Assessment and Management

The ED may be the first point of contact with a medical provider for an individual experiencing psychosis. The patient may walk into the ED of their own accord or at the urging of an outpatient provider, they may be brought to the ED by a concerned family member or friend, or they may be transported from the community via EMS or the police. The presenting symptoms may be varied, ranging from a young adult who is brought in by parents because he has begun to talk to himself to someone with a known history of schizophrenia who has stopped taking medications or an 80-year-old with a new acute onset of psychotic symptoms.

Regardless of the presentation, the first step in the initial management is a rapid safety assessment. It is vital to ensure that the patient is not an imminent danger to self or others. Protecting the safety of the patient, staff, and bystanders is paramount. If it is determined that the patient is an acute danger to self or others, the patient should be placed in a room, free from means to inflict harm, under constant observation.

Patients who are acutely agitated need to be rapidly de-escalated in order to ensure their safety, the safety of those around them, and to allow for a medical evaluation. This initial assessment may entail verbal or nonpharmacologic de-escalation or the administration of sedative–hypnotic or antipsychotic medications or, as a last resort, physical restraints. De-escalation should occur nearly simultaneously with the initial medical assessment of the patient.

Initial Medical Assessment

The initial medical assessment begins, as with all patients presenting to the ED, with a primary survey and a focus on the ABCs of emergency management. Namely, are the patient's airway, breathing, and circulation intact? This evaluation includes vital signs, a glucose finger stick, and an initial rapid diagnostic physical exam. There are multiple causes of acute psychosis, and many of these can be evaluated with the initial emergency assessment. These include the following:[24,25]

Vital sign abnormalities

- Tachycardia—infection, sepsis, hypovolemic shock, thyroid disease, alcohol or benzodiazepine withdrawal, anticholinergic toxicity, sympathomimetic toxicity, serotonin syndrome
- Tachypnea—infection, sepsis, sympathomimetic toxicity
- Hypotension—infection, sepsis, hypovolemic shock
- Hypertension—alcohol or benzodiazepine withdrawal, sympathomimetic toxicity, intracranial abnormality, serotonin syndrome
- Hypothermia—infection, sepsis, intracranial abnormality
- Hyperthermia—infection, sepsis, substance intoxication or overdose, intracranial abnormality, anticholinergic toxicity, serotonin syndrome, neuroleptic malignant syndrome
- Hypoxia—infection, sepsis, substance intoxication or overdose

Glucose finger stick abnormalities

- Abnormal blood glucose—hypoglycemia, diabetic ketoacidosis, hyperglycemic hyperosmolar state

Primary physical survey abnormalities

- Head trauma
- Injury causing significant blood loss

This initial assessment can quickly help narrow the differential for the etiology of the psychosis. The presence of any of the above clearly warrants further medical workup and treatment.

Further Evaluation

Once immediate safety is established and the initial risk and medical assessments are complete, the next step is to triage the patient: Do they require further medical workup or is it appropriate to transition to focus more on a psychiatric etiology of the patient's presenting symptoms? Although a psychiatric etiology is a diagnosis of exclusion after medical etiologies have been thoroughly considered, the differential should be prioritized based on both presenting and historical symptoms. A patient's presentation should be put in the context of known history, although without anchoring to a primary psychiatric diagnosis.

Collecting a History

Collecting an accurate history from a patient who is experiencing acute psychosis can be a challenge. The patient may be internally preoccupied with auditory hallucinations. Paranoia may inhibit the patient from conversing with medical personnel. Thought disorganization may impede the presentation of an accurate history. And trepidation regarding the medical system may decrease the patient's willingness to share personal information in an emergency setting, particularly if they have already experienced marginalization due to race, ethnicity, gender, homelessness, or mental illness.

Although there can certainly be challenges involved with talking to an acutely psychotic patient, there are ways in which this can be a more productive and less upsetting conversation for either party involved. It is important to remain calm and speak slowly in a non-confrontational tone. Do not block doorways but also do not place yourself in the room such that you could not exit rapidly if needed. Maintain a relaxed pose, and consider sitting in a chair or leaning casually against a wall to convey a calm and nonthreatening attitude. Validate the patient's experience of their reality. It is rarely helpful to either challenge the rationality of their beliefs or reinforce any delusional thought content. Assure the patient that they are safe, and attempt to gather information with clear and specific questions. If the patient begins to become distressed or agitated with certain questions, simply change lines of inquiry or politely terminate the interview.

Regardless of whether an accurate, reliable history can be collected from the patient, gathering collateral information from other sources can be useful. Often, the first point of contact with a patient experiencing psychosis occurs in the community when police, EMS, or a mobile crisis team responds to a call from a concerned family member or bystander. In these circumstances, it is important to gather as much information as possible to aid in the evaluation, treatment, and disposition of the patient. For example, the following questions may be asked:

- Where was the patient found?
- What were the circumstances surrounding the call?
- Were there any substances, drug paraphernalia, or empty pill bottles on the patient or in their belongings?

- Were any firearms or other weapons found on the patient or in their home?
- What medications, if any, did the patient receive in route to the hospital?

It can be equally as important to gather collateral information from family members and friends closest to the patient. Jurisdiction and state policies dictate who can be contacted in the event of a psychiatric emergency. Providers in emergency settings should be aware of the local regulations where they practice.

Collateral information from family members or close relationships can be paramount in making an accurate diagnosis. Important information to gather includes the following:

- Did the patient experience a rapid and acute change from baseline?
- Has the patient been complaining of any recent physical symptoms?
- Has the patient been using any substances or alcohol?
- Does the patient have a known psychiatric disorder?
- Have there been any recent medication changes?
- Has the patient experienced recent mood changes, difficulty with sleep, or difficulty caring for their basic needs?
- Has the patient been agitated at home? Have they threatened suicide or homicide?
- Does the patient have access to any weapons?

It may be difficult to talk about psychosis to the patient's family, particularly given the persistent stigma involved with mental illness. When speaking with them, it is important to share that the patient is often not aware that their psychotic symptoms are unusual or concerning; to the patient, their experiences are their reality, and as such, the patient may not be aware that they need to seek help. Often, family or friends may feel guilty for bringing the patient to the attention of medical providers, especially if the patient is upset and resistant to medical care. In these circumstances, recognize the family members' distress and reassure them that they were acting in the patient's best interest. It may be helpful to present potential causes of the psychosis. Be careful not to label the patient with a diagnosis if the diagnosis is at all unclear. If appropriate, explain why further medical workup may be needed and discuss initial treatment approaches.

When possible, accessing the patient's previous medical and behavioral health records may be helpful. The patient's primary care physician, outpatient psychiatrist, or case manager can provide important information about medical and social history, prior and current medication trials, medication allergies or intolerances, and connection to outpatient care. Again, this is all important information as one starts to narrow down the differential diagnosis and consider the first steps in treatment and disposition.

Physical Examination

Following the initial safety assessment, evaluation of the ABCs, and after gathering information from the patient and collateral sources, a thorough physical exam is typically warranted if it can be conducted safely. Not only can the physical exam help elucidate potential medical causes of the patient's psychosis but also individuals with primary psychotic illnesses have higher rates of chronic physical conditions and substance use disorders than the general population.[26] These chronic medical conditions contribute to individuals with schizophrenia living 9–12 years fewer than the general population, and they frequently go undetected by psychiatrists and non-psychiatrist physicians.[27]

A head-to-toe physical exam in the ED may be one of the few that patients with psychosis receive given barriers to accessing medical care and the stigma of mental illness that continues to penetrate even the medical profession. Just as vital sign abnormalities may point to certain etiologies of the patient's psychotic symptoms, so too can physical exam findings.

Routine Laboratory Testing

The utility of routine laboratory testing for patients who present to the ED with psychosis has been debated. Studies have demonstrated little value in routine lab testing for adult patients presenting with psychosis with otherwise no medical complaints or focal findings on the physical exam.[28] The American College of Emergency Physicians (ACEP) clinical policy guidelines provide recommendations that laboratory testing not be ordered routinely on patients presenting with acute psychosis but, rather, should be guided by medical and psychiatric history and physical exam.[29] The clinical policy does note, however, that routine laboratory testing may be beneficial in those at higher risk for disease, including the elderly, those who are immunosuppressed, those who are intoxicated, and those with new-onset psychosis. Although certainly not necessary for all patients presenting with psychotic symptoms, laboratory testing—including complete blood count (CBC), basic metabolic panel, liver function tests, thyroid-stimulating hormone (TSH), urinalysis, and urine toxicologic screen—does indeed have utility at times and can point toward various etiologies of a patient's psychosis.

Routine Head Imaging

For adults with new-onset psychosis but without focal neurological symptoms, ACEP clinical policy guidelines advise that the need for imaging be based on the provider's assessment of patient risk factors.[29] Similarly, National Institute for Health and Care Excellence guidelines do not recommend routine magnetic resonance imagining for patients with new-onset psychosis.[30]

Differential Diagnosis

When encountering someone who is displaying psychotic symptoms, skepticism is crucial. Although early diagnoses of etiology of altered mental status are moderately accurate,[31] it is important not to rush to a diagnosis of a primary psychotic disorder. There are many potential causes of psychotic symptoms. Some people who are experiencing auditory or visual hallucinations may be concerned that they have "gone crazy" or have a permanent psychotic disorder. Families and friends of people experiencing psychotic symptoms may also assume that their loved one has a severe psychiatric illness. Innumerable people have been told they have "schizophrenia" but, in fact, what they have are psychotic symptoms whose etiology has not yet been elucidated. In encountering an individual with psychotic symptoms, be curious and avoid reductive thinking. Even in the absence of other medical causes of psychosis, not everyone who has a brief psychotic episode develops a primary psychotic disorder, and primary brief psychotic episodes account for only 9% of first-episode psychosis.[3]

If you are unsure of the etiology of psychotic symptoms, consider recording in the chart a diagnosis of *unspecified psychotic disorder* or *unspecified psychotic episode*.

Providers can use the *specified psychotic disorder* diagnosis if they proceed to describe distinguishing features—for example, *specified psychotic disorder, intermittent olfactory hallucinations for 3 months*. This requires more work but helps clarify what exactly is occurring, especially if the person is seen again for similar symptoms in the future. If someone has a long-standing, documented diagnosis of schizophrenia, this of course should be recorded as such. However, even if a primary psychotic disorder such as schizophrenia is strongly suspected, for multiple reasons, it is inadvisable to label someone with this in the emergency encounter.

First, emergency encounters are just that—emergencies. People can present very differently during a crisis as opposed to during their day-to-day life and may appear far more psychotic than they actually are. Do not underestimate the power of regression during crises. For example, people with borderline personality disorder can experience some psychotic symptoms during an acute crisis but should not be diagnosed with a primary psychotic illness. Diagnoses with life-changing implications, such as schizophrenia, should be confirmed by providers with longer term relationships with the patient. In the absence of diagnostic "tests" for psychiatric illnesses, restraint is advised in diagnosis in general. Consider diagnosing someone with cancer: Even if a provider is certain something "looks like" cancer, without confirmatory pathology, imaging, and assessment, this diagnosis is withheld until certainty is obtained. The same patience should be exercised in diagnosing someone with a primary psychotic disorder. Another way of documenting a suspected psychotic disorder in the chart is to label it "provisional"—for example, *schizophrenia (provisional)*. This allows the degree of uncertainty to be preserved in the medical record.

Second, if the primary psychotic illness diagnosis later turns out to be incorrect, a patient may have trouble having the original diagnosis removed from their chart. The patient may have been inadvertently and incorrectly labeled with a severe psychotic spectrum illness that can have a lasting impact on future care. Finally, being labeled with a psychotic spectrum disorder can itself be detrimental to the individual being diagnosed. Care is warranted in explaining diagnoses to patients. Consider stating something such as "I suspect you may have a psychotic illness but at this point, but only time will tell. I recommend follow up with a mental health provider." Remember confounders. Marijuana, for example, may be associated with psychosis, but differentiating between a primary psychotic illness and a substance-induced psychosis is difficult as long as the substance continues to be used. Consider telling the patient, "I also recommend that you stop using [e.g.] marijuana to see if that helps your symptoms. It may help you to determine if the [e.g.] marijuana is causing your symptoms or if you are trying to treat your symptoms with the marijuana."

Toxins/Substances

When evaluating someone with psychotic symptoms, immediately consider toxins and substances. According to the fifth edition of the *Diagnostic and Statistical Manual of Mental Disorders* (DSM-5),[3] among those presenting for a first episode of psychosis, between 7% and 25% of cases are due to a substance or medication. Many people take prescribed medications that are known to potentially cause psychosis. These include stimulants such as methylphenidate, cyclosporine, tacrolimus, corticosteroids,[32] and even anticholinergics such as diphenhydramine, among many others.

Although it may be difficult to distinguish whether someone has a primary psychotic disorder while the individual is using substances, one study attempted to separate the two conditions. Fraser et al.[33] found that among young people with first-episode psychosis and concurrent substance use, those who were eventually determined to have a substance-induced psychotic disorder were more likely to have hostility, anxiety, and more insight into their presentation. They also more commonly used marijuana and stimulants and were more likely to have had contact with the legal system or to have had a history of trauma. Those with a primary psychotic disorder were more likely to have had a family history of psychosis. These distinguishing characteristics help suggest whether an individual might be having a substance-induced or primary psychotic episode. Either way, until the substance is stopped, and time unfurls, a definitive diagnosis is impossible.

Sample substances include the following:

- Alcohol withdrawal can lead to alcohol hallucinosis or delirium tremens. In the former, hallucinations occur within 12–24 hours of the last drink. In the latter, hallucinations are part of a more serious constellation of symptoms called delirium tremens that can be fatal and usually occurs approximately 3 days after the last drink.
- Cocaine intoxication can be associated with psychosis, especially tactile hallucinations, classically of bugs on or in the skin, also known as formication.
- Methamphetamine intoxication can cause psychosis including paranoia, delusions, and hallucinations. For some individuals, methamphetamine can also lead to a prolonged psychotic state that lasts long after the acute period of intoxication. This is often referred to as a persistent methamphetamine-induced psychotic disorder.
- LSD and psilocybin famously cause hallucinations. People who have used a considerable amount of LSD may have hallucinogen persisting perception disorder, in which they experience flashbacks or other perceptual disturbances far after the period of use.

Although it is important to test the urine for substances, it is essential to remember that not all psychosis-inducing substances are revealed in a standard or even an extended urine drug screen. Synthetic marijuana, which can cause psychosis, comes in many formulations and is rarely detectable in urine.[34] PCP and ketamine, both of which can cause psychosis, must be tested for specifically.

By contrast, just because someone tests positive for a substance does not mean that the substance is causing the psychosis. For example, there is at least one case of a woman who had peripartum psychosis but also tested positive for methamphetamines, making the etiology of the psychosis unclear.[35] Still others take prescribed medications that can cause false-positive drug-screen results.

Other Medical Conditions

Psychosis can be caused by multiple medical conditions or states. Sometimes psychiatrists or mental health providers call these psychotic disorders due to another medical condition. This is because primary psychotic disorders are also medical conditions. If we were to say "psychosis due to medical condition," this would imply that psychosis itself is not a medical condition. Hence the somewhat confusing terminology.

The possible other medical causes of psychosis are manifold and are more common as people age. By contrast, most, but not all, primary psychotic disorders usually appear in young adulthood to middle age. A selection of other medical causes of psychosis includes the following:

- Psychosis can be due to various neurocognitive disorders.[36] People with dementia can have fully formed visual hallucinations, especially in Lewy body dementia. People with Parkinson's disease can also experience hallucinations, delusions, or other psychotic symptoms. Treating psychosis in those with Parkinson's disease can be particularly challenging due to the fact that antipsychotics further reduce dopamine and can worsen parkinsonism. Quetiapine or clozapine, two atypical antipsychotics with lower antidopaminergic activity, are the preferred antipsychotics in the treatment of psychosis in Parkinson's disease. The American Psychiatric Association provides practice guidelines on the use of antipsychotics to treat agitation in those with dementia.[37]
- Tumors in different parts of the brain, especially frontal meningiomas, can cause psychotic symptoms.
- Hyperthyroidism, particularly thyrotoxicosis, can be associated with psychosis. Given this, it is important to check a TSH level if a patient is having other signs or symptoms of thyroid disease.
- Infections such as meningitis and encephalitis can be associated with psychosis as well. Consider a lumbar puncture if the patient is displaying altered mental status, including psychosis, and any signs or symptoms of infection, an acute onset of symptoms, potential infectious exposure, or risk of infectious disease. Viruses, bacteria, or fungi in the brain or meninges can all cause psychosis.
- Some autoimmune diseases can also cause psychotic symptoms. Limbic encephalitis—for example, anti-NDMA receptor encephalitis—can present with psychotic symptoms or altered mental status, and it should be considered if a patient has any neurological symptoms or if there is an acute onset. The prevalence is considerably higher in females, and particular consideration should be given in young adult and middle-aged women.[38] Systemic lupus erythematosus (SLE) can also be associated with psychotic symptoms when someone is experiencing neuropsychiatric SLE; however, this is fairly uncommon.
- Epilepsy can present with altered mental states and hallucinations, including visual, olfactory, or tactile auras, and should be considered as an etiology of psychosis in anyone with a history of seizure or recurrent transient episodes of the aforementioned. Psychosis can occur in the preictal, ictal, or postictal phases, with postictal being the most common.[3] Importantly, antipsychotics can lower seizure threshold, so caution is important when utilizing these medications in those with epilepsy.[39]
- Even migraine headaches can be associated with visual hallucinations, or scotoma, that may be mistaken for psychosis.

The point to remember is that not all psychosis is due to a primary psychotic disorder. Considering a wide breadth of other medical causes of psychosis is crucial to accurate diagnosis and appropriate treatment. Box 9.1 provides a list of additional conditions that can cause psychosis.

Box 9.1 A Selection of Other Medical Causes of Psychosis

Autoimmune disorders
    Systemic lupus erythematous
    Anti-NDMA receptor encephalitis or other limbic encephalidities
Delirium due to any cause
Electrolyte disturbances
    Severe derangements of calcium, magnesium, potassium, sodium
Endocrine disorders
    Hyper- or hypothyroidism
    Hyper- or hypoparathyroidism
    Hyper- or hypocortisolism
Neoplastic
    Paraneoplastic syndromes
    Brain tumors of all kinds, especially meningiomas in the frontal area
Neurocognitive disorders
    Alzheimer's disease
    Frontotemporal dementia
    Huntington's disease
    Lewy body dementia
    Parkinson's disease
Neurologic
    Central nervous system infections (HIV, syphilis, herpes simplex encephalitis)
    Epilepsy, especially temporal lobe epilepsy
    Migraine
    Multiple sclerosis

Psychiatric Conditions

Mood Disorders

Some mood disorders can have psychotic features. People with major depression can have psychotic symptoms, in which case they are diagnosed with *major depressive disorder with psychotic features*. These psychotic symptoms are typically auditory hallucinations that express the same depressed mood as the individual. For example, the auditory hallucinations may tell the person that they are worthless and might as well die. The psychotic symptoms occur only during the depressive episode, never otherwise.

People with bipolar I disorder have episodes of both mania and depression. They can also have psychotic features associated with their mood episodes. If a person with bipolar disorder experiences psychotic symptoms during a mood episode, they are automatically diagnosed with bipolar I, as opposed to bipolar II, due to the severity of the illness. In bipolar I, the psychotic symptoms tend to be mood congruent and can occur during the manic or depressive phases but can never occur without a mood component. For example, when an individual with bipolar I disorder with psychotic features is in a manic episode, the voices they hear are likely happy or irritable, underscoring the manic mood. By contrast, if the individual is in a depressive episode, the voices they hear are typically depressed and negative in tone.

Schizoaffective disorder, depressive type and *schizoaffective disorder, bipolar type* indicate that the individual sometimes has psychotic symptoms in the absence of mood symptoms, but they do have mood symptoms at times during their illness. For instance, someone with schizoaffective disorder, depressive type has both depression and psychosis, although the psychotic features sometimes occur in the absence of depressive symptoms.

Although this may all sound like semantics, it is important for prognosis and treatment planning. Overall, those with schizoaffective disorder are thought to have a primary psychotic illness, whereas those with major depressive disorder with psychotic features and those with bipolar I with psychotic features are thought to have mood disorders.

Psychotic Disorders

The DSM-5 distinguishes several types of psychotic spectrum illnesses. The classifications are designed to help with ascertaining prognosis and treatment. Schizoaffective disorder, depressive and bipolar types are two of these illnesses. The other psychotic disorders are schizophrenia, schizophreniform disorder, brief psychotic disorder, and delusional disorder.

Schizophrenia

Only 1% of people have schizophrenia, although working in an emergency setting means that this population may be encountered more frequently than in other settings. In summary, individuals with schizophrenia have positive, and also often negative, symptoms of psychosis for a period of at least 6 months. The DSM-5 outlines specific criteria that ensure that schizophrenia is not confused with other psychotic spectrum or mood disorders. It is vital that the diagnosis is appropriately given because it will likely mean a lifetime of treatment.

In order to be diagnosed with schizophrenia, individuals must have at least one positive symptom (hallucinations, delusions, or disorganized speech) and at least two symptoms overall. Many who are ultimately diagnosed with schizophrenia have a preceding social withdrawal, or *prodromal period*, that may initially be attributed to depression or to teenage mood changes. These negative symptoms are in fact prodromal psychotic symptoms. Most men are diagnosed with schizophrenia in their late teens to mid-20s. Women tend to have a later age of onset and are typically diagnosed in their late 20s to 30s. Most individuals with schizophrenia have lifelong symptoms and impairments. These symptoms may plateau, with many reaching a certain level of negative symptoms and cognitive impairment that persists throughout their life span. Conversely, positive symptoms may improve with medication and with age. Some individuals with schizophrenia get progressively worse, and few recover entirely.[3]

Schizophreniform Disorder

Schizophreniform disorder is similar to schizophrenia, but symptoms have not yet lasted more than 6 months. The duration of symptoms is between 1 and 6 months; once an individual has experienced symptoms for more than 6 months, the diagnosis becomes schizophrenia. Symptoms that have lasted less than 1 month may be termed brief psychotic disorder. A diagnosis of schizophreniform disorder also assesses the presence or absence of negative symptoms that are not included in assessment or diagnosis of brief psychotic disorder, possibly because negative symptoms of short duration are fairly common and can be confused with other problems. The reason it is important to distinguish between schizophreniform disorder and schizophrenia is that one-third of people with schizophreniform disorder recover and do not go on to be diagnosed with schizophrenia.[3] This is very important to share with patients and families. Do not rush to a diagnosis of schizophrenia unless you are sure symptoms have been present for at least 6 months.

Brief Psychotic Disorder

Brief psychotic disorder is diagnosed when an individual has at least one positive symptom of psychosis for at least a day but less than 1 month. These episodes may be due to a major life stressor such as loss or trauma and can be qualified as brief psychotic disorder with marked stressors. The psychotic episode cannot be a culturally normed reaction to a stressor. After the episode, the individual returns to their prior level of functioning with no residual symptoms. Brief psychotic disorder is thought to be more common in women than men.[3] The risk of recurrence of brief psychotic disorder is significantly less than the risk of a second episode of schizophrenia after a first.[40]

Delusional Disorder

Delusional disorder is diagnosed when an individual has a delusion, or a fixed false belief, for at least 1 month. The delusion may interfere with one's ability to function well in society, but typically there are no other psychotic symptoms present. Often, there is no evidence of any overt psychosis when the individual is not discussing their delusion; the provider may then be surprised when the individual begins talking about how they are married to the president or that someone has been breaking into their apartment to set up little hairballs. Delusions may seem hypothetically possible but are highly unlikely.

People may have isolated delusions that a celebrity is in love with them, that someone is moving things around in their house, or that they are being gang-stalked, among others. Delusions can be difficult to treat and are not as responsive to antipsychotics compared to other positive psychotic symptoms. Pure delusional disorders are fairly uncommon, with a lifetime prevalence of approximately 0.2%.[3]

Delusion types include the following:

- *Erotomanic*—beliefs that someone, for instance a celebrity, is in love with the affected individual despite evidence to the contrary
- *Grandiose*—beliefs that include a false or overexaggerated sense of one's own greatness
- *Jealous*—usually relating to beliefs that a loved one is cheating on the individual despite all contrary evidence
- *Persecutory*—includes beliefs of being followed or targeted
- *Somatic*—false beliefs regarding one's own bodily functions

Catatonia

Catatonia is a syndrome that is listed in the DSM-5 in the "schizophrenia spectrum and other psychotic disorders" chapter for historical reasons. Individuals with catatonia can appear agitated or extremely withdrawn, and behavior can appear psychotic. They may not eat or drink, stand in odd positions, repeat words or phrases, or stare vacantly. Their behavior appears motiveless. In many ways, catatonia is like delirium; patients can have agitated catatonia or hypoactive catatonia.

Also, like delirium, there is always an etiology to catatonia. Catatonia can be caused by almost any medical disorder, especially ones that cause inflammation such as cancer, head trauma, or central nervous system infections. In those who are medically ill, catatonia is most likely caused by a medical illness and not a psychiatric one, especially if the patient has no prior psychiatric history.[41] Catatonia can also be caused by decompensated schizophrenia or other psychotic disorders, bipolar disorders, or depressive disorders.

In general, the treatment of catatonia, again like delirium, is to address the underlying cause. However, the mainstay of treatment for the symptoms of catatonia is a benzodiazepine. Lorazepam is most used, both for treatment and for diagnostic purposes. If there is a concern for catatonia based on symptoms present, a lorazepam challenge can validate the diagnosis. For the lorazepam challenge, 1 or 2 mg of lorazepam is administered intravenously. If, after 5 minutes, there is no response, a second dose can be administered. A positive response to the challenge is a reduction in catatonic signs and symptoms of at least 50%, usually occurring within 10 minutes of the lorazepam administration.[42]

Zolpidem, memantine, and amantadine are other treatment options.[43] If these medications fail to resolve the catatonic symptoms after the underlying cause has been addressed, the definitive treatment is electroconvulsive therapy (ECT). Unfortunately, antipsychotics can worsen catatonic symptoms, so these medications tend to be held, at least initially, even in those experiencing both psychosis and catatonia. ECT may be an alternative treatment for those with acute decompensated schizophrenia and catatonia. Screening for catatonia and tracking of symptom can be done in various ways. The Bush–Francis Catatonia Rating Scale is most commonly used, but others, such as the DSM-5 catatonia criteria, Rosebush criteria, Barnes criteria, and Lohr criteria, are available as well.

Treatment

The choice of medication depends to an extent on the cause of the psychotic symptoms. For instance, if the psychosis is due to alcohol withdrawal, antipsychotics should largely be avoided because they can mask the symptoms of worsening withdrawal and delay the appropriate treatment; instead, benzodiazepines are the mainstay of treatment for alcohol withdrawal.[44] If delirium is the etiology of the psychotic symptoms, the cause of the delirium needs to be addressed.

First-Generation Antipsychotics

When an antipsychotic is required, the choice of medication is based largely on prior response and side effects to medication trials, as well as on the side effect profile of a particular medication. Of course, patient preference regarding medication choice should be honored whenever possible.

First-generation or "typical" antipsychotics have antagonism at several different types of receptors, including (1) D_2 dopamine receptors in the nigrostriatal system, (2) H_1 histamine receptors, (3) α_1 norepinephrine receptors, and (4) M_1 muscarinic receptors.[45]

The activity at these receptors leads to both the acute and the chronic side effects of the first-generation antipsychotics.

Dopamine antagonism can lead to extrapyramidal symptoms (EPS) or medication-induced movement disorders. These include akathisia or a sense of uncomfortable motor restlessness; acute dystonia or involuntary muscle contractions; and parkinsonism or symptoms resembling those of Parkinson's disease, such as tremor, rigidity, and slowed movements. Chronically, antagonism at the dopamine receptors can lead to tardive dyskinesia or involuntary movements of various muscles, including orofacial, tongue, truncal, and extremity muscles. Antagonist activity at H_1 histamine receptors can lead to sedation and weight gain, whereas activity at α_1 norepinephrine receptors can cause hypotension. Antagonistic binding of M_1 muscarinic receptors can contribute to constipation, urinary retention, dry mouth, blurred vision, and mental slowing.

Administration of antipsychotic medication may also lead to neuroleptic malignant syndrome (NMS). NMS is a rare but critical complication related to antipsychotic administration, with a prevalence of approximately 1 case per 1,000 people. The mortality rate is as high as 10%.[46] Primary symptoms of NMS include severe muscle rigidity, hyperpyrexia, altered mental status, and autonomic instability. Abnormal lab values associated with NMS include leukocytosis and elevated creatine phosphokinase typically greater than 1,000 IU/L.

Although the exact etiology remains unknown, potential causes of NMS include dopaminergic D_2 blockade and a toxicity on musculoskeletal fibers.[46] Risk factors for NMS include recent initiation or dose change, high doses, as well as intramuscular or intravenous administration of antipsychotic medications. Other risk factors include high-potency first-generation antipsychotics and concurrent use of more than one antipsychotic. If NMS is suspected, antipsychotic medication should immediately be discontinued; supportive management to reduce fever, manage autonomic lability, and correct electrolyte imbalances should be initiated. Other treatment options include dantrolene, bromocriptine, and ECT.

In general, the higher the potency or affinity for the D_2 receptor, the higher the risk for EPS as well as NMS. Conversely, the lower potency antipsychotics have a lower risk for EPS and NMS, but they a higher risk of sedation and hypotension. Commonly used first-generation antipsychotics, their relative potency, side effect profile, and typical daily dosing are presented in Table 9.1.

Second-Generation Antipsychotics

Second-generation or "atypical" antipsychotics act as both dopaminergic antagonists, with varying degrees of affinity for the D_2 receptor, and serotonergic $5HT_{2A}$ antagonists. The atypical antipsychotic aripiprazole, sometimes considered a third-generation antipsychotic, acts as a D_2 receptor partial agonist. Like first-generation antipsychotics, atypical antipsychotics additionally are antagonists at H_1 histamine receptors, α_1 norepinephrine receptors, and M_1 muscarinic receptors, all of which contribute to side effects.

Generally, the atypical antipsychotics have significantly lower risk of EPS compared to typical antipsychotics. However, atypical antipsychotics are associated with higher rates of metabolic side effects, including weight gain, dyslipidemia, cardiovascular disease, and diabetes. Due to antagonism at the H_1, α_1, and M_1 receptors, side effects such as sedation, hypotension, constipation, and urinary retention may also be present at varying

Table 9.1 First-Generation Antipsychotic Side Effect Profile and Typical Dosing

Drug	Potency	Sedation	Hypotension	EPS	Average Daily Dose (mg)	Acute Agitation Dosing (mg)
Fluphenazine (Prolixin)	High	+	+	+++	2–12	—
Haloperidol (Haldol)	High	+	+	+++	2–20	PO: 2–10 q6h prn, max 30/day IM: 2–10 q15min–q2h prn, max 20/day
Perphenazine (Trilafon)	Mid	++	+	++	12–24	—
Loxapine (Loxatine)	Mid	++	+	++	20–80	—
Chlorpromazine (Thorazine)	Low	+++	+++	+	400–600	IM: 25 × 1, then 25–50 q4–6h prn, max 200/day

EPS, extrapyramidal symptoms; IM, intramuscular.

Sources: Cohen[45] and Jibson.[47]

degrees for the different antipsychotics. Table 9.2 presents commonly used atypical antipsychotics, common side effects, and average daily dosing.

Clozapine

Clozapine was the first atypical antipsychotic formulated, and there are special considerations associated with this medication. Clozapine has been found to be superior to other first- and second-generation antipsychotics for treatment-resistant schizophrenia.[48] It has also been shown to reduce the risk of suicidal behavioral in individuals with schizophrenia or schizoaffective disorder. However, clozapine has multiple serious side effects, including agranulocytosis, myocarditis, bowel obstruction, and seizures, as well as orthostatic hypotension. Due particularly to the risk of severe neutropenia, there are restrictions for prescribing clozapine. Specifically, it is part of a Risk Evaluation Mitigation Strategy (REMS) program, which requires regular monitoring of the absolute neutrophil count (ANC).

If, in an emergency setting, a patient is found to be taking clozapine at home, it is important to confirm the dose as well as when the patient took the last dose, either with the patient, family members, or outpatient provider. A CBC with differential should also be checked. If dosing has been interrupted for more than 48 hours, clozapine will need to be re-titrated, starting again at 12.5 or 25 mg daily, to reduce the risk of hypotension, bradycardia, and syncope. During this titration period, the patient may need an additional antipsychotic in order to control their symptoms of psychosis. If dosing has been interrupted for fewer than 2 days, clozapine can be reinitiated at the prior home dose, after ensuring that the ANC is ≥1,500/mm^3. Note that there are different values for those with benign ethnic neutropenia, and the most up-to-date ANC values can be found on the Clozapine REMS website (https://www.newclozapinerems.com/home#).

Table 9.2 Atypical Antipsychotic Side Effect Profile and Typical Dosing

Drug	Metabolic Risk	Sedation	Average Daily Dose (mg)	Acute Agitation Dosing (mg)
Aripiprazole (Abilify)	Low	+	10–30	—
Ziprasidone (Geodon)	Low	++	80–160	IM: 10 q2h or 20 q4h, max 40/day
Risperidone (Risperdal)	Moderate	++	2–8	PO: 1–2 q2h, max 6/day
Paliperidone (Invega)	Moderate	++	6–12	—
Quetiapine (Seroquel)	Moderate	+++	400–900	—
Olanzapine (Zyprexa)	High	+++	10–30	PO: 5–10 q2h, max 30/day IM: 5–10 q2-4h, max 30/day
Clozapine (Clozaril)	High	+++	150–900	—

IM, intramuscular.
Sources: Cohen[45] and Jibson.[47]

Side Effect Medications

Given the side effects associated with typical and atypical antipsychotic medications, it is important to also be aware of medications to target these iatrogenic symptoms. Particularly important are anticholinergic medications such as benztropine. Anticholinergics specifically target parkinsonism, as well as other forms of EPS. Akathisia is one type of EPS that does not respond as readily to an anticholinergic medication. Instead, it tends to respond better to the addition of a β-blocker, such as propranolol, or a benzodiazepine. Acute dystonia can be treated with the administration of either an anticholinergic or an antihistaminergic medication such as diphenhydramine. Frequently, benztropine or diphenhydramine is administered concurrently with a typical antipsychotic medication, particularly when administered in an intramuscular formulation, in order to prevent acute dystonia. There are also medications, such as valbenazine, that have been approved by the U.S. Food and Drug Administration for the treatment of tardive dyskinesia.

Adjunctive Treatment Strategies

Although medication tends to be the mainstay of treatment for acute agitation and psychosis in an emergency setting, psychosocial interventions are an important adjunctive treatment for a primary psychotic disorder such as schizophrenia, in an inpatient as well as community setting.[49] Among the evidence-based interventions is cognitive–behavioral therapy, which has been shown to reduce both positive and negative symptoms and to improve overall functioning in individuals with schizophrenia. Additional psychosocial interventions include family psychoeducation; substance use disorder (SUD) treatment for comorbid SUDs; weight management; and assertive community treatment programs, which provide psychiatric services, case management, and out-reach to the individual in the community.

Conclusion

Medical assessment, acute stabilization, and determination of disposition are paramount when an individual experiencing psychotic symptoms presents to an ED. Emergency providers and staff are often the first point of contact with the medical system, particularly for those with new-onset psychosis. They can additionally serve an important role in connecting patients with psychotic disorders to outpatient treatment, not only to behavioral health services but also to a primary care physician, which is particularly important given the common comorbid medical conditions. The process of excellent medical care as well as psychoeducation and support to both patients and family members can also occur in the ED and may in fact form the foundation of patients' future relationship with behavioral health providers and the medical system as a whole.

References

1. Mental illness. National Institute of Mental Health. Published 2019. Accessed February 16, 2020. https://www-nimh-nih-gov.proxy.hsl.ucdenver.edu/health/statistics/mental-illness.shtml

2. Mental health by the numbers. National Alliance on Mental Illness. Published 2019. Accessed February 16, 2020. https://www.nami.org/mhstats

3. American Psychiatric Association. *Diagnostic and Statistical Manual of Mental Disorders*. 5th ed. American Psychiatric Publishing; 2013.

4. Linscott RJ, van Os J. An updated and conservative systematic review and meta-analysis of epidemiological evidence on psychotic experiences in children and adults: On the pathway from proneness to persistence to dimensional expression across mental disorders. *Psychol Med*. 2013;43(6):1133–1149.

5. Hooker EA, Mallow PJ, Oglesby MM. Characteristics and trends of emergency department visits in the United States (2010–2014). *J Emerg Med*. 2019;56(3):344–351.

6. Theriault K, Rosenheck R, Rhee T. Increasing emergency department visits for mental health conditions in the United States. *J Clin Psychiatry*. 2020;81(5):20m13241 .

7. Peltzer-Jones J, Nordstrom K, Currier G, Berlin JS, Singh C, Schneider S. A research agenda for assessment and management of psychosis in emergency department patients. *West J Emerg Med*. 2019;20(2):403–408.

8. Stahl S, Munter N. *Stahl's Essential Psychopharmacology*. 4th ed. Cambridge University Press; 2013.

9. Sauve G, Brodeur M, Shah J, Lepage M. The prevalence of negative symptoms across the stages of the psychosis continuum. *Harv Rev Psychiatry*. 2019;27(1):15–32.

10. Gournellis R, Tournikioti K, Touloumi G, et al. Psychotic (delusional) depression and completed suicide: A systematic review and meta-analysis. *Ann Gen Psychiatry*. 2018;17:39–39.

11. Hor K, Taylor M. Suicide and schizophrenia: A systematic review of rates and risk factors. *J Psychopharmacol*. 2010;24(4 Suppl):81–90.

12. Tiihonen J, Wahlbeck K, Lönnqvist J, et al. Effectiveness of antipsychotic treatments in a nationwide cohort of patients in community care after first hospitalisation due to schizophrenia and schizoaffective disorder: Observational follow-up study. *BMJ*. 2006;333(7561):224.

13. Yates K, Lång U, Cederlöf M, et al. Association of psychotic experiences with subsequent risk of suicidal ideation, suicide attempts, and suicide deaths: A systematic review and meta-analysis of longitudinal population studies. *JAMA Psychiatry*. 2019;76(2):180–189.

14. Betz M, Boudreaux E. Managing suicidal patients in the emergency department. *Ann Emerg Med*. 2016;67:276–282.

15. Furin M, Eliseo L, Langlois B, et al. Self-reported provider safety in an urban emergency medical system. *West J Emerg Med*. 2015;16(3):459-464.

16. Roppolo LP, Morris DW, Khan F, et al. Improving the management of acutely agitated patients in the emergency department through implementation of Project BETA (Best Practices in the Evaluation and Treatment of Agitation). *J Am Coll Emerg Physicians Open*. 2020;1(5):898–907.

17. Phillips J. Workplace violence against health care workers in the United States. *N Engl J Med*. 2016;374:1661–1669.

18. Pompeii L, Dement J, Schoenfisch A, et al. Perpetrator, worker and workplace characteristics associated with patient and visitor perpetrated violence (Type II) on hospital workers: A review of the literature and existing occupational injury data. *J Saf Res*. 2013;44:57–64.

19. Volavka J. Triggering violence in psychosis. *JAMA Psychiatry*. 2016;73(8):769–770.

20. Douglas K, Guy L, Hart S. Psychosis as a risk factor for violence to others: A meta-analysis. *Psychol Bull*. 2009;135(5):679–706.

21. Wilson MP, Pepper D, Currier GW, Holloman GH Jr, Feifel D. The psychopharmacology of agitation: Consensus statement of the American Association for Emergency Psychiatry Project Beta Psychopharmacology Workgroup. *West J Emerg Med*. 2012;13(1):26–34.

22. Zeller S, Citrome L. Managing agitation associated with schizophrenia and bipolar disorder in the emergency setting. *West J Emerg Med*. 2015;17(2):165–172.

23. Wilson M, Nordstrom K, Anderson E, et al. American Association for Emergency Psychiatry Task Force on Medical Clearance of Adult Psychiatric Patients. Part II: Controversies over medical assessment, and consensus recommendations. *West J Emerg Med*. 2017;18(4):640–646.

24. McKee J, Brahm N. Medical mimics: Differential diagnostic considerations for psychiatric symptoms. *Ment Health Clin*. 2016;6(6):289–296.

25. Griswold KS, Del Regno PA, Berger RC. Recognition and differential diagnosis of psychosis in primary care. *Am Fam Physician*. 2015;91(12):856–863.

26. Šprah L, Dernovšek MZ, Wahlbeck K, Haaramo P. Psychiatric readmissions and their association with physical comorbidity: A systematic literature review. *BMC Psychiatry*. 2017;17(1):2.

27. Lambert T, Velakoulis D, Pantelis C. Medical comorbidity in schizophrenia. *Med J Aust*. 2003;178:S67–S70.

28. Parmar P, Goolsby CA, Udompanyanan K, Matesick LD, Burgamy KP, Mower WR. Value of mandatory screening studies in emergency department patients cleared for psychiatric admission. *West J Emerg Med*. 2012;13(5):388–393.

29. Brown MD, Byyny R, Diercks DB, et al. Clinical policy: Critical issues in the diagnosis and management of the adult psychiatric patient in the emergency department. *Ann Emerg Med*. 2017;69(4):480–498.

30. Borgwardt S, Schmidt A. Implementing magnetic resonance imaging into clinical routine screening in patients with psychosis. *Br J Psychiatry*. 2018;211(4):192–193.

31. Sporer K, Solares M, Durant E, Wang W, Wu A, Rodriguez R. Accuracy of the initial diagnosis among patients with an acutely altered mental status. *Emerg Med J*. 2013;30:243–246.

32. Corbett B, Nordstrom K, Vilke G, Wilson M. Psychiatric emergencies for clinicians: Emergency department diagnosis and management of steroid psychosis. *J Emerg Med*. 2016;51(5):557–560.

33. Fraser S, Hides L, Philips L, Proctor D, Lubman D. Differentiating first episode substance induced and primary psychotic disorders with concurrent substance use in young people. *Schizophr Res*. 2012;136:110–115.

34. Skryabin V, Vinnikova M. Clinical characteristics of synthetic cannabinoid-induced psychotic disorders: A single-center analysis of hospitalized patients. *J Addict Dis*. 2018;37(3–4):135–141.

35. Zaydlin M, Tamargo C. Organic vs stimulant-induced psychosis in the peripartum period. *Cureus*. 2020;12(9):e10718.

36. Kales H, Gitlin L, Lyketsos C. Assessment and management of behavioral and psychological symptoms of dementia. *BMJ*. 2015;350:h369.

37. Reus V, Fochtmann L, Eyler A, et al. The American Psychiatric Association practice guideline on the use of antipsychotics to treat agitation or psychosis in patients with dementia. *Am J Psychiatry*. 2016;173(5):543–546.

38. Kayser M, Kohler C, Dalmau J. Psychiatric manifestations of paraneoplastic disorders. *Am J Psychiatry*. 2010;167(9):1039–1050.

39. Kanner A. Management of psychiatric and neurological comorbidities in epilepsy. *Nat Rev Neurol*. 2016;12(2):106–116.

40. Fusar-Poli P, Cappucciati M, Bonoldi I, Hui M, Rutigliano G, Stahl D. Prognosis of brief psychotic episodes: A meta-analysis. *JAMA Psychiatry*. 2016;73(3):211–220.

41. Oldham M. The probability that catatonia in the hospital has a medical cause and the relative proportions of its causes: A systematic review. *Psychosomatics*. 2018;59(4):333–340.

42. Sienaert P, Dhossche DM, Vancampfort D, De Hert M, Gazdag G. A clinical review of the treatment of catatonia. *Front Psychiatry*. 2014;5:181–181.

43. Beach S, Gomez-Berna F, Huffman J, Fricchione G. Alternative treatment strategies for catatonia: A systematic review. *Gen Hosp Psychiatry*. 2017;48:1–19.

44. Wolf C, Curry A, Nacht J, Simpson S. Management of alcohol withdrawal in the emergency department: Current perspectives. *Open Access Emerg Med*. 2020;12:53–65.

45. Cohen B. *Theory and Practice of Psychiatry*. Oxford University Press; 2003.

46. Tse L, Barr AM, Scarapicchia V, Vila-Rodriguez F. Neuroleptic malignant syndrome: A review from a clinically oriented perspective. *Curr Neuropharmacol*. 2015;13(3):395–406.

47. Jibson M. First generation antipsychotic medications. UpToDate. Published 2021. https://www.uptodate.com/contents/first-generation-antipsychotic-medications-pharmacology-administration-and-comparative-side-effects#!

48. Asenjo Lobos C, Komossa K, Rummel-Kluge C, et al. Clozapine versus other atypical antipsychotics for schizophrenia. *Cochrane Database Syst Rev*. 2010;2010(11):CD006633.

49. Dixon LB, Dickerson F, Bellack AS, et al. The 2009 schizophrenia PORT psychosocial treatment recommendations and summary statements. *Schizophr Bull*. 2010;36(1):48–70.

10

Emergency Psychiatry Evaluation and Treatment of Mood Disorders

Katherine Maloy

Prevalence and Comorbidity of Mood Disorders in the Emergency Department

Mood-related complaints are among the most common reasons for presentation to an emergency psychiatric setting, along with anxiety disorders and substance-related disorders.[1] Mood disorders, particularly depression, are highly prevalent and highly comorbid with both medical disorders and substance use disorders. Based on Substance Abuse and Mental Health Services data, the 12-month prevalence of major depressive disorder in 2017 was estimated to be 7.1% for adults and 13.3% for adolescents.[2] The rate of visits to the emergency department (ED) for depression increased more than 25% from 2006 to 2014.[3] Although we frequently think of a depressed patient in the ED presenting because of the primary issue of a suicide attempt or suicidal ideation, depression is frequently comorbid with or underlies non-psychiatric ED presentations. A 2012 review of the National Hospital Ambulatory Medical Care Survey estimated that depression-related visits accounted for 2% of all ED visits and that approximately 59% of all depression-related visits were not associated with suicidal ideation or self-harm.[3] Bipolar disorder is less prevalent than depression but not insignificant: A 2016 review showed a 12-month population prevalence of 1.5% for bipolar I and lifetime prevalence of 2%.[4]

Depression is frequently hiding in plain sight. A 2012 study in which patients presenting to the ED with non-psychiatric complaints using a screening tool (the Mini-International Neuropsychiatric Interview) found the most common diagnoses for patients screening positive for a mental illness were major depression (24%), general anxiety (9%), and drug abuse (8%).[5] In 2008, a prospective observational study in two EDs used criteria from the fourth edition of the *Diagnostic and Statistical Manual of Mental Disorders* (DSM) and found a prevalence of 21.6% of depressive symptoms in 505 patients screened.[6]

Mood disorders are also highly associated with increased suicide risk, and many fewer people are able to access and receive adequate care for their mood disorder than suffer from clinically significant symptoms. According to a 2019 review of National Epidemiologic Survey data, two-thirds of people with major depressive disorder had no treatment in the last 12 months, and that increased to three-fourths of patients who lacked insurance coverage.[7] As is the case with other chronic illnesses, lack of outpatient follow-up—whether due to financial barriers, shortages of available treatment facilities, or stigma—can cause increased morbidity and can lead to unnecessary or avoidable ED presentations. Long wait times to access outpatient care may also lead to patients presenting to the ED because they simply cannot wait weeks or months to start treatment.

Mood disorders can also be difficult to diagnose definitively in the hyperacute setting of the ED, which provides only a single snapshot of a patient's symptoms. In geriatric patients, for example, comorbid medical illness leading to delirium or undiagnosed cognitive decline may present as behavioral change, disinhibition, or apathy that may lead to a psychiatric referral for someone who needs a more thorough medical or neurologic workup. Even in younger populations, drug intoxication or the early stages of an acute autoimmune encephalitis may be difficult to distinguish from a new onset of mania. Further complicating the ED's ability to manage these issues is that in the absence of acute dangerousness leading to the patient requiring emergency inpatient admission or monitoring, referral to immediate aftercare may not be readily available. In the absence of immediate referral to aftercare, the emergency psychiatric clinician may be reluctant to initiate pharmacologic treatment that may not be followed up.

Mood disorders are, however, highly treatable, particularly if recognized early and if the patient is able to be engaged in the importance of follow-up. Recognizing a mood disorder and providing psychoeducation and referral may be an opportunity for the emergency clinician to have a profound positive impact on the future course of a patient's interaction with mental health services and the prognosis of their illness. A positive therapeutic interaction in the ED, even if brief or part of a single visit, can set the stage for engagement in longer term treatment that has the potential to greatly improve the course of illness.

Depression

Depression is highly prevalent and causes a great deal of collateral morbidity, including lost days of work, impact on care of dependent children, increased risk of suicide, co-morbidity of substance use disorders, and poorer outcomes of major medical illnesses. A 2015 study of patients presenting to a major academic medical center ED enrolled 999 patients, of which 27% screened positive for major depressive disorder, which then conveyed a 61% increase in the rate of ED visits, as well as a 2.5-fold increase in rate of hospitalization.[8] Patients may present to the ED for depression because they are acutely in crisis, have nowhere else to seek care, or have presented for some other medical issue as their first priority. The chief complaint, however, of "I am depressed," although a common reason for emergency psychiatric consultation, is not particularly specific in terms of a diagnosis or prognosis. Although depressed mood and/or anhedonia (loss of interest or pleasure in life) are necessary diagnostic criteria for a depressive episode, a diagnosis of a depressive episode requires additional information and the ruling out of associated medical conditions.

Case Example

Mr. M is a 42-year-old man, employed as a truck driver, who presents to the ED with worsening headaches during the past several months. Today, he left work due to the headache, which is not associated with any other neurologic symptoms. He was told to be medically evaluated before returning to work, so he presented to the emergency room. When discussing his symptoms, he spontaneously reports multiple ongoing stressors, including marital and financial difficulties. His headache remits with a dose of naproxen and Imitrex, but he also reports multiple other complaints, including diffuse musculoskeletal pain, fatigue, reduced exercise tolerance, and poor appetite. He has screened positive on routine questions administered on triage, noting depressed mood, anhedonia, and occasional passive suicidal thoughts. Due to difficulty sleeping, he has been drinking a few glasses of whiskey at bedtime for the past several months. He feels guilty about his financial issues and ruminates at night about possibly losing his house. He is obese and has a large, short, neck; his wife has stopped sleeping in bed with him because of his snoring. He becomes suddenly tearful, then ashamed, when asked about suicidal thoughts, immediately brushing off the doctor, stating "I'm fine, really" and then asking for discharge and a letter for the company at which he works to inform it that he is safe to return to work. His random glucose is 134, so additional labs are ordered. He refuses to provide a sample for urinalysis, expressing concern over who would see the results, alluding to marijuana use as recommended by a friend for his "chronic pain issues." Mr. M is referred to see the ED social worker, who is tasked with referring him to outpatient psychiatric care. He scoffs at this idea and becomes angry that he might have to stay longer to speak with a psychiatrist. "I just filled out that paperwork wrong, I didn't understand it," he states, when asked about his answers on the initial screening questionnaire. "I'll just see my doctor next week, I promise."

Mr. M's presentation is designed to highlight the difficulties in reaching a diagnosis and obstacles to initiating treatment. There are multiple factors that could be contributing to Mr. M's low mood. He could have an "organic" cause to his physical complaints—migraine, tension headache, arthritic or musculoskeletal process leading to his body pain, and undiagnosed sleep apnea. He may meet criteria for an alcohol use disorder, given his daily intake of liquor is more than what would be considered the threshold for problematic alcohol use. His marijuana use for pain may be worsening apathy and social withdrawal. Even if Mr. M could be diagnosed as meeting criteria for clinical depression, is this a true depressive episode or are his marital and financial difficulties causing stress that would better describe his condition as an adjustment disorder? Given all of the factors above, and his clear affective reaction to discussion of suicidality, does he warrant further evaluation? What are his risk factors for suicide?

Mr. M also illustrates some of the frustration of trying to sort out these issues in the ED. Does he warrant being forced to stay longer for a more detailed psychiatric consultation, if one is even available? Should he have more thorough medical studies before he leaves? Should someone be contacted for collateral information to assess his risk more thoroughly? What kind of "routine" screening can or should be done at intake to a medical visit? Even if he was clearly meeting criteria for a depressive episode, would it be safe to start any medication given how much he is drinking at home? Is he in fact "safe" to return to work?

Diagnostic Criteria and Clinical Presentation

The diagnosis of major depressive disorder, as per DSM-5 criteria, requires at least 2 weeks of at least five of the criteria symptoms occurring nearly every day, with at least one being prominent depressed mood or anhedonia (loss of interest or pleasure in activities). Depressed mood (i.e., a person appears constantly dysphoric or tearful but does not identify feeling "depressed") may be self-reported or reported by others. The criteria symptoms other than depressed mood and anhedonia include significant change in appetite; disruption of sleep (insomnia or hypersomnia); fatigue or loss of energy; feelings of worthlessness or excessive guilt; diminished ability to think, concentrate, or make decisions; persistent thoughts of death or suicide; and psychomotor agitation or retardation.[9] Many people do not immediately present to treatment; thus, patients may have trouble specifying an exact 2 weeks duration, but timing is important in ruling out an acute dysregulation of mood caused by an acute stressor. Particularly in patients with chronic personality pathology or problems with affective regulation, rapid swings of mood over a period of a few hours or a few days may be difficult to distinguish from a depressive episode without getting a detailed time frame. It is unlikely to have a full-blown depressive episode of only a few hours or days duration, for example, and would be reasonable to manage such a short, acute mood disruption with supportive treatment rather than changing or initiating medications. An acute disruption of a relationship, perceived abandonment, or other interpersonal dispute may precipitate feelings of low mood that are very intense but brief and temporally related to the stressor itself. This is not to minimize the risk of self-harm or suicide attempt in an acutely dysregulated patient with an acute stressor, but the treatment approach may be different. Similarly, patients experiencing major depressive episodes are frequently overdiagnosed with personality pathology and may exhibit poor coping strategies or a negativistic attitude that dissipates when the acute episode is adequately treated. Collateral from providers and family or friends about the longitudinal course of the patient's symptoms and their behaviors can therefore be essential in assessing risk, and it can also clarify whether the presentation represents an acute episode or a lifelong pattern of poor coping and mood regulation.

Depression as a symptom is also frequently cited by patients with other psychiatric disorders, including psychosis, and depression itself can of course be accompanied by psychotic symptoms. Patients with psychosis may become depressed by their delusions or hallucinations, or they may experience apathy and inability to engage with the world as depression. Patients with post-traumatic stress disorder (PTSD) frequently experience emotional numbing, depressed or irritable mood, or suffer from a comorbid depressive disorder. Screening for a trauma history or prior episodes of psychosis and whether they are associated with mood symptoms can help clarify some of these diagnostic issues.

In general, patients with major depressive disorder with psychotic features experience mood-congruent psychotic symptoms that have a depressive feel to them, although DSM-5 does permit for a specifier of "mood-incongruent psychotic features." Typical mood-congruent depressive psychosis symptoms include the patient believing they are unloved, that friends and family have given up on them, that they are dying or severely ill, their body has stopped working, or even more frank paranoia that people are after them or they have made some kind of grave or unforgivable mistake. A psychotic level of ambivalence, with inability to make even simple decisions or carry out simple tasks, may be an indicator of more significant psychosis developing. Delusions can be difficult to elicit because they are associated with a great deal of shame and guilt. Even without frank delusions, many depressed patients suffer from cognitive distortions that can contribute to suicide risk and may sound very plausible. The depressed person, for example, who believes that nobody cares about them and that everyone is disappointed in them may be surprised or disbelieving when they learn that their spouse is worried about them and is not in fact planning to leave them or angry at them about some kind of perceived transgression. In summary, the clinical assessment should investigate the possibility of psychosis and cognitive distortion in all patients presenting to the ED with mood symptoms, in a manner that is open and non-stigmatizing. Collateral from friends, family, or treaters can also help clarify both the time frame and the overall course of symptoms, as well as the veracity of depressive cognitions.

Anxiety and depression are highly comorbid, and the presence of symptoms such as panic attacks can increase risk of suicide attempts. The 2015 World Health Organization survey reported that 45.7% of individuals with lifetime major depressive disorder had a lifetime history of one or more anxiety disorders.[10] The highly anxious person presenting to the ED may have a comorbid depressive episode, and the person with a highly anxious depressive episode is at increased risk for poor prognosis and comorbid substance abuse. Depressive episodes with anxious features can present with subjective feelings of agitation, insomnia, and hypervigilance that are intensely distressing.

Risk Assessment

As mentioned above, cognitive distortion or psychosis can worsen suicidality, in that it provides a framework for the patient to believe the world is better off without them. Psychosis can also be very frightening in itself. Comorbid substance use also increases risk, due to both disinhibition of behavior and worsening of mood symptoms caused by the substance itself. History of prior attempts is important to consider, particularly a pattern of escalating lethality or high-risk past attempts. Static epidemiologic risk factors for suicide not unique to depression include age, gender, race or ethnicity, and religion, with higher risk in Whites, men, those older than age 65 years, those with a family history of mental illness, and those with prior suicide attempts.[11] Higher risk was also associated with being separated or divorced and lack of access to social support.[12] Access to firearms is a potentially modifiable risk factor, as well as social support and access to treatment. Comorbid anxiety symptoms also increase the risk of suicide in the depressed patient, as do hopelessness and drug use.[13] Other risk factors that should be considered in the assessment, but should not be treated as definitive evidence of suicide risk, include the presence or absence of a plan and the lethality of that plan. It is important to remember that there is no one screening tool that can ascribe certainty to a prediction regarding suicidality in any psychiatric disorder, including depression. The ability to "contract for safety," in which a patient is asked if they can "promise" that they will not act on suicidal thoughts or feelings, is not a reliable predictor of safety and should not be routinely used either in clinical documentation or as a method of clinical assessment of risk.

Special Populations

Pediatric psychiatric emergencies are discussed in Chapter 15, but in general, children and adolescents may have a more atypical presentation of depressive symptoms, with prominent irritability as opposed to neurovegetative symptoms. Children also may express their symptoms somatically, such as complaints of stomachaches, headaches, or school avoidance due to feeling ill.

Post-/peripartum psychiatric emergencies are discussed Chapter 18, but clinicians should be alert to depression during pregnancy and in the postpartum period. Mood and anxiety symptoms are associated with a great deal of shame and stigma because the pregnant patient is expected to be happy and preparing joyfully for birth. It is important for providers to actively seek out information about pregnant and postpartum patients' mood and not assume that it will be volunteered. Pregnant and nursing patients also may hide symptoms due to fear of medication treatment and its potential complications.

Geriatrics is discussed in more detail in Chapter 16, but it is important to remember that elderly patients with depression typically have a higher rate of melancholic presentations. They may show neurovegetative slowing, "pseudodementia" or cognitive impairment related to poor effort on memory testing, poor oral intake, and social withdrawal. It can be very difficult to determine a clear etiology of depression versus a dementing process in an elderly, slowed, withdrawn patient who is having difficulty attending to a mini-mental exam without collateral input from family or providers who know them well. The presence of psychosis can be even more difficult to distinguish between a dementing process and an acute mood episode.[14] In addition, antidepressants are more likely to cause complications such as the syndrome of inappropriate antidiuretic hormone secretion, hypotension, or falls in the elderly. ED providers may also be more reluctant to ask elderly patients about substance abuse. Careful consideration of medical comorbidity is very important in this population.

Comorbidity: Substance Use Disorders and Medical Issues

Probably the most significant confounding factor in the emergency evaluation of mood disorder is the influence of substances. Apart from the specific effects of each substance, the course of addiction can be financially and personally devastating, causing estrangement from family and other sources of support. Although the term "self-medication" is overused and oversimplified, many patients with heavy substance use do have some comorbid mood or anxiety disorder. Substance abuse complicates the treatment of those disorders and makes accessing care more difficult because providers may be reluctant to take on the patient with a comorbid substance use disorder, and substance abuse–specific programs may be reluctant or unable to provide pharmacotherapy for mood disorders.

Alcohol use disorder has an extremely high prevalence in the general population, is highly comorbid with depression, and increases risk of suicide. Major depressive disorder is the most common co-occurring psychiatric disorder among people with DSM-IV alcohol use disorder.[15] Although antidepressants may be less effective in someone who is actively abusing alcohol, withholding them due to alcohol use and expecting cessation of drinking behavior to result in mood remission is unlikely to be effective either. Studies regarding efficacy in patients using alcohol have found that medications are more effective than placebo.[16] People presenting with symptoms of depression and heavy alcohol use likely have a combination of both disorders and warrant treatment that can address both issues. It is important to try to get patients to be as specific as possible about how much they are drinking because what is perceived as "normal" or "social" drinking can vary highly between patients, and it is frequently well above what constitutes national guidelines about "problem" drinking. Patients who are highly intoxicated may not be able to make an informed decision about hospitalization and decide they want to leave as soon as they sober up or begin craving alcohol again. It is also important to note that very heavy drinkers may begin to exhibit signs of withdrawal before even reaching a zero alcohol level, so waiting until someone is "completely sober" or using alcohol levels to determine sobriety before evaluating them may not be possible.

Cocaine and stimulant abuse can precipitate depressive symptoms—most notably the "crash" at the end of a period of bingeing on cocaine or amphetamines, which can include irritability somnolence, decreased oral intake, depressed mood, and even frank suicidality. With cocaine, even after heavy use, symptoms may remit somewhat within a day or two, but prolonged amphetamine or methamphetamine abuse, particularly if resulting in psychosis, can take significantly longer to clear. Even occasional stimulant abuse can lead to rebound depressed mood and anxiety the following day.

Pain, opioid abuse and dependence, and depression and anxiety are highly intertwined. Chronic pain is highly associated with depression, and the majority of patients with chronic pain disorders have at least two comorbid psychological factors.[17] Depression and anxiety are risk factors for opioid abuse. Prescription opiate use is also a risk factor for opioid abuse and dependence, particularly in patients with a history of comorbid depression and those with a family or personal history of substance use disorders. Thus, it is reasonable to consider screening patients presenting with depression for misuse of opiates and vice versa. Even if the patient is compliant with a pain management program and not abusing their prescribed opiates, chronic pain is an independent risk factor for depression. Opiates are also highly lethal in overdose, and the availability of a significant quantity of opiates in a depressed patient should be considered a potential risk factor for completed suicide. Comorbid benzodiazepine use increases this risk as well due to synergistic effects with opiates in respiratory suppression.

Heavy regular marijuana use can also lead to symptoms consistent with depression, in that patients may become socially withdrawn, apathetic, or exhibit cognitive slowing. Abruptly stopping heavy marijuana use, although not known to cause a clinically dangerous syndrome in the way that alcohol or benzodiazepine use can, may cause irritability, anxiety, or depressed mood as well. Finally, it is important to consider that in some states, marijuana can be prescribed for certain mood or anxiety conditions such as PTSD, and clinicians must be alert for unintended side effects of that use.

With ketamine, MDMA, and hallucinogens such as psilocybin garnering more media attention as potential treatments for depression, patients who do not have access to those treatments in a structured or research setting may experiment with use in the community. Given the lack of standardization of illicitly obtained substances, this attempt at self-medication can have unforeseen consequences, including psychosis or other adverse reactions that may lead to ED presentations. Other substances that may be used illicitly for depression include kratom, micro dosing of LSD, cannabidiol (some preparations of which may contain THC as well, but absent THC is unlikely to have many adverse effects), and ayahuasca. Given that in most states these substances are still illegal, patients may be reluctant to disclose their use.

The medical differential for depression is wide, but in an otherwise healthy person, checking a baseline set of metabolic labs, complete blood count, thyroid function, and B_{12}/folate levels is a reasonable place to start. If the patient is on any QTc-prolonging medications, a baseline electrocardiogram should be obtained before starting medications. If urine toxicology can be obtained, it may be helpful in clarifying whether substance use is involved if the patient is not forthcoming about their use. It is rare to find a clear solely medical cause of a classic depressive episode with any cognitive impairment or confusion, but the need to rule out any comorbid medical issues increases in older and more medically complex patients. For patients who are of reproductive age, baseline pregnancy testing before starting medication can help patients make an informed decision about any risk but should not preclude starting routine antidepressants such as selective serotonin reuptake inhibitors (SSRIs) as long as a clear conversation about risks and benefits can be conducted.

Treatment

First-line pharmacologic treatment of depression most typically involves treatment with an SSRI. A 2018 *Lancet* study examined available evidence for all antidepressants on the market in the United Kingdom and found that all were more effective than placebo, with highest acceptability as measured by lowest dropout rates for agomelatine (not available in the United States), citalopram, escitalopram, fluoxetine, sertraline, and vortioxetine.[18] Given that all but vortioxetine are available as generics, there are multiple options to choose from that could be accessible. If the patient has no significant comorbid anxiety symptoms, bupropion is also a reasonable choice. It may have a lower risk of sexual side effects, but it does carry a risk of seizures in patients with seizure history or with active eating disorders. Referral to psychotherapy for mild to moderate cases of depression can also be helpful because there are studies that show significant response particularly to cognitive–behavioral therapy. In patients with significant insomnia or loss of appetite, mirtazapine may be a good first choice because it does have some sedation in lower doses and can stimulate appetite. In the short term, use of a sleep aid such as zolpidem may help with insomnia, but it should be avoided in patients with comorbid alcohol or benzodiazepine use issues.

There are a few specific concerns in initiating an antidepressant in the emergency setting. One is that it will not work immediately; thus, if the patient is to be discharged, follow-up needs to be sufficient to address supportive treatment and psychosocial support. In addition, the black box warning for increased suicidal thinking must be noted and the patient advised to have a safety plan in place in case suicidal thinking develops or worsens. Antidepressants also can cause akathisia in early initiation, which is an extremely unpleasant sensation that can exacerbate or cause suicidality. Finally, emergence of precipitated mania, although not common, is a possibility, and patients with a family history of bipolar disorder may be at higher risk. Adequate counseling of the patient regarding potential risks as well as providing a resource for them to contact if complications develop are essential. Initiation of treatment prior to a first appointment, however, can help bridge the patient to treatment and may allow for them to have some earlier relief of their symptoms. In these cases, on-site "crisis clinic" or walk-in after care clinics may be most helpful in bridging patients to longer term treatment. Although many primary care physicians are comfortable prescribing and managing antidepressants, not all are, and coordination with the primary care physician, if possible, can help clarify what resources are or are not available. In a 2016 study of ED patients, depressed patients most commonly reported work conflicts, difficulty with transportation, and difficulty finding a responsive clinician as barriers to treatment, and greater severity of depression was correlated with greater perceived barriers.[19] Thus, making care as accessible as possible and anticipating barriers to follow-up should be prioritized in this population, even those who appears "functional," compared to more severely mentally ill patients.

In terms of emerging treatments, ketamine has been studied as a possible ED-based intervention for acute depressive episodes, particularly in patients with acute suicidality who do not have comorbid psychotic symptoms. Studies have been mixed, with one retraction of an early paper that showed promise. Studies have been limited by small sample size and varying doses and modes of administration. A study investigating a lower dose 5-minute infusion, for example, which might be more feasible in an ED setting than a 40-minute infusion, showed that 88% of treatment-arm subjects had resolution of suicidal ideation at 90 minutes compared to 33% of the placebo arm, but each arm only had nine subjects.[20] Currently, use of intravenous ketamine in the acute setting is likely still limited to facilities with ongoing research studies or that have more experience initiating and monitoring the treatment, as a 2021 review paper found only three non-retracted studies in the ED setting with mixed results.[21] However, given the approval of esketamine, the inhaled form of ketamine, and the emergence of outpatient ketamine "clinics" in many metropolitan areas, more patients are asking about this option and how to be referred to treatment. Ideally, ketamine could potentially be used to provide rapid relief of suicidality and depressive symptoms, shortening or deferring inpatient admissions or allowing time for maintenance medications to take effect. Currently, it is not widely available in the emergency setting and requires more study.

In cases of severe depression with acute suicidality, or with severe impairment of function including patients who are not eating or drinking or who are exhibiting severe psychomotor retardation or catatonia, electroconvulsive therapy (ECT) in the hospital may be indicated. Patients who have had ECT in the past are likely to require it again for relapse of similar symptoms. Patients who are medically compromised from their depression, pregnant, experiencing psychosis, postpartum, or unable to tolerate antidepressant medications may also benefit from ECT, and this may be an indication for inpatient admission even in the absence of acute suicidality. Although ECT is generally safe and can in some cases be initiated in an outpatient setting, frequently an initial hospitalization may be appropriate for a patient who is new to the procedure or who is medically ill.

Case Outcome

The social worker eventually persuades Mr. M to allow her to call his wife to verify his primary care doctor and insurance information and to get some collateral about how he has been doing. She is able to get some information about how he is doing at home and the wife's concerns about his overall low mood, headaches, and irritability. His wife has never known him to express any suicidal thinking but has been concerned that he is more withdrawn from her and drinking more heavily. The social worker is also able to reach the primary care doctor's office and secure him an appointment the following day and provide the patient with a note for work excusing him to attend the appointment. The patient consents to having the emergency room visit records including the social worker's notes sent to his primary care doctor, and he agrees to attend the appointment the next day, with the encouragement that his headaches and muscle tension may be related to his mood and can respond to treatment. The social worker also notifies Mr. M that she will be following up to find out if he attended his appointment, and if he does not, she may consider crisis outreach services for him. Given all the wraparound services provided, Mr. M is able to be discharged from the ED.

Mania

Bipolar disorder is less prevalent than depression, both in community samples and in presentations to the ED, but presentations of acute mania can be particularly challenging to manage in the ED, particularly if there is no dedicated psychiatric space available. Although the typical florid, euphoric manic episode is the most common picture that comes to mind in emergency psychiatry, manic patients can also be irritable, hostile, and angry, and most notably turn from one to the other in seconds. Disinhibited behavior, such as uncharacteristic drug use or risk-taking, may be difficult to recognize as stemming from a mood episode if the patient's baseline personality and level of functioning are unknown. As with any presentation to the ED, medical comorbidity and acute intoxication should be considered and ruled out, particularly in patients who have no prior known history of mood episodes. In addition, manic patients may become medically compromised due to dehydration, poor nutrition, excessive exercise, stimulant use, or agitated catatonia.

Case Example

Mrs. S, a 28-year-old married woman, presents to the ED via emergency medical services from her workplace. After several days of increasingly erratic behavior, atypical for such a diligent and well-respected human resources employee at a local department store, Mrs. S showed up to work late today, dressed in a bizarre outfit and accompanied by a young man whom she had not met before that morning, who reported he worked as a barista at the coffee shop she frequented. She had been behaving so oddly that he thought he should make sure she got to work. Mrs. S proceeded to have the young man sit in her office while she played music loudly. When approached by concerned staff, she locked herself in the office crying and called several of her colleagues from her desk phone, asserting they had a plot to get her fired. No one was able to locate her emergency contact information, so after pleas for her to open the door were not successful, 911 was called. After a protracted negotiation, Mrs. S was escorted to the hospital but refused to cooperate with triage. She disrobed and began singing loudly. When staff approached her to ask her to put on a hospital gown, she punched one of them in the face, screaming "You smell terrible!" She was eventually sedated.

Mrs. S's husband was contacted. He reports that she had not slept in about a week. She had initially been anxious about their plan to purchase a home and had started staying up late researching various mortgage rates and neighborhood statistics, and then she did not sleep at all for several days. He notes she had been talking very fast and not making very much sense. He also notes that she left before he woke up this morning, and she had taped a note to the bathroom mirror that stated, "I know what you did." He denies that she has a history of drug abuse but notes she had been drinking the past few nights to "calm down." "I think she said her grandmother was in a mental ward a few times," he notes.

Diagnostic Criteria and Clinical Presentation in Evaluation of Bipolar Disorder

Mania is the defining criteria for bipolar disorder, type I. It is characterized by periods of increased energy; decreased need for sleep; rapid, pressured speech; flight of ideas;

grandiosity; impulsivity; behavioral disinhibition; and hypersexuality. Hypomania is similar but less severe, and it does not, by definition, include psychosis. A patient does not need to have a history of depressive episodes to meet criteria for bipolar disorder, although most do. Manic patients typically present to the ED when their behavior has become so extreme that they put themselves or someone else in danger, and patients who are manic tend to lack insight into their behavior in a profound and alarming way. Delusions associated with mania frequently have a grandiose or spiritual nature, with themes of a grand unification of the universe, special powers, healing, or massive destruction.

Mania can swing rapidly from euphoric unity to irritability, anger, and rage. Profound irritability can be extremely unpleasant for the patient and may lead them to seek treatment. However, lack of insight can persist in irritable mania as well, and it is not uncommon for the families of these patients to assure the clinician "they really aren't like this normally at all, they're a nice person" after an irritable, angry manic patient has viciously insulted them. It is important to not overdiagnose personality pathology in the acutely manic patient because frequently the person looks and sounds nothing like the way they did in their acute episode once it has resolved.

Manic episodes—either of first onset or in a patient with a known history of prior episodes—are frequently associated with changes in sleep patterns. Insomnia may be a trigger and/or an early warning sign of an impending episode; therefore, acute psychosocial stressors triggering anxiety and thus insomnia, changes in routine, travel across time zones, or use of stimulant drugs to prolong wakefulness can all be risk factors for a slip into mania. Emergency psychiatry clinicians frequently speak of the emergency of mania in the spring and summer months, corresponding to increasing daylight hours, and there has been some evidence to support this cyclical recurrence.[22]

Time course is important in separating bipolar disorder from more acute episodes of affective dysregulation and chronic psychotic processes such as schizoaffective disorder. In an acute manic presentation in the ED, when evaluating someone presenting with psychotic symptoms and manic symptoms, it may not be possible to fully distinguish between bipolar I and schizoaffective disorder. A person who was "otherwise normal" a few weeks ago, is well-related at baseline, and has a rapid onset of mood elevation or lability followed by a progression into behavioral disinhibition and then eventually psychosis is more likely to be having a new onset of a bipolar illness. Someone who has had psychotic symptoms in the absence of acute mood symptoms, or who has had a more chronic and latent prodromal course of psychosis, may in fact have schizoaffective disorder. In either case, the treatment of the acute episode is similar, and only time can distinguish the longer term clinical course. It is also important to note that historically, there has been racial bias in the diagnosis of mood versus psychotic disorders, with a tendency to overdiagnose African American individuals with psychotic illness versus a primary mood disorder.[23]

Similar to patients with depression who can present as negativistic or help-rejecting, an irritable, hostile, and grandiose hypomanic patient is at risk of being overdiagnosed with a personality disorder, when those symptoms may disappear or not be clinically significant when the patient is treated for the acute episode. The converse is also true: A patient with antisocial personality disorder or psychopathy engaging in criminal or "disinhibited" behavior may be diagnosed with hypomania or mania inappropriately. Patients with borderline personality disorder experiencing acute affective dysregulation may present as highly irritable, aggressive, disinhibited, and even at times somewhat psychotic but not experiencing a manic episode. In the acute setting, getting more information about time course is the most prudent option, and if the patient's behavior is dangerous enough, the patient may warrant admission for stabilization even if the true etiology cannot be fully determined. In settings in which short-term emergency observation is feasible, such as an extended observation unit, it may be more probable to clarify diagnosis.

Certain dementias of early onset, particularly frontotemporal dementia, may also present with disinhibition, risk-taking, and inappropriate affect. Mania is not generally associated with cognitive deficits, so any true cognitive problem should raise red flags for a dementing process or a delirium.

Bipolar disorder does have a strong genetic component, but a family history is not necessary to make the diagnosis. The age of onset is typically in early adulthood. Some patients may present later, particularly if they have had episodes of depression in early adulthood with mild hypomanic episodes that may have been missed because they were not severe enough to be distressing or led to periods of increased productivity. Patients presenting very late in life with new onset of mania are rare, and particularly in geriatric populations, medical issues, dementia, or delirium should be considered first.

True mixed episodes are rare, and DSM-5 allows for a depressive episode with mixed features outside of a bipolar disorder diagnosis. Whether the person is meeting full criteria for a mixed episode or not, the presence of intense irritability, agitation, and subjective feelings of restlessness is concerning and can increase risk for suicide or violence.

Comorbid substance use is highly prevalent in bipolar disorder. A 2004 study frequently cited indicated that at least 50% of adults with bipolar disorder have issues with impulsivity and substance use disorders at some point in their lives.[15] Substances may be used by patients to manage irritability and agitation (alcohol, sedatives, and marijuana) or to enhance alertness and euphoria in mania (stimulants, cocaine, and MDMA). They may also be used by patients who do not typically use any substances as part of their behavioral disinhibition. It may be difficult in the acute setting to separate acute intoxication, particularly on a stimulant, with a manic episode, and the sleeplessness caused by a prolonged stimulant binge can precipitate mania in a vulnerable patient. In general, drugs and alcohol wear off, so if there is an option for a period of observation to clarify the diagnosis if substances are suspected, that can help, as can additional collateral from friends, family, and providers. A patient with no history of substance use who is suddenly engaging in high-risk substance use behaviors may have an underlying mania, and so clinicians should look for other symptoms or evidence of disinhibition.

Steroid use can also precipitate mania, and patients undergoing steroid therapy for another condition can present with new onset of insomnia, irritability, and even frank psychosis. It is highly unlikely for steroid psychosis to persist after steroid taper, however. In the short term, if steroid withdrawal would be life-threatening due to the underlying condition being treated, symptom management would involve use of similar agents, including antipsychotics and benzodiazepines, and behavioral management.

In patients with a genetic predisposition toward bipolar disorder, it is possible for antidepressant medication to precipitate hypomania or mania. In a patient who has recently been started on an antidepressant and is presenting with intense irritability, insomnia, disinhibition, or euphoria, this possibility should be considered and the antidepressant tapered accordingly.

Medical conditions to rule out include hyperthyroidism, which can precipitate agitation, intense affect, and insomnia, as well as acute NMDA receptor encephalitis.

Anti-NMDA encephalitis can unfortunately, in its early stages, closely mimic an acute manic episode, including agitation, psychosis, and disinhibited behavior. Although NMDA encephalitis should be accompanied by neurologic signs, the differential can be challenging, particularly before frank neurologic signs such as seizures develop. In general, mania should not be accompanied by seizures or memory loss. Neurologic signs such as movement disorders or dyskinesias in pediatric or young patients with no exposure to neuroleptics would raise suspicion of an encephalitic process. Unfortunately, no clear psychiatric phenotype that would immediately indicate an encephalitis has been found, and many symptoms overlap with new onset of a manic episode.[24] In the elderly, delirium from a simple urinary tract infection can look much like mania, in terms of the presence of agitation, disorganized behavior, and irritability, so medical causes should be considered early in vulnerable populations. In developmentally delayed or nonverbal autistic patients, physical distress from a medical complaint can lead to aggression, irritability, insomnia, or disinhibition, and occult medical complaints should be investigated before making a diagnosis of a manic episode.

Special Populations

Unfortunately, patients do not outgrow bipolar disorder: Mania can present late in patients who might have had a history of depressive episodes or mild hypomania in the past, and cycling of mood episodes can worsen over the life span. Patients who have been maintained for years on lithium and cannot tolerate it anymore due to renal or thyroid complications may be much more difficult to manage, particularly given the risk of antipsychotic use in geriatric patients. It is a rare finding to have an entirely new onset of mania in an elderly patient, and all other causes, particularly delirium, should be ruled out first. Frontotemporal dementia, in particular, may present with behavioral disinhibition like a manic episode, although the onset would be more gradual.

Post-/peripartum psychiatric emergencies are addressed in Chapter 18, but postpartum psychosis is highly associated with bipolar disorder. The postpartum period is high risk for patients with mood disorders, given lack of sleep and massive hormonal changes. Pregnant patients are frequently told to stop their psychiatric medications due to perceived or real risk to the fetus but are no less vulnerable to relapse than if they were not pregnant, so they should be monitored closely. Untreated mania is dangerous for the patient and her fetus and should be treated aggressively. ECT can sometimes be the best option for rapid resolution of symptoms without use of agents contraindicated in pregnancy.

The diagnosis of bipolar disorder is children is complex, and pediatric emergencies are discussed in Chapter 15. In general, it is a rare finding for a child to have a frank manic episode, but risk increases through the teens into adulthood. In young children, developmental issues, trauma, anxiety, and acute environmental or social stressors are more likely to cause behavioral changes compared to evolving bipolar illness.

Risk Assessment

Bipolar disorder has the highest rate of suicide of all psychiatric conditions, and there are no validated suicide risk assessment tools specifically for bipolar disorder.[25] Many of the risk factors are the same as those for depression (male gender, social isolation, divorce, White, and elderly). Substance use is also significantly associated with suicidality in bipolar disorder.[26] Per a 2020 review article, approximately one-third to one-half of bipolar patients attempt suicide ate least once in their lifetime, and approximately 15–20% die of suicide.[27] Depressive and mixed episodes are more highly associated with suicide compared with mania or hypomania, but when assessing risk in an acute manic or hypomanic episode, it is important to consider behavior and indicators of danger outside of strictly whether the patient is "suicidal" or "homicidal." Manic patients frequently take unnecessary risks that put themselves or others in danger without any suicidal or violent intent. Driving recklessly, engaging in dangerous sexual behavior with strangers, getting into fights, or uncharacteristic criminal behavior may be indicators of acute dangerousness. The patient's baseline level of functioning and behavior is also vitally important in assessing risk, as well as a timeline of the change in behavior and function. Collateral information from family or other contacts can help establish a pattern of behavior in these cases. It is also important to remember that even patients with more typically "euphoric" presentations may be considering suicide, particularly if it fits into the delusional process.

Risk can also increase after the mania subsides. Although some patients sink into a post-manic depressive episode that can be severe, even in the absence of depressive symptoms, coming to terms with the consequences of a manic episode can be difficult to tolerate, with intense shame regarding one's behavior or reckoning with financial losses and disruption of important relationships.

Treatment

In the ED, initial treatment should focus on rapid management of agitation, regulation of sleep, and behavioral management. If the patient is acutely dangerous and requires sedation, antipsychotics and/or benzodiazepines are typically used, with the caveat that administration of parenteral benzodiazepines in combination with parenteral olanzapine carries a black box warning for excessive sedation. Atypical antipsychotics are better tolerated in terms of risk of dystonia and extrapyramidal symptoms, but availability varies. Severe mania with psychosis can be treated with a combination of mood stabilizers and antipsychotic medication, but addition of a benzodiazepine for sleep at night can also be helpful in the acute period.

ECT can also be used for treatment of mania, particularly if the patient is medically compromised, exhibiting catatonia, pregnant, postpartum, or otherwise unable to tolerate titration of medication. If the patient is known to need ECT in the past to treat their mania, this may also be an indication that inpatient admission will be necessary.

If the patient has an existing relationship with a psychiatrist who can treat them rapidly or adjust an existing medication regimen, inpatient admission might be avoidable, but experienced providers know how overconfident and difficult manic patients can be. It is important to not collude with the patient who is presenting themself as better than they actually are or to prematurely discharge the patient who is so frankly unpleasant and annoying that the clinician hopes for any possible way to send them home. The laser-like focus that manic, irritable patients can have in determining and exploiting a clinician's points of weakness can be quite remarkable and difficult to defend against. Even seasoned clinicians can find themselves exhausted by the endless energy of the manic patient or carried along by their euphoria.

Case Outcome

Mrs. S was calmer when she awoke from sedation but reported that during the past 3 days she had discovered a global plot to control her finances and that she had developed the power to read minds. She underwent a full medical workup and was admitted to an inpatient psychiatric unit for stabilization. Additional collateral from her family was obtained: Her grandmother took lithium for most of her life, and so Mrs. S was started on that medication as well.

Catatonia

Although catatonia has historically been associated with psychotic disorders, it also occurs in mood disorders, autism spectrum disorders, and delirium. DSM-5 recognizes catatonia as an independent syndrome that may be associated with psychotic disorders, mood disorders, general medical conditions, autism spectrum disorder, or even obsessive–compulsive disorder, whereas *International Classification of Diseases, Tenth Revision*, only permits diagnosis of catatonia as a result of schizophrenia or an organic brain syndrome.[27] Clinicians who have seen catatonia know that it is certainly not just associated with schizophrenia and that it does occur in mood disorders, most notably in geriatric patients but can also occur in children and adolescents. Catatonia is most often thought of as a combination of posturing, negativism, and waxy flexibility, but other symptoms are important to consider. It can be difficult in the emergency setting to distinguish between neuroleptic malignant syndrome, serotonin syndrome, and catatonia because some features can overlap, particularly in malignant catatonia, in which vital sign changes including autonomic instability, fever, and rigidity and be present. Catatonia-like behavior can also be precipitated by drugs of abuse such as phencyclidine and synthetic cannabinoids.

The classic motor feature of catatonia is stupor, or unresponsiveness while appearing awake, and waxy flexibility, which can be illustrated by moving a limb of the catatonic patient as if manipulating a wax figure and then leaving it in place—for example, lifting the arm over the head and watching the patient not put it down. Catatonic patients also frequently appear "stuck" in fixed postures. Extremes of this include the "psychological pillow" sign, in which the patient reclines, suspended a couple of inches off the bed. Speech abnormalities may be present, such as echolalia or perseveration. Ambivalent behaviors are also described, in which the patient begins and reverses a movement, such as reaching out to shake a hand and then pulling their hand back. Stereotypies and persistent mannerisms may be present, such as miming unbuttoning or buttoning a shirt. Echopraxia or mimicking the evaluator's actions, may occur, as can "automatic obedience," in which the patient exhibits exaggerated cooperation with the examiner's commands. "Gegenhalten" is resistance to pressure equal and opposite to the pressure applied—for example, the clinician moves the patient's arm and the patient pushes back with equal force. It is important to also consider catatonic excitement; if an agitated patient is engaging in rapid, perseverative, or stereotypic movements, it may be a sign of catatonia.[28]

In contrast, neuroleptic malignant syndrome (NMS) is characterized by muscle rigidity, not the waxy, pliable postures of the catatonic patient, and features of autonomic instability are present. However, malignant catatonia also can present with muscle rigidity, hyperthermia, and autonomic instability, and it has a mortality rate of 12–20%.[29] The two syndromes may be clinically indistinguishable, although NMS is more commonly associated with use of antipsychotic medication and most commonly occurs in the first month of starting treatment but can occur at any time. The treatment for both syndromes is supportive—that is, managing the autonomic symptoms, monitoring electrolytes, and treatment with benzodiazepines and ultimately ECT if necessary. In the ED setting, it is most important to recognize the severity of the syndrome and initiate appropriate supportive care.

Severely depressed patients with psychomotor retardation may look as if they are lapsing into catatonia without meeting full criteria—for example, becoming "stuck" in various places for extended periods of time. Occasionally, however, a patient who appears catatonic once treated with a benzodiazepine may be unmasked as truly manic, appearing more agitated.

Catatonia is treated first with benzodiazepines, typically lorazepam, titrated to relieve symptoms without excess sedation. As the underlying disorder is treated, the lorazepam can be slowly tapered. Some studies have proposed use of zolpidem, memantine, or amantadine as adjunctive treatments.[28] In severe cases in which oral intake is compromised or physical complications have become too severe, such as autonomic dysregulation or development of rhabdomyolysis, ECT is rapidly effective and may be indicated emergently.[30]

Malignant catatonia is a true medical emergency, and patients can deteriorate quickly if it is not recognized. ECT is the treatment of choice if benzodiazepines are not rapidly effective. Patients who have a history of malignant catatonia may require admission to an inpatient setting before their symptoms deteriorate severely, given the high mortality rate once the syndrome progresses.

Conclusion

Mood disorders are highly prevalent and a common cause of ED psychiatric evaluation. The assessment in the emergency setting can be most thorough and diagnostically helpful if it focuses on time course and specificity of symptoms, consideration of substance use comorbidity, and risk assessment based not just on the patient's immediate clinical presentation but also historic risk factors and collateral from people who know the individual well. The possibility of having a positive impact on someone who may have an improvement in other health outcomes if their mood disorder is recognized and treated early can help inform how emergency providers approach these disorders.

Currently, in the later stages of the COVID-19 pandemic, with vaccines available and the United States starting to "re-open," the full impact of the pandemic on psychiatric illness and morbidity remains to be seen. It is already clear to clinicians who routinely work in acute care settings or with severely mentally ill individuals that the pandemic had a profound effect on access to services, including availability of acute care beds during surges in hard-hit areas. EDs have been overwhelmed with COVID cases, and patients have been fearful to present unless they are in extreme distress to an emergency room that may be packed with COVID patients. The long-term trauma from the extent of death and illness is unfolding. In addition, the economic impact of unemployment and disruption in ability to work due to child care or other dependent care needs has been an immense stressor, particularly for families who were already stretched to their limit before the pandemic began. Early studies have already shown an increase in rates of mood illness since the beginning of the pandemic.[31] Although the increased prevalence of telepsychiatry access and relaxation of rules around its provision may help increase access long term, emergency providers should expect an increase in presentations going forward.

References

1. Kuo D, Tran M, Shah A, Matorin A. Depression and the suicidal patient. *Emerg Med Clin*. 2015;33(4):765–778. https://doi.org/10.1016/j.emc.2015.07.005

2. Substance Abuse and Mental Health Services. Key substance use and mental health indicators in the United States: Results from the 2017 National Survey on Drug Use and Health. Published 2018. https://www.samhsa.gov/data/sites/default/files/cbhsq-reports/NSDUH FFR2017/NSDUHFFR2017.pdf

3. Ballou S, Mitsuhashi S, Sankin L, et al. Emergency department visits for depression in the United States from 2006–2014. *Gen Hosp Psychiatry*. 2019;59:14–19.

4. Blanco C, Compton W, Saha T, et al. Comorbidity of bipolar and substance use disorders in national surveys of general populations, 1990–2015: Systematic review and meta-analysis. *J Affect Disord*. 2016;206:321–330. doi:10.1016/j.jad.2016.06.051

5. Downey L, Zun L, Burke T. Undiagnosed mental illness in the emergency department. *J Emerg Med*. 2012;43(5):876–882. doi:10.1016/j.jemermed.2011.06.055

6. Hoyer D, David E. Screening for depression in emergency department patients. *J Emerg Med*. 2012;43(5) 786–789. doi:10.1016/j.jemermed.2008.05.004

7. Olfson M, Blanco C, Wall M, Liu S-M, Grant B. Treatment of common mental disorders in the United States: Results from the National Epidemiologic Survey on Alcohol and Related Conditions–III. *J Clin Psychiatry*. 2019;80(3):18m12532.

8. Beiser D, Ward C, Bu M, Laiteerapong N, Gibbons R. Depression in emergency department patients and association with health care utilization. *Acad Emerg Med*. 2019;26(8):878–888. doi:10.1111/acem.13726

9. American Psychiatric Association. *Diagnostic and Statistical Manual of Mental Disorders*. 5th ed. American Psychiatric Publishing; 2013.

10. Kessler R, Sampson A, Berglun P, et al. Anxious and non-anxious major depressive disorder in the World Health Organization World Mental Health Surveys. *Epidemiol Psychiatr Sci*. 2015;24(3):210–226. doi:10.1017/S2045796015000189

11. Ronquillo L, Minassian A, Vilke G, Wilson M. Literature-based recommendations for suicide assessment in the emergency department: A review. *J Emerg Med*. 2012;43(5):836–842. http://dx.doi.org/10.1016/j.jemermed.2012.08.015

12. Baldessarini R. Epidemiology of suicide: Recent developments. *Epidemiol Psychiatr Sci*. 2020;29:e71. https://doi.org/10.1017/S2045796019000672

13. Hawton K, Comabella C, Haw C, Saunder K. Risk factors for suicide in individuals with depression: A systematic review. *J Affect Disord*. 2013;147:17–28. http://dx.doi.org/10.1016/j.jad.2013.01.004

14. Wagner G, McClintock S, Rosenquist P, McCall WV. Major depressive disorder with psychotic features may lead to misdiagnosis of dementia: A case report and review of the literature. *J Psychiatr Pract*. 2011;17(6):432–438. doi:10.1097/01.pra.0000407968.57475.ab

15. Grant B, Stinson F, Dawson D. Prevalence and co-occurrence of substance use disorders and independent mood and anxiety disorders: Results from the National Epidemiologic Survey on Alcohol and Related Conditions. *JAMA Psychiatry*. 2004;61(8):807–816.

16. McHugh RK, Weiss R. Alcohol use disorder and depressive disorders. *Alcohol Res*. 2019;40(1):arcr.v40. doi:10.35946/arcr.v40.1.01

17. Wilsey B, Fishman S, Tsodikov A, Ogden C, Symreng I, Ernst A. Psychological comorbidities predicting prescription opioid abuse among patients in chronic pain presenting to the emergency department. *Pain Med*. 2008;9(8):1107–1117. doi:10.1111/j.1526-4637.2007.00401.x

18. Cipriani A, Funukawa T, Salanti G, et al. Comparative efficacy and acceptability of 21 antidepressant drugs for the acute treatment of adults with major depressive disorder: A systematic review and network meta-analysis. *Lancet*. 2018;3891:1357–1366. http://dx.doi.org/10.1016/S0140-6736(17)32802-7

19. Abar B, Hong S, Aaserude E, Holub A, DeFlienzo V. Access to care and depression among emergency department patients. *J Emerg Med*. 2016;53(1):30–37. http://dx.doi.org/10.1016/j.jemermed.2016.11.029

20. Domany Y, Shelton R, McCullumsmith C. Ketamine for acute suicidal ideation: An emergency department intervention: A randomized, double-blind, placebo-controlled, proof-of-concept trial. *Depression Anxiety*. 2020;37:224–233. https://doi.org./10.1002/da.22975

21. Maguire L, Bullard T, Papa L. Ketamine for acute suicidality in the emergency department: A systematic review. *Am J Emerg Med*. 2021;43:54–58. doi:10.1016/j.ajem.2020.12.088

22. Baowu W, Chen, D. Evidence for seasonal mania: A review. *J Psychiatr Pract*. 2013;19(4):301–308. doi:10.1097/01.pra.0000432600.32384.c5

23. Schwartz R, Blankenship D. Racial disparities in psychotic disorder diagnosis: A review of empirical literature. *World J Psychiatry*. 2014;4(4):133–140. doi:10.5498/wjp/v4.i4.133

24. Graus F, Titulaer M, Balu R, et al. A clinical approach to the diagnosis of autoimmune encephalitis. *Lancet Neurol*. 2016;15(4) 391–404.

25. Miller J, Black D. Bipolar disorder and suicide: A review. *Curr Psychiatry Rep*. 2020;22: Article 6. https://doi.org/10.1007/s11920-020-1130-0

26. Messer T, Lammers G, Muuler-Siecheneder F, Schmidt R-F, Latifi S. Substance abuse in patients with bipolar disorder: A systematic review and meta-analysis. *Psychiatry Res*. 2017;253:338–350. http://dx.doi.org/10.1016/j.psychres.2017.02.067

27. Walther S, Strik W. Catatonia. *CNS Spectr*. 2016;21:341–348. doi:10/1017/S1092852916000274

28. Francis A. Catatonia: Diagnosis, classification and treatment. *Curr Psychiatry Rep*. 2010;12:180–185. doi:10.1007/s11920-0010-0113-y

29. Kroll K, Kroll D, Pope J, Tibbles C. Catatonia in the emergency department. *J Emerg Med*. 2012;43(5):843–846.

30. Rajagopal S. Catatonia. *Adv Psychiatr Treat*. 2007;13:51–59. doi:10.1192/apt.bp.106.002360

31. Ettman C, Abdalla S, Cohen G. Prevalence of depression symptoms in US adults before and during the COVID-19 pandemic. *JAMA Network Open*. 2020;3(9):e2019686. doi:10.1001/jamanetworkopen.2020.19686

11

Anxiety, Post-Traumatic Stress Disorder, and Other Trauma-Related Disorders

Anna K. McDowell and Scott A. Simpson

Introduction

Patients with anxiety and trauma-related disorders present frequently to the emergency department (ED).[1] Indeed, anxiety, depressive, and trauma-related presentations constitute the most common behavioral health presentation in emergency settings. Emergency clinicians should be prepared to identify anxiety, exclude life-threatening diagnoses, assess for suicide and violence risk, and intervene acutely upon anxiety.

In the fifth edition of the *Diagnostic and Statistical Manual of Mental Disorders* (DSM-5), anxiety disorders and trauma-related disorders are classified as separate diagnostic categories.[2] In clinical practice, these categories have many overlapping symptoms and presentations. However, the differences between categories are worth highlighting because they guide risk assessment and treatment planning in the ED. The patient with an anxiety disorder is frequently experiencing fear related to an anticipation of danger rather than an imminent or current stressor. Although patients with trauma-related disorders also experience anticipatory fear and anxiety, the content and quality of this anxiety differ in that they relate to one or more past traumatic exposures. Some patients can present with both anxiety and trauma-related disorder symptoms.

This chapter reviews common presentations for patients with anxiety and trauma-related disorders in the ED and approaches to assessment and management in the emergency psychiatry setting.

Presentations of Anxiety in Emergency Settings

Anxiety manifests in different ways for ED patients. Most explicit and easiest to recognize are patients who describe worry and fear driving their presentation. Patients may describe panic symptoms, such as a racing heartbeat and fears of something terrible happening. Other patients share concerns that a physical ailment may be a harbinger of deadly disease. Family and friends may coax a patient to the ED out of concern that the patient is too scared to leave the home or fretting constantly to the point of missing work or school. In these examples, the need for treatment is readily apparent. An anxiety disorder diagnosis is likely present.

Other presentations of anxiety are more subtle and require elicitation by an attentive provider. In these cases, anxiety complicates needed medical and psychiatric treatment. For example, a patient who is non-adherent with primary care but presents repeatedly to the ED for refills may have unaddressed fears related to taking medication or accepting the need for medical treatment. Patients with chronic pain syndromes often experience anxiety related to a number of ongoing life stressors and their perceived inability to cope. Those stressors can often feel far removed from the ED visit—which is focused on a specific chief complaint—yet signal the need for more comprehensive mental health services. For these examples, clinicians can often surmise the presence of problematic anxiety but defer further action or referrals out of lack of urgency. However, forgoing the opportunity for treatment may result in the patient experiencing unnecessary discomfort or even adverse outcomes due to lack of treatment.

Finally, EDs are stressful places, where patients are experiencing acute illness, uncertainty if not terror, and life-changing decisions. Some degree of anxiety is normal and expected. Just like its more pathologic versions, normal anxiety may cause patients to feel easily overwhelmed, emotionally labile, and have difficulty making decisions. Patients with normal anxiety are readily receptive to assurance and supportive statements. Clinicians should reconnect patients with supportive persons who can help with decision-making and provide a calming presence. Normal anxiety is unlikely to interfere with treatment.

Medical Assessment

There is a dictum among psychotherapists that "anxiety is uncomfortable, not dangerous." Although that is generally sage advice, emergency settings pose an exception. Life-threatening conditions may present with anxiety, including toxidromes and withdrawal syndromes, tachyarrhythmias, and metabolic disorders including hyperthyroidism and hypoglycemia. Box 11.1 describes a brief medical differential of anxiety for the ED patient. Patients with anxiety and post-traumatic stress disorder (PTSD) frequently exhibit somatic complaints in the absence of underlying somatic disease.[3] In all cases, the emergency clinician—regardless of specialty and training—should maintain a high suspicion for concurrent medical illness. Patients who have incident anxiety during prolonged ED courses or boarding may warrant repeat investigation; for example, a patient who has remained in the ED for more than 12 hours after arriving intoxicated on alcohol may begin exhibiting anxiety as the first sign of alcohol withdrawal. The medical workup for psychiatric presentations is described in Chapter 3."

Although medical etiology underlying psychiatric presentations to the ED can be readily uncovered with assessment, the need for ongoing medical management does not stop at the exclusion of delirium. Anxiety conveys risk for chronic medical conditions, including cardiac and pulmonary disease, chronic pain, and neurologic disorders.[4] This relationship may depend on common pathologic processes, sustained hyperinflammatory states, or altered health behaviors. Mortality from undermanaged medical illness and accidents far outweighs that from suicide even among ED patients with suicidal ideation; emergency psychiatric clinicians must consider the need for ongoing medical management in any treatment plan for anxious and distressed patients.[5,6]

The Differential of Psychiatric Anxiety

After excluding somatic etiologies of anxiety, the first step in distinguishing among DSM-5 anxiety disorders rests in identifying a patient's most important source of anxiety.

Box 11.1 A Brief Differential of Medical Conditions Manifesting as Anxiety in the Emergency Department

---

Cardiac
Arrhythmia
Myocardial infarction
Metabolic
Hyperthyroidism
Hyperparathyroidism
Hypoglycemia
Pheochromocytoma
Neurologic
Epilepsy
Migraines with auras
Pulmonary
Asthma
Chronic obstructive pulmonary disease
Toxidromes and withdrawal
Alcohol or benzodiazepine withdrawal
Stimulant intoxication

DSM-5 diagnoses contain many criteria, duration specifiers, and symptom combinations. A prudent first step is not a checklist of all these criteria. Instead, a briefer focus on the patient's most distressing thoughts can rapidly narrow the differential. The following questions should be asked:

- "When you say you are anxious, what is it that you are most worrying about?"
- "What is it that goes through your mind when you are anxious?"
- "You seem worried right now. If I could read your mind right now, what would I hear you telling yourself?"
- "What is the single most important thing you worry about?"

Often, the patient will then describe a "hot thought" or the most prominent anxiety-provoking perseveration. The source of anxiety then prioritizes the differential. For example, a patient who fears "having another panic attack" is more likely to have panic disorder; a patient who reports "being in another car accident, last time that was so scary" evinces concern for PTSD. The differential may extend beyond anxiety disorders. For example, some patients share bizarre or delusional content more consistent with a psychotic disorder: "Aliens are monitoring my thoughts, this is the only place I'm safe." Or, a patient may share, "I am scared of gaining weight," which would be more suggestive of an eating disorder. Figure 11.1 illustrates an approach to discerning some anxiety disorders by hot thoughts.

The clinician should be mindful that almost any psychiatric disorder—related to psychosis, depression, or substance intoxication or withdrawal—is associated with anxiety at some point in the illness course. This overlap of anxiety across all diagnoses speaks to the

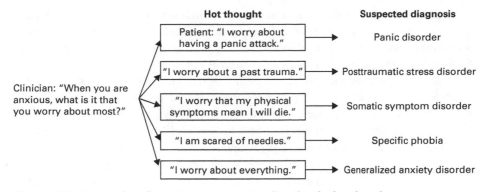

Figure 11.1 Approach to discerning some anxiety disorders by hot thoughts.

universality of experiencing anxiety, including in the absence of psychopathology. Again, anxiety only constitutes a psychiatric disorder when it causes significant impairment in functioning for the patient. In the following sections, we describe common anxiety diagnoses in the emergency setting. For each presentation, we discuss its features, review implications for risk assessment, and provide guidance on emergency management.

Panic Attacks, Panic Disorder, and Generalized Anxiety

Panic attacks are brief, self-limited episodes of intense anxiety accompanied by physical symptoms. The DSM-5 criteria for a panic attack include an abrupt surge of intense fear or discomfort that peaks in minutes and includes several characteristic symptoms. These symptoms include palpitations, sweating, fear of losing control or "going crazy," and the fear of dying; Box 11.2 enumerates a complete list of panic symptoms. It is important to clarify the patient's definition of a panic attack—the criteria for a panic attack and the patient's use of the term are not always equivalent. Panic attacks may be a feature of many other disorders, in which case the diagnosis is recorded with panic as a specific (e.g., generalized anxiety disorder with panic attacks). Panic may be either the primary reason for an ED visit—for example, driving a medical workup for chest pain—or occur during the course of a visit, such as when the patient receives bad news. However, panic attacks do not always have a clear precipitant.

Box 11.2 DSM-5 Panic Attack Symptoms

Palpitations	Feeling dizzy or faint
Sweating	Chills or heat sensations
Trembling or shaking	Paresthesia
Shortness of breath	Derealization or depersonalization
Feelings of choking	Fear of losing control or "going crazy"
Chest pain	Fear of dying
Nausea or gastrointestinal distress	

Panic disorder is a syndrome in which patients maladaptively change their behavior in relation to attacks; for example, they stop going to work or school for fear of others seeing them have a panic attack. Patients can have panic attacks without panic disorder if these maladaptive behavioral changes are not present.

In the ED, patients with panic symptoms benefit from brief psychotherapy and symptom-guided pharmacotherapy. Brief behavioral interventions including mindfulness, verbal de-escalation,[7] and coping tools can be highly effective. EDs might have a "comfort cart" with fidget spinners, scented lotions, and squeeze balls. Use of behavioral aids not only provides patients symptomatic relief but also reinforces a sense of self-efficacy and resilience. Patients who are not responsive to brief behavioral interventions may be offered medication. In specialized psychiatric emergency settings with available trained staff, a medication order may be written "as needed for anxiety not responsive to 30 minutes of coping skills practice." Appropriate initial agents include hydroxyzine for less intense anxiety and short-acting benzodiazepines (e.g., lorazepam 2 mg oral or intravenously) for more severe symptoms. Patients with concurrent suicidal ideation should be monitored according to local protocol.

Panic is an intense hyper-autonomic experience but not dangerous itself (contrary to patients' intense beliefs otherwise). After the attack passes, patients can be embarrassed and minimize the severity of the impairment. In these cases, clinicians should validate the patient's very real symptoms, distress, and impairment due to panic attacks. Panic attacks are by definition transient and do not require additional investigation in the absence of other symptoms.

Generalized anxiety disorder (GAD) is characterized by excessive, uncontrollable, and impairing anxiety and worry most days. Patients experience restlessness, fatigue, difficulty concentrating, irritability, and sleep disturbances (Box 11.3). When asked, the patient with GAD will frequently have difficulty describing one specific worry or even set of worries. The emergency psychiatric clinician in turn feels easily overwhelmed and frustrated during the assessment and treatment planning stages with these patients. Unlike patients with discrete panic attacks, patients with GAD may experience something more akin to relentless and diffuse anxiety without a discrete hot thought.

ED visits provide an opportunity to intervene effectively upon the chronic course of generalized anxiety and panic disorder. Like most chronic illnesses, anxiety disorders have a varying course with periods of heightened anxiety and longer periods of symptom control. A suicide risk assessment should be completed, given the heightened risk of

---

Box 11.3 DSM-5 Symptoms of Generalized Anxiety Disorder

Uncontrollable worry over a number of events more days than not with three or more of the following:
Restlessness
Fatigue
Difficulty concentrating
Irritability
Muscle tension
Sleep disturbance

suicide and self-harm among patients with panic;[8] the absence of suicidal ideation is not necessarily reassuring because most patients who die by suicide after an ED visit deny suicidality while in the ED.[5] An approach to risk assessment is described in Chapter 4. As with any emergency psychiatric interview, a helpful starting point is identifying the precipitants for the patient's visit. A focused interview on the events prompting the visit will help both the patient and the clinician focus the brief emergency encounter.

Providing psychoeducation is an invaluable intervention for helping patients maintain longer term symptom control of panic and generalized anxiety. With panic disorder and panic attacks, patients often fear they are dying when having a panic attack. Reinforcing the reality that patients did not in fact die during their ED visit and promoting the use of behavioral treatments can challenge patients' cognitive distortions related to panic. The cognitive distortions include self-talk that "I'm going to die" or "The world is going to end" when a panic attack occurs. Patients should be referred to cognitive–behavioral therapy (CBT); online CBT is freely available and effective.[9] Exercise is also an effective intervention for reducing anxiety.[10]

Generalized anxiety and panic are treated long term with serotonergic medication, typically selective serotonin reuptake inhibitors (SSRIs). If the patient is medication naive or does not have established follow-up, it is advisable to either refer the patient back to their outpatient psychiatrist or engage in warm hand off to the psychiatry care team for follow-up care. In one small study, there was evidence that prescribing an SSRI for patients with panic disorder resulted in improved follow-up treatment adherence.[11] However, the optimal long-term medication regimen for panic remains uncertain.[12]

Benzodiazepines are highly effective for treating acute anxiety in the ED and are unlikely to be problematic in that controlled environment. However, anxious patients should not be prescribed benzodiazepines upon discharge. Benzodiazepines do not improve the outcome of anxiety disorders—or even reduce anxiety long term—and increase the risk of suicide while also putting patients at risk of use disorder.[13] Moreover, benzodiazepines reduce the effectiveness of other medication and psychotherapeutic interventions for depression and anxiety.[14] Behavioral disinhibition related to benzodiazepines may increase the risk of self-harm, dangerous behaviors, or substance use in the time after discharge. Should the clinician be inclined, patients may be provided a document with coping skills to use and as needed hydroxyzine or propranolol for short-term use. But even these medications should not be prescribed with regularity from the ED, and the patient should preferably be referred to definitive psychotherapy and mental health treatment. In general, no medication treatment should be initiated out of the ED without an explicit follow-up arrangement to an ongoing care provider who can monitor treatment.

Acute and Post-Traumatic Stress Disorders

Most people experience one or more traumatic events throughout their lives. Many of these people will recover without developing persistent mental health symptoms relating to past traumatic experiences.[15] Characteristics supportive of recovery from traumatic events include lower number of lifetime traumatic events, absence of comorbid mental health disorder, and good social support.[16]

An understanding of trauma and traumatic reactions is necessary for multiple reasons in the ED. First, the events that bring ED patients to medical treatment may themselves be experienced as traumatic—for example, an accident or episode of violence. Traumatic reactions to these events may complicate care. Second, there may be opportunities in emergency psychiatry to mitigate the risk that traumatic reactions progress to more chronic trauma-related anxiety, in essence, PTSD. Finally, the role of complex trauma in the lives of patients can make EDs uniquely triggering locations. Patients' history of trauma can complicate medical treatment, and trauma-informed approaches can improve emergency care for survivors of trauma.

Although anxiety is a normal reaction after a traumatic event, some patients experience symptoms of intense anxiety accompanied by unwanted re-experiencing of the traumatic event and mood symptoms. Patients often describe a hot thought related to recent trauma. Difficulty concentrating, irritability, and discomfort are common. When these symptoms persist beyond 3 days after the trauma, acute stress disorder (ASD) should be considered. Diagnostic criteria for ASD include exposure to a traumatic event and multiple symptoms in the intrusive, negative mood, dissociative, avoidance, and arousal domains (Table 11.1). ASD symptoms last from 3 days to 1 month after traumatic experience.

If ASD symptoms persist beyond 1-month, PTSD may be present. PTSD is diagnosed when patients have exposure to a traumatic event and patients similarly meet diagnostic criteria in the intrusive, avoidance, negative mood, and arousal domains. Unlike for ASD, dissociative symptoms are not considered specifically when making a diagnosis of PTSD, although patients with PTSD may still have dissociative symptoms. As noted above, also differentiating ASD from PTSD is length of time that symptoms have persisted, with PTSD symptoms persisting for at least 1 month after the traumatic exposure.

The approach to the traumatized patient in the ED is predicated on helping the patient rebuild a sense of safety. Standardized therapies for approaching trauma survivors include psychological first aid and trauma-informed interventions. (These are described in Chapter 22.) The goals of these interventions include ameliorating acute discomfort and reducing the risk that the patient's symptoms progress to ASD and PTSD. These trauma-informed approaches share several common principles. The clinician should orient patients to the ED setting and time course of evaluation, reassure patients as to their physical safety, help patients reconnect with social supports, reinforce the use of healthy coping skills, and provide clear guidance on how to seek professional services in

Table 11.1 DSM-5 Symptoms of Acute Stress Disorder

Symptom Cluster	Examples
Intrusive symptoms	Unwanted thoughts Nightmares Flashbacks
Negative thoughts and mood	Inability to experience positive emotions
Dissociative symptoms	Altered sense of reality Inability to remember the trauma
Avoidance symptoms	Avoiding places or situations associated with trauma
Hyperarousal	Exaggerated startle response Hypervigilance Changes in concentration or sleep

the future at a time of their choosing. Critical incident debriefing is discouraged because it may exacerbate the risk of incident PSTD. Clinicians can reassure patients that recovery after traumatic events is not only possible but also common.[17] These approaches are different than the cognitive–behavioral approaches to anxiety and panic, although tenets of trauma-informed care have value for all patients.

Medications for acutely agitated and extremely anxious patients are sometimes indicated. If the patient has a standing anxiolytic regimen from their outpatient provider, continuing this as necessary is reasonable. A sedating antihistamine or oral benzodiazepine may be helpful for acute anxiety not responsive to brief therapeutic techniques. There is inadequate evidence for medication administration after a traumatic event, such as a benzodiazepine or β-blocker, in the prevention of ASD or PTSD.[18,19] Benzodiazepines are considered contraindicated for ongoing treatment of PTSD due to the concurrent risk of problematic alcohol use and lack of efficacy.

Risk assessment for the trauma-exposed patient should take into account potential exposure to reminders of trauma as well as strength of coping skills, availability of supportive people, and ability to safety plan. Trauma anniversaries are often a time of increased suicidal thoughts and risk as well. Finally, consideration of substance use history and impact on risk is important given comorbidity with PTSD.

The primary treatments for PTSD are exposure-based psychotherapies such as prolonged exposure or cognitive processing therapy. Psychoeducation regarding the availability of treatment may be helpfully provided by the emergency clinician. Coaching patients in the access of coping skills developed to support an exposure therapy is appropriate in the ED; provision of exposure therapy is not.

EDs and crisis psychiatry services can be chaotic, challenging places for patients to receive care—and for clinicians to work. Trauma-informed care recognizes the risk that health care settings pose to the clinicians who work in these environments. Trauma-informed care principles can thus be incorporated in all emergency settings to the benefit of building better clinician–patient relationships.

Adjustment Disorders and Medically Ill Patients

Many patients visit the ED in the context of significant life stressors—unemployment, medical illness, or the death of a loved one. Sometimes the ED visit itself is the precipitant for such life changes. Distress related to these events may result in anxiety, depressed mood, lack of energy, or a feeling of listlessness. Patients with poor coping skills may experience somatization that becomes the focus of emergent evaluation. In these ways, the ED visit may be both a symptom and a cause of patients' significant life events.

One common life stressor experienced in all medical environments is anxiety related to medical illness. Patient may face uncertainty about what is wrong with them, when or if they will get better, whether or not they will die, how they will continue to provide for themselves, and how clinicians perceive them. Often, patients with these natural reactions will be referred to the emergency psychiatry clinician after completion of a medical assessment.

Anxiety in response to stressful life events and medical illness is normal. But in more extreme forms, these symptoms impair patients' ability to cope with stressors and problem-solve. Patients with such impairment may have an adjustment disorder. Adjustment disorders comprise emotional or behavioral symptoms in clear relation to a specific stressor. The symptoms cause distress out of proportion to the precipitant and cause significant impairment in the patient's life; symptoms can be anxious, depressive, conduct, and/or emotional in nature. Unlike ASD and PTSD, adjustment disorders occur in the absence of a life-threatening trauma, disappear after resolution of the stressor, and less frequently include dissociation or reexperiencing symptoms.

Simply helping the patient recognize the presence of adjustment disorder is therapeutic. Even in the absence of a diagnosis, the clinician's suggestion that the patient consider how their life stressors may be affecting their mood, anxiety, and somatic symptoms can be a first and necessary therapeutic step. Patients with adjustment disorder often have difficulty ascribing reasons for their symptoms, even when the correlation to an acute stressor may be obvious to others. Naming these symptoms' cause and validating the patient's distress helps orient the patient to seeking out and engaging in treatment. Supportive psychotherapy should emphasize practical problem-solving approaches, and a brief single session of psychotherapy can mitigate acute reactions and inform risk assessment.[20] Little evidence supports long-term psychotherapy or medication treatment for adjustment disorder.

Although adjustment disorders are often considered less severe pathology than other anxiety and trauma-related disorders, the diagnosis carries appreciable risk for suicidal thoughts and behaviors,[21] and patients with medical illness also experience elevated risk of suicide.[22] Safety assessment and safety planning should not be overlooked. Substance use and its impact on symptoms must be assessed and addressed. Lethal means counseling for the medically ill anxious patient should consider the patient's access to medications that might be means of suicide, including not only benzodiazepines and opioids but also insulin, anticoagulants, and antiarrhythmic agents.

Stressed patients in the ED may also be grieving. Grief is a reaction to loss. Grief may be common during periods of significant death rates such as pandemics, natural disasters, and terrorist attacks.[23] Grief occurs in the context of bereavement, the period after a loss in which grief is processed. Many cultures have bereavement rituals to assuage grief, such as funeral rites. Like anxiety, grief and bereavement are normal parts of life and should not be pathologized.[24] However, persistent complex bereavement disorder may be present if the patient experiences impairment related to persistent longing for the deceased, intense emotional pain, preoccupation with the deceased, or preoccupation with the circumstances of death. As with adjustment disorder, naming and validating the patient's distress in the setting of bereavement can be helpful. Risk assessment and safety planning of the bereaved patient should be comprehensive and take into account the elevated risk for suicidal behavior, particularly among patients who have lost a loved one to suicide or another sudden, unexpected event.[25] For these patients, anniversaries of loss should be taken into account when safety planning because these events may pose transient periods of heightened risk.

Somatization

Anxiety in response to medical illness is natural. Normal anxiety in this context is typically responsive to reassurance by clinicians. However, perseverative thoughts that are intense, resistant to reassurance, and introduce impairment may be the result of an illness anxiety or somatic symptom disorder.

Illness anxiety disorder, related to the prior diagnosis of hypochondriasis, is characterized by a patient's recurrent and impairing anxiety that their symptoms represent a disabling or fatal outcome. Patients may repeatedly request medical tests that are not indicated. Illness anxiety is an example of a somatic symptom disorder, a category of psychiatric syndromes characterized by anxiety related to somatic complaints more generally. These disorders include illnesses in which the patient experiences anxiety and disability related to chronic pain or medically unexplained symptoms. Somatic symptom patients are often highly attuned to physical sensations, which are suspected to be dangerous pathology. Patients' commitments to these thought distortions often border on delusional in their intensity.

If the clinician suspects illness anxiety or a somatic symptom disorder, treatment should begin with a physical exam and due diligence to exclude underlying medical illness. Care should be taken that excessive testing and imaging are minimized and that iatrogenic procedures are avoided. A physical exam should be performed and a report of normal test results provided. Patients' anxiety and experience should be validated. This validation not only mitigates anxiety but also reinforces the therapeutic alliance in order to facilitate a referral to treatment. The clinician should provide psychoeducation as to the relationship between the patient's anxiety and somatic experiences. Definitive treatment for somatic symptom disorders is psychotherapy, particularly CBT. Some patients benefit from an SSRI, tricyclic antidepressant, or other medication treatments. As-needed benzodiazepines should be avoided.

Other Anxiety Disorders

Other anxiety disorders are less commonly implicated in ED treatment. The most common anxiety disorder is specific phobia, in which patients fear a specific activity, place, or thing—for example, snakes or spiders. Needle phobia may be of most pertinence in medical settings, but the phobic patient's fear can typically be overcome by reassurance, behavioral coping skills or distraction, or, in very rare instances, the use of anxiolytic medication for a brief procedure.

Obsessive–compulsive disorder (OCD) is anxiety characterized by ritualized thoughts or activities. Examples of compulsions are handwashing and counting behaviors. OCD may be the cause of injury or other complications leading to an ED visit, as with a patient who has compulsions to self-harm or cellulitis from picking behaviors. When OCD is suspected, a suicide risk assessment and treatment referral should be completed because the diagnosis is a strong risk factor for suicide and carries substantial morbidity.[26]

Social anxiety disorder is an intense fear of being humiliated in front of others; patients with severe disease may be reclusive. Social anxiety is uncommon in ED settings. However, severely ill patients may be brought in by family members or encountered by mobile crisis and prehospital clinicians in the community. When brought to care, patients with severe social anxiety should be assessed for safety as well as their ability to maintain self-care. Are they obtaining food? Do they have safe shelter? An acute deterioration in functioning may herald comorbid illness or changes in the patients' social system that hinder self-care—for example, a supportive family member has stopped paying the patient's rent. Specific social stressors should be addressed, but severe impairment resulting in an inability to care for oneself may require hospitalization.

Conclusion

There are numerous causes of anxiety for patients in the ED—if only because anxiety is a normal part of life and being a patient in the ED is stressful. However, when anxiety becomes resistant to normal reassurance or a source of impairment itself, the clinician should consider the presence of an anxiety or stressor-related disorder. Emergency clinicians are well positioned to treat these disorders with brief psychotherapy, psychoeducation, thoughtful suicide risk intervention, medications, and referrals to ongoing care.

References

1. Weiss AJ, Barrett ML, Heslin KC, Stocks C. Trends in emergency department visits involving mental and substance use disorders, 2006–2013. HCUP Statistical Brief No. 216. Agency for Healthcare Research and Quality. Published 2016. Updated December 6, 2016. Accessed June 2, 2020. https://www.hcup-us.ahrq.gov/reports/statbriefs/sb216-Mental-Substance-Use-Disorder-ED-Visit-Trends.jsp

2. American Psychiatric Association. *Diagnostic and Statistical Manual of Mental Disorders*. 5th ed. American Psychiatric Publishing; 2013.

3. Gupta MA. Review of somatic symptoms in post-traumatic stress disorder. *Int Rev Psychiatry*. 2013;25(1):86–99.

4. Niles AN, Dour HJ, Stanton AL, et al. Anxiety and depressive symptoms and medical illness among adults with anxiety disorders. *J Psychosom Res*. 2015;78(2):109–115.

5. Simpson SA, Goans C, Loh R, Ryall K, Middleton MCA, Dalton A. Suicidal ideation is insensitive to suicide risk after emergency department discharge: Performance characteristics of the Columbia-Suicide Severity Rating Scale Screener. *Acad Emerg Med*. 2021;28(6):621–629.

6. Goldman-Mellor S, Olfson M, Lidon-Moyano C, Schoenbaum M. Association of suicide and other mortality with emergency department presentation. *JAMA Netw Open*. 2019;2(12):e1917571.

7. Simpson SA, Sakai J, Rylander M. A free online video series teaching verbal de-escalation for agitated patients. *Acad Psychiatry*. 2020;44(2):208–211.

8. Scheer V, Blanco C, Olfson M, et al. A comprehensive model of predictors of suicide attempt in individuals with panic disorder: Results from a national 3-year prospective study. *Gen Hosp Psychiatry*. 2020;67:127–135.

9. McDonald A, Eccles JA, Fallahkhair S, Critchley HD. Online psychotherapy: Trailblazing digital healthcare. *BJPsych Bull*. 2020;44(2):60–66.

10. Smits JA, Berry AC, Rosenfield D, Powers MB, Behar E, Otto MW. Reducing anxiety sensitivity with exercise. *Depress Anxiety*. 2008;25(8):689–699.

11. Wulsin L, Liu T, Storrow A, Evans S, Dewan N, Hamilton C. A randomized, controlled trial of panic disorder treatment initiation in an emergency department chest pain center. *Ann Emerg Med*. 2002;39(2):139–143.

12. Bighelli I, Trespidi C, Castellazzi M, et al. Antidepressants and benzodiazepines for panic disorder in adults. *Cochrane Database Syst Rev*. 2016;2016(9):CD011567.

13. Garakani A, Murrough JW, Freire RC, et al. Pharmacotherapy of anxiety disorders: Current and emerging treatment options. *Front Psychiatry*. 2020;11:595584.

14. Lim B, Sproule BA, Zahra Z, Sunderji N, Kennedy SH, Rizvi SJ. Understanding the effects of chronic benzodiazepine use in depression: A focus on neuropharmacology. *Int Clin Psychopharmacol.* 2020;35(5):243–253.

15. Kessler RC, Aguilar-Gaxiola S, Alonso J, et al. Trauma and PTSD in the WHO World Mental Health Surveys. *Eur J Psychotraumatol.* 2017;8(Suppl 5):1353383.

16. Kroll J. Posttraumatic symptoms and the complexity of responses to trauma. *JAMA.* 2003;290(5):667–670.

17. Bryant RA. Acute stress disorder as a predictor of posttraumatic stress disorder: A systematic review. *J Clin Psychiatry.* 2011;72(2):233–239.

18. Steenen SA, van Wijk AJ, van der Heijden GJ, van Westrhenen R, de Lange J, de Jongh A. Propranolol for the treatment of anxiety disorders: Systematic review and meta-analysis. *J Psychopharmacol.* 2016;30(2):128–139.

19. Gelpin E, Bonne O, Peri T, Brandes D, Shalev AY. Treatment of recent trauma survivors with benzodiazepines: A prospective study. *J Clin Psychiatry.* 1996;57(9):390–394.

20. Simpson SA. A single-session crisis intervention therapy model for emergency psychiatry. *Clin Pract Cases Emerg Med.* 2019;3(1):27–32.

21. Fegan J, Doherty AM. Adjustment disorder and suicidal behaviours presenting in the general medical setting: A systematic review. *Int J Environ Res Public Health.* 2019;16(16):2967.

22. Juurlink DN, Herrmann N, Szalai JP, Kopp A, Redelmeier DA. Medical illness and the risk of suicide in the elderly. *Arch Intern Med.* 2004;164(11):1179–1184.

23. Mayland CR, Harding AJE, Preston N, Payne S. Supporting adults bereaved through COVID-19: A rapid review of the impact of previous pandemics on grief and bereavement. *J Pain Symptom Manage.* 2020;60(2):e33–e39.

24. Shear MK, Ghesquiere A, Glickman K. Bereavement and complicated grief. *Curr Psychiatry Rep.* 2013;15(11):406.

25. Hamdan S, Berkman N, Lavi N, Levy S, Brent D. The effect of sudden death bereavement on the risk for suicide. *Crisis.* 2020;41(3):214–224.

26. Fernandez de la Cruz L, Rydell M, Runeson B, et al. Suicide in obsessive–compulsive disorder: A population-based study of 36,788 Swedish patients. *Mol Psychiatry.* 2017;22(11):1626–1632.

12

Personality Disorders

Joseph B. Bond and Nicole R. Smith

Introduction

In addition to mood, thoughts, and behaviors, the field of psychiatry is concerned with how an individual views themself and interacts with the world. *Personality* is a stable and enduring set of characteristics that are distinct to an individual and predict how that individual will interact with their environment. Although not strictly defined, personality is thought to have both developmental and environmental origins. When the personality traits of an individual differ significantly from what is typically or culturally expected such that they are impaired in some area of functioning, such as cognition, emotions, relationships, or impulse control, then that individual might be diagnosed with a personality disorder (PD). The fifth edition of the *Diagnostic and Statistical Manual of Mental Disorders* (DSM-5) defines 10 specific PDs as well as PDs due to another medical condition or not otherwise specified.[1]

Regardless of the clinical specialty, all clinicians are likely to encounter patients with PDs; the prevalence is estimated to be approximately 10% of the general population in the United States[2] and approximately half of patients in psychiatric settings.[3] A PD diagnosis is predictive of high utilization of psychiatric emergency services,[4,5] as well as prolonged length of stay in the emergency department (ED).[6] Although patients may not necessarily have a chief complaint of a PD, PDs are, by definition, pervasive and thus frequently affect areas of health and well-being. For example, patients diagnosed with a PD are more likely to also be diagnosed with chronic medical conditions such as hypertension,[7] diabetes,[8] and obesity,[9] and they are more likely to present to the ED and be hospitalized overnight for non-psychiatric medical reasons than the general population.[10,11] Patients with PDs have shorter life spans overall than those without comorbid PDs.[12] These are often the most difficult patients physicians see, and so an understanding of the etiology, epidemiology, and common features of PDs can help improve patient care and reduce misunderstandings that often lead to conflict in clinical settings.

Patients with PDs often elicit emotional reactions from members of their care team. The goal of this chapter is to teach clinicians how to recognize those emotions as diagnostic tools for identifying PD traits that affect patient care and care team well-being. Recognizing these traits and the patterns that they follow paves the way for better patient and self-care. An understanding of the etiology of PDs makes it easier to provide compassionate care for these difficult patients. That is, people are rarely disruptive for the fun of it; humans have various ways to ensure that their needs are met, and disruptive behaviors, even those behaviors that become counterproductive, serve a purpose—to fulfill a need for safety, reassurance, or comfort. Often, what the patient needs or is seeking is hidden behind challenging behaviors, but a clinician who has learned the skills to recognize patterns in these behaviors is capable of recognizing those needs. Many of the factors that can negatively affect care team morale, such as non-adherence, disruptive behaviors, and frequent ED utilization, can be exacerbated by a disconnect between what the patient needs and what the clinical team provides (even with the best intentions).

Remember, a patient seen in the ED may be having the worst day of their life so far, so they may behave in a dysfunctional or regressed way. Although it is important to recognize disordered personality traits, it may not be helpful or even possible to diagnose a PD from an isolated ED encounter. The clinician evaluating patients in an emergency setting should be aware of the patterns that occur within PDs but should avoid diagnosing a PD without evidence that the observed behaviors are stable and pervasive. Some patients with specific PDs will become high utilizers of emergency services and medical care. In those circumstances, it can be very valuable to include PDs in the differential diagnosis and treatment planning because there are specific treatments and approaches that can benefit patients with certain PDs.

The 10 named PDs have classically been divided into three clusters for ease of discussion (Table 12.1). These clusters are meant to be descriptive, but there is no genetic or etiologic link identified within clusters at this time. As evidence of this, one person may have co-occurring PDs from different clusters. A common mnemonic to differentiate the three clusters is the weird (Cluster A), the wild (Cluster B), and the worried (Cluster C).

Table 12.1 Summary of Personality Disorders

Personality Disorder	Predominant Traits	Function of Behaviors
Paranoid personality disorder	Paranoia and mistrust of others	An attempt to feel safe or secure
Schizoid personality disorder	Prefers solitude, few emotional connections, and flattened affect	An attempt to find comfort, to relieve distress
Schizotypal personality disorder	Odd beliefs, behaviors, and appearance; a schizophrenia spectrum disorder	An attempt to explain sensory and perceptual disturbances
Antisocial personality disorder	Disregard for the autonomy of others, lack of empathy	An attempt to have needs/desires fulfilled by using others as tools
Borderline personality disorder	Unstable emotions and impulsive behaviors	An attempt to avoid feelings of abandonment and to feel understood
Histrionic personality disorder	Dramatic and attention-seeking	An attempt to gain nurturance through attention and praise
Narcissistic personality disorder	Grandiosity, need for admiration, lack of empathy	An attempt to mask a fragile sense of self through external validation
Avoidant personality disorder	Social inhibition, feelings of inadequacy, hypersensitivity to negative evaluation	An attempt to avoid rejection
Dependent personality disorder	Submissive and clinging behavior	An attempt to elicit caregiving due to lack of self-efficacy
Obsessive–compulsive personality disorder	Rigid need for order and perfection	An attempt to maintain control, predict the environment, and avoid failure

Cluster A Personality Disorders

Cluster A PDs include paranoid personality disorder, schizoid personality disorder, and schizotypal personality disorder. Individuals with these disorders are unlikely to present with a chief complaint related to their PD and often fail to present with medical illness or present later in the course of the disease due to symptoms of the Cluster A PD. These patients may be oddly related to resistant and may underreport symptoms to avoid further interaction. This cluster is the most highly correlated with schizophrenia spectrum illnesses.

Paranoid Personality Disorder

Paranoid PD is characterized by suspiciousness of others. A person with paranoid PD mistrusts the motives of others in multiple contexts (not just health care). The patient demonstrates at least four of the following seven diagnostic symptoms: (1) suspects that others are trying to deceive or hurt them, (2) doubts the trustworthiness or loyalty of other people, (3) hesitates to confide in others for fear that information will be used against them, (4) infers insulting or threatening meaning from benign comments, (5) bears grudges or is unable to forgive, (6) retaliates against others for perceived offenses, and (7) is suspicious that romantic partners are unfaithful without evidence. In addition, these symptoms must not be better explained by another condition, such as a psychotic disorder or substance use. As with all PDs, these symptoms should be part of a persistent pattern and not a one-time occurrence to be considered a PD.

Clinical Considerations

This condition may affect academic, career, and social functioning and begin in childhood. Few data exist about suicide risk in people with paranoid PD. Having a relative with a psychotic disorder may increase the risk of developing a paranoid PD, but the link is not as well characterized as it is with schizotypal PD discussed later in this chapter.[13]

Paranoid PD typically does not require additional treatment, but other causes of paranoia might. Although paranoia is a common feature of psychotic disorders (e.g., schizophrenia), psychotic disorders involve a constellation of other positive symptoms (e.g., hallucinations, delusions, and disorganized thoughts) and negative symptoms (e.g., avolition, social withdrawal, and blunted affect) that differentiate them from paranoid PD, in which those other symptoms are absent. Paranoid PD may also be confused with substance-induced paranoia or delirious paranoia, so an infectious workup and toxicology may help differentiate the etiology of a patient's paranoia.

Epidemiology

The prevalence of paranoid PD is estimated to be 2.3–4.4% of the population, and it is diagnosed more frequently in males.[14,15]

Case Example

John, a 51-year-old man with no known past medical history and taking no medications, presents to the ED with chest pain. Nitroglycerine and aspirin are ordered for John while awaiting confirmatory lab work. When the nurse offers the medications, he initially declines to take them. "What are these for? Did the cardiologist say to take these? I haven't even seen a cardiologist yet." He does eventually take them after some reassurance. Electrocardiogram (ECG) is indicative of non-ST segment elevation myocardial infarction. When discussing these results with the emergency physician, John asks, "Are you sure those were my lab results? There are a lot of patients here and you could have gotten them confused." The physician indicates that they are, in fact, his results, to which John states, "The nurse checked my name and date of birth before giving me those pills, but you didn't check that stuff. Do you even know that you're supposed to do that?" To appease John, the physician asks him to confirm his name and date of birth. However, John gives the wrong name and birthday to see if she double-checks. The physician is initially startled, thinking that maybe she did walk into the wrong room. She checks his wristband, which lists his correct name and birth date. She confronts John about giving false information, and he states, "I need a different doctor, one who knows what they are doing. There is no way I could trust you after you made such an error." The physician feels frustrated with John but also has some doubts about herself and wonders if maybe she should have done something differently. Soon after, John's wife approaches the physician. She had been waiting in the lobby outside of the ED. She says,

> John would be mad if I told you this, but he has been having that chest pain for a few days now. He saw his doctor yesterday and the doctor told him to go to the emergency room then, but he would not go, because he was convinced that his doctor was trying to run up a higher bill. Please don't tell him I talked to you. I am really worried about him, I think he might be having a heart attack, but he gets so upset if I talk about him behind his back. He wouldn't hurt a fly, but he just has a hard time trusting people, you know.

John's case is a good example of how individuals with personality disorders can incite doubt and confusion in medical staff. His care was delayed because of his distrust of others. Once in the appropriate treatment setting, John creates conflict by speaking down to the staff and becoming argumentative. One can easily see how the staff would believe John is trying to manipulate them. John is scared, as anyone would be when told that they are having a heart attack. He genuinely believes that his actions will help him feel safe, but, in fact, they are counterproductive.

Personality Pearls

As with other PDs discussed in this chapter, many of the thought and behavior patterns observed in those with paranoid personality traits can be understood as a maladaptive way to serve some function. In this case, that function is to create a sense of safety. For that reason, the symptoms of paranoid PD are often worse in times of stress, such as in the ED. Patients with paranoid PD view the world as hostile. Consequently, they tend to mistrust medical professionals and may project that mistrust onto a clinician who is trying to help them. Clinicians will avoid projective identification by remaining predictable and professional.

Schizoid Personality Disorder

Schizoid PD is characterized by disconnection from and disinterest in social relationships and activities. Someone with schizoid PD demonstrates at least four of the following seven symptoms: (1) disinterest in having or forming close relationships, (2) preference for solitude, (3) limited or no interest in romantic or sexual relationships, (4) limited or no interest in activities, (5) few or no friends or confidants (excluding first-degree relatives), (6) indifference to the opinion of others, and (7) blunted emotional/affective range. In addition, these symptoms must not be better explained by another condition, such as a psychotic disorder or substance use. As with all PDs, these symptoms should be part of a persistent pattern and not a one-time occurrence.

Clinical Considerations

Those with this condition may appear to live an isolated life, but people with schizoid PD are not typically distressed by their symptoms and so rarely report other psychiatric symptoms. Schizoid PD is not known to increase the risk of death from suicide. There may be an increased prevalence of schizoid PD in the first-degree relatives of those with schizophrenia, but this link is not as strong as it is with schizotypal PD (discussed later).[13]

There is no specific treatment for schizoid PD, and people who have it are not typically distressed by it. However, schizoid PD can be confused with other conditions that do have specific treatments. The social withdrawal and disinterest in relationships are similar to the negative symptoms described in schizophrenia, but unlike schizophrenia, schizoid PD is not associated with cognitive or functional decline or positive symptoms (e.g., hallucinations or delusions). Schizoid PD also has some similarities to autism spectrum disorder (ASD) but lacks the sensory symptoms, motor symptoms, or developmental delays associated with autism.

Epidemiology

Because people with schizoid PD tend to avoid interactions with other people, they are not commonly seen in a clinical setting. The infrequent presentation makes it difficult to state the prevalence of schizoid PD, but some sources estimate that between 3% and 5% of people meet the diagnostic criteria.[14,15]

Case Example

Jeff, a 38-year-old man with no significant medical history, presents to the ED, where he drove himself from his home 30 miles away, reporting right arm pain. On examination, it is clear that his humerus was broken a few days ago. Jeff is wearing a homemade sling around his right arm. Brittany, the triage nurse assessing him, becomes quickly frustrated by his brief, monosyllabic answers:

"So what happened to your arm?"
"Skiing."
"The injury must have been a few days ago. And did you try to fix it yourself?"
"Yeah."
"The doctor will probably want an X-ray to know where exactly the break is. To get the best angle for the X-ray, we may need to move your arm a bit. I imagine that could be painful. Would you like to take some medication for pain now so that it can start to work before you get the X-ray?"
"Okay."

Brittany goes on to explain that the pain medication may make Jeff feel tired or loopy, so he may need someone to help drive him home after he is X-rayed and casted. Brittany asks if there is someone who Jeff can call to get a ride home in a couple of hours, but Jeff says there is no one. He lives alone and has no close friends in the area. He does freelance web design from his home, so he also has no work colleagues.

Brittany and the rest of the medical team find themselves in a quandary because they do not want to manipulate his arm without providing some pain medication, but neither do they want him to drive home after taking an opioid pain reliever. Jeff also presented later after the injury than he might have had he not had symptoms of schizoid PD. In Jeff's case, this could lead to less-than-ideal approximation and healing. People with schizoid PD may avoid or delay medical care until the disease process is at an advanced stage, and they may have limited or no social support.

Personality Pearls

The function of the schizoid behaviors is to create a comfortable environment, generally solitude, so these patients rarely present to the ED. They may not have close personal relationships, but family involvement (when possible) can be a valuable resource. If no social supports can be identified, it may be necessary to consult social work to assist with a disposition plan (e.g., a cab ride home).

These patients may be difficult to connect with and may not demonstrate expected reciprocal social responses. This can make the interviewer feel distant or disengaged. Long silences and the interpersonal distance may feel uncomfortable for the clinician, but it is what the patient with schizoid PD needs to feel comfortable. Tolerating one's own discomfort can lead to a more productive interview.

Schizotypal Personality Disorder

Schizotypal PD is characterized by deficits in social functioning, unusual thoughts or perceptions, and eccentric behavior. A patient with schizotypal PD demonstrates at least five of the following nine symptoms: (1) thoughts that events are directly linked to or influenced by them (ideas of reference), (2) unusual beliefs or superstitions that are not explained by cultural or religious norms (magical thinking), (3) misinterpretation of sensory experiences (illusions), (4) unusual thought processing and/or speech, (5) mistrust of others, (6) incongruent affect, (7) eccentric dress or appearance, (8) lack of close relationships, and (9) social anxiety often due to mistrust of others. In addition, these symptoms should not be the result of a thought disorder, mood disorder, or ASD.

Clinical Considerations

Schizotypal PD, more so than other PDs, is associated with future development of other psychiatric conditions. In fact, the DSM-5 also includes schizotypal PD in the chapter on schizophrenia spectrum disorders. There appears to be a genetic component linking schizotypal PD to other schizophrenia spectrum disorders, as evidenced by its increased prevalence among those with a first-degree relative with a schizophrenia spectrum disorder and vice versa.[16–18] Given the increased risk for developing a schizophrenia spectrum disorder, those diagnosed with schizotypal PD are at an increased risk to die from suicide.[19]

Epidemiology

The prevalence of schizotypal PD in the general population appears to be approximately 3.9%.[20] However, the prevalence in clinical settings is lower than that (0–2%).[1] This could be due to the fact that symptoms that reach clinical significance often progress to schizophrenia, which then "overrides" the diagnosis of schizotypal PD.

Case Example

Stella, a 22-year-old woman with a past medical history of asthma, presents to the ED reporting worsening depression during the past few weeks. She is well groomed but wearing multiple pieces of crystal jewelry that she reluctantly surrenders when changing into a hospital gown. She states,

> I'm a Pisces, so I guess I have always been gloomy, an old soul you could say, but this feels different. I just don't feel motivated or excited about anything, and I am tired all the time. I was planning to call my primary care doctor, but I guess I never did, and tonight I started wishing that I was dead. Nothing against my doctor, of course; she is lovely, but I just couldn't make the call for some reason. Maybe I was afraid of what she might do, my doctor, not my mom. My mom came here, well, was brought here by the police once. I was worried that my doctor might call the police on me. I'm kind of nervous around the police. They never did anything to me, it's just all the stuff on the news. You can't really trust anyone, can you?

She continues to speak tangentially, as if telling a story out of order, but is not pressured. She insists that she is not feeling suicidal and has no plan or intent to die but feels that she would rather be dead than to feel the way she does. She describes how she used to enjoy her work as a school librarian and how she made some extra money over the summer reading tarot cards for shoppers at a local farmer's market, but none of those things have been pleasurable for the past few weeks. She wishes that she had someone to talk to about her recent feelings but finds that people do not "stick around for long." When asked about hallucinations, she describes "an electrical sensation" that allows her to sense other people's thoughts sometimes but denies ever hearing voices or sounds that no one else can and denies any visual hallucinations. The psychiatry resident assessing Stella believes that she meets criteria for major depressive disorder, but also found that Stella made him feel uncomfortable and scattered.

Stella demonstrates many of the traits that define schizotypal PD, but she also describes symptoms of depression that are not explained by schizotypal PD alone. She even tries to explain her depression symptoms through her system of beliefs. Stella's case is meant to illustrate that those with a PD are not immune to other psychiatric disorders. Those with schizotypal PD, unlike other Cluster A PDs, may be distressed by their limited social connectedness. The resident feels uncomfortable and scattered around Stella; this is a good representation of how those with schizotypal PD might make others feel and why it is difficult for them to maintain relationships. These feelings can be important diagnostic tools, but it is also important to listen empathically and to avoid acting cold or distant because this could worsen paranoid thoughts.

Personality Pearls

Some of the symptoms of schizotypal PD function to create a narrative that explains some of the sensory and perceptual symptoms that those with schizotypal PD experience, not unlike early civilizations creating myths to explain natural phenomena. It is unnecessary and unhelpful to try to dissuade the patient from their odd beliefs. As noted in the case, patients with schizotypal PD may generate a feeling of discomfort or a disconnect from the clinician. This countertransferential feeling is similar to that experienced by clinicians interviewing patients with psychotic disorders. However, recognizing the symptoms of schizotypal PD and the correlation with other schizophrenia spectrum disorders can help mental health clinicians form a treatment plan that includes follow-up assessments. Some patients with schizotypal PD may fail to meet the criteria for a psychotic disorder at one time but then meet criteria later in the course of the disease process. In high-risk patients (e.g., those with a strong family history), it may even be beneficial to consider treatment of psychotic symptoms even if they do not meet criteria for schizophrenia yet, because schizotypal PD symptoms can significantly lower quality of life and ability to function.[21] In addition to psychotic disorders, patients with schizotypal PD are also at higher risk for depression. Of note, belief systems that are congruent with a patient's own culture or religion (e.g., the belief in life after death in some religions) do not indicate a schizotypal PD, so it may be helpful to perform a cultural assessment or to ask about spirituality or religion.

Cluster B Personality Disorders

Cluster B includes four different personality disorders: antisocial PD, borderline PD, histrionic PD, and narcissistic PD. These PDs are related to an individual's sense of self and their ability to form connections with others. These PDs can lead people to react in ways that seem out of context to observers. As a result, Cluster B PDs are associated with a higher risk of suicide than the other clusters.[22,23] When interviewing a patient with Cluster B PD, the patient may derail the process with unrelated details and emotionally laden behaviors. This may lead the clinician to feel overwhelmed, frustrated, or that they have lost control of the conversation. However, an understanding of the function these behaviors serve can help recenter the clinician with empathy and direction.

Antisocial Personality Disorder

Antisocial PD is a pervasive disregard for the autonomy of others. Although antisocial PD, like other PDs, is not usually diagnosed in children or adolescents, symptoms must begin by age 15 years and include at least three of the following seven diagnostic symptoms: (1) disregard for social norms and institutions (e.g., breaking laws), (2) dishonesty—especially deception for personal gain, (3) impulsive behaviors, (4) irritability and aggressive behaviors, (5) disregard for the safety and well-being of others, (6) failure to follow through with obligations, and (7) lack of remorse or empathy. These symptoms must be part of a pattern and not only present as a feature of another psychiatric disorder such as schizophrenia or mania.

Clinical Considerations

Symptoms of antisocial PD begin in childhood or adolescence. Children and adolescents who display antisocial PD traits are often diagnosed with conduct disorder. If the antisocial traits persist into adulthood, then the conduct disorder diagnosis is converted to a diagnosis of antisocial PD. Not every child diagnosed with conduct disorder will meet criteria for antisocial PD in adulthood. Both conduct disorder and antisocial PD patients are more likely to have experienced childhood abuse or trauma or a head injury, but none of those are required to make a diagnosis.[24] There is evidence indicating that those with maldevelopment of the limbic system are more likely to be diagnosed with antisocial PD.[25] Terms such as "sociopath" and "psychopath" have been used to describe people with antisocial PD, but the DSM-5 makes no distinction. There is a correlation between antisocial PD and substance use disorder,[26,27] as well as increased likelihood to be arrested and incarcerated for various charges, both misdemeanor and criminal.[28] Those with more arrests are more likely to be affected by antisocial PD. Those with antisocial PD have shorter life spans and are more likely to die of suicide.[22]

Epidemiology

Whereas conduct disorder has a relatively high prevalence at approximately 9.5%,[29] the prevalence of antisocial PD is relatively low at 0.2–3%. Antisocial PD is diagnosed in men approximately three times more often than in women, but some studies suggest that this difference may not be entirely genetic but also associated with cultural factors.[30,31] It is estimated that in an incarcerated population, up to 60% of inmates meet criteria for antisocial PD.[30] Interestingly, antisocial PD may be more common among corrections workers in prisons as well.[32]

Case Example

Michael is a 44-year-old man with a past medical history of attention-deficit/hyperactivity disorder (ADHD), alcohol use disorder, cannabis use disorder, and opioid use disorder who was brought in by police for suicidal ideation (SI). A local restaurant owner called the police when Michael tried to leave without paying his bar tab. When police arrived, they checked his record and found that there were multiple warrants out for his arrest, so they prepared to arrest him. When Michael was handcuffed and placed into the police car, he stated that he was feeling suicidal and needed to go to the hospital. At the hospital, an officer waits outside of his room while the doctor enters to evaluate him. Michael says, "I am too tired to talk now, come back later."

The doctor replies, "I understand that, but I do need to make sure that you are safe. Are you having suicidal thoughts?"

Michael shrugged and said,

Yeah, I feel like I might jump off a bridge or something. Look, I can't really focus on this right now. I have ADHD and haven't had any Adderall in a few days. Someone stole mine and my doctor won't give me a new prescription because she doesn't understand how important it is to treat my ADHD. If you get me some Adderall, I'll answer all of your questions. I take 30 mg, two of them. And turn the lights out when you leave so I can get some rest.

The doctor tried to engage Michael again, but Michael rolled over in the stretcher and would not answer. Given that Michael reported suicidal ideation with a plan, the doctor asked security and the waiting police officer to collect Michael's belongings and to have him change into a hospital gown. When security asked Michael to change and surrender his belongings for search and safekeeping, he refused and became hostile. He demanded to be discharged and recanted his suicidal thoughts. "I'm fine now forget it. There aren't even any bridges in town anyway."

The doctor is faced with a dilemma: Michael lied, but at which point in time. That is, was he lying about having SI or lying about the SI having abated? In reviewing Michael's chart, the doctor found multiple similar encounters wherein Michael came to the hospital and demanded pain medication, sleeping medication, or stimulants but left soon after being denied those things. Given this information and the fact that Michael would be discharged into police custody, the doctor felt comfortable signing his discharge papers.

Cases such as Michael are not uncommon in EDs. Michael has a pattern of manipulating others to have his needs met (e.g., delaying incarceration and getting stimulants). Recognizing this pattern was helpful when the doctor was deciding on a safe disposition. Michael was benign (just wanting to rest) but showed a rapid shift in tone and changed his story when asked to do something that he did not want to do. This can also be a helpful clue that the patient may have antisocial PD traits and may help inform the clinician's approach.

Personality Pearls

Patients with antisocial PD trigger strong emotional responses in others, so it is important to recognize these emotions when they occur and to treat the patient according to best practices rather than with sympathy or anger. The clinician must not be coerced into providing care that is counter-therapeutic or harmful, but neither should the clinician completely dismiss the concerns of those with antisocial PD. Specifically, those with antisocial PD are more likely to have co-occurring substance use, so if they will be in the hospital for an extended time, it may be necessary to monitor for withdrawal from alcohol and benzodiazepines or barbiturates, which can become a medical emergency. Although opioid withdrawal is not lethal, it is generally considered the standard of care to monitor and treat symptoms of opioid withdrawal, even when the patient may be manipulative. In addition, although suicidal statements may be made to manipulate others, those with antisocial PD are at an increased risk to die from suicide, so a suicide risk assessment tool such as the Columbia-Suicide Severity Rating Scale[33] can be helpful. Patients with antisocial PD may be more likely to demonstrate malingered symptoms or symptoms that do not have a physiologic cause. Various rating scales are available to assist in the evaluation of general or specific malingering symptoms (e.g., depression, hallucinations, and memory deficits).[34]

Borderline Personality Disorder

Borderline PD is characterized by unstable relationships, sense of self, and emotions as evidenced by erratic and sometimes harmful behaviors. People with borderline PD demonstrate at least five of the following nine symptoms: (1) frantic efforts to avoid abandonment; (2) unstable interpersonal relationships that vacillate between extremes (love or hate, idealization or devaluation); (3) unstable identity or self-image; (4) at least two different impulsive and potentially harmful behavior patterns (self-harm, substance use, unsafe sex, unsupported spending, disordered eating, etc.); (5) self-harm or recurrent suicidal behaviors, threats, or gestures; (6) unstable and reactive mood with labile affect; (7) feelings of emptiness; (8) intense or inappropriate feelings of anger; and (9) paranoia or dissociative symptoms especially when under stress. The final symptom (paranoia or dissociation) led to the name of the disorder because it was thought that the reaction to stress was on the borderline between psychotic and neurotic defense mechanisms. The behaviors that are hallmark to borderline PD often evoke a strong response from others. These behaviors may re-create the emotional turmoil that these patients feel inside. These symptoms may occur in adolescence, but borderline PD is generally not diagnosed until early adulthood or when the pattern has proven to be pervasive and enduring.

Clinical Considerations

Borderline PD has gained cultural relevance recently as more celebrities and public figures share their experiences with the diagnosis to raise awareness. Although not a part of the diagnostic criteria, many cases of borderline PD are preceded by trauma. There is evidence linking trauma and borderline PD through changes in the hypothalamic–pituitary–adrenal axis, glucocorticoid signaling, and gene methylation.[35,36] Symptoms typically arise in adolescence or early adulthood and may fluctuate in severity throughout early and middle adulthood before generally decreasing in severity by middle to late adulthood. In fact, there are even data indicating that up to 85% of patients with borderline PD achieve complete remission of symptoms after 10 years (remission is defined by no longer meeting criteria for the disorder for at least 12 months).[37]

Symptoms tend to worsen around times of stress and may result in "self-sabotaging" behaviors wherein the person's borderline PD symptoms undermine their own goals or accomplishments. This is an important consideration because those with borderline PD may be at the highest risk to die from suicide in the weeks following an inpatient hospitialization.[38] Compared to the general population, those with borderline PD are at an increased risk to die from suicide. It is estimated that between 8% and 10% of those with borderline PD will die from suicide.[39,40] Those with borderline PD are also at risk for substance use, physical violence, sexual violence, and poverty, which can all negatively affect health. Although there are therapies meant to address the symptoms of other PDs, dialectical behavioral therapy (DBT) was developed specifically for and shows efficacy in treating borderline PD.[41] DBT is the gold standard, but even a single session of psychoeducation can reduce symptom severity,[42] so even in regions where DBT is not readily accessible, other therapeutic interventions can still help reduce symptom burden.

Epidemiology

The prevalence of borderline PD is estimated to be as low as 1.6% in the general population but as high as 20% in the inpatient psychiatry population. There is a general idea that borderline PD is more common in women, but recent studies suggest that men are just as likely to meet criteria for borderline PD but also have behaviors consistent with antisocial PD and so are diagnosed with that instead (even though the two are not mutually exclusive). Women are more likely to have treatment including pharmacology and psychotherapy, whereas men are more likely to develop a substance use disorder and to be arrested.[43]

Case Example

Abbie, a 19-year-old woman, is brought to the ED by emergency medical services (EMS) after her ex-girlfriend called 911 stating that Abbie was texting her about her plans to take an intentional overdose of her home quetiapine in a suicide attempt. EMS arrived before she took any medication, but she continued to state that she could not be safe from her suicidal thoughts and requested to be transported to the ED. Abbie has a medical history of fibromyalgia and migraine headaches but has no pain complaints on this presentation. She is prescribed topiramate for migraines; quetiapine for sleep, mood, and anxiety; and gabapentin for her fibromyalgia.

Abbie was seen first by the emergency medicine (EM) resident, Dr. Cunningham. When Dr. Cunningham saw Abbie's name show up on the patient list, he thought, "Ugh, her again." Abbie is a high utilizer of emergency services at Dr. Cunningham's hospital. Dr. Cunningham and other members of the staff are familiar with Abbie from previous ED visits. She frequently presents with similar suicidal thoughts and has presented with four previous suicide attempts by overdosing on medications. She often stays in the ED overnight but feels safe to return home the next morning. Occasionally, she becomes disruptive in the ED (refusing to stay in her room, insisting on being seen immediately, etc.), but she has not been physically aggressive. There have been discussions about creating a behavioral plan for Abbie's ED visits, but this has not been created yet. Dr. Cunningham's first call is to the psychiatry resident. He implies that Abbie should be admitted, but the psychiatry resident is hesitant to commit to admit her without speaking with her outpatient team. She has been admitted approximately 10 times in the 2 years that Dr. Cunningham has worked in the ED. Dr. Cunningham finds himself feeling irritated and even angry as he prepares to argue with the psychiatry resident to admit Abbie.

Patients with borderline PD can be among the most difficult to treat in emergency settings. Like Abbie, they are likely to be high utilizers of emergency services. Like most physicians, Dr. Cunningham feels job satisfaction in treating patients and watching their health improve through his efforts, so it is easy to see why patients such as Abbie, who present to the ED for care multiple times but never seem to improve, can elicit feelings of cynicism—a defense for Dr. Cunningham. Another difficulty when caring for these patients is that they may behave in a way that forces others to feel what they are feeling. That is, when these patients feel angry, they are able to make those around them feel angry as well. They can also cause discord through behaviors that facilitate splitting among team members (as seen between Dr. Cunningham and the psychiatry resident).

Personality Pearls

People generally do not choose to behave in these dysfunctional ways. Rather, the patterns of behavior seen in borderline PD are repeated because they serve a function, or they did at some point in time. For example, although dissociation is detrimental in daily life, it may be advantageous or protective during times of trauma. The primary function of borderline PD behaviors is to avoid feelings of abandonment, but there are also secondary functions to avoid or diffuse intolerable emotions or to make others experience the emotions that the person with borderline PD is experiencing; that is, the symptoms are a way to feel understood.

Many of these individuals will present to the ED after self-harming by cutting, head-banging, swallowing objects, or various other forms of self-mutilation. This nonsuicidal self-injury (NSSI) is separate from suicidal behavior. It is essential to do a full safety assessment when a patient presents with self-harm to differentiate between NSSI and a suicide attempt. Motivations vary, but frequently patients will say that physical pain is a distraction from emotional pain; although they cannot control the emotional pain, they believe that they can control the physical pain from NSSI. Emptiness is a common symptom of borderline PD, so some might want to "just feel something" by inducing pain. There are, in fact, neurophysiological effects from self-harm that individuals may find pleasurable. Studies have shown that there are lower baseline levels of endogenous opioids in individuals who engage in NSSI, possibly related to effects of chronic stress such as childhood trauma. It is theorized that individuals who engage in these behaviors do so to achieve a release of endogenous opioids that can regulate emotions.[44,45] No matter the motivation, the primary reason is an inability to use other coping skills for emotional pain.

Clinicians should guard against the tendency to react with strong emotions to these patients because this can reinforce the borderline PD symptoms. On the other hand, apathy is also counter-therapeutic because it may result in symptom escalation due to feelings of not being heard or understood. Symptom escalation due to negative interactions between the patient and staff can increase the need for potentially avoidable medical interventions (restraints and intramuscular medications). Instead, the clinician can create a holding environment for the patient and model distress tolerance.

The first priority in the psychiatric emergency setting is safety. For acutely agitated patients, verbal de-escalation should take precedence to minimize excessive use of medical interventions. Benzodiazepines and antipsychotics can be used but carry the risk of side effects such as sedation, as well as paradoxical disinhibition with benzodiazepines or extrapyramidal symptoms with antipsychotics. Physical restraints should only be used in the most extreme circumstances in which there is imminent risk of harm to the patient or others and all other efforts to maintain safety have failed.

In deciding whether to admit or discharge a patient with borderline PD from the ED, it is essential to collaborate with the patient's outpatient care team. If the patient receives care at a community mental health center, they may have a case manager who can coordinate services. If possible, family or other loved ones should be involved. Importantly, encouraging active participation in care planning from the patient can help reestablish an internal locus of control, thus increasing self-efficacy.

It can be difficult to feel alignment with a patient who is actively trying to hurt or kill themself. It may even feel as if the physician is at odds with the patient with borderline PD. Understanding the functions of these behaviors and that the etiology often involves an adaptation to trauma can be helpful in replenishing empathy for these patients. Although these patients may be high utilizers of emergency services during periods of their lives, there is hope in the fact that the majority of people diagnosed with borderline PD will no longer meet the criteria after 10 years. In addition, unlike many of the other PDs, borderline PD has a treatment modality that is efficacious and evidence-based (when done according to the model)—DBT.[41] This form of therapy may not be readily available to all patients, but if the patient does have a DBT team, the team can be invaluable in helping risk stratify and safety plan with the patient (even after hours).

Histrionic Personality Disorder

Histrionic PD is characterized by exaggerated emotionality and attention-seeking behaviors. Patients with histrionic PD are most comfortable as the center of attention and when they feel an emotional connection to those around them. These individuals show a pattern of at least five of the following traits: (1) discomfort when not the center of attention; (2) seductive or provocative behaviors; (3) shallow and rapidly changing emotions; (4) use of physical appearance to draw attention; (5) impressionistic speech with few factual details; (6) dramatic, theatrical displays of emotion; (7) being impressionable; and (8) believing relationships to be closer than they are. These traits must be present from early adulthood and present in multiple domains. Combined, these traits can result in a person who expresses emotion over substance and seeks attention over intimacy.

Clinical Considerations

There is a significant amount of overlap between histrionic PD and borderline PD, in which individuals can also express rapidly shifting emotions and attention-seeking behavior. Borderline PD is distinguished by an intense negative view of the self and chronic feelings of emptiness and loneliness, whereas those with histrionic PD do not necessarily have a low view of themselves. This pattern of rapidly shifting emotions may also be confused for the lay use of the term "bipolar." However, histrionic PD distinguishes itself from true bipolar affective illness in that the mood swings typically occur in response to something in the environment and thus can be changed through external influence. That is, mood swings in those with bipolar affective disorder occur independent of environmental factors and last for longer periods of time (often days to weeks), whereas mood swings in histrionic PD are strongly influenced by external factors and can change within minutes to hours. Those with antisocial PD or narcissistic PD may also treat a new acquaintance with the intimacy usually reserved for a close friend or display sexually provocative behaviors. Histrionic PD can be differentiated by the goal of attaining attention and validation rather than exploitation. As may be expected, those with histrionic PD are at an increased risk to attempt suicide.[46]

Epidemiology

The prevalence of histrionic PD is thought to be 1.84% of the population in the United States.[14] There was once a sense that histrionic PD was more common in women than in men, but more recent population-based studies found no difference in frequency between genders.[47] These data suggest a probable ascertainment bias because many of the "emotional" traits of histrionic PD were once thought to be more feminine.

Case Example

Nikki is a 55-year-old woman with no known medical problems who is brought into the ED by EMS. In the hallway before entering the exam room, she is sitting up on the gurney exclaiming, "I'm dying!" She's dressed in a low-cut evening gown wearing bright red lipstick and a colorful hat and has captured the attention of other patients and staff. Once in the exam room, she tells the EM physician, Dr. Wilson, "I cannot do it anymore. My heart has arrested. There is not enough oxygen in the room." She squints and looks at his nametag, "Jeremy. Can I call you Jeremy?" Dr. Wilson asks if she is having any chest pain and she replies, sobbing, "I've been stabbed in the chest and ripped open!" He listens to her heart and asks if she is having any palpitations. "Only when you get close to me like that, darling," she responds with a smile.

Dr. Wilson orders an ECG, which shows normal sinus rhythm. Troponins are negative. Nikki is oxygenating well on room air. Physical exam is normal.

Nikki's friend Blake arrives and explains that they are actors and the reviews have just come out for their recent show. Upon seeing the unfavorable reviews earlier in the night, Nikki began hyperventilating, grabbed her chest, complained of numbness in her extremities, and began to speak of doom and death.

Dr. Wilson determines that Nikki has had a panic attack and provides reassurance.

Nikki has several features consistent with histrionic PD. Upon arrival, she makes herself the center of attention by exclaiming loudly and theatrically for everyone to hear. She displays dramatic, rapid shifts in emotions as she goes from sobbing to flirting. She describes her symptoms with very little detail, instead using vague and exaggerated statements such as "I'm dying!" Like the bold brush strokes of impressionist art, her impressionistic speech serves to capture the essence and feelings of her experience rather than an accurate portrayal of reality. Patients with histrionic PD use physical appearance and sexuality as a tool for external validation and attention; this can be seen in her style of dress and her flirtatiousness with her doctor. Attention garnered in this way can serve as an ego boost to correct underlying low self-esteem. Similarly, patients with histrionic PD may overvalue interpersonal connectedness by imagining relationships to be more intimate than they are, such as when Nikki uses Dr. Wilson's first name with familiarity and refers to him by the term of endearment "darling."

Personality Pearls

Rapid, shallow shifts in emotion may seem to the outside observer to be inauthentic or fake; however, these emotions feel completely real for people with histrionic PD. Deception is not the goal but, rather, empathy and compassion. When a patient with histrionic PD is flirtatious or sexually provocative, it is important for the clinician to set firm boundaries. Although it may seem counterintuitive, enforcing normative boundaries can be incredibly reassuring for these patients, who may feel overwhelmed or out of control in the ED. These patients frequently display somatization and may present to the ED with exaggerated concerns for their physical health. That is, the strong emotions they experience may also have bodily manifestations such as chest tightness with anxiety or limb numbness with depression. Again, a lack of physiologic explanation for these symptoms does not indicate manipulation or deceit but is instead an opportunity for the physician to acknowledge what the patient is feeling and reassure them of their safety.[48]

Narcissistic Personality Disorder

Narcissistic PD is characterized by grandiosity, a need for admiration, and lack of empathy. It is diagnosed by five or more of the following traits: (1) inflated sense of self-importance; (2) preoccupation with or fantasies of success, power, or beauty; (3) a belief of being unique or special; (4) need for constant admiration; (5) a sense of entitlement or expectation of compliance from others; (6) exploitation of others; (7) a lack of empathy; (8) envy of others or belief that others are envious of them; and (9) arrogance. These symptoms must occur by early adulthood and be present in multiple domains.

Clinical Considerations

Women with narcissistic PD are slightly more likely than the general population to also have a diagnosis of an anxiety disorder or bipolar affective disorder, type II. Men with narcissistic PD are more likely than the general population to have a co-occurring substance use diagnosis, obsessive–compulsive PD, or histrionic PD. Regardless of gender, people with narcissistic PD are more likely to carry a diagnosis of bipolar affective disorder, type I, post-traumatic stress disorder, schizotypal PD, or borderline PD and less likely to be diagnosed with dysthymia (persistent depressive disorder). Narcissistic PD is associated with an increased risk of death from suicide. Interestingly, those with narcissistic PD are less likely to make impulsive, low-lethality suicide attempts but are more likely to attempt suicide by more lethal means, and thus they are more likely to die from their suicide attempts.[49] In contrast to other psychiatric disorders associated with increased suicide risk, those with narcissistic PD may have low or no intent while also having a very well-formed plan or even steps of furtherance.[50] For this reason, asking "Do you want to die?" may be insufficient to assess risk, and the clinician should also ask about any plans for suicide.

Epidemiology

Narcissistic PD occurs in approximately 6.2% of the population, with slightly more men than women meeting the diagnostic criteria (7.7% compared to 4.8%).[51]

Case Example

Ron is a 65-year-old man presenting to the ED brought in by one of his employees. The employee tells the triage desk that he is concerned about Ron's safety. Apparently, the two were playing squash together earlier that afternoon at Ron's club. Ron became winded and performed poorly during the game. After the employee won, Ron became visibly frustrated and started to say things such as "I might as well kill myself." The employee was not sure what to do, so he brought Ron to the nearest hospital. When the ED resident enters the room, she introduces herself, "Hi, my name is Dr. Thomas. Can you tell me what brought you into the hospital?"

Initially, Ron states his chief complaint as shortness of breath. He explains that he became more winded than usual while playing squash. When Dr. Thomas asks about the suicidal statements that the employee mentioned, Ron becomes defensive:

> What are you talking about? That's ridiculous! I would never do something like that! I am the CFO of a multi-billion-dollar organization, I can get any woman I want and take her to an island resort on a company jet! You would kill to be me for a day. I would never kill myself! Call the medical director of the hospital. He knows me. We play golf together. Such an upstanding guy—hope he runs this hospital better than he plays golf.

Dr. Thomas again tries to ask about the suicidal statement: "That does sound like a very nice life. I wonder what could have happened tonight to make your friend concerned about your safety. Help me to understand what happened." Ron answered,

> Let me tell you. I started playing squash when I was a young boy—I was taught by the best, it's true—and all my life when I play people say, Ron, you are the best squash

player there is. I could beat anybody. And that's how I became so good at business. My father always said, you wake up an hour before everyone else, go to sleep an hour after. That's how you succeed in life, young lady. Hard work. You have to beat people and be ready for the game.

Dr. Thomas finds herself getting bored and losing track of the conversation. She looks at her notes and realizes this tangent has been going on for nearly a minute. She decides to redirect the conversation back to her question and repeats it.

"Look. This is enough. I'm ready to leave. This place is full of idiots. When am I going to see the doctor?"

Ron exhibits multiple symptoms common among those with narcissistic PD: inflated sense of self-importance ("CFO of a multi-billion-dollar organization"), preoccupation with success/power ("best squash player"), belief that he is unique and special ("I could beat anybody"), a sense of entitlement (asking to speak to the medical director), exploitation of others (implication that to succeed in life, one has to beat others), assumption that others are jealous of him ("You would kill to be me for a day"), and arrogant behavior throughout the interaction with Dr. Thomas. Although not a diagnostic criterion, devaluing others is also a common trait among patients with narcissistic PD (assuming that Dr. Thomas is not the doctor). The techniques that Dr. Thomas used were helpful in preventing an escalation and redirecting Ron toward the pertinent information. For example, she was able to model empathy and humility even when it was difficult for Ron to demonstrate those traits, thus avoiding a power struggle. Dr. Thomas experienced a feeling of boredom when listening to Ron describe himself and his career. She maintained a sense of direction, which prevented her from getting overwhelmed by Ron's extraneous details. Dr. Thomas was wise to continue to ask about safety even when Ron attempted to change the topic because patients with narcissistic PD are at an increased risk to die from suicide even though they may not make many nonlethal attempts that might indicate a "cry for help" in other psychiatric conditions.

Personality Pearls

In a medical setting, the risk to the patient's health can be a narcissistic threat because it represents a possible loss in control, power, or beauty. For example, patients with narcissistic PD may struggle more with symptoms of angina or shortness of breath or problems that cause disfigurement because these symptoms limit functioning and therefore negatively impact the patient's vulnerable self-worth.[52] In this vulnerable state, the symptoms of narcissistic PD may be more prevalent—devaluing others in order to elevate the patient's self-worth, non-adherence to exert a sense of control, demanding unnecessary tests or consultations, or threatening litigation. Although it can be tense, it is important to remember that a patient's demand is not typically a medical justification for specific testing or treatments. An alternative approach to bolster their self-worth and to give them back a sense of control without subjecting them to unwarranted and potentially harmful interventions would be to involve them in the decision-making discussions. Clinicians can validate how the patient feels—if the patient feels understood, then they can begin to regain a sense of autonomy (without the need for a power struggle). Clinicians can avoid adversarial encounters by remaining imperturbable and communicating effectively—even apologizing if the situation warrants because this can diffuse some of the tension inherent in such cases. For example, acknowledging that a patient waited too long to see the doctor and apologizing for the fact of the wait (without taking direct responsibility) can help create an alliance. "Oh! You are right, ma'am, you have been waiting over an hour. That would make anyone upset. I appreciate how patient you have been, and I am ready now to do everything I can to help."

As discussed in the case of Ron, common countertransferential feelings when treating a patient with narcissistic PD can range from a sense of boredom to hatred of the patient. An awareness of one's own countertransference allows the clinician to maintain compassion despite the tendency toward projective identification. For example, a patient who assumes that their doctor does not care about them may engender a sense of indifference in the doctor by their behaviors.

A patient with narcissistic PD who is having suicidal thoughts may feel ashamed, and they may attempt to hide that shame by avoiding the topic and focusing instead on topics that bolster their self-esteem. Like the case of Ron, these patients may defend against that discomfort by derailing the conversation or adding distracting information about more comfortable topics. However, patients with narcissistic PD remain at an elevated risk to die from suicide, so it is important that the clinician persevere in assessing both intent and the presence of a plan for suicide.

Cluster C Personality Disorders

Cluster C personality disorders include avoidant PD, dependent PD, and obsessive–compulsive PD. Those with Cluster C PDs are notable for having worries that compel them to behave in a certain way that relieves or delays the cause of those worries. As such, although these PDs are unlikely to be the presenting complaint in an ED, they can affect both psychiatric and medical presentations. These patients may seem hesitant and indecisive, requiring reassurance throughout the clinical interview. There are not as much data describing the risk for suicide among those with Cluster C PDs compared to some of the Cluster B PDs; however, some data suggest that patients with comorbid depression and Cluster C PDs are more likely to describe suicidal ideation than those with depression alone.[53]

Avoidant Personality Disorder

Avoidant PD is characterized by a general sense of inadequacy and hypersensitivity to criticism, resulting in restricted social engagement. Avoidant PD symptoms must be present from early adulthood and include four of the following seven symptoms: (1) avoidance of jobs or activities that involve interpersonal contact, (2) fear of not being "liked," (3) hesitance to enter an intimate relationship for fear of rejection, (4) preoccupation with criticism or rejection in social settings, (5) feelings of inadequacy that limit social interactions, (6) view of self as inferior, and (7) reluctance to participate in activities that could result in embarrassment.

Clinical Considerations
Cluster C PDs are associated with other psychiatric comorbidities, including depressive disorders, anxiety disorders, and eating disorders. The symptom profile of avoidant PD is similar to that of social anxiety disorder. Some have even suggested that the two may

exist on a continuum; however, avoidant PD is differentiated by symptoms affecting self-image and inadequacy and a debilitating, deep fear of embarrassment. That is, someone with avoidant PD may feel unsafe because they are inadequate, whereas someone with social anxiety disorder may feel unsafe because the world is judgmental. Of course, the two may also be comorbid—the patient feels inadequate and feels that other people are judgmental. More than one-third of people with social anxiety disorder may also meet the criteria for avoidant PD.[54]

Epidemiology
Approximately 2.36% of the U.S. population are estimated to meet criteria for avoidant PD.[14]

Case Example

Dan is a 20-year-old man with diabetes mellitus type 1, depression, social anxiety, and obsessive–compulsive disorder (OCD). He is brought to the ED by his parents, who found him confused, shaky, and sweaty early this morning. In the ED, he is oriented to self but not to place, time, or situation. He complains of weakness, dizziness, and headache. He is notably irritable, anxious, and diaphoretic. His blood glucose is found to be 45. After the ED physician stabilizes his hypoglycemia, she considers the possibility of an intentional insulin overdose given his psychiatric history and calls a psychiatry consult from Dr. Hong.

On interview, Dan is reserved and restrained when speaking with Dr. Hong. His parents explain to Dr. Hong that Dan has been waking up sweating and anxious in the middle of the night most nights for the past 6 months. He has not seen his endocrinologist or gotten any blood work done due to anxiety about blood draws, despite encouragement for the past year. His parents describe him as an introvert with few friends. They struggle to get him to leave the house with them to go places and note that sometimes it takes him hours to work up the courage to take the dog on a walk because he is afraid of being embarrassed. They have tried to encourage him to join extracurricular activities in his college, but he has declined due to fears of embarrassing himself and feeling like no one will like him.

On interview alone, Dan tells Dr. Hong, "You must think I'm so stupid." He explains that the last time he saw his endocrinologist, he had been told that he would likely need a continuous glucose monitor due to his fluctuating glucose levels. He states, "I know I should follow up but . . . I know he's judging me. I can't do anything right. I can't even keep my blood sugars stable. It's humiliating. You must think I'm such an idiot for messing this up." Dr. Hong responds empathically, stating, "It must be really hard having to manage that every day." She assesses him for depression, and he stops himself frequently mid-sentence, biting his nails and sighing in frustration. "I'm sorry. I don't want to waste your time. I just . . . I don't want to tell you the wrong thing." She assures him that he is in a safe place. He denies depressed mood, suicidal ideation, or intentional insulin overdose (which is supported by his normal C peptide level). She conducts a full safety assessment with collateral from his family and his therapist and determines that he is safe for discharge with therapy follow-up but would also benefit from medications for anxiety, so she also places a referral for a psychiatrist and emphasizes the importance of following up with his endocrinologist.

In this case, Dan meets several criteria for avoidant PD, which is apparent in his repeated statements of his own sense of inadequacy and failure. Although some might label him a "noncompliant patient" and feel annoyed at his perplexing lack of follow-up, understanding that he avoided medical care due to his debilitating fear of being criticized by his doctor makes it easier to understand his inaction. In fact, Dan very much wanted to control his diabetes but felt too embarrassed by his disease progression to discuss it with his endocrinologist. Dr. Hong's use of reassurance relieved some of his anxiety, allowing him to complete the interview. Some clues that this is avoidant PD rather than just his social anxiety disorder come from his parents' collateral information regarding the depth and extent of his fears of embarrassment and his own self-efficacy pervading all aspects of his life.

Personality Pearls

As seen in the case of Dan, patients with avoidant PD may be so impeded by their own symptoms as to obfuscate the interview. These patients may retract their own reports, withhold pertinent information, or minimize their own suffering to avoid further interactions with clinicians. The patient's goal is not to deceive but, rather, to relieve distress by avoiding prolonged interactions. While caring for such patients, clinicians might notice that they feel boredom or exasperation. It can be helpful to set the expectation that you are listening nonjudgmentally and most concerned with the patient's safety and well-being. An expert interviewer may even be able to speak with the patient in such a way as to bolster their confidence and enhance the therapeutic alliance. On the other hand, a patient who senses judgment from the clinician may begin to demonstrate even more severe symptoms of hesitance, mistrust, and general avoidance, further derailing the interview process. For this reason, it is important to be aware of one's own reaction to these patients to avoid showing emotions that could be interpreted as impatience or criticism.

Also seen in the case of Dan, those with avoidant PD may feel embarrassment at their own clinical symptoms and so delay care for fear that they might be blamed or reprimanded for their symptoms. As such, they may present later in the course of an illness or delay until symptoms are too severe to continue avoiding care. Even when they are able to attend physician appointments, they may avoid other situations that involve social interactions. Imagine a patient who is prescribed a benzodiazepine but is too afraid of his pharmacist judging him for being on such a medication to go in for his refill. This patient might present to the ED with benzodiazepine withdrawal symptoms that were precipitated by his avoidant PD.

Dependent Personality Disorder

Dependent PD is characterized by a pervasive need to be cared for, leading to pathologic passivity and fear of separation. A person can be diagnosed with dependent PD if they demonstrate five of the following eight symptoms: (1) inability to make decisions without advice or reassurance, (2) ceding most responsibilities to others, (3) hesitation to disagree with others for fear of losing approval, (4) difficulty initiating tasks due to lack of self-confidence, (5) willingness to do unpleasant things to receive nurturance from others, (6) fear of being alone or being unable to care for themself, (7) a frantic need for a new relationship when another relationship ends, and (8) preoccupation with fears of being left to care for themself. These symptoms should be present by early adulthood and should be inappropriate in some way. That is, a person with difficulty standing from a wheelchair may ask another shopper at the grocery store to reach for a high item for him. Although this behavior does show some dependence on another, it is appropriate to the situation and so would not indicate a dependent PD.

Clinical Considerations

Individuals with dependent PD are highly likely to seek medical care and therefore comprise a significant portion of patients presenting to the ED.[55,56] Dependent PD is associated with an increased risk for both suicide attempts and death from suicide. Dependent PD is prevalent in elderly populations but is also associated with suicide attempts earlier in life. Specifically, dependent PD is associated with increased suicidal behaviors in all genders but most notably in males. In depressed men who attempted suicide, almost three-fourths reported symptoms of dependent PD (specifically related to self-worth).[57,58]

Dependent PD and avoidant PD overlap in both presentation and comorbidity. Both involve a sense that others are more capable and a fear of rejection from others. However, the two differ in the motivations for these symptoms. Those with dependent PD fear being left alone to their own insufficient resources, whereas those with avoidant PD fear that they will be judged by others for their inadequacies. There is also some overlap with borderline PD, and 30–40% of those diagnosed with borderline PD will also meet criteria for dependent PD.[59] The symptoms of dependent PD may appear, at first, similar to anhedonia. However, the two are distinct in that someone with anhedonia does not perform tasks due to lack of motivation, whereas someone with dependent PD does not perform tasks due to lack of self-efficacy. It could be important in an emergency setting to recognize that those with dependent PD are more likely to be victims of intimate-partner violence (as this may be the presenting problem).[60] In addition, males with more dependent traits may be more likely to be physically assaultive toward female partners.[61,62]

Although passivity and submission are among the diagnostic criteria, when faced with the fear of losing a caregiving spouse or partner, behaviors can rapidly shift to more assertive and even violent means to avoid abandonment.

Epidemiology

The prevalence of dependent PD is thought to be 0.49% of the population in the United States, and it is diagnosed more often in women.[14] There is also a high prevalence in the elderly.[58]

Case Example

Jack is a 30-year-old man with a history of depression who presents to the ED with a chief complaint of "I won't survive!" He has a history of childhood abuse and one psychiatric admission following a suicide attempt by overdose on his home sertraline after his divorce last year. His therapist recently left for a 1-week vacation.

Jack is seen by the emergency psychiatrist Dr. Brown. Jack states, "I can't function without my therapist! I know she said she's on vacation, but she is not answering when I call. I just . . . don't know how to get by without her." He denies suicidal ideation, plan, or intent; he simply has the feeling that he cannot survive if he cannot speak with his therapist.

He repeatedly asks Dr. Brown what she thinks he should do and whether she thinks he needs to be in the hospital. "You're so much smarter than me, Dr. Brown. I can tell that you understand. I'll trust you whatever you say. So, do you think I need to be admitted?"

Jack explains that he is also going through a breakup right now with his girlfriend, Susan. "She just broke up with me out of the blue, and I don't know what to do without her. I love her so much. Here, let me call her so you can talk to her." Without waiting for a response from Dr. Brown, Jack pulls out his phone and dials.

Jack says, "Susan, I am in the emergency room again, and my doctor needs to talk to you." After Dr. Brown introduces herself warily, Susan states,

> I haven't seen him for a month, so I really don't know how he's been doing. We broke up a month ago. We'd only been dating 6 weeks and then I noticed he couldn't do anything without me. He is so clingy. I told him I couldn't be his mom anymore and that he needed to talk to a professional.

Meanwhile, Jack's mother, Lucille, enters the exam room. She states, "I think we have been here long enough, don't you, sweetie? I will have you talk to my therapist in the morning and see if he can start seeing you instead."

As they go to leave, Jack thanks Dr. Brown, "You're so helpful. Can you be my psychiatrist outside the hospital?" Dr. Brown notices that in response to his shy and childlike demeanor, she is reminded of her young son, and she almost agreed to see Jack as an outpatient before considering that this may be crossing a boundary because she already has a long wait-list of other patients waiting to see her in her clinic.

For patients with dependent PD, others in their lives become an important fixture and the patient may feel lost or out of control when those people are unavailable—like Jack's therapist or ex-girlfriend. Jack feels incapable of making any decision on his own, and so he has been depending on others whom he views as more competent than himself to make decisions for him. These patterns are common in patients who are frequent care utilizers. Dr. Brown likely found it difficult to assess Jack's safety given his chief complaint and the general vagueness. Although Jack may believe that he could not survive while his therapist is on a 1-week vacation, there does not appear to be any threat of suicide or self-harm. This is reassuring to Dr. Brown, although she is also aware that those with dependent PD are at an increased risk for suicide attempt. Jack's relationship with his mother seems enmeshed, but it can also be protective. That is, that relationship is the purview of his psychiatrist, not the ED.

Personality Pearls

Patients with dependent PD can invoke in some physicians an urge to parent or to protect or even to do favors for the patient. Although this may initially make the physician providing care feel good about the work they are doing, it often leads to feelings of frustration in the clinician who is compelled to cross their own boundaries. One could easily imagine how it might feel good to a doctor to know that a patient trusted and relied on them. However, this pattern can breed an unhealthy codependency and resentment. If the doctor continues to go out of their way to meet the dependent patient's needs, a pattern may develop in which the dependent patient continues to rely on the doctor's efforts and the doctor continues to cross boundaries to feel helpful (e.g., offering appointments outside of normal clinic time or answering messages on days off). Imagine the patient who pleads for an appointment outside of regular clinic hours. It might feel good for the clinician to be able to offer this service to an appreciative patient, but this may reinforce the cycle of dependency.

Other physicians may feel an aversion toward patients with dependent traits. Patients with dependent PD are very sensitive to social cues, and if they sense that the physician does not like them, it may reinforce the needy and clingy behaviors out of a feeling of rejection. In turn, this increase in dependent behaviors amplifies the aversion.

If the physician is aware of their own reaction when working with patients with dependent PD, they are more likely to be able to regulate their own behaviors to prevent worsening of the dependent symptoms in the patient. Because the function of dependent PD traits is to elicit caregiving behaviors from others, it is important for the physician to avoid falling into a codependency trap by offering too much care and also important to avoid worsening the patient's dependent symptoms by showing disinterest.

Obsessive–Compulsive Personality Disorder

Obsessive-compulsive PD involves a widespread preoccupation with order and control. It includes patterns of perfectionism and rigidity to the detriment of efficiency and interpersonal relationships. A patient with obsessive–compulsive PD will demonstrate at least four of the following eight symptoms: (1) preoccupation with details, order, rules, or schedules such that the point of the activity is lost; (2) perfectionism that interferes with task completion; (3) excessive devotion to work or responsibilities to the detriment of interpersonal relationships (excluding circumstances of financial necessity); (4) a rigid system of rules or values; (5) inability to discard objects that are no longer needed; (6) hesitance to delegate without strict oversight; (7) frugal spending habits; and (8) general rigidity and stubbornness. These symptoms should be present by early adulthood.

Clinical Considerations

Although obsessive–compulsive PD is unlikely to be the chief complaint, many other psychiatric conditions may be complicated by symptoms of obsessive–compulsive PD.

There are, as one might suspect, similarities between OCD and obsessive–compulsive PD, including compulsions, rigid thinking patterns, checking behaviors, need for completion, perfectionism, and hoarding. Although the colloquial use of the term "OCD" often refers to those who have obsessive–compulsive PD traits, the two clinical diagnoses are distinct. One way to differentiate the two (OCD and obsessive–compulsive PD) is to consider the level of distress caused by these symptoms. Patients with OCD are distressed by the intrusive thoughts that drive them to compulsions (ego-dystonic). Patients with obsessive–compulsive PD often do not find their symptoms distressing; that is, symptoms of obsessive–compulsive PD are aligned with the patient's own worldview and values (ego-syntonic). The distress in obsessive–compulsive PD often comes from the consequences of their symptoms on their relationships. Another distinction is that obsessive–compulsive PD does not include motor compulsions.

Obsessive–compulsive PD may have some symptoms in common with ASD, including restrictive behaviors, rigidity, perfectionism, and over-conscientiousness. There is a high concurrence between ASD and obsessive–compulsive PD in clinical populations and among family members, leading some to believe that there may be a neurodevelopmental link between the two.[63] Obsessive–compulsive PD does not include the sensory symptoms associated with ASD. Some of the social/interpersonal symptoms appear to be more pervasive in ASD than obsessive–compulsive PD. As a PD, obsessive–compulsive PD is typically only diagnosed in adults, whereas the majority of ASD diagnoses are in childhood or adolescence.

Obsessive–compulsive PD is often comorbid with eating disorders. Approximately one in seven patients in treatment for an eating disorder also meet criteria for obsessive–compulsive PD.[64]

Along with the other Cluster C PDs, obsessive–compulsive PD is associated with an increased risk for suicidal behavior. Suicide risk may be masked by obsessive–compulsive PD symptoms. A person with obsessive–compulsive PD may appear rigid and in control, hiding vulnerability and making it difficult for clinicians and family members to recognize the seriousness of the patient's depression.[65] Patients with obsessive–compulsive PD may also seem emotionally cold, distant, and controlling, which can make it more difficult for loved ones and clinicians to empathize with them or recognize their distress.

Epidemiology
The prevalence of obsessive–compulsive PD is thought to be 7.88% of the population in the United States, making it the most prevalent PD.[14] It is diagnosed more often in men but thought to be about equally prevalent.

Case Example

Amanda is a 23-year-old woman with a history of generalized anxiety disorder and anorexia nervosa, in remission, who presents to the ED at the recommendation of her clerkship director. Amanda is a third-year medical student currently on her Ob/Gyn rotation. At presentation, Amanda is extremely drowsy and difficult to interview, so her clerkship director provides collateral. Apparently, Amanda reported to her inpatient obstetrics rotation for rounds this morning but was slurring her words and falling asleep during patient handoff from the on-call team. Amanda's clerkship director is the inpatient attending this week, and so, when she noticed this, she asked Amanda to step outside to talk. At first, Amanda tried to deny that anything was wrong, but she could not stand and fell to the floor unexpectedly. The clerkship director was able to get a wheelchair and take Amanda down the hallway to the emergency room for an evaluation.

Amanda's vital signs are unremarkable (HR 60, BP 105/65, RR 9, O_2 97%) at evaluation, but she is somnolent and sobbing while saying, "I'm sorry." She is dressed in scrubs and clinging to a notebook containing her patient lists from the past week along with meticulous notes on each patient. After her vitals are taken and labs are drawn, she starts to clear and becomes more alert. After reviewing her vitals and labs, everything appears normal except that her urine toxicology is positive for benzodiazepines. The emergency physician goes back to Amanda's room to try to understand more about what is going on. At first, Amanda reports, "I am fine. I just made a mistake, but it's fine now." She tries to get up and leave, but the emergency physician is concerned about her safety and asks Amanda to tell him more about what happened. Amanda reluctantly tells him that she got her scores back from the shelf exam from her previous rotation this morning and did not do as well as she needed to high pass. In her frustration with herself, she took the remainder of her bottle of clonazepam that had been prescribed for panic attacks. She thinks there were approximately 10 1-mg pills in the bottle when she took them approximately 6 hours ago. She stops crying, composes herself, continues to insist that she is fine now, and tries to leave. Although she can provide a coherent response and present a stoic confidence that she is "fine" and "I need to get back to rounds, because I have two more patients to present before noon conference," the emergency physician does not believe that she should leave before talking to psychiatry to assess her suicide risk.

The psychiatry consultant arrives and speaks with Amanda's roommate for collateral. Amanda's roommate is surprised to hear that Amanda is in the ED. She says,

> She has never seemed depressed or anything like that. I mean, she is the top of the class and makes it look easy. I have never known her to show any signs of being upset or down or anything. It seems like she always has everything completely under control. I thought she was doing really well, because she is already studying for Step 2. She already has a study calendar and everything. She is kind of a champ at that stuff . . . it bugs the hell out of me sometimes.

In this case, Amanda fits many criteria for obsessive–compulsive PD. She sets a high standard of perfection, and failure to meet that standard causes unmanageable distress—in this case even leading to a suicide attempt. Amanda displays self-criticism about the "stupid mistake" of making a "failed" suicide attempt rather than distress from the underlying psychosocial stress. Therefore, when assessing her, the psychiatric consultant might feel a disconnect between the presenting symptom (e.g., her recent suicide attempt) and the well-appearing person in front of them.

Personality Pearls

The functions of behaviors in obsessive–compulsive PD are to maintain control, predict the environment, and avoid failure. A factor to keep in mind when assessing patients with obsessive–compulsive PD, particularly in a crisis, is that their symptoms of obsessive–compulsive PD often obscure other psychiatric symptoms. They may be so well-practiced at maintaining emotional control that they do not show their underlying emotional turmoil. In the interview, they may try to avoid directly confronting vulnerable topics, and the clinician may need to redirect the patient to the present, utilizing empathy and validation to help the patient feel safe and comfortable. Addressing functional impairment may reveal the severity of symptoms. A clinician may identify with the hardworking and high-achieving obsessive–compulsive PD patient, but it is important to remain unbiased in assessing safety. As always, there are various tools that can help the clinician to stratify suicide risk. To avoid making a potentially fatal misdiagnosis and underestimating these patients, the clinician should be aware of this potential disconnect and consider facts of the case objectively.

Conclusion

In the emergency setting, staff will encounter patients with PDs and traits presenting with various clinical concerns. These individuals are more at risk for chronic illness and die sooner than those without a PD, so small targeted interventions in the ED can have cascading effects. This patient population is especially vulnerable, but their symptoms can also affect others (including friends, family, and caregivers), so it is important for clinicians to protect themselves from exhaustion and empathy depletion. It is hoped that, in reading this chapter, you have learned not only how to identify personality disorders but also to recognize an underlying need behind the PD symptoms. For each of the 10 PDs discussed in detail, we have illustrated through a case and our own experience that PD symptoms can serve a function for the patient. A clinician who can address that need in a more effective and less disruptive way can have a powerful impact on the patient's health outcomes. The patient is not the only one who benefits from these interventions. It is also hoped that the topics discussed in this chapter will reduce the stress associated with seeing patients with PDs and allow clinicians to feel confident and competent in their work. A clinician who is able to reflect on their own experiences and emotions is better able to understand a patient in crisis and the factors that can lead to care disruption.

References

1. American Psychiatric Association. Diagnostic and Statistical Manual of Mental Disorders. 5th ed. American Psychiatric Publishing; 2013.

2. Lenzenweger MF. Epidemiology of personality disorders. *Psychiatr Clin North Am*. 2008;31(3):395–403. doi:10.1016/j.psc.2008.03.003

3. Zimmerman M, Chelminski I, Young D. The frequency of personality disorders in psychiatric patients. *Psychiatr Clin North Am*. 2008;31(3):405–420. doi:10.1016/j.psc.2008.03.015

4. Richard-Lepouriel H, Weber K, Baertschi M, DiGiorgio S, Sarasin F, Canuto A. Predictors of recurrent use of psychiatric emergency services. *Psychiatr Serv*. 2015;66(5):521–526. doi:10.1176/appi.ps.201400097

5. Slankamenac K, Heidelberger R, Keller DI. Prediction of recurrent emergency department visits in patients with mental disorders. *Front Psychiatry*. 2020;11:48. doi:10.3389/fpsyt.2020.00048

6. Warren MB, Campbell RL, Nestler DM, et al. Prolonged length of stay in ED psychiatric patients: A multivariable predictive model. *Am J Emerg Med*. 2016;34(2):133–139. doi:10.1016/j.ajem.2015.09.044

7. El-Gabalawy R, Katz LY, Sareen J. Comorbidity and associated severity of borderline personality disorder and physical health conditions in a nationally representative sample. *Psychosom Med*. 2010;72(7):641–647. doi:10.1097/PSY.0b013e3181e10c7b

8. Pelizza L, Pupo S. Brittle diabetes: Psychopathology and personality. *J Diabetes Complications*. 2016;30(8):1544–1547. doi:10.1016/j.jdiacomp.2016.07.028

9. Gerlach G, Loeber S, Herpertz S. Personality disorders and obesity: A systematic review. *Obes Rev*. 2016;17(8):691–723. doi:10.1111/obr.12415

10. Fok ML-Y, Chang C-K, Broadbent M, Stewart R, Moran P. General hospital admission rates in people diagnosed with personality disorder. *Acta Psychiatr Scand*. 2019;139(3):248–255. doi:10.1111/acps.13004

11. Wagner JA, Pietrzak RH, Petry NM. Psychiatric disorders are associated with hospital care utilization in persons with hypertension. *Soc Psychiatry Psychiatr Epidemiol*. 2008;43(11):878–888. doi:10.1007/s00127-008-0377-2

12. Fok ML-Y, Hayes RD, Chang C-K, Stewart R, Callard FJ, Moran P. Life expectancy at birth and all-cause mortality among people with personality disorder. *J Psychosom Res*. 2012;73(2):104–107. doi:10.1016/j.jpsychores.2012.05.001

13. Kendler KS, McGuire M, Gruenberg AM, O'Hare A, Spellman M, Walsh D. The Roscommon Family Study: III. Schizophrenia-related personality disorders in relatives. *Arch Gen Psychiatry*. 1993;50(10):781–788. doi:10.1001/archpsyc.1993.01820220033004

14. Grant BF, Hasin DS, Stinson FS, et al. Prevalence, correlates, and disability of personality disorders in the United States: Results from the National Epidemiologic Survey on Alcohol and Related Conditions. *J Clin Psychiatry*. 2004;65(7):948–958.

15. Lenzenweger MF, Lane MC, Loranger AW, Kessler RC. DSM-IV personality disorders in the National Comorbidity Survey Replication. *Biol Psychiatry*. 2007;62(6):553–564. doi:10.1016/j.biopsych.2006.09.019

16. Asarnow RF, Nuechterlein KH, Fogelson D, et al. Schizophrenia and schizophrenia-spectrum personality disorders in the first-degree relatives of children with schizophrenia: The UCLA family study. *Arch Gen Psychiatry*. 2001;58(6):581–588. doi:10.1001/archpsyc.58.6.581

17. Kendler KS, Gruenberg AM, Strauss JS. An independent analysis of the Copenhagen sample of the Danish Adoption Study of Schizophrenia: II. The relationship between schizotypal personality disorder and schizophrenia. *Arch Gen Psychiatry*. 1981;38(9):982–984. doi:10.1001/archpsyc.1981.01780340034003

18. Siever LJ, Silverman JM, Horvath TB, et al. Increased morbid risk for schizophrenia-related disorders in relatives of schizotypal personality disordered patients. *Arch Gen Psychiatry*. 1990;47(7):634–640. doi:10.1001/archpsyc.1990.01810190034005

19. Palmer BA, Pankratz VS, Bostwick JM. The lifetime risk of suicide in schizophrenia: A reexamination. *Arch Gen Psychiatry*. 2005;62(3):247–253. doi:10.1001/archpsyc.62.3.247

20. Pulay AJ, Stinson FS, Dawson DA, et al. Prevalence, correlates, disability, and comorbidity of DSM-IV schizotypal personality disorder: Results from the Wave 2 National Epidemiologic Survey on Alcohol and Related Conditions. *Prim Care Companion J Clin Psychiatry*. 2009;11(2):53–67.

21. Cramer V, Torgersen S, Kringlen E. Personality disorders and quality of life: A population study. *Compr Psychiatry*. 2006;47(3):178–184. doi:10.1016/j.comppsych.2005.06.002

22. Bosman HS, van Rensburg CJ, Lippi G. Suicide risk of male State patients with antisocial personality traits. *S Afr J Psychiatr*. 2020;26:1543. doi:10.4102/sajpsychiatry.v26i0.1543

23. Oldham JM. Borderline personality disorder and suicidality. *Am J Psychiatry*. 2006;163(1):20–26. doi:10.1176/appi.ajp.163.1.20

24. Holmes SE, Slaughter JR, Kashani J. Risk factors in childhood that lead to the development of conduct disorder and antisocial personality disorder. *Child Psychiatry Hum Dev*. 2001;31(3):183–193. doi:10.1023/a:1026425304480

25. Raine A, Lee L, Yang Y, Colletti P. Neurodevelopmental marker for limbic maldevelopment in antisocial personality disorder and psychopathy. *Br J Psychiatry J Ment Sci*. 2010;197(3):186–192. doi:10.1192/bjp.bp.110.078485

26. Krueger RF, Markon KE, Patrick CJ, Benning SD, Kramer MD. Linking antisocial behavior, substance use, and personality: An integrative quantitative model of the adult externalizing spectrum. *J Abnorm Psychol*. 2007;116(4):645–666. doi:10.1037/0021-843X.116.4.645

27. Windle M. A longitudinal study of antisocial behaviors in early adolescence as predictors of late adolescent substance use: Gender and ethnic group differences. *J Abnorm Psychol*. 1990;99(1):86–91. doi:10.1037//0021-843x.99.1.86

28. Black DW, Gunter T, Loveless P, Allen J, Sieleni B. Antisocial personality disorder in incarcerated offenders: Psychiatric comorbidity and quality of life. *Ann Clin Psychiatry*. 2010;22(2):113–120.

29. Nock MK, Kazdin AE, Hiripi E, Kessler RC. Prevalence, subtypes, and correlates of DSM-IV conduct disorder in the National Comorbidity Survey Replication. *Psychol Med*. 2006;36(5):699–710. doi:10.1017/S0033291706007082

30. Alegria AA, Blanco C, Petry NM, et al. Sex differences in antisocial personality disorder: Results from the National Epidemiological Survey on Alcohol and Related Conditions. *Personal Disord.* 2013;4(3):214–222. doi:10.1037/a0031681

31. Moran P. The epidemiology of antisocial personality disorder. *Soc Psychiatry Psychiatr Epidemiol.* 1999;34(5):231–242. doi:10.1007/s001270050138

32. Holland TR, Heim RB, Holt N. Personality patterns among correctional officer applicants. *J Clin Psychol.* 1976;32(4):786–791. doi:10.1002/1097-4679(197610)32:4 <786::aid-jclp2270320409>3.0.co;2-f

33. Posner K, Brown GK, Stanley B, et al. The Columbia-Suicide Severity Rating Scale: Initial validity and internal consistency findings from three multisite studies with adolescents and adults. *Am J Psychiatry.* 2011;168(12):1266–1277. doi:10.1176/appi.ajp.2011.10111704

34. Miller HA. The Miller-Forensic Assessment of Symptoms Test (M-Fast): Test generalizability and utility across race literacy, and clinical opinion. *Crim Justice Behav.* 2005;32(6):591–611. doi:10.1177/0093854805278805

35. Cattane N, Rossi R, Lanfredi M, Cattaneo A. Borderline personality disorder and childhood trauma: Exploring the affected biological systems and mechanisms. *BMC Psychiatry.* 2017;17(1):221. doi:10.1186/s12888-017-1383-2

36. Martín-Blanco A, Ferrer M, Soler J, et al. Association between methylation of the glucocorticoid receptor gene, childhood maltreatment, and clinical severity in borderline personality disorder. *J Psychiatr Res.* 2014;57:34–40. doi:10.1016/j.jpsychires.2014.06.011

37. Gunderson JG, Stout RL, McGlashan TH, et al. Ten-year course of borderline personality disorder: Psychopathology and function from the Collaborative Longitudinal Personality Disorders study. *Arch Gen Psychiatry.* 2011;68(8):827–837. doi:10.1001/archgenpsychiatry.2011.37

38. Kullgren G. Factors associated with completed suicide in borderline personality disorder. *J Nerv Ment Dis.* 1988;176(1):40–44.

39. Paris J. Suicidality in borderline personality disorder. *Medicina.* 2019;55(6):223. doi:10.3390/medicina55060223

40. Pompili M, Girardi P, Ruberto A, Tatarelli R. Suicide in borderline personality disorder: A meta-analysis. *Nord J Psychiatry.* 2005;59(5):319–324. doi:10.1080/08039480500320025

41. Lynch TR, Trost WT, Salsman N, Linehan MM. Dialectical behavior therapy for borderline personality disorder. *Annu Rev Clin Psychol.* 2007;3(1):181–205. doi:10.1146/annurev.clinpsy.2.022305.095229

42. Biskin RS. The lifetime course of borderline personality disorder. *Can J Psychiatry.* 2015;60(7):303–308. doi:10.1177/070674371506000702

43. Sansone RA, Sansone LA. Gender patterns in borderline personality disorder. *Innov Clin Neurosci.* 2011;8(5):16–20.

44. Bresin K, Gordon KH. Endogenous opioids and nonsuicidal self-injury: A mechanism of affect regulation. *Neurosci Biobehav Rev.* 2013;37(3):374–383. doi:10.1016/j.neubiorev.2013.01.020

45. Stanley B, Sher L, Wilson S, Ekman R, Huang Y, Mann JJ. Non-suicidal self-injurious behavior, endogenous opioids and monoamine neurotransmitters. *J Affect Disord.* 2010;124(1–2):134–140. doi:10.1016/j.jad.2009.10.028

46. Ansell EB, Wright AGC, Markowitz JC, et al. Personality disorder risk factors for suicide attempts over 10 years of follow-up. *Personal Disord Theory Res Treat.* 2015;6(2):161. doi:10.1037/per0000089

47. Nestadt G, Romanoski AJ, Chahal R, et al. An epidemiological study of histrionic personality disorder. *Psychol Med.* 1990;20(2):413–422. doi:10.1017/s0033291700017724

48. Morrison J. Histrionic personality disorder in women with somatization disorder. *Psychosomatics.* 1989;30(4):433–437. doi:10.1016/S0033-3182(89)72250-7

49. Blasco-Fontecilla H, Baca-Garcia E, Dervic K, et al. Specific features of suicidal behavior in patients with narcissistic personality disorder. *J Clin Psychiatry.* 2009;70(11):1583–1587. doi:10.4088/JCP.08m04899

50. Chu C, Buchman-Schmitt JM, Joiner TE, Rudd MD. Personality disorder symptoms and suicidality: Low desire and high plans for suicide in military inpatients and outpatients. *J Personal Disord.* 2017;31(2):145–155. doi:10.1521/pedi_2016_30_241

51. Stinson FS, Dawson DA, Goldstein RB, et al. Prevalence, correlates, disability, and comorbidity of DSM-IV narcissistic personality disorder: Results from the Wave 2 National Epidemiologic Survey on Alcohol and Related Conditions. *J Clin Psychiatry.* 2008;69(7):1033–1045. doi:10.4088/jcp.v69n0701

52. Geringer ES, Stern TA. Coping with medical illness: The impact of personality types. *Psychosomatics.* 1986;27(4):251–261. doi:10.1016/S0033-3182(86)72700-X

53. Dervic K, Grunebaum MF, Burke AK, Mann JJ, Oquendo MA. Cluster C personality disorders in major depressive episodes: The relationship between hostility and suicidal behavior. *Arch Suicide Res.* 2007;11(1):83–90. doi:10.1080/13811110600992928

54. Cox BJ, Pagura J, Stein MB, Sareen J. The relationship between generalized social phobia and avoidant personality disorder in a national mental health survey. *Depress Anxiety.* 2009;26(4):354–362. doi:10.1002/da.20475

55. Soeteman DI, Hakkaart-van Roijen L, Verheul R, Busschbach JJV. The economic burden of personality disorders in mental health care. *J Clin Psychiatry.* 2008;69(2):259–265. doi:10.4088/jcp.v69n0212

56. Wilberg T, Hummelen B, Pedersen G, Karterud S. A study of patients with personality disorder not otherwise specified. *Compr Psychiatry.* 2008;49(5):460–468. doi:10.1016/j.comppsych.2007.12.008

57. Bolton JM, Belik S-L, Enns MW, Cox BJ, Sareen J. Exploring the correlates of suicide attempts among individuals with major depressive disorder: Findings from the National Epidemiologic Survey on Alcohol and Related Conditions. *J Clin Psychiatry.* 2008;69(7):1139–1149. doi:10.4088/jcp.v69n0714

58. Szücs A, Szanto K, Aubry J-M, Dombrovski AY. Personality and suicidal behavior in old age: A systematic literature review. *Front Psychiatry.* 2018;9:128. doi:10.3389/fpsyt.2018.00128

59. Bornstein RF, Becker-Matero N, Winarick DJ, Reichman AL. Interpersonal dependency in borderline personality disorder: Clinical context and empirical evidence. *J Personal Disord.* 2010;24(1):109–127. doi:10.1521/pedi.2010.24.1.109

60. Loas G, Cormier J, Perez-Diaz F. Dependent personality disorder and physical abuse. *Psychiatry Res.* 2011;185(1–2):167–170. doi:10.1016/j.psychres.2009.06.011

61. Berk S, Rhodes B. Maladaptive dependency traits in men. *Bull Menninger Clin.* 2005;69(3):187–205. doi:10.1521/bumc.2005.69.3.187

62. Murphy CM, Meyer SL, O'Leary KD. Dependency characteristics of partner assaultive men. *J Abnorm Psychol.* 1994;103(4):729–735. doi:10.1037//0021-843x.103.4.729

63. Gadelkarim W, Shahper S, Reid J, et al. Overlap of obsessive–compulsive personality disorder and autism spectrum disorder traits among OCD outpatients: An exploratory study. *Int J Psychiatry Clin Pract.* 2019;23(4):297–306. doi:10.1080/13651501.2019.1638939

64. Halmi KA, Tozzi F, Thornton LM, et al. The relation among perfectionism, obsessive–compulsive personality disorder and obsessive–compulsive disorder in individuals with eating disorders. *Int J Eat Disord*. 2005;38(4):371–374. doi:10.1002/eat.20190

65. Raja M, Azzoni A. The impact of obsessive–compulsive personality disorder on the suicidal risk of patients with mood disorders. *Psychopathology*. 2007;40(3):184–190. doi:10.1159/000100366

13

Deception in the Emergency Setting

Malingering and Factitious Disorder

Laura W. Barnett and Eileen P. Ryan

Malingering

Malingering involves purposeful deception and can be "pure" malingering (faking and/ or making up a disorder or symptoms), "partial" malingering (exaggerating genuine symptoms), and/or false imputation (when real symptoms are ascribed to a cause the individual knows is unrelated to the symptoms).[1] Many medical illnesses, including psychiatric disorders, can be malingered, some more easily than others. Exaggeration and outright deceit are not the exclusive purview of antisocial individuals but, rather, are pervasive in society.[2] In the emergency psychiatry setting, external benefits may be found in the form of temporary shelter, food, hospitalization as a respite from homelessness, and/or a safe, warm place to detox from drugs and/or alcohol. However, a desire for longer term food and shelter in the form of inpatient hospitalization, medications such as benzodiazepines, or to avoid legal consequences or responsibilities (e.g., an upcoming examination or occupational requirement) may also precipitate feigned or exaggerated psychiatric symptomatology.

Malingering is a medical diagnosis but is not recognized as a mental disorder in the fifth edition of the *Diagnostic and Statistical Manual of Mental Disorders* (DSM-5). However, it does have a V code as one of the "Other Conditions That May Be a Focus of Clinical Attention" and indicates that malingering should be "strongly suspected if any combination of the following is noted":[3]

1. Presentation in a medicolegal setting (referred by an attorney or oneself) for examination in the context of a criminal case or civil litigation
2. A significant discrepancy between the individual's stated distress/disability and objective findings and the clinician's observations
3. Lack of cooperation with the evaluation and the recommended treatment
4. The presence of antisocial personality disorder

Feigned mental illness has been known for ages. Ulysses was confronted by Palamedes for "pretending madness" by ploughing the seashore with salt in an effort to avoid being recruited for the attack on Troy. Palamedes put Ulysses' infant son in the path of the horses, and Ulysses' diversion of the plough unmasked his deception.[4] Shakespeare's Hamlet would likely be considered to have a genuine mental illness (major depressive disorder) by today's standards, but he feigns madness so as to confuse Claudius and divert the king's suspicions away from himself.[5] The purposeful exaggeration of mental illness for external gain is a form of malingering and is not uncommon in psychiatric emergency settings. Many patients who exaggerate or fake psychiatric symptoms in the emergency setting also have a diagnosable mental illness, confounding efforts to distinguish which symptoms are currently genuine versus what may have been genuine in the past.

There is a paucity of well-designed studies on malingering in clinical settings generally, let alone the psychiatric emergency setting. It is frustrating that such a vexing issue for emergency psychiatrists would merit such little scholarship, but perhaps not so surprising. Deception may be difficult to determine. Seasoned clinicians may struggle with the diagnosis of malingering, and the stresses and time constraints of the emergency setting may make differentiating the distinctions between malingering and genuine mental illness, let alone distinguishing the nuances between malingering and factitious disorder, less than straightforward.

Prevalence of Malingering

The prevalence of malingering in the general population or even in general medical or clinical psychiatric practice is unknown, but malingering is accepted to be higher in forensic populations (including criminal defendants and civil litigants). Forensic psychiatrists should always consider the possibility of feigned or exaggerated symptomatology when conducting a forensic evaluation. The feigning of disabling illness for the purpose of disability compensation is common in disability examinations, estimated to occur in 30–60% of adult cases.[6,7] For forensic psychiatrists, consideration of malingering is critical for every legal or civil evaluation because there is clear external gain identified by the very nature of the proceedings. Individuals who successfully feign psychosis may end up being hospitalized versus imprisoned (although note that the insanity defense is raised in less than 1% of felony cases and successful for only 15–25% of defendants who raise it).[8] Far more common is the litigant who feigns or exaggerates physical or mental distress in an effort to be awarded a large sum in damages. In the clinical arena, it is appropriate and necessary for physicians to have a higher threshold for considering that a patient is engaging in deceitful behavior. The emergency setting confers additional challenges given the higher level of acuity of patients presenting for evaluation and care and also the time constraints inherent in emergency evaluation and treatment. Unfortunately, these constraints can make the emergency department (ED) fertile ground for deception and exaggeration of symptomatology. Resnick[9] noted with respect to malingering that "no other syndrome is so easy to define but so difficult to diagnose."

Yates et al.[10] found that 13% of 227 patients evaluated over a 2-month period in the psychiatric emergency services of an urban community hospital were moderately, strongly, or definitely suspected of malingering. Reasons for feigned symptoms included seeking food and/or shelter, seeking to avoid jail, seeking to obtain medications, and attempting to avoid work commitments. As the authors hypothesized, most of the patients suspected of malingering had a genuine mental disorder. A 2018 study of 405 patients presenting to an urban psychiatric emergency program over the course of 1 month by Rumschik and Appel[11] used questionnaires after completed psychiatric evaluations to assess for the prevalence, predictors, and outcomes of malingering. Malingering was suspected in one-third of patients, and it was strongly or definitely suspected in 20% of patients. Among the patients strongly or definitely suspected of admission, 4% were admitted to the hospital; however, the likelihood of discharge did correspond to the increased suspicion of malingering. Variables increasing the likelihood of admission among suspected malingerers included malingering suicidal ideation, seeking social work or housing assistance, and seeking admission to the hospital. Rissmiller et al.[12] approached 58 consecutively admitted suicidal patients to a suburban community hospital inpatient psychiatric unit to participate in a study utilizing psychological testing (the Minnesota Multiphasic Personality Inventory [MMPI]) and an anonymous questionnaire asking if they had lied or exaggerated their suicidality; 40 of the patients agreed to participate. Four patients (10%) reported that they had malingered their suicidality. None of the MMPI-2 validity scores correlated with self-reported malingering. Although the clinicians detected malingerers with 100% sensitivity, the specificity rates were only 58% for the blinded psychiatrist and 32% for the blinded psychologist. Despite the small sample size, the study demonstrated the difficulty in diagnosing malingering either clinically or by psychological testing. A replication study on 50 consecutively admitted (different) patients found similar results—12% of patients admitted for suicidal ideation had fabricated or grossly exaggerated their suicidality.[13]

Obstacles to Diagnosing Malingering

Identifying a patient as a malingerer should not be undertaken lightly and may have serious ramifications. If in error, needed treatment may be withheld; a lawsuit could result. However, avoiding the diagnosis (or at least considering it as a rule-out) when, after a thorough evaluation and thoughtful consideration, the physician has sufficient information to indicate the presence of malingering confers other risks. Patients who feign or exaggerate psychiatric disorders present significant financial and emotional cost to the health care system as well as potential harm to themselves, including exposure to unnecessary medications with potential side effects. In addition, duplicitous behavior is reinforced. Physicians may be reluctant to diagnose malingering for a number of reasons, including fear of misdiagnosis and the pejorative consequences that follow.[14] The physician's caveat, "First do no harm," adds to a physician's reluctance to indicate that a patient is essentially lying. In addition, there may be fear of litigation on the clinician's part because "defamation of character" may not be covered by physicians' malpractice insurance policies.[15] Psychiatrists and other clinicians may fear being assaulted by patients who become angry at the diagnosis. Some payer sources will not reimburse for a malingering diagnosis. Furthermore, with the 21st Century Cures Act regulations making notes viewable to patients in real time (barring concerns related to dangerousness), there may be additional safety concerns.[16]

Hospitals in urban areas with high rates of malingering are also academic centers, and residents often feel uncomfortable diagnosing patients with malingering without concrete data to support the diagnosis.[17] However, some clinicians in emergency psychiatry settings may be too quick to determine that an individual is malingering, particularly with respect to patients who present to the psychiatric emergency setting repeatedly, and a rush to judgment confers different risks. Potential consequences of misdiagnosing malingering may include refusal of needed care and unwarranted stigma. Malingering does not confer immunity against genuine mental illness, and many patients who feign or exaggerate psychopathology have legitimate psychiatric diagnosis.[10] Inexperienced and/or exhausted clinicians may be biased by the diagnosis into performing an inadequate assessment of the patient's new complaints. A retrospective study by Humphreys and Ogilvie[18] found 3 out of 10 patients previously diagnosed with malingering met criteria for schizophrenia approximately 20 years following their malingering diagnoses. Electronic health records may perpetuate the diagnosis in problem lists long after the diagnosis has come into question or even been disproved.

Emergency psychiatry services frequently encounter patients whose social situations are difficult. The most comprehensive examination of homelessness in the United States, by the U.S. Department of Housing and Urban Development in 2015, found that 564,708 people were homeless on a given night in the United States, and at a minimum, 25% of these people were seriously mentally ill (most frequently with schizophrenia or bipolar disorder, and at least 45% had some form mental illness).[19] Homelessness and harsh weather conditions may precipitate a mentally ill person's presentation to the psychiatric emergency service (PES). Individuals with alcohol and substance use disorders may also present anticipating hospitalization or an extended stay in the ED due to a variety of factors, including genuine despair and suicidal ideation regarding their condition, withdrawal symptoms, and/or difficult social and economic situations. A rush to judgment that is more emotive than thoughtful can result in missed opportunities for therapeutic engagement and recognition of new and treatable symptoms or an additional disorder. However, ignoring and not addressing malingering, and hospitalizing an individual on the basis of malingered symptomatology, lowers that person's threshold for engaging in the behavior again and makes future unnecessary treatment and hospitalization more likely.

A diagnosis of malingering requires confirmation by either observation or inference.[14] Observation may involve being "caught in the act" while being unknowingly observed or engaging in activities that they claim are impossible because of an infirmity. Observation can be in a controlled environment (e.g., observation of behaviors in the ED, observation area, or inpatient unit) or in a real-world environment (e.g., when a litigant in a disability claim indicates that he is unable to work because his agoraphobia precludes his leaving the home is videotaped by a private investigator leaving his house and bowling in a crowded bowling alley or shopping in a mall). Inference is based on information from the patient or collateral sources that conflicts with the professed level of distress or dysfunction. An example of inference is the patient who repeatedly comes to the ED claiming auditory hallucinations telling the patient to kill themself and others, but collateral sources report that the patient has told them that they go to the hospital for admission when they are homeless and have run out of money, previous inpatient hospitalizations have been unproductive, and the patient is noncompliant with medications or outpatient treatment recommendations. Definitive diagnosis can also be made in the lucky but infrequent circumstance in which a patient admits to malingering.

Factitious Disorder

The DSM-5 saw a major reorganization of disorders of somatization with a de-emphasis from the DSM-IV's organization around the lack of a medical etiology for symptoms to the individual's distress and pathological thoughts, feelings, and behaviors related to the symptoms. The DSM-IV specifically noted that the gain was to be in the patient role,[20] but the diagnosis of DSM-5 indicates that the symptoms occur in the "absence of obvious

> ## Box 13.1 DSM-5 Diagnostic Criteria for Factitious Disorder
>
> Factitious disorder imposed on self
> A. Falsification of physical and/or psychological symptoms/signs or induction of injury or disease associated with identified deception.
> B. The patient presents themself as ill, injured, or impaired.
> C. The patient's deceptive behavior is evident in the absence of any obvious external reward.
> D. The behavior is not better explained by another medical or mental health disorder (especially another delusional or psychotic disorder).
>
> Adapted from the DSM-5.[2]

external rewards."[3] However, this reconceptualization did little to clarify the diagnostic criteria or the differentiation of factitious disorder, although one of the purposes of the reorganization of the DSM-IV somatoform disorders was to make them more useful for other medical specialists (Box 13.1).[21]

Malingering can be very difficult to distinguish from factitious disorder (more so in an emergency setting) because both are consciously feigned (Figure 13.1). The determination of external benefit is necessary for differentiating malingering from factitious disorder. Patients with factitious disorder consciously create or feign physical or psychological symptoms, but there is no obvious external gain. Therefore, differentiating malingering from factitious disorder requires assessment for the presence of obvious external incentives, but this is obviously very difficult to discern in a psychiatric emergency setting, unless the individual has a well-documented history of factitious disorder. Malingering patients are intentionally reporting/faking symptoms in search of external incentives—for example, in the form of shelter, food, disability, medication, etc.

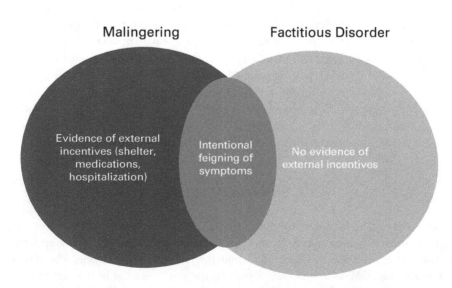

Figure 13.1 Broad comparison of malingering versus factitious disorder.

The prevalence of factitious disorder is unknown. The DSM-5 indicates that in hospital settings, the prevalence is approximately 1%; however, the prevalence may be higher.[3,22,23] Factitious disorder imposed on another is beyond the scope of this chapter, but it is the diagnosis given to an individual (the perpetrator, not the victim) who falsifies illness in another (children, adults, or pets).[3]

Reich and Gottfried[24] studied 40 patients diagnosed with factitious disorder over a 10-year period, of which 33 were directly confronted that their disorders were self-induced and none of them signed out of the hospital against medical advice (AMA) or became suicidal. Only 13 patients acknowledged inducing their own simulated illnesses, but most improved after the confrontation and 4 of the most chronic became asymptomatic. However, the authors note that these were inpatients on medical and surgical wards from 1970 to 1980, predominantly women, and none had a comorbid mental disorder or antisocial personality disorder or traits. Also, the confrontations were described as nonpunitive and supportive and explained to the patients and families as a "cry for help." However, Krahn et al.[25] advised against direct confrontation. Their later retrospective study of 93 medically ill patients diagnosed with factitious disorder over 21 years found that 22% (16 of the 71 patients confronted) acknowledged factitious behavior, but 18 patients left the hospital AMA. The patients in this study had more comorbid psychopathology, including alcohol or substance use disorder.

Malingering and Factitious Disorder in the Emergency Setting

The most effective assessment and management of suspected deception in the emergency setting begins with the assumption that the patient has a legitimate need for presenting to the ED and that the patient presented to the ED with the belief that it is the most optimal setting for getting their needs met. However, the reality is that it is fairly easy for individuals to access diagnostic criteria for all psychiatric disorders on the internet, and the diagnosis of mental illness lacks laboratory or imaging findings to assist in diagnosis. Some disorders are easier to feign than others, and clinicians' familiarity with the phenomenology of common psychiatric disorders is helpful in distinguishing genuine from deceptive presentations (Table 13.1).

The Clinical Interview

1. Even if the patient is a "known malingerer" who has presented to the ED multiple times, approach the patient in an open and empathic manner. As previously noted, many patients who feign or exaggerate psychiatric symptoms also have a genuine mental disorder. Starting off the evaluation with a dismissive attitude is likely to be met with defensiveness and hostility, resulting at best in a shutdown interview in which the patient provides little other than one- or two-word answers. This will make it difficult to detect genuine psychiatric symptoms in a patient who also has a history of deception. Also, if the patient is malingering, disengaging the patient at the outset of the evaluation will make it difficult to obtain the information needed to justify your decision to discharge and to develop a crisis plan, which may be

Table 13.1 Clues to Malingering

Example	Clinician Statement or Question	Patient Response and/or Behavior
Conditional suicidal threats	How can we develop a safety plan so that you're better able to manage these disturbing thoughts?	"If you discharge me, I'm going to walk into traffic, and when I'm dead or paralyzed, it's on you."
Vagueness or inability or unwillingness to provide specific information	What do the voices say? Is it a man's or woman's voice? Do you recognize the voices? When did this begin?	"I don't know." "I forgot." Irritable, annoyed by questioning. Will not engage in the interview.
Behavior inconsistent with level of professed distress	How much do these symptoms interfere with your ability to function at home or work?	"I can't do anything—the voices are constant; I'd rather be dead than put up with this." "I haven't been able to get out of bed for days." Patient observed to be watching TV, making frequent requests for food, and asking to use the phone. Refusing labs and urine toxicology screen.
Inconsistency in descriptions of symptoms	How long have you been having suicidal thoughts? When did you first start hearing voices?	"Since this morning when the pain started," and telling a different clinician "since last week when I got kicked out of my apartment." "They started when I woke up this morning," and telling a different clinician "since I was 7 years old."
Information withheld regarding housing, behavior, and/or legal situation, or differs from that of collateral sources	Has anything happened recently in your life that's been particularly stressful?	"Nope, just these voices telling me to run into traffic"; collateral sources indicate that the patient recently incurred domestic abuse charges, is now homeless, and has a warrant out for his arrest.

problematic in the event of a lawsuit. A respectful and accepting tone may cultivate more honest and open responses from the patient.

2. Review the medical record prior to the evaluation, especially the most recent discharge summary for patients who have been previously admitted to the hospital.

3. Start the interview with open-ended questions. This will not only convey your interest in what the patient is experiencing but also is more likely to produce information that will help you uncover evidence of malingering, as you may uncover inconsistencies with respect to what the patient has spontaneously told you and what is said in response to specific questions.

4. Although the psychiatric ED is not the most convenient or appropriate setting for a prolonged interview, recognize that deception can be exhausting. It is often difficult, if not impossible, to maintain the deception for a prolonged period of time. For example, a patient who appears to be responding to internal stimuli at the beginning of an interview may unconsciously drop the facade 15–20 minutes into

an evaluation. Nursing staff may inform the team that the same person who is too distressed to participate in an evaluation a short while ago is watching television, requesting snacks, and talking calmly with visitors or other patients. It is understandable and appropriate for patients unknown to the emergency psychiatry team who report symptoms of a severe mental illness such as psychosis, disabling depression, suicidal ideation, or claiming to have engaged in suicidal behavior, despite suspicions of malingering, to be hospitalized out of an abundance of caution. It is more difficult to sustain deception over the course of a hospital stay, and the inpatient team should document the specifics of deceptive behavior and the diagnosis of malingering (at least provisionally) when indicated. This will assist the psychiatric emergency clinicians with discharge if appropriate.

5. Listen carefully for inconsistencies with respect to symptomatology as well as the patient's narrative with respect to the onset and evolution of symptoms. Listen for symptoms or symptom clusters that are rare or unusual. After an open-ended exploration of the patient's symptoms, proceed to specific questions. It may be helpful to follow-up with specific questioning about implausible symptoms. For example,
   a. Do plants ever tell you to harm yourself or someone else?
   b. When people talk to you, do you see the words they speak spelled out?[26]
   c. Do the voices ever tell you to eat roadkill when you are driving?

6. Listen carefully during the interview for references to individuals (family, friends, therapists, case managers, or others) who are aware that the patient is exhibiting psychiatric symptomatology, and indicate that you will need to contact them to complete your evaluation. This does not have to be an exhaustive process; even one collateral informant can be helpful, especially in determining disposition. A possible clue to malingering is when a patient can provide no information regarding an individual who may be able to assist the clinical in understanding how the patient has been struggling and functioning during the past few weeks. The clinician may ask, "It's usually very helpful to get additional information from someone who has observed you struggling over the last week or two; who can I call?" Malingerers will often claim either that no one can provide information or that they do not know how to contact individuals they have mentioned in the evaluation as having knowledge of their symptom exacerbation. For any patient presenting to a psychiatric emergency setting endorsing suicidal or homicidal ideation, permission from the patient to contact collateral sources for information is not necessary. Disclosing that the patient is in the ED in order to obtain that information, even without the patient's consent, is not a violation of the Health Insurance Portability and Accountability Act (HIPAA) because the patient is indicating that they present a serious and imminent threat to their safety or the safety of others.[27]

7. The evaluating physician or clinician should be open with the patient in discussing that individuals present to the ED for numerous important reasons and that some needs can be met in the emergency setting and others cannot, but that the team will do what they can to be of assistance (obtain shelter resources, link the patient with appropriate resources, assist with transportation especially during harsh weather conditions, etc.).

8. If feasible, it may be helpful to have a suspected malinger (one who has presented to the same facility repeatedly) initially assessed by a clinical social worker. Clinical social workers are more familiar with resources and may have insights as to

whether the information that a patient provides with respect to their housing situation is suspect. (For example, a patient may complain there are no shelter beds available when a call to a shelter for a previous patient indicated that there are beds; a call to the patient's last shelter may indicate that the patient was aggressive or stole from others.) Case managers and social workers are often better able to address underlying needs, such as shelters, free clinics, safe houses, and other social service agencies.

Additional Clues to Feigned Psychosis

There are some hints or clues to the possible presence of deception, and they are best considered within the totality of the history and examination, especially given the fact that many, if not most, individuals who present for emergency psychiatric services have a genuine mental disorder. Therefore, it is critical to obtain enough information from the patient so that it can be compared to how major mental illness typically presents. McCarthy-Jones and Resnick[1,28] provide useful indicators of possible malingered psychosis while noting that the diagnosis can be difficult and is made by careful analysis of the information available from not only the current assessment but also collateral information for others and corroborating evidence from prior presentations and the medical record.[9]

1. Consider symptom inconsistency in the patient's report.
   a. For example, a patient may be able to give very specific information about a variety of topics but become confused when asked to provide specific information about their symptoms (onset, evolution, quality, frequency, etc.).
   b. Inconsistency between what is reported and observed: For example, a patient may describe extreme distress in the form of frightening command hallucinations that cannot be ignored but during the interview does not appear to be distressed or distracted by internal stimuli.
   c. Inconsistency between what the patient reports and the phenomenology of how the symptoms present: For example, a patient may complain of hearing voices constantly without reprieve or describe voices that speak in a stilted manner, such as saying "Commit a murder."
   d. Inconsistency between known history and patient behavior: For example, a patient who has graduated from high school and has completed some college is unable to do simple math.
2. Evaluate hallucinations thoroughly.
   Individuals who malinger hallucinatory phenomena frequently expect their complaints of hearing voices to harm themselves or others to automatically gain them admission to the hospital and may be surprised when questioned about their evolution, quality, intensity, etc. Although patients with genuine psychotic or neurologic pathology, as well as those who are intoxicated or withdrawing from alcohol or other substances, can present with atypical hallucinatory phenomena, the emergency psychiatric clinician is well served by knowing how perceptual abnormalities for various disorders typically present. One must be cautious, however, about using phenomenology as a litmus test for feigned hallucinations. Atypicality is best considered as a part of the whole, combined with additional data gleaned from

interview, observation, and collateral sources with respect to assessing the genuineness of atypical hallucinations.

Goodwin et al.[29] studied hallucinatory phenomena in 116 patients with a variety of diagnoses, including schizophrenia, affective psychosis, and alcohol withdrawal. The study is dated 1971, and it is unclear as to how many of the patients diagnosed with schizophrenia in the study would be diagnosed as such according to DSM-IV or DSM-5 criteria. Nayani and David[30] administered a comprehensive semi-structured questionnaire to 100 psychotic patients who had experienced auditory hallucinations. Their findings indicated that psychotic individuals typically experience repetitive and emotive voices that are context dependent. They found that 38% of patients experienced the voices as coming from inside their heads, and 49% perceived them as coming from outside their heads and through their ears. Many patients retain some degree of control of their hallucinations. A more recent survey of auditory hallucinations by McCarthy-Jones et al.[31] of 199 inpatients diagnosed with a psychotic disorder (81% of whom had schizophrenia) only partially replicated previous phenomenological findings. The theme or content of the voices was always the same in 45%; 39% reported that the voices appeared to be replays of memories of prior conversations, and 55% indicated that new voices have the same theme or content as previous voices. The investigators also did not find evidence to support the fact that voices emanating from either inside or outside a person's head are atypical, as 38% of patients experienced the voices as emanating from both inside and outside their heads, 34% experienced voices as coming only from inside, and 28% experienced voices as coming only from outside. With the caveat that the clinician should not rely exclusively on the phenomenology of hallucinatory because more research is needed, aspects of hallucinations that may raise suspicion include the following:

a. Vague messages: Patients with genuine auditory hallucinations are generally clear on what messages they are receiving, although they may be embarrassed to repeat the content, particularly if it is of a sexual nature. Suspect evasiveness and malingering if the patient indicates that they "can't make out" the content, particularly if they are indicating that they are significantly distressed by the hallucinations. However, individuals with genuine hallucinations also may experience individual auditory hallucinations (which they can decipher) accompanied by indistinct background noise or mumbling.[32]

b. Visual hallucinations that are in black and white: In the Goodwin et al.[29] study, visual hallucinations were almost always in color, and only one patient who would have been classified today as personality-disordered experienced hallucinations in black and white. There is a paucity of research on hallucinatory phenomena in general, but less on visual than auditory hallucinations.

c. Command hallucinations in the absence of delusional ideation or non-command hallucinations.[9]

d. Hallucinations that are not altered or diminished with activity: Most individuals retain some control over their auditory hallucinations.[31]

3. Evaluate suicidal ideation and homicidal ideation thoroughly every time a patient presents to the ED, even those with a history of malingering. Suicide and violence risk assessment is beyond the scope of this chapter and is covered elsewhere; however, recall that personality disorders that are associated with malingering, including borderline and antisocial personality disorders, are also associated with

an increased risk of suicidal behavior and suicide.[33] Suicide risk is increased in patients with substance use disorders, particularly in women.[34] Suicide risk is especially heightened in those with alcohol use disorder, opioid use disorder, and/or comorbid alcohol use disorder with a mood disorder.[35] As noted previously, patients with these disorders commonly present to the ED malingering with the goal of finding a comfortable and safe place to detox or obtain medications.

Psychological Testing to Detect Malingering

Although a number of instruments designed to detect malingering are available, they are best utilized in settings outside of the ED, such as in forensic settings. Testing is limited in the ED mostly due to time restrictions, but other factors are considerations, such as cost and the validity of instruments applied to emergency patients. Two malingering instruments that have been mentioned as possible screening tools are the Structured Interview of Reported Symptoms (SIRS)[36] and the Miller Forensic Assessment of Symptom Test (M-FAST).[26,37] The SIRS questionnaire is well validated; however, it takes 30–40 minutes to administer the 172-item assessment. The M-FAST may be a better option to study in the emergency psychiatric setting because it only takes 5–10 minutes to administer the 25-item assessment. Zubera et al.[38] suggested that the M-FAST could be used as a malingering screener in the ED, and if there is high suspicion for malingering, the SIRS can then be administered given its high specificity. However, given the time constraints of the emergency setting, unless such a project was undertaken as a research study and the instruments were administered by clinicians not tasked with the assessment and management of patients (and trained in the tests' administration), it is difficult to envision how to incorporate such instruments into routine emergency psychiatric practice.

Management of Deception in the Emergency Setting

Briefly, one may consider three types of deceptive patients:

1. A patient strongly suspected of deception presents with suicidal or homicidal ideation, but for whom no collateral sources of information exist (or are accessible to the clinician), nor is there any institutional history with the patient. This patient will likely be admitted out of an abundance of caution. The main task in the PES is helping trainees and staff (and the inpatient team) deal with their frustration around the admission.
2. A patient strongly suspected of deception presents with suicidal or homicidal ideation complaining of symptoms of a mental illness but then tires of the wait and wants to be discharged. In this case, a psychiatric evaluation and risk assessment must be completed, with the note delineating risk factors as well as mitigating factors (the patient's plan to pick up their Supplemental Security Income check or go to another hospital that they perceive as more accommodating, the fact that they are no longer intoxicated, etc.). Specific quotes from the patient at the time of discharge that contrast with earlier complaints may be useful.
3. A patient presents with suicidal or homicidal ideation complaining of symptoms of a mental illness with clear history of malingering and frequent similar

presentations to hospital EDs for whom the decision is made that inpatient hospitalization is not appropriate and the patient should be discharged. This is the most challenging situation with respect to documentation and is discussed in greater detail below.

There is scant research on the management of deception in the psychiatric emergency setting. Direct confrontation of deceptive patients has been advocated by some, but this is fraught with danger. Accusing a patient of being a liar, fraud, or fake is never productive and potentially puts the examiner in danger of violence. Although some clinicians might defend this approach as blunt or direct in the press of a busy emergency setting, it may be a product of the clinician's anger, frustration, and resentment. It also precludes any chance of using an empathic and therapeutic stance in the development of a safety plan. Kontos et al.[39] noted that although confrontation of a patient might stem from a clinician's frustration and desire to "pick a fight," some patient confrontations are worth having, provided they are done in an empathic but firm and direct manner. They proposed three questions to help physicians "choose a 'good fight' and fight it well":

1. Is the patient prioritizing health? Many patients, especially those experiencing an exacerbation of mental illness, may present with behavior that is unpleasant, nasty, or demanding. Confrontation of these patients based solely on objectionable behavior is not appropriate. However, consider a patient who frequently presents to the emergency room complaining of suicidal ideation and hallucinations who has had numerous inpatient hospitalizations and does not follow up with medications or outpatient linkage. Honest, direct, and empathic confrontation, regardless of whether hospitalization is indicated at that time, is not only permissible but also necessary.

2. Is confrontation ethically permissible? If the patient is continually making decisions that compromise health, a physician may choose to confront the patient about those decisions. In addition, in the psychiatric ED, deceptive patients are utilizing finite resources, which may compromise the care of other patients (consider EDs that must divert patients when overcrowded or the busy PES with agitated, psychotic, and/or suicidal patients awaiting evaluation).

3. Is confronting the patient emotionally gratifying? Kontos et al. note that the physician's self-reflection regarding their own thoughts and feelings can be useful in considering their role in responding to patients. An abusive deceptive patient who has symptoms of a genuine mental illness (e.g., depression and amphetamine-induced psychotic symptoms) may threaten to kill themself if they are not hospitalized despite a history of not following through with treatment. The clinician, while recognizing their frustration and/or anger at the attempt at extortion, should not ignore the patient's unacceptable behavior in an effort to "keep the peace." Instead, a more therapeutic approach may be for the clinician to recognize their own negative thoughts and feelings toward the patient in that moment and directly and calmly point out the unreasonable, disruptive, and self-defeating aspects of the patient's presentation. The physician can then communicate the desire to be helpful and work with the patient, as well as a willingness to not continue to work with the patient if the patient continues to make it impossible to do so.

The "therapeutic discharge" has been advocated as a safe and effective intervention in inpatient settings with deceptive patients, but it can also be adapted to the emergency setting.[40,41] Therapeutic discharge may be thought of as an intervention like a medication or procedure in that it has its own indications, contraindications, risks, and benefits. The only contraindication to a therapeutic discharge is if the patient has an actual indication requiring an inpatient level of care; this is more commonly seen in cases of factitious disorder in which patients induce their own physical illness. Once the decision has been made to discharge a deceptive patient, it is advisable to not inform the patient until a discharge plan is in place because the patient may "up the ante" and escalate deceptive and possibly dangerous behavior.[40]

Documentation of the rationale for discharging a patient presenting with serious complaints that could merit hospitalization were the patient not believed to be feigned is a critical skill for the emergency psychiatrist (Box 13.2). The following should be considered in the preparation of the discharge note or plan section in the assessment:

1. The history of present illness (HPI) in the context of deception does not lend itself well to the use of drop-down boxes in which symptoms are clustered on the basis of diagnostic entities (e.g., depression or psychosis). Instead, documentation should clarify inconsistencies as well as the fact that multiple sources of information were utilized in decision-making (collateral sources of information, the medical record, etc.).

2. The past medical (psychiatric) history should be briefly reviewed with a focus on documenting the specific symptoms that are suspected of being fabricated or exaggerated and clarifying why they raise suspicion of malingering. For example, the patient may indicate a history of multiple suicide attempts by overdose, but the record indicates that none of them were serious enough to merit hospitalization, toxicology was negative, and the attempts and the aftermath were unwitnessed. Documentation of the number of presentations to the ED for similar complaints, lack of follow-through with treatment recommendations, etc. is helpful to include. Risk factors for malingering, such as antisocial personality disorder, should be documented.

3. The mental status exam (MSE) that is documented may reflect the variability over time in the patient's presentation (e.g., noting that the patient is complaining of constant command auditory hallucinations but is watching television and eating and appears in no distress). Documentation of affect may note that the patient is initially calm and cooperative but becomes hostile when the examiner begins to ask more specific questions and/or it appears that hospitalization is not a given. Documentation of the patient's cognitive status might note complaints of confusion, but there is no evidence of distractibility and the patient is able to provide very specific information in those areas that are designed to convince the examiner of a need for hospitalization, medication, etc. Alternatively, the patient may be quite able to articulate their needs for food choices, phone use, etc. to staff but claim to be unable to cooperate with the physician due to the level of their distress. This level of inconsistency should be clearly documented.

4. Documentation of the plan should include recommendations of treatments and resources recommended or provided to the patient for comorbid psychiatric conditions, including substance use.

5. A suicide and violence risk assessment should be performed and documented with special attention as to why the individual is being discharged.

6. Documentation of the assessment and plan should be bolstered by the information in the HPI and MSE. Someone else reading the chief complaint, HPI, and

Box 13.2 Sample Assessment Summary and Plan

I believe that this patient's current presentation, evaluation, and past presentations reflect deception in an effort to be hospitalized for food and shelter. There is no evidence that he is experiencing auditory hallucinations; rather there is evidence to the contrary. Mr. Jones presented to this emergency service last night complaining of voices telling him to jump into traffic. He has presented five times in the past 3 months with a similar complaint requesting hospitalization and threatening to kill himself if discharged. He has also presented three times in the past month to another emergency department with similar complaints. Mr. Jones has received varying diagnoses over the past 10 years, including schizophrenia, schizoaffective disorder, cocaine use disorder, cannabis use disorder, alcohol use disorder, and psychosis due to cocaine intoxication. He is homeless. His most recent hospitalization at our facility was 2 months ago. At discharge he was diagnosed with malingering and amphetamine-induced psychosis, with a rule-out diagnosis of schizophrenia. During that hospitalization he was prescribed risperidone and linked with a case manager in the community as well as outpatient mental health services, including psychiatry, and housing. He reportedly assaulted another resident at the group home, and is currently homeless again. He did not follow through with his outpatient appointments and stopped his medication immediately after discharge, claiming it was stolen. However, he did not engage his case manager or the community mental health center, which has walk-in availability, in an attempt to obtain medication. A review of his record indicates a history of noncompliance with outpatient treatment. Last night, after expressing his suicidal intent and being moved to the PES, Mr. Jones promptly fell asleep. When the social work clinician tried to rouse him, he angrily told her he was too tired to cooperate. He awoke two times after that to request food and another blanket and to use the bathroom. He was congenial with other patients and select staff. He denied any alcohol or substance use, and his vital signs remained normal. His urine drug screen revealed the presence of cocaine, amphetamine/methamphetamine, and cannabinoids. He refused to provide blood for an alcohol level. After several hours of sleep, he awoke and asked to see a doctor because he needed to be admitted, but refused to engage meaningfully with the social work clinician, telling him that his questions were "stupid." With the psychiatrist, he was vague about onset and quality of all of his symptoms with the exception of voices that tell him to run into traffic, which he claims are constant, but there was no evidence of attending to them or even distress during the evaluation. He became belligerent as the evaluation progressed, finally indicating he was "done," and closing his eyes, rolling over, and feigning sleep. Collateral information from his case manager indicates that he came by the mental health center earlier in the week requesting to be placed in a group home, but refusing assistance with accessing shelters. She did not observe any symptoms of psychotic decompensation. Mr. Jones is not evidencing any symptoms of alcohol withdrawal. Although he has difficult life circumstances and likely has experienced symptoms compatible with a major mental illness or substance use, there is no indication that he requires inpatient hospitalization or even that it will be therapeutic for him. He appears to be feigning both the hallucinations and his suicidal ideation in an attempt to be hospitalized, and this is an established pattern for him. He has a chronically elevated risk for suicide by virtue of his depression, chronic substance use, and homelessness. However, he has been resistant to modalities that are designed to mitigate his risk. Discharge with information for shelters and accessing community mental health is recommended. His case manager is willing to see him tomorrow morning at 8 a.m., and we offered to provide transportation to a local shelter with beds, but the patient refused. He was escorted out by security, threatening that we would "read about him in the papers," and he would "sue our a -- es."

MSE should not think, "How could they have discharged this patient?" or even "I wonder why this patient was not hospitalized?"

7. Informal consultation with a colleague or the hospital's legal counsel (in the event of homicidal threats) regarding a particularly challenging patient may also be helpful and can be documented in the record. However, it is important to recognize that risk assessment and decision-making is a critical skill within the purview of the general psychiatrist, and requesting a formal forensic consultation is not the norm.

Pillow et al.[42] conducted a study in which a multidisciplinary team identified the top 50 most frequent ED visitors in one ED. The team constructed care plans for these patients that consisted of a summary of the patients' pertinent history, relevant psychosocial issues leading to frequent ED utilization, and recommended treatment plans for the patients. Of note, this study only identified 20% of those top ED utilizers as carrying a malingering diagnosis. However, the study did show that utilization of care plans showed a downward trend in ED visits, although readmission rates did not decrease.

Conclusion

The reality that it is not possible to be absolutely sure that a patient is malingering in the psychiatric emergency setting should not result in a passive approach to the malingering patient, nor in a pejorative and frustrated approach. The skills required to evaluate and manage deception in the emergency setting are critical ones for all psychiatrists and psychiatric residents to acquire. Confidence in the evaluation and management of deception will help clinicians work with these patients in an empathic and thoughtful manner, with the hope of steering them in the direction of more appropriate ways to get their very real needs met.

References

1. Resnick PJ. Defrocking the fraud: The detection of malingering. *Isr J Psychiatry Relat Sci.* 1993;30(2):93–101.

2. Ford CV, King BH, Hollender MH. Lies and liars: Psychiatric aspects of prevarication. *Am J Psychiatry.* 1988;145(5):554–562. doi:10.1176/ajp.145.5.554

3. American Psychiatric Association. *Diagnostic and Statistical Manual of Mental Disorders.* 5h ed. American Psychiatric Publishing; 2013:726–727.

4. Nunez AP, Pena AG, Pleteiro JMP, Arribi MM, Vazquez, JMA. Pseudodementia, malingering, and revenge in ancient Greece: Odysseus and Palamedes. *Neurosci History.* 2016;2(2):47–50.

5. Wilson JR, Fradella HF. The Hamlet syndrome. *Law Culture Humanities.* 2020;16(1):82–102.

6. Mittenberg W, Patton C, Canyock EM, Condit DC. Base rates of malingering and symptom exaggeration. *J Clin Exp Neuropsychol.* 2002;24(8):1094–1102. doi:10.1076/jcen.24.8.1094.8379

7. Chafetz M, Underhill J. Estimated costs of malingered disability. *Arch Clin Neuropsychol.* 2013;28(7):633–639. doi:10.1093/arclin/act038

8. Cirincione C, Steadman HJ, McGreevy MA. Rates of insanity acquittals and the factors associated with successful insanity pleas. *Bull Am Acad Psychiatry Law.* 1995;23(3):399–409.

9. Resnick PJ. The detection of malingered psychosis. *Psychiatr Clin North Am.* 1999;22(1):159–172. doi:S0193-953X(05)70066-6

10. Yates BD, Nordquist CR, Schultz-Ross R. Feigned psychiatric symptoms in the emergency room. *Psychiatr Serv.* 1996;47(9):998–1000. doi:10.1176/ps.47.9.998

11. Rumschik SM, Appel JM. Malingering in the psychiatric emergency department: Prevalence, predictors, and outcomes. *Psychiatr Serv.* 2019;70(2):115–122. doi:10.1176/appi.ps.201800140

12. Rissmiller DJ, Wayslow A, Madison H, Hogate P, Rissmiller FR, Steer RA. Prevalence of malingering in inpatient suicide ideators and attempters. *Crisis.* 1998;19(2):62–66. doi:10.1027/0227-5910.19.2.62

13. Rissmiller DA, Steer RA, Friedman M, DeMercurio R. Prevalence of malingering in suicidal psychiatric inpatients: A replication. *Psychol Rep.* 1999;84(3 Pt 1):726–730. doi:10.2466/pr0.1999.84.3.726

14. LoPiccolo CJ, Goodkin K, Baldewicz TT. Current issues in the diagnosis and management of malingering. *Ann Med.* 1999;31(3):166–174. doi:10.3109/07853899909115975

15. Weiss KJ, Van Dell L. Liability for diagnosing malingering. *J Am Acad Psychiatry Law.* 2017;45(3):339–347. doi:45/3/339

16. Bonamici S. 21st Century Cures Act. 114th Congress; 2016.

17. Zubera A, Raza M, Holaday E, Aggarwal R. Screening for malingering in the emergency department. *Acad Psychiatry.* 2015;39(2):233–234. doi:10.1007/s40596-014-0253-1

18. Humphreys M, Ogilvie A. Feigned psychosis revisited—A 20 year follow up of 10 patients. *Psychiatr Bull.* 1996;20(11):666–669. doi:10.1192/pb.20.11.666

19. U.S. Department of Housing and Urban Development. 2015 annual homelessness assessment report: Part 1. Point-in-time estimates of homelessness in the U.S. U.S. Department of Housing and Urban Development, Office of Community Planning and Development; 2015.

20. American Psychiatric Association Task Force on DSM-IV. *Diagnostic and Statistical Manual of Mental Disorders DSM-IV-TR.* Text rev. American Psychiatric Association; 2000.

21. Ross CA. Problems with factitious disorder, malingering, and somatic symptoms in DSM-5. *Psychosomatics.* 2019;60(4):432–433. doi:10.1016/j.psym.2018.11.003

22. Wallach J. Laboratory diagnosis of factitious disorders. *Arch Intern Med.* 1994;154(15):1690–1696.

23. Fliege H, Scholler G, Rose M, Willenberg H, Klapp BF. Factitious disorders and pathological self-harm in a hospital population: An interdisciplinary challenge. *Gen Hosp Psychiatry.* 2002;24(3):164–171. doi:S0163834302001718

24. Reich P, Gottfried LA. Factitious disorders in a teaching hospital. *Ann Intern Med.* 1983;99(2):240–247. doi:10.7326/0003-4819-99-2-240

25. Krahn LE, Li H, O'Connor MK. Patients who strive to be ill: Factitious disorder with physical symptoms. *Am J Psychiatry.* 2003;160(6):1163–1168. doi:10.1176/appi.ajp.160.6.1163

26. Miller HA. *M-FAST Interview Manual.* Psychological Assessment Resources; 2001.

27. U.S. Department of Health and Human Services. HIPAA privacy rule and sharing information related to mental health. n.d. https://www.hhs.gov/sites/default/files/hipaa-privacy-rule-and-sharing-info-related-to-mental-health.pdf

28. McCarthy-Jones S, Resnick PJ. Listening to voices: The use of phenomenology to differentiate malingered from genuine auditory verbal hallucinations. *Int J Law Psychiatry.* 2014;37(2):183–189. doi:S0160-2527(13)00106-4

29. Goodwin DW, Alderson P, Rosenthal R. Clinical significance of hallucinations in psychiatric disorders: A study of 116 hallucinatory patients. *Arch Gen Psychiatry*. 1971;24(1):76–80. doi:10.1001/archpsyc.1971.01750070078011

30. Nayani TH, David AS. The auditory hallucination: A phenomenological survey. *Psychol Med*. 1996;26(1):177–189. doi:10.1017/s003329170003381x

31. McCarthy-Jones S, Trauer T, Mackinnon A, Sims E, Thomas N, Copolov DL. A new phenomenological survey of auditory hallucinations: Evidence for subtypes and implications for theory and practice. *Schizophr Bull*. 2014;40(1):231–235. doi:10.1093/schbul/sbs156

32. Bosman HS, van Rensburg CJ, Lippi G. Suicide risk of male State patients with antisocial personality traits. *S Afr J Psychiatr*. 2020;26:1543. doi:10.4102/sajpsychiatry.v26i0.1543

33. Schneider B, Schnabel A, Wetterling T, Bartusch B, Weber B, Georgi K. How do personality disorders modify suicide risk? *J Pers Disord*. 2008;22(3):233–245. doi:10.1521/pedi.2008.22.3.233

34. Lynch FL, Peterson EL, Lu CY, et al. Substance use disorders and risk of suicide in a general US population: A case control study. *Addict Sci Clin Pract*. 2020;15(1):14. doi:10.1186/s13722-020-0181-1

35. Davis L, Uezato A, Newell JM, Frazier E. Major depression and comorbid substance use disorders. *Curr Opin Psychiatry*. 2008;21(1):14–18. doi:10.1097/YCO.0b013e3282f32408

36. Green D, Rosenfeld B. Evaluating the gold standard: A review and meta-analysis of the structured interview of reported symptoms. *Psychol Assess*. 2011;23(1):95–107. doi:10.1037/a0021149

37. Vitacco MJ, Jackson RL, Rogers R, Neumann CS, Miller HA, Gabel J. Detection strategies for malingering with the Miller Forensic Assessment of Symptoms Test: A confirmatory factor analysis of its underlying dimensions. *Assessment*. 2008;15(1):97–103. doi:10.1177/1073191107308085

38. Zubera A, Raza M, Holaday E, Aggarwal R. Screening for malingering in the emergency department. *Acad Psychiatry*. 2015;39(2):233–234. doi:10.1007/s40596-014-0253-1

39. Kontos N, Querques J, Freudenreich O. Fighting the good fight: Responsibility and rationale in the confrontation of patients. *Mayo Clin Proc*. 2012;87(1):63–66. doi:10.1016/j.mayocp.2011.07.002

40. Taylor JB, Beach SR, Kontos N. The therapeutic discharge: An approach to dealing with deceptive patients. *Gen Hosp Psychiatry*. 2017;46:74–78. doi:S0163-8343(17)30053-1

41. Kontos N, Taylor JB, Beach SR. The therapeutic discharge II: An approach to documentation in the setting of feigned suicidal ideation. *Gen Hosp Psychiatry*. 2018;51:30–35. doi:S0163-8343(17)30366-3

42. Pillow MT, Doctor S, Brown S, Carter K, Mulliken R. An emergency department-initiated, web-based, multidisciplinary approach to decreasing emergency department visits by the top frequent visitors using patient care plans. *J Emerg Med*. 2013;44(4):853–860. doi:S0736-4679(12)01086-4

14

Eating Disorders

Claire Drom

Introduction

Patients with eating disorders present psychiatric and medical practitioners with a unique subset of clinical challenges (Box 14.1). By and large, patients are often prompted to seek treatment for the management of medical complications of disordered eating behavior or for stabilization of psychiatric comorbidities rather than for primary management of the eating disorder. It is not uncommon for patients to conceal or actively deceive examiners to avoid detection of the underlying eating disorder psychopathology. Further adding to the complexity of management, patients may often present in a nonvoluntary fashion, either due to coercion by others or by means of an involuntary mental health law. Eating disorders are underdiagnosed, and clinicians in the emergency setting are very likely to treat patients with covert or known eating disorder pathology. This chapter reviews the historical and physical findings that should prompt the treating clinician to hold a low threshold for suspicion of disordered eating behaviors.

General Epidemiology

Epidemiologic data regarding eating disorders should be interpreted with caution. Studies of eating disorder incidence and prevalence are confounded by changes in diagnostic criteria, numerous sources of bias, and the variable quality of information collected. It is widely accepted by epidemiologists that eating disorders are underdiagnosed, leading to falsely low estimates of eating disorder incidence and prevalence. With the change from the fourth edition of the *Diagnostic and Statistical Manual of Mental Disorders* (DSM-IV) to the fifth edition (DSM-5), the criteria of both bulimia nervosa (BN) and anorexia nervosa (AN) were broadened with the hope of reflecting a larger spectrum of pathological behavior. In AN, secondary amenorrhea was removed as a criterion because this erroneously excluded males, premenarchal females, and those taking hormones from meeting criteria for the disorder. The frequency of bingeing in BN was decreased from at least twice to once weekly.

Anorexia Nervosa

Surveys have estimated a lifetime prevalence of AN to be approximately 1% in women and approximately 0.3% in men.[1] Incidence is the highest in women aged 15–19 years.[1] AN in children younger than age 13 years is rare but does occur.

Box 14.1 Implications of Eating Disorders in the Emergency Department

Patients with disordered eating behaviors

- have high rates of emergency department and health care utilization;
- are more likely to present for treatment of physical ailments or comorbid psychiatry disorders, rather than the eating disorder itself;
- may make efforts to conceal behaviors or actively deceive medical investigation; and
- may present as distinctly "nonvoluntary" secondary to coercion or involuntary psychiatric treatment laws.

Bulimia Nervosa

The lifetime prevalence of BN is estimated to be slightly higher at 1–1.5% in women and 0.1–0.5% among men. In the United States, rates of BN are higher in Latinos and African Americans than among non-Latino Whites.[1]

Binge Eating Disorder

Binge eating disorder (BED) is the most common eating disorder. Internationally, the lifetime prevalence of BED among women is approximately 2%. The prevalence of BED is higher in the United States, compared to international data, with up to 3.5% of adult women and 2% of adult men meeting diagnostic criteria.[1]

Demographic and Cultural Influences

DSM-5 eating disorders may be conceptualized as culture-bound syndromes. Eating disorders, as described in the DSM-5, are essentially nonexistent in non-Western cultures. Globally, data reveal that rates of diagnosed eating disorders increase with modernization of a society and the influx of Western beauty ideals. Studies comparing rates of eating disorders across cultures suggest that cultures that do not value thin bodies as representative of ideal beauty standards may be protective against the development of eating disorders.[2] Additional studies have shown that migration to a Western culture is associated with the development of an eating disorder.[1] Studies across ethnicities have found no significant difference in the age of onset of the eating disorder, prevalence, or risk factors.

Additional key demographic risk factors for the development of an eating disorder have been identified. Both BN and BED are more common among women, students, and individuals with a higher body mass index (BMI).[3] Although eating disorders are most often thought to be an affliction of young women, attention is increasingly turning toward populations typically considered to be free from eating disorder psychopathology, including males and older adults. A 2016 Australian report surveyed nearly 500 men aged 40–75 years. More than half reported a history of purging behaviors, including overexercise, and 6.8% reported the presence of active eating disorder symptoms.[4] Men are also more likely than women to endorse overeating behaviors.[5] Similarly, international surveys have found the prevalence of eating disorder symptoms in adults older than age 65 years to parallel those in younger cohorts. BED, BN, and unspecified eating disorder occur at rates in women older than age 40 years comparable to those of younger women. The rate of AN in this older female population, however, is very low.[6]

Suicide and Mortality

Morbidity and mortality across all eating disorders are high, with AN being the deadliest psychiatric disorder. Individuals with AN have a mortality rate of approximately 5% per decade or 0.5% per year. Most deaths are a direct consequence of the physical complications of the disorder; however, approximately one-fifth to one-third of deaths in AN can be attributed to suicide.[1] Like the general population, risk factors for suicide attempts in those with AN include alcohol use, anxiety and panic, post-traumatic stress disorder (PTSD), and Cluster B personality traits. Suicide attempts are more common among those with the binge/purge subtype of AN, and many patients with a history of AN and suicide attempts tend to display an anxious–impulsive personality profile. Noted that in individuals with AN, attempts are more likely to be associated with a strong desire to die and a higher degree of expected lethality.[7]

Mortality and suicide rates in the other eating disorders lack more detailed studies. The death rate in BN is approximately 0.1–0.2% per year. Suicide attempts among patients with BN are common; approximately one-third of patients with BN attempt suicide during their lifetime. One 20-year study on mortality data in BN revealed that 23% of patients died by suicide.[1] Purging behaviors and impulsivity are associated with suicide attempts in both AN and BN.[8] In BN, the use of laxatives, but not the presence of a mood disorder, has proven to be a statistically significant predictor of suicide attempts.[8] Mortality data in BED are limited, and many reported deaths in this population are thought to be associated with obesity-related physical complications.[1] The rate of suicidal ideation among individuals with BED is high, with prevalence estimates ranging from roughly 25–50%. Estimates of suicide attempts and completed suicides vary widely (2.3–34%). Suicidal ideation and suicide attempts are increased in individuals with BED who are younger, prone to high degrees of alexithymia and neuroticism, and have comorbid mood or substance use diagnoses.[9]

Diagnosis and Clinical Features

The DSM-5 defines the eating disorders as disturbances of eating behaviors leading to nutrient intake patterns that impair physical health or psychosocial function. Most diagnoses are intended to be mutually exclusive to aid in stratification of clinical treatment and outcomes.[10] Diagnostic criteria for pica (the consumption of nonfood substances), rumination disorder (repeated regurgitation of food), and avoidant/restrictive food intake disorder are outlined in the DSM-5 but not included in this discussion.

Anorexia Nervosa

The DSM-5 outlines three core features of the diagnosis of AN: (1) the intentional re-striction of calories to achieve a significantly low body weight; (2) fear of gaining weight or engagement in behavior that prevents weight gain; and (3) a distorted view of body's shape, weight, and/or denial of one's impaired health status. Two predominant patterns of behavior have been described in AN: binge eating/purging (AN-BP) and restricting (AN-R). Over the course of the illness, it is common for individuals to alternate be-tween restricting and binge eating/purging. The severity of AN is graded based on a patient's BMI.[10,11]

The onset of AN often follows a stressful life event and most commonly occurs in older adolescent or young adult women. Onset later in life is associated with a longer course of illness that may best be conceptualized as a chronic, relapsing and remitting condition.[10] In those with less severe forms of illness, remission can be achieved within 5 years of onset.

A diagnosis of AN is often made in adults or older adolescents after an observable loss in weight occurs. In children, however, clinicians may often see a patient fail to gain weight or begin to fall below the expected developmental trajectory rather than overt weight loss.[10] In those with AN, the fear of weight gain is not ameliorated with weight loss. Some patients, especially younger adolescents and children, may not consciously express a fear of weight gain, leaving the clinician to infer this criterion. Aberrant per-ception of body image can be expressed by frequent "checking behaviors" (looking in the mirror, measuring body parts, weighing, etc.). Self-esteem is rigidly linked to weight status, with weight gain equating to failure and weight loss to discipline and achievement. Furthermore, many individuals fail to recognize or express that they acknowledge the significant medical consequences of their malnourished stated.[10] Patients often engage in high levels of maladaptive rationalization and may disguise their disordered habits as "healthy" or philosophically directed lifestyle choices. For example, they may endorse nu-merous dietary allergies or intolerances, leading to a very restrictive diet, or may follow a very limited vegan diet in the name of ethical principles. Most patients with AN present at the behest of family or friends. A patient may self-present with somatic or psychological complaints. "Weight loss" is rarely the chief complaint of a voluntary patient with AN.[10]

Bulimia Nervosa

Similar to the description of AN, the DSM-5 identifies three core features in the diag-nosis of BN: binge eating episodes, engagement in inappropriate behaviors to prevent weight gain, and a view of one's self that is heavily dependent on body weight or shape. A "binge" is characterized by both eating more food during a period of time than most would consume and a perceived loss of control over food intake.[10]

Classically, an underweight BMI is not consistent with BN. Severity of BN is deter-mined by the frequency of compensatory behaviors per week. Binge episodes may be planned or unplanned, and the types of foods consumed vary but are typically foods a person would otherwise avoid.[10] Patients frequently report a negative mood preceding the binge episode in addition to shame following the binge. Many take efforts to conceal their behaviors. Between binges, individuals commonly select for low-calorie or "diet" foods and consciously monitor and restrict calorie consumption.

Compensatory purging behaviors include vomiting (the most common), laxative and diuretic abuse, exercise, fasting, abuse of orlistat (a weight loss supplement), thyroid hormone abuse, and insulin manipulation (discussed later), among others. Most patients engage in multiple purging modalities.

As for AN, the typical age of onset is later adolescence or young adulthood (mean 20 years), and onset usually follows a stressful event and/or a concerted effort to lose weight or "diet."[3] Reviews of several studies suggest that the age of onset of BN may be trending toward younger, but it is unclear if this trend is in fact an artifact of earlier age of detection.[1] Symptoms fluctuate but appear to minimize in frequency and severity over time. BN persists for a mean of 6.5 years in afflicted individuals,[3] and over a lifetime, a patient may diagnostically crossover between AN, BN, and BED. BMI is the defining diagnostic separator between BN and AN-BP: Those with BMI < 18.5 are diagnosed with AN-BP.[11]

Binge Eating Disorder

Binge eating disorder is defined by the presence of a binge episode at least once per week for 3 months. The same definition of a binge is used as in BN, and patients experience marked distress following the binge. A binge is usually triggered by a negative mood state and is associated with much shame and secrecy. In contrast to BN, however, no compensatory behaviors are utilized.[10]

Data surrounding the development of BED are limited, but age of onset is similar to that for other eating disorders (mean age 23 years). Patients are more likely to be older at the time that they seek treatment and may experience a more persistent illness course through the life span compared to those with AN and BN.[3]

Most individuals with BED are normal to overweight. It is important to note that obesity does not indicate the presence of BED. However, in those seeking weight loss surgery, as many as one in five may meet criteria for BED.[12]

Others

Other Specified Feeding or Eating Disorder

The DSM-5 added several subtypes to this class of disorders, defined under the other specified feeding or eating disorder category, including atypical anorexia nervosa (AAN), purging disorder, night eating syndrome, and subthreshold binge eating and bulimia nervosa.[10] Although not commented upon in this chapter, these psychopathologies are worth noting because they are hypothesized to affect many patients, frequently evade detection, and are associated with a great deal of distress and psychiatric comorbidity.

Although clear epidemiologic data are lacking, AAN is not infrequently encountered in the community and in those with higher degrees of psychiatric and medical comorbidity. The diagnostic criteria of AAN are the same as for AN, except that "significant weight loss" may happen without the person reaching an abnormally low BMI. The cognitive distortions and intrapsychic distress experienced by these individuals separate them from those who restrict calories for nonpathological weight loss alone.[13] Because these patients appear "normal" or even overweight, severely pathological eating behaviors may go undetected. They may be just as likely to experience medical consequences of caloric restriction, most notably electrolyte disturbances and refeeding syndrome.[11] Indeed, AAN accounts for nearly one-third of admissions to eating disorder treatment.[14]

New Directions

Muscularity-Oriented Disordered Eating

Muscularity-oriented disordered eating (MODE) was initially conceptualized as a "reverse anorexia" experienced by bodybuilders because these individuals displayed behavioral and cognitive processes similar to those classically attributed to AN.[15] Diagnostic criteria were first suggested in the 1990s and included a preoccupation with being sufficiently muscular and/or lean, even though the person is more muscular than average. The preoccupation results in significant impairment or distress.[16] Indeed, muscle dysmorphia was added in the DSM-5 as a subtype of body dysmorphic disorder. Obsessive checking behaviors are characteristic of the psychopathology, sparking a debate as to whether its inclusion with obsessive–compulsive disorder (OCD) would be more appropriate. Among individuals with muscularity-disordered eating, the use of overexercise, diets, and anabolic steroids is common.[15]

Global estimates of anabolic steroid use are approximately 3%, with rates higher among men than women. Anabolic steroid use may be more common among gay and bisexual men, with surveys reporting approximately 10–15% of gym-going men using anabolic steroids with the goal of achieving a more muscular physique.[17] There is a strong association between anabolic steroid use and the presence of eating disorder symptoms.[17]

Like the classic stereotype of a young woman with anorexia, individuals experiencing MODE may wear baggy clothes and avoid swimming pools. Many will follow a diet focused on high-protein and low-fat content. Deviation from this strict diet is followed by compensation with exercise, and the person may be intensely anxious or distressed until able to exercise.[16] Individuals may also become similarly distressed if unable to engage in a desired, regular pattern of weight training. Spending excess sums of money on supplements and devoting time to weightlifting can cause significant difficulties in a person's life.[16] Many affected persons may also engage in frequent mirror-checking, weigh themselves often, and routinely seek reassurance from others regarding their physique.[16] A high number of individuals who meet criteria for MODE have met criteria for BN or AN in the past; this is especially true among women bodybuilders. Men with MODE have higher rates of comorbid mood and anxiety disorders, substance use, and past suicide attempts.[18] The degree of distress, body dissatisfaction, and impaired social and occupational functioning that accompanies MODE distinguishes it as a pathological entity, separate from the hobby of bodybuilding.[16] A validated screening scale, the Muscle Appearance Satisfaction Scale, has been developed.

Insulin Manipulation ("Diabulimia")

An emerging concept in the field of eating disorder research is the diagnosis of "diabulimia," which has earned the infamous title of "the world's most dangerous eating disorder" in popular culture. In this condition, individuals with insulin-dependent diabetes mellitus (DM) intentionally restrict insulin to avoid gaining weight. Although some may represent this pattern of behavior as a distinct disorder, insulin manipulation is currently classified as a type of purging behavior. The practice of restricting insulin for weight loss may be very common, with as many as 40% of affected men and 20% of women reporting intentionally restricting insulin to avoid weight gain at some point in their lives.[19] Although this practice is most often seen in patients with type 1 DM, those with type II DM are also at an increased risk of exhibiting this behavior. These patients are typically older in age and have an existing history of BED. Eating disorders, in general, are estimated to be twice as prevalent in type I DM compared to the general population, with up to 20% of women with type I DM meeting criteria for an eating disorder.[20,21] Overall, women with type 1 DM aged 15–30 years are at the highest risk of persistent and more significant insulin manipulation for weight loss. Risk factors for the development of sustained insulin misuse include a history of trauma and psychiatric diagnoses, high perceived stress, and isolation.[21] In susceptible individuals, the necessary focus on weight and nutrition as part of medical management of diabetes becomes a nidus for maladaptation. Emerging studies suggest that the manipulation of insulin parallels behaviors seen in addictive disorders and self-harming habits, in that insulin is used as a means of coping to aversive stimuli and directing control over one's physiology.[20] Patients are at increased risk of accelerated end organ damage from hyperglycemia, including blindness, neuropathy, vascular disease, and amputations. Mortality is increased threefold in this population,[21] and these individuals may have a history of frequent eating disorder presentations for diabetic ketoacidosis, poor glycemic control, and unexplained weight loss, as well as bouts of hypoglycemia when insulin is overdosed in order to justify or prepare for a binge.

Psychiatric Comorbidity

Eating disorders rarely occur in isolation, and patients experience high rates of both medical and psychiatric comorbidity. Studies of international populations routinely cite the presence of at least one co-occurring psychiatric diagnosis in 20–95% of individuals with eating disorders.[22] Reporting of prevalence data is biased by methodology, patient characteristics (e.g., outpatient versus inpatient), and diagnostic criteria used. Most current data reflect the co-occurrence of psychiatric disorders in the setting of DSM-IV eating disorder criteria. With the broadening of criteria in DSM-5, current prevalence rates of comorbid disorders are likely underestimated. Historically, patients with AN-restricting subtype experience the lowest rate of comorbid psychiatric disorders, whereas those with BN or BED experience the highest rate.[22]

Mood Disorders

The starvation state of AN can induce numerous changes in both cognition and mood, leading to symptoms that resemble a depressive episode. Low mood, withdrawal, fatigue, reduced sex drive, insomnia, and irritability are common in individuals suffering from starvation. The presence of suicidal ideation and significant anhedonia are not necessarily considered secondary to starvation and would be suggestive of a comorbid mood disorder. Depression associated with starvation clears within a few weeks of refeeding.[10]. Depressive disorders are highly comorbid in BN and AN, with rates ranging from 20% to nearly 100%,[11] and a major depressive episode may precede the development of AN or BN.

Several decades of research suggest that bipolar disorder and disordered eating overlap considerably. The prevalence of bipolar disorders in eating disorder pathology ranges from 0% to 64%, depending largely on diagnostic criteria.[23] Specifically, rates of BN and BED are increased in patients with bipolar disorder. A more recent study of patients with bipolar disorder found that using DSM-5 criteria, 15% met criteria for BN, 12% for BED, and 0.2% for AN.[24] This study also noted a correlation between BN and increased suicidality and mood instability, whereas BED was associated with increased anxiety symptoms. Patients with co-occurring eating disorders and bipolar disorders are more likely to be female and White and to experience elevated degrees of suicidality, mood instability, substance abuse, and overall psychiatric distress.[24,25]

Anxiety Disorders

Anxiety disorders are highly comorbid with eating disorders, and estimated prevalence varies widely from 25% to 75%.[26] Anxiety symptoms are often noted to precede the development of the disordered eating behavior. Social anxiety and OCD tend to have the highest rates of comorbidity. However, generalized anxiety, PTSD, and specific phobias are also common.[26] Prognosis for recovery tends to be worse in patients with both an eating disorder and an anxiety disorder, particularly OCD. These patients tend to experience greater psychiatric distress and more refractory illness courses.

There exists considerable overlap between the cognitive distortions and compulsive behavior seen in eating disorders, especially AN, and OCD. Indeed, many individuals with AN display obsessive thoughts and behaviors involving food and weight. In those who are malnourished, these thoughts are amplified by the starvation state.[10] The prevalence of OCD in AN and BN varies across studies from 0% to 60%. Patients with AN are more likely to experience OCD than those with BN.[27] The converse is also true: The prevalence of eating disorders co-occurring with OCD is elevated and is estimated to be 3–13%.[28] Female patients with OCD are more likely than males to experience some degree of disordered eating and should be considered higher risk for development of an eating disorder.[28] When distinguishing between OCD and an eating disorder, a diagnosis of OCD may be appropriate if a patient displays symptoms not related to the eating disorder (i.e., not involving food, weight, or body shape). The preoccupation with food and shape seen in AN is usually ego-syntonic, representing a further distinction from the ego-dystonic obsessions of OCD.[26]

Attention has increasingly turned towards character traits of perfectionism, rigidity, and inflexibility as being risk factors for the development of disordered eating. Obsessive–compulsive personality traits occur frequently in patients with eating disorder psychopathology, especially in individuals with AN.[26] Perfectionism has a stronger association with any eating disorder compared to OCD. Perfectionism coupled with obsessive–compulsive personality disorder (OCPD) seems to represent a particularly strong vulnerability for the development of disordered eating behaviors.[27] OCPD has a stronger association with restrictive eating patterns compared to purging behaviors.[27]

Rates of co-occurring PTSD and eating disorders are poorly understood. However, sexual abuse and trauma are strongly associated with the development of disordered eating behaviors, especially BN.[26]

Substance Use Disorders

The psychopathology of disordered eating overlaps strongly with that seen in addictive disorders. Many patients with eating disorders display compulsive use and cravings, affective dysregulation, impulsivity, and novelty-seeking.[10,29] Substance use disorders are highly comorbid with eating disorders. Some studies estimate the presence of a use disorder in upwards of 50% of patients with an eating disorder.[30] However, most surveys suggest approximately one-fourth to one-third of eating disorder patients will qualify for an addictive disorder during their lifetime.[31] Substance use disorders correspond more directly with bingeing and purging behaviors, as opposed to restrictive patterns.[30] The highest rates of co-occurrence are found in BN; nearly 30–40% of patients with BN meet criteria for a use disorder at some point in their lifetime.[10,31]

Several decades of research has established that food deprivation (either voluntarily or involuntarily) increases the risk of self-administration of psychoactive substances. Psychologically, the use of substances to soothe negative affective states can be equated to the use of disordered eating behaviors to achieve the same effect.[30] In addition, abusable substances may become tools for maintaining the eating disorder; specifically, nicotine, caffeine, and stimulants may potentially be misused in order to suppress appetite or induce vomiting.[31] In studies of women who abuse methamphetamine, nearly one-third reported that their substance use began as a means of controlling weight. Many women also cite concern for weight gain as a deterrent for achieving sobriety.[31]

Childhood adversity and trauma not only contribute to the development of substance use disorders but also increase the risk of developing an eating disorder. Maladaptive personality traits and coping patterns of impulsivity and rigid perfectionism are associated with comorbid alcohol use disorder and eating disorder.[31] In studies of women recovering from both PTSD and addiction, individuals expressed high concern about weight gain and approximately 14% met criteria for an eating disorder.[31]

Medical Complications Associated with Disordered Eating Behavior

Associated with Food Restriction

Cardiovascular
Cardiovascular complications are the most common in the setting of caloric restriction, occurring in up to 80% of patients, and range from bradycardia, arrhythmias, hypotension, and syncope to sudden cardiac death (Table 14.1).[32] Cardiac complications are the cause of one-third of deaths due to anorexia. Bradycardia is common across all subtypes of AN.[33] Slowing of the heart rate is caused by increased vagal tone and reduced metabolic rate and can occur early in the course of the illness.[34] In addition, in patients with more chronic courses of illness, reduced muscle mass and capacity of the left ventricle causes a physiologic reduction in heart rate.[35-37] Patients with AN-R are also at an

Table 14.1 Medical Complications of Food Restriction, Vomiting, and Laxative Abuse

Physiologic System	Starvation	Vomiting	Laxative Use
Cardiovascular	Bradycardia and other arrhythmias Hypotension Mitral valve prolapse Complaints of syncope and chest pain Sudden cardiac death Cardiomyopathy[a]	Arrhythmia from electrolyte abnormalities Ipecac-associated cardiac toxicity	Arrhythmia from electrolyte abnormalities
Hepatic	Transaminitis (ALT > AST) Acute liver failure		Acute liver failure (Senna abuse)
Hematologic	Leukopenia Anemia		
Gastrointestinal	Delayed gastric emptying Superior mesenteric artery syndrome[a]	Esophagitis Reflux, increased rates of Barrett's esophagus Intussusception,[a] rectal prolapse,[a] esophageal rupture,[a] pneumomediastinum[a]	Colonic dysmotility and melanosis coli (stimulant laxative abuse)
Endocrine	Blunted growth Osteopenia and osteoporosis Hypogonadism (amenorrhea and low testosterone) Sick euthyroid syndrome	PCOS[a]	Osteomalacia (phenolphthalein abuse)
Electrolytes and nutrients	Hyponatremia Low prealbumin Vitamin deficiencies	Hypochloremic metabolic alkalosis Hypokalemia	Hyperchloremic metabolic alkalosis Hypokalemia Hypermagnesemia (magnesium-containing laxatives)
Renal		Renal failure	Renal calculi formation

[a]Rare complication.
PCOS, polycystic ovarian syndrome.

increased risk of mitral valve prolapse (MVP); MVP is diagnosed in 30–50% of severe AN.[36] MVP risk resolves once weight is restored.[37] QT interval prolongation and sudden cardiac death risk have long been associated with eating disorders due to pro-arrhythmic electrolyte imbalances, namely hypokalemia and hypomagnesemia. QT intervals >600 ms are more strongly associated with sudden cardiac death from ventricular arrhythmias. More recently, studies of QT prolongation in the setting of eating disorders suggest that the degree of QT interval dispersion, combined with poor heart rate variability, is the source of increased cardiac death risk, rather than prolonged QT alone.[32] QT interval is longer in AN-BP and BN patients compared to AN-R subtype, although these patients are also at increased risk for QT prolongation.[33] There are rare case reports of Takotsubo cardiomyopathy developing in patients with AN in the setting of a catecholamine surge triggered by hypoglycemia.[32]

Hepatic

More than 50% of patients with AN develop mild to moderate elevations of aspartate aminotransferase (AST) and alanine aminotransferase (ALT), with ALT often being greater than AST. Bilirubin and alkaline phosphatase are usually within the normal range.[38] A patient may present without laboratory abnormalities, but transaminase elevation can occur during the refeeding process, peaking around day 27 with ALT often rising more so than AST. Starvation leading to autophagy and apoptosis is the proposed mechanism for hepatic cell death.[33] Overt hepatic dysfunction is rare but not unheard of. Coagulopathies have been reported, as have cases of acute liver failure with encephalopathy.[39] Hypoglycemia from defective glycogen synthesis is rare and is considered a very poor prognostic indicator.

Electrolytes and Nutrients

Electrolyte abnormalities are common across all eating disorders. In patients with restrictive behaviors, hyponatremia is approximately twice as common in AN (both restricting and binge/purge) compared to BN, with rates estimated to be 16% or 17%.[33] Patients may also drink excess water before a planned weigh-in to artificially increase the weight; hyponatremia may be an indicator of this behavior. Severe hyponatremia can lead to significant neurological consequences.[35] Hypophosphatemia is infrequently found on initial labs and tends to emerge during weight restoration, a hallmark of refeeding syndrome.[33] Albumin levels are usually unremarkable; prealbumin serves as a more reliable measure of overall nutritional status in cases of AN.[33] Deficiencies of vitamins and other essential nutrients can occur, with vitamin D deficiency being quite frequent.

Hematologic

Leukopenia is the most common hematologic abnormality in AN (~30–40% of patients). Appropriately 10% of patients with AN will have anemia.[33]

Neurocognitive

Severe AN can lead to loss of brain tissue volume. Reports on the degree and persistence of cognitive deficits vary in the literature. During acute starvation, cognitive processing may be severely altered. For many patients, cognitive function will normalize with weight restoration.[35]

Gastrointestinal

Ongoing caloric restriction may cause an adaptation of delayed gastric emptying, leading to complaints of bloating, constipation, fullness, reflux, and pain.[35] Significant weight loss can also lead to the formation of superior mesenteric artery (SMA) syndrome, in which the distal duodenum is compressed between the aorta and the SMA. Patients present with symptoms of early satiety, bilious vomiting, and severe abdominal pain.

Endocrine

Growth

The development of an eating disorder at a younger age, especially AN-R subtype, increases the risk of growth disruption that may result in permanent loss of height attainment.[34] Irreversible growth loss is more pronounced in patients who develop AN prior to puberty onset.[35] As an individual ages, they are at increased risk of osteopenia and osteoporosis, as well as increased rates of nontraumatic fracture. Osteoporosis is more common in women with anorexia and develops over time from consistently low estrogen levels and low body mass. Patients receive very little benefit from estrogen supplementation as a means of correcting the bone abnormality.[37]

Sex Hormones

Hormonal signaling across the hypothalamic–pituitary axis is diffusely disrupted. Levels of estrogen and testosterone are low in women and men, respectively, secondary to aberrant gonadotropin-releasing hormone release. Hypothalamic hypogonadotropic hypogonadism develops, leading to amenorrhea in women and low testosterone levels in men.[35,37]

Thyroid Hormones

Patients may also present with laboratory findings consistent with sick euthyroid syndrome (abnormal thyroid hormone levels in a clinically euthyroid patient), indicating the presence of systemic illness, rather than thyroidal pathology. Thyroid laboratory abnormalities resolve with weight restoration.[35]

Associated with Purging

Purging behaviors are most commonly endorsed in young women; lifetime estimates of purging in women are approximately 16%, and they are approximately 3% among men.[38] Regarding frequency of behaviors, vomiting is more commonly reported than laxative use, and diuretic abuse is the least common modality.[38] Hypokalemia from volume losses occurs frequently in AN-BP (estimated rates ~40%) and can lead to cardiac conduction abnormalities and renal failure. A metabolic hypochloremic contraction alkalosis can emerge in cases of AN-BP.[33] Dehydration leads to increases in serum aldosterone, resulting in wasting of potassium in the urine and elevated serum sodium and bicarbonate levels as the kidneys attempt to maintain intravascular volume.[33] This pattern of metabolic alkalosis is termed "pseudo-Bartter syndrome" and may be the sole indicator of surreptitious purging behaviors. Urine chloride concentrations will be low, helping differentiate from other causes of hypokalemic metabolic alkalosis.

Self-Induced Vomiting

Characteristic physical exam findings that may indicate self-induced vomiting include lesions on the backs of hands (Russell's sign), subconjunctival hemorrhages, and parotid gland swelling. Parotid sialadenitis usually develops after cessation of vomiting, can be quite painful, and may or may not be associated with elevated serum amylase. Esophageal pathology is common, including esophagitis, gastroesophageal reflux disease, hoarseness, and impaired esophageal motility. Rates of Barrett's esophagus may be increased and, along with it, there may be an increased risk of esophageal cancer.[38] Rare complications include rectal prolapse, gastroesophageal intussusception, hiatal hernia, subcutaneous emphysema, and hyoid bone fracture. Ipecac use is associated with cardiac toxicity, including heart failure, hypotension, and death.[38] BN has been associated with polycystic ovarian syndrome and hirsutism. Although causation has not been established, the theorized mechanism is through alterations in levels of follicle-stimulating hormone, luteinizing hormone, and estrogen. Recurrent vomiting may also have a direct effect on the hypothalamic–pituitary axis.[35]

Laxative and Diuretic Abuse

Several types of laxative agents are available for purchase—bulking and osmotic agents, stool softeners, and lubricant laxatives. Osmotic agents increase fluid content in stool and can lead to electrolyte imbalances if used long-term. Stimulant laxatives are more prone to abuse due to rapid onset of action. Long-term use can lead to colonic motility dysfunction and the development of pathognomonic tissue changes such as melanosis coli.[38] Because both diuretics and laxatives cause significant fluid shifts, laboratory and renal complications are common. Whereas patients who self-induce vomiting develop a hypochloremic metabolic alkalosis, patients abusing laxatives may develop a *hyper*chloremic metabolic acidosis.[35] This distinction in acid–base status can aid in the identification of the purging method. Furosemide abuse can lead to tubulointerstitial nephritis, and laxatives can lead to the formation of ammonium urate calculi. Cases of acute liver failure have been associated with Senna abuse. Phenolphthalein, an acid–base indicator with laxative properties, has been abused and can result in hypocalcemia and hypophosphatemia, leading to the development of osteomalacia.[38]

Other

Abuse of thyroid medication can cause nervousness, anxiety, and insomnia, as well as more severe cardiac consequences, including hypertension, arrhythmia, and heart failure. As discussed previously, some patients may manipulate insulin dosing in an effort to avoid weight gain; as such, these individuals present to the emergency department with hyperglycemia and associated acute and chronic complications.

Associated with Binge Episodes

Patients rarely seek emergent treatment for a binge episode alone. Although rare, acute gastric dilatation and rupture following a binge episode have been reported.[32]

Emergency Room Assessment and Differential Diagnosis

Findings on History and Physical Exam

Patients may often appear "well," thus conferring a false sense of reassurance. During the patient assessment, the astute clinician may detect subtle clues suggestive of disordered eating. Patients often present with common and nonspecific complaints, such as syncope, chest pain, and abdominal pain.[40] Self-induced vomiting can lead to hoarseness or complaints of a sore throat. As mentioned previously, this purging technique, when used over long periods of time, can lead to poor dentition, salivary gland enlargement, and Russell's sign.[40] Subconjunctival hemorrhages may also indicate more recent vomiting. Malnourished patients may develop lanugo on their back, abdomen, and forearms. These patients may also complain of feeling cold, constipated, or amenorrheic.

Screening Questions

When screening for disordered eating, it is important to consider that shame, denial, and symptom minimization are inherent to the psychopathology. Direct lines of questioning in an open and nonjudgmental stance will be the most fruitful for clinician and patient alike. When appropriate, ask permission to gather collateral information to bolster rapport.

Several brief validated screening tools for disordered eating exist. The most commonly utilized are the SCOFF (Table 14.2) and the Eating Disorder Screen for Primary Care.[41,42] A new screening tool that is more sensitive to the detection of BED, the Screen for Disordered Eating (SDE), has also been validated (Box 14.2).[43] For both SCOFF and SDE, two or more positive responses are considered a "positive" screen and should prompt further evaluation.

The following are the best questions to rule out an eating disorder:[44]

- Does your weight affect the way you feel about yourself?
- Are you satisfied with your eating patterns?

In a patient who has screened positive for an eating disorder, the clinician should explore the patient's thoughts on weight, assess daily caloric and liquid intake, and screen for and describe bingeing and purging activities. Suggested questions to ask the patient are detailed in Box 14.3.

Differential Diagnoses

Numerous systemic illnesses may cause drastic weight loss, the inability to maintain sufficient weight, or episodes of disordered eating activity. The key to differentiating between eating disorders and other conditions lies in the clinician's ability to discern

Table 14.2 SCOFF Eating Disorder Screen[a]

S	Do you make yourself *sick* (vomit) because you feel uncomfortably full?
C	Do you worry that you have lost *control* over how much you eat?
O	Have you recently lost more than *one* stone (15 pounds) in a 3-month period?
F	Do you believe yourself to be *fat* when others say you are thin?
F	Would you say that *food* dominates your life?

[a]A score of 2 or more positive responses qualifies as a positive screen and prompts further evaluation.
Adapted from Morgan et al.[42]

Box 14.2 Screen for Disordered Eating

---

1. Do you often feel the desire to eat when you are emotionally upset or stressed?
2. Do you often feel that you can't control what or how much you eat?
3. Do you sometimes make yourself throw up (vomit) to control your weight?
4. Are you often preoccupied with being thinner?
5. Do you believe yourself to be fat when others say you are thin?

Adapted from Maguen et al.[43]

---

a patient's evaluation of the problem (Table 14.3). Patients with eating disorders will express a preoccupation with weight and shape, suggesting a psychological origin for a low body weight or abnormal eating behaviors.

Important systemic causes of weight loss that must not be overlooked occur across organ systems. Gastrointestinal disorders may reduce appetite, lead to malabsorption, or cause excessive losses through diarrhea. Malignancy, infections, and endocrinopathies may first present with weight loss as the chief complaint. Many patients suffering from advancing and chronic pulmonary and renal diseases often experience weight

---

Box 14.3 Suggested Questions to Ask Patients with Strong Suspicion of an Eating Disorder

---

Thoughts on body weight
   What is your desired body weight?
   What is the most you would feel comfortable weighing?
   What has been your lowest weight?
   How often do you weigh yourself?
Daily food intake
   Do you count calories? If so, how?
   How many calories do you eat in a day?
   What are the most calories you will allow in a day?
   Do you have any dietary allergies or food intolerances?
   Do you follow a limited diet for personal beliefs, such as vegetarianism or veganism?
Binge episodes
   Do you ever eat to the point of feeling uncomfortably full?
   Do you ever experience a loss of control when you eat?
   What kind of foods do you eat when you binge?
   What happens after a binge? How do you feel?
Purging behaviors
   Do you ever restrict fluids in order to lose weight?
   Have you ever used laxatives or diuretics to lose weight?
   How much would you exercise if it didn't burn calories?
   How much time do you spend exercising? Do you miss activities because of exercise?
   "Do you exercise alone or in groups?

Table 14.3 Differential Diagnoses

For patients presenting with low body weight and/or weight loss	
Infections—TB, hepatitis, HIV/AIDS, parasites	Endocrinopathies—hyperthyroidism, primary adrenal insufficiency, new type 1 diabetes mellitus
Gastrointestinal disorders—celiac sprue, inflammatory bowel disease, ulcers	Advanced lung disease
Malignancy	Neurological disorders—post-stroke, ALS, MS, Parkinson's disease, muscular dystrophy
Esophageal pathology	Psychiatric disorders—OCD, MDD, psychosis, phobias
Drug and alcohol abuse	

For patients presenting with a history suggestive of bingeing or purging episodes

Kleine–Levin syndrome

Major depressive disorder with atypical features

Cannabis hyperemesis syndrome

Somatic symptom disorder, factitious disorder

ALS, amyotrophic lateral sclerosis; MDD, major depressive disorder; MS, multiple sclerosis; OCD, obsessive-compulsive disorder; TB, tuberculosis.

loss and have difficulty maintaining adequate nutrition. Esophageal and neurological disorders that impair a patient's ability to swallow and feed themself can severely limit caloric intake.[10]

Psychiatric conditions may also present with weight loss as part of the clinical syndrome. In major depressive disorder, a patient may experience loss of appetite. These patients, however, will not express a fear of weight gain or a desire for weight loss. Delusions surrounding food and eating behaviors are not uncommon in those experiencing psychosis or neurocognitive disorders. Similar to depressive disorders, these patients will not express cognitive distortions surrounding body image and weight gain. Severe social phobia may cause an individual to fear eating in public and may limit that person's caloric intake to the point of weight loss. OCD should be included in the differential as well. Whereas the cognitions of AN closely mirror OCD, those with OCD alone will experience obsessions and compulsions unrelated to food and body image.

Those in the throes of severe addiction may experience such functional impairment that they are unable to meet their caloric needs. The abuse of stimulants is classically associated with weight loss, sometimes to an extreme degree. In all patients with addiction and weight loss or low body weight, the clinician must screen for fear of weight gain or desire of weight loss as being contributing factors to the substance use.

Diagnoses that may mimic bingeing/purging patterns of behavior are less diverse and tend to fall within neurological and psychiatric categories. Patients with somatic symptom disorder and factitious disorder may present with mysterious episodes of vomiting or diarrhea. As in patients with disordered eating, they may appear non-distressed by these episodes, but these patients will not express concerns about body image or weight gain. Cannabis use may lead to a hyperemesis syndrome. More common in younger men, patients may present with alternating episodes of severe vomiting and abdominal pain interspersed with periods of hyperphagia or excess food intake while intoxicated on cannabis. Symptoms classically dissipate after taking a hot bath or shower.[45] Kleine–Levin syndrome is a rare sleep disorder, primarily affecting adolescents, that presents with episodes of hypersomnia; psychiatric and cognitive symptoms; and behavioral changes, including hyperphagia.[46] Patients suffering from major depressive disorder with atypical features may become hyperphagic but will not endorse concerns around body image or weight and will not engage in compensatory behaviors after an episode of overeating.

Medical and Psychiatric Stabilization

Medical Workup and Management in the Emergency Department

Physical Exam
The examining clinician should pay particular attention to the cardiac, abdominal, and endocrine systems.[47] In addition to routine vital signs (heart rate, blood pressure, temperature, and oxygen saturation), a set of orthostatic vital signs should be obtained. Patients should be weighed in a hospital gown because underweight individuals may wear bulky clothing or have heavy objects in pockets to artificially increase weight.[48]

Laboratory and Other Studies
Investigations should be clinically guided (Table 14.4). In all patients with an eating disorder (both strong clinical suspicion for and confirmed cases), a complete blood count, basic electrolytes, liver enzymes, magnesium, phosphorus, and confirmation of pregnancy status should all be collected. All patients should have a spot electrocardiogram (ECG) or be placed on telemetric monitoring while in the emergency department. Specific complaints of chest pain should be assessed at each presentation with an ECG, chest X-ray, and telemetry monitoring.[40] A transthoracic echocardiogram may be indicated in very underweight patients, especially those presenting with peripheral edema or other signs of heart failure, although this evaluation is usually completed on medical inpatients rather than emergency department admissions.[47]

Abnormal Vital Signs
Bradycardia represents a physiologic adaptation to increased vagal tone and does not necessarily require treatment. Symptomatic hypotension and bradycardia, however, should be addressed in the emergency department and may warrant medical admission.

Laboratory Abnormalities
Elevated hepatic markers may be found on laboratory testing. Imaging and biopsy are usually of low diagnostic yield. An extensive workup is generally not recommended unless there are conditions besides an eating disorder that may be contributing to this abnormality. An acetaminophen level, however, should be drawn in all patients with elevated liver enzymes and a comorbid eating disorder. In very ill patients, tests of hepatic synthetic function may also be abnormal, including a prolonged prothrombin time and hypoglycemia.

Hydration Status
Large boluses of intravenous (IV) fluids should be avoided in all patients with disordered eating. In patients with AN, the cardiac muscle will not be able to accommodate

Table 14.4 Recommended Medical Workup in the Emergency Department

All patients should receive	
Comprehensive metabolic panel	
Complete blood count	
Magnesium	
Phosphorous	
Confirmation of pregnancy status	
ECG or telemetric monitoring	
By clinical indication	
Chest pain	Continuous telemetry
	Chest X-ray
Transaminitis	Acetaminophen level
	PT and INR
Bone pain or point tenderness	Radiographic imaging of affected area
Severe constipation	Abdominal X-ray

ECG, electrocardiogram; INR, international normalized ratio; PT, prothrombin time.

the increased workload, leading to acute development of heart failure. IV fluids should be adjusted for weight and given at a dose of 15–20 mL/kg.[36] Patients who self-induce vomiting may present with contraction alkalosis. Because the adrenal glands perceive the intravascular fluid compartment as being dehydrated, aldosterone will continue to be secreted until fluid status is restored, resulting in ongoing alkalosis and hypokalemia. Thus, gentle fluid support (normal saline at a rate of 50 mL/hr) will correct the hypokalemia and alkalosis.[36]

Aggressive fluid hydration may also precipitate significant edema in patients with both AN and BN due to low serum oncotic pressure and aberrant aldosterone signaling, respectively. Edema can be incredibly distressing and physically uncomfortable in these patients. The fear of edema may even prevent patients from seeking medical treatment, especially if they have had prior negative experiences with this side effect of treatment. In the medical setting, edema typically resolves within 3 weeks and is managed with spironolactone (an aldosterone antagonist), leg elevation, compression stockings, and a low-sodium diet.[36]

Physical Complaints

Patients with AN are at risk of developing osteoporosis and may experience fractures spontaneously or from low-impact injuries. Complaints of bone or joint pain may warrant radiographic imaging to assess for fracture. Symptoms of constipation, bloating, diarrhea, and abdominal discomfort are common and may represent physiologic adaptations to minimal caloric consumption. In the setting of laxative abuse, patients may experience significant rebound constipation. Abdominal imaging may be helpful in assessing for stool burden and origins of changes in bowel behaviors.[36] Particularly severe gastrointestinal pain may warrant a workup for SMA syndrome[35] or acute gastric dilatation or rupture. Although rare, Boerhaave syndrome (esophageal rupture) should be considered in any patient with an eating disorder who presents with a history or evidence of frequent vomiting, chest pain (classically worse with yawning), tachycardia, tachypnea and shortness of breath, and severe distress.[40] Pneumomediastinum, another rare complication, can occur spontaneously in malnourished individuals but is more commonly associated with forceful vomiting. Patients present with chest pain and distress and may have elevated heart rate.[40]

Management of Refeeding Syndrome

Although not generally an active concern early in a patient's hospital course, the consequences of refeeding can be dire, and the emergency clinician has to take preventative steps. The refeeding syndrome consists of marked abnormalities in serum electrolytes and fluid compartments. As the body begins to metabolize glucose, phosphate is rapidly utilized, leading to acute cellular adenosine triphosphate depletion. Direct physiologic consequences include delirium and cardiovascular collapse. The risk of developing refeeding syndrome peaks at weeks 2 and 3 of treatment.[37] Risk factors for refeeding syndrome include <70% ideal body weight, little to no nutritional intake for 10 days prior to admission, and abnormal electrolytes at time of presentation.[36]

Management of Psychiatric Risk

As reviewed previously, individuals who suffer from disordered eating behaviors are at an inordinately increased risk of death by suicide. The ethical and medicolegal implications of involuntary treatment in eating disorders are reviewed below. In general, the risk assessment of the patient presenting with eating disorder symptoms does not differ from any other. The clinician should carefully screen for co-occurring psychiatric diagnoses and substance abuse. Past suicide attempts should be assessed for the degree of impulsivity and expected medical significance. Some patients may report that the disordered behaviors (e.g., purging or starvation) are suicidal in intent. It is worth reiterating that individuals with AN tend to make suicide attempts of higher lethality and with strong intent to be dead. They may impress an examiner with their seemingly rational and reassuring statements regarding imminent dangerousness. In this case, risk assessment should rely more heavily on past patterns of suicidal behaviors, other historical risk factors, and comorbid conditions rather than the patient's report of intent or imminence. Verifying external protective factors, such as employment and financial stability, is also prudent. When allowed by the patient, engaging their social supports and collecting collateral information may be beneficial. To avoid iatrogenic harm, a careful review of outpatient medications should be conducted. The clinician may advise implementing additional safeguards around dangerous medications in this population, such as stimulants, bupropion, and lithium. The patient's outpatient treatment team should be contacted regarding their presentation, ideally with the patient's permission. Consent for this communication, however, is not required by law. The clinician should weigh the risks and benefits of this decision considering that concealment of the patient's emergency presentation is not likely to be helpful to their care in the long term.

Triage to Appropriate Treatment Setting

Admission for medical stabilization is recommended if body weight is <70–75% of ideal weight, in the event of arrhythmias or symptomatic hypotension, and when the heart rate is <35–40 beats per minute.[37] Patients may also be eligible for referral to residential or day treatment programs. Many of these programs will have strict criteria regarding the patient's weight and voluntariness to eat.

Staff Behavioral Approach

Invariably, strong reactions and countertransference are evoked toward this patient population. Patients often continue to engage in the same behaviors that led to their emergency presentation and may consciously (or unconsciously) cause rifts within staff teams. The appearance of a very underweight patient may be shocking and disturbing to staff. Alternatively, staff may self-identify with patients with more normal-range or overweight BMIs and minimize the severity of the pathology. Close nursing supervision is recommended to monitor for attempts at overexercise (pacing or fidgeting), purging (vomiting into the toilet), or throwing away/hiding food or liquids. Toilet bowls should be checked before flushing. Risk of self-injury may be elevated, and safety precautions should be implemented based on risk assessment.

Ethical and Legal Considerations

Involuntary treatment of individuals with eating disorders is a long-debated and complicated topic among experts in medical ethics. A full review of the subject is beyond the scope of this chapter. On a general level, those with BN and BED are more likely to voluntarily engage in treatment due to high degrees of associated shame and distress from binge episodes. Patients with AN, however, are significantly less likely to voluntarily seek treatment. Some consider this treatment avoidance and ambivalence to be an expected symptom of AN, attributable to the ego-syntonic nature of the pathologic cognitions. Patients with AN account for the majority for whom involuntary eating disorder treatment is considered. The emergency department clinician will likely, at some point, encounter a person who is refusing life-saving nutritional support. Removing a person's autonomy is not to be taken lightly. In the case of forced feeding, it is not difficult to imagine that implementing this intervention may be incredibly traumatizing to both the patient and the staff, who will likely need to use physical and chemical restraints in order to administer the nutrition. Indeed, forced feeding has been declared "inhumane" by international human rights organizations.[49] Ethical practices dictate that a patient's choice be entirely voluntary and made while free of coercion. Many clinicians fear rupturing an already tenuous therapeutic alliance by forcing treatment. Treatment is further complicated by clinician frustration and disengagement, family dynamics, and perceptions of treatment futility.[50,51]

In an obviously starved and medically ill person refusing treatment, it is the duty of the clinician to assess for any suicidal intent behind the refusal of nutrition and for decision-making capacity to refuse nutritional supplementation. Many patients who have severe medical complications secondary to disordered eating behaviors deny suicidal intent behind their actions and acknowledge that unchecked continuation of their current practices may lead to death. However, they will often point out that death will come at some unspecific time in the future or that they will be able to control the behaviors before "letting it get that far." In this situation, the clinician may be placed in a particularly challenging position with a patient who, apart from body image and eating behaviors, appears rational and is not expressing *imminent* danger to themselvf.[52]

Determination of Capacity to Refuse Treatment

A discussion of capacity and competency to refuse treatment in long-standing cases of severe AN is not attempted in this chapter. However, the bulk of legal literature consists of case law wherein the court is deciding a person's competency to refuse continued treatments and instead pursue hospice care. By and large, the courts (both in the United States and internationally) have found these patients with chronic, treatment-resistant AN to be incompetent to make decisions regarding food intake.[49]

In the clinical setting, decision-making capacity is predominantly assessed via tests of functional cognitive abilities.[49] The standards of capacity include the ability to express a choice, understand information, appreciate the consequences of a decision as it applies to an individual's case, and use reasonable logical processes to manipulate information. It is not uncommon for patients to be found to lack specific, focal capacity regarding decisions surrounding food intake and weight[51] while retaining decision-making capacity for all other health care choices. In legal critiques of cases declaring incompetency on the basis of anorexia, scholars have noted the "circular logic" employed by the courts—namely that courts and clinicians "treat anorexia as a cause of its own diagnostic symptoms" and declare that a person lacks capacity due to the anorexia. By this rationale, a person with anorexia will refuse treatment. The person's refusal of treatment (an inherent element of anorexia) is both the evidence of incapacity and the effect of incapacity.[49] A method of assessing capacity to refuse nutrition in AN that would avoid this circular logic has been proposed:[49]

- The patient may endorse undeniably factually incorrect beliefs about the quality or adequacy of food provided to them in an effort to restrict their diet to effective starvation. The clinician may then note that the person is making decisions based on clearly incorrect beliefs and, thus, lacks capacity for those decisions (i.e., the required elements of understanding and reasoning are unmet).
- The patient may not be able to apply medical and nutritional facts to their current health status, even when presented with overwhelming objective evidence and expert medical opinion. A patient may, on the surface, recognize that starvation can have numerous detrimental effects but will deny that they will fall victim to these. They may say, "It won't happen to me because I am fat and not thin enough" or "I do not feel like I am that underweight or that ill." A patient relying on these beliefs to decide lacks an appreciation for their current situation and would not have the capacity to refuse nutritional supplementation.

Civil Commitment for Eating Disorder Treatment

In the United States, a patient may be legally force-fed against their will based on the determination of incapacity to make health care decisions or via involuntary civil commitment for treatment of a mental disorder. The measures for assessing decision-making capacity were reviewed above. Involuntary civil commitment laws can vary considerably from state to state, and treatments allowed under these statutes are, classically, more restrictive than the treatments allowed by declaration of incapacity for health care decision-making. In general, the laws broadly define "mental disorders" and are meant to be enacted when the effect of the person's behaviors and symptoms poses a danger to themselves or others,[52] meaning that the *intent* behind the behaviors is under less scrutiny than the consequences of the behavior. By no substantial stretch of the imagination, then, would eating disordered behaviors, especially those leading to severe medical complications, qualify for involuntary psychiatric treatment. Despite this, the majority of psychiatric clinicians (both in the United States and internationally) rarely invoke involuntary treatment for patients with severe eating disorders. Clinicians generally pursue civil commitment in cases of significant starvation with severe, life-threatening medical conditions. In these instances, the courts have been receptive to arguments that the person qualifies for civil commitment based on "grave disability" or an "inability to meet basic needs" secondary to the eating disorder.[52]

The Decision to Pursue Involuntary Treatment

When contemplating involuntary eating disorder treatment, by means of either civil commitment or declaration of incapacity, the clinician must consider several elements:

- What is the goal of treatment? Is the goal of the recommended treatment acute medical stabilization and prevention of imminent death, restoration to ideal body weight, or correction of the psychological distress? The clinician must accept that refeeding or restoring weight may stabilize a person, medically, but is not likely to impact long-term outcomes or modify the pathological psychological processes.[53] Depending on the treatment stance (e.g., purely medical versus purely psychological), clinicians may find themselves with opposing views regarding involuntary treatments. Psychologically, involuntary treatment is counterproductive by removing autonomy and invalidating a person's experiences, thus reinforcing the entrenched negative schema within the patient.[53]
- Are therapeutic gains likely? In some cases, the gain may be as simple and significant as preventing imminent death.[52]
- Is the proposed treatment accessible? Even though a patient may meet criteria for involuntary treatment, the proposed treatment must be both logistically and legally accessible.[52]
- What are the expected implications to the therapeutic alliance?

Several practical steps to deciding whether to pursue involuntary treatment have been suggested and parallel those used by clinicians who treat diseases of addiction:

1. Consider the patient's stage of change. If a person is in the precontemplative stage (not yet willing or able to see a need for change) and is at acute medical risk, involuntary treatment may be necessary. If, however, a patient is contemplative or determined to seek treatment, involuntary treatment should be avoided because invoking this route risks jeopardizing treatment engagement and overall health status significantly.[53]

2. All efforts to encourage voluntary treatment should be exhausted prior to pursuing involuntary treatment.[52] At the same time, the treatment team should be distinctly aware of the existence of coercion in these efforts.

3. Medical "red flags" for involuntary treatment vary slightly from the indications for hospitalization and include rapid weight loss (>15 pounds in 4 weeks or less), seizures, renal dysfunction, tetany, syncope, bradycardia, exercise-induced chest pain, and arrhythmias.[52]

References

1. Smink FRE, Van Hoeken D, Hoek HW. Epidemiology of eating disorders: Incidence, prevalence and mortality rates. *Curr Psychiatry Rep.* 2012;14:406–414. doi:10.1007/s11920-012-0282-y

2. Cheng ZH, Perko VL, Fuller-Marashi L, Gau JM, Stice E. Ethnic differences in eating disorder prevalence, risk factors, and predictive effects of risk factors among young women. *Eat Behav.* 2019;32:23–30. doi:10.1016/j.eatbeh.2018.11.004

3. Kessler RC, Berglund PA, Chiu WT, et al. The prevalence and correlates of binge eating disorder in the World Health Organization World Mental Health Surveys. *Biol Psychiatry.* 2013;73(9):904–914.

4. Mangweth-Matzek B, Kummer KK, Pope HG. Eating disorder symptoms in middle-aged and older men. *Int J Eat Disord.* 2016;49(10):953–957. doi:10.1002/eat.22550

5. Striegel-Moore RH, Rosselli F, Perrin N, et al. Gender difference in the prevalence of eating disorder symptoms. *Int J Eat Disord.* 2009;42(5):471–474. doi:10.1002/eat.20625

6. Mangweth-Matzek B, Hoek HW. Epidemiology and treatment of eating disorders in men and women of middle and older age. *Curr Opin Psychiatry.* 2017;30(6):446–451. doi:10.1097/YCO.0000000000000356

7. Bulik CM, Thornton L, Pinheiro AP, et al. Suicide attempts in anorexia nervosa. *Psychosom Med.* 2008;70(3):378–383. doi:10.1097/PSY.0b013e3181646765

8. Franko DL, Keel PK. Suicidality in eating disorders: Occurrence, correlates, and clinical implications. *Clin Psychol Rev.* 2006;26(6):769–782. doi:10.1016/j.cpr.2006.04.001

9. Conti C, Lanzara R, Scipioni M, Iasenza M, Guagnano MT, Fulcheri M. The relationship between binge eating disorder and suicidality: A systematic review. *Front Psychol.* 2017;8:2125. doi:10.3389/fpsyg.2017.02125

10. Walsh BT. Eating disorders. In: *Diagnostic and Statistical Manual of Mental Disorders.* 5th ed. American Psychiatric Publishing; 2013:326–360.

11. Micula-Gondek W, Guarda, AS. Eating disorders. In: Levenson J, ed. *The American Psychiatric Association Publishing Textbook of Psychosomatic Medicine and Consultation-Liaison Psychiatry.* 3rd ed. American Psychiatric Association Publishing; 2019;341–376.

12. Dawes AJ, Maggard-Gibbons M, Maher AR, et al. Mental health conditions among patients seeking and undergoing bariatric surgery: A meta-analysis. *JAMA.* 2016;315(2):150–163. doi:10.1001/jama.2015.18118

13. Forney KJ, Brown TA, Holland-Carter LA, Kennedy GA, Keel PK. Defining "significant weight loss" in atypical anorexia nervosa. *Int J Eat Disord.* 2017;50(8):952–962. doi:10.1002/eat.22717

14. Garber AK, Cheng J, Accurso EC, et al. Weight loss and illness severity in adolescents with atypical anorexia nervosa. *Pediatrics*. 2019;144(6):e20192339. doi:10.1542/peds.2019-2339

15. Nieuwoudt JE, Zhou S, Coutts RA, Booker R. Muscle dysmorphia: Current research and potential classification as a disorder. *Psychol Sport Exerc*. 2012;13(5):569–577. doi:10.1016/j.psychsport.2012.03.006

16. Pope HG, Gruber AJ, Choi P, Olivardia R, Phillips KA. Muscle dysmorphia: An underrecognized form of body dysmorphic disorder. *Psychosomatics*. 1997;38(6):548–557. doi:10.1016/S0033-3182(97)71400-2

17. Griffiths S, Murray SB, Dunn M, Blashill AJ. Anabolic steroid use among gay and bisexual men living in Australia and New Zealand: Associations with demographics, body dissatisfaction, eating disorder psychopathology, and quality of life. *Drug Alcohol Depend*. 2017;181:170–176. doi:10.1016/j.drugalcdep.2017.10.003

18. Cafri G, Olivardia R, Thompson JK. Symptom characteristics and psychiatric comorbidity among males with muscle dysmorphia. *Compr Psychiatry*. 2008;49(4):374–379. doi:10.1016/j.comppsych.2008.01.003

19. Torjesen I. Diabulimia: The world's most dangerous eating disorder. *BMJ*. 2019;364:l982. doi:10.1136/bmj.l982

20. Staite E, Zaremba N, Macdonald P, et al. "Diabulima" through the lens of social media: A qualitative review and analysis of online blogs by people with type 1 diabetes mellitus and eating disorders. *Diabet Med*. 2018;35(10):1329–1336. doi:10.1111/dme.13700

21. Coleman SE, Caswell N. Diabetes and eating disorders: An exploration of "diabulimia." *BMC Psychol*. 2021;8(1):101. doi:10.1186/s40359-020-00468-4

22. Ulfvebrand S, Birgegård A, Norring C, Högdahl L, von Hausswolff-Juhlin Y. Psychiatric comorbidity in women and men with eating disorders: Results from a large clinical database. *Psychiatry Res*. 2015;230(2):294–299. doi:10.1016/j.psychres.2015.09.008

23. McElroy SL, Kotwal R, Keck PE Jr. Comorbidity of eating disorders with bipolar disorder and treatment implications. *Bipolar Disord* 2006;8:686–695.

24. McElroy SL, Crow S, Blom TJ, et al. Prevalence and correlates of DSM-5 eating disorders in patients with bipolar disorder. *J Affect Disord*. 2016;191:216–221. doi:10.1016/j.jad.2015.11.010

25. McElroy SL, Crow S, Biernacka JM, et al. Clinical phenotype of bipolar disorder with comorbid binge eating disorder. *J Affect Disord*. 2013;150(3):981–986. doi:10.1016/j.jad.2013.05.024

26. Swinbourne JM, Touyz SW. The co-morbidity of eating disorders and anxiety disorders: A review. *Eur Eat Disord Rev*. 2007;15(4):253–274. doi:10.1002/erv.784

27. Halmi KA, Tozzi F, Thornton LM, et al. The relation among perfectionism, obsessive–compulsive personality disorder and obsessive–compulsive disorder in individuals with eating disorders. *Int J Eat Disord*. 2005;38(4):371–374. doi:10.1002/eat.20190

28. Bang L, Kristensen UB, Wisting L, et al. Presence of eating disorder symptoms in patients with obsessive–compulsive disorder. *BMC Psychiatry*. 2020;20(1):1–10. doi:10.1186/s12888-020-2457-0

29. Harrop EN, Marlatt GA. The comorbidity of substance use disorders and eating disorders in women: Prevalence, etiology, and treatment. *Addict Behav*. 2010;35(5):392–398. doi:10.1016/j.addbeh.2009.12.016

30. Dennis AB, Pryor T. The complex relationship between eating disorders and substance use disorders—Eating disorders catalogue. Published 2019. Accessed March 16, 2021. https://www.edcatalogue.com/complex-relationship-eating-disorders-substance-use-disorders

31. Killeen T, Brewerton TD, Campbell A, Cohen LR, Hien DA. Exploring the relationship between eating disorder symptoms and substance use severity in women with comorbid PTSD and substance use disorders. *Am J Drug Alcohol Abus.* 2015;41(6):547–552. doi:10.3109/00952990.2015.1080263

32. Jáuregui-Garrido B, Jáuregui-Lobera I. Sudden death in eating disorders. *Vasc Health Risk Manag.* 2012;8(1):91–98. doi:10.2147/VHRM.S28652

33. Mehler PS, Blalock D V., Walden K, et al. Medical findings in 1,026 consecutive adult inpatient-residential eating disordered patients. *Int J Eat Disord.* 2018;51(4):305–313. doi:10.1002/eat.22830

34. Katzman DK. Medical complications in adolescents with anorexia nervosa: A review of the literature. *Int J Eat Disord.* 2005;37(Suppl 1):S52–S59. doi:10.1002/eat.20118

35. Peebles R, Sieke EH. Medical complications of eating disorders in youth. *Child Adolesc Psychiatr Clin N Am.* 2019;28(4):593–615. doi:10.1016/j.chc.2019.05.009

36. Mascolo M, Trent S, Colwell C, Mehler PS. What the emergency department needs to know when caring for your patients with eating disorders. *Int J Eat Disord.* 2012;45(8):977–981. doi:10.1002/eat.22035

37. Mehler P. Diagnosis and care of patients with anorexia nervosa in primary care settings. *Ann Intern Med.* 2001;134:1048–1059

38. Forney KJ, Buchman-Schmitt JM, Keel PK, Frank GKW. The medical complications associated with purging. *Int J Eat Disord.* 2016;49(3):249–259. doi:10.1002/eat.22504

39. Rosen E, Bakshi N, Watters A, Rosen HR, Mehler PS. Hepatic complications of anorexia nervosa. *Dig Dis Sci.* 2017;62(11):2977–2981. doi:10.1007/s10620-017-4766-9

40. Ernest S, Kuntz HM. Emergency department management of eating disorder complications in pediatric patients. *EB Med.* 2020;17(2):1–16.

41. Hill LS, Reid F, Morgan JF, Lacey JH. SCOFF, the development of an eating disorder screening questionnaire. *Int J Eat Disord.* 2010;43(4):344–351. doi:10.1002/eat.20679

42. Morgan JF, Reid F, Lacey JH. The SCOFF questionnaire: Assessment of a new screening tool for eating disorders. *Br Med J.* 1999;319(7223):1467–1468. doi:10.1136/bmj.319.7223.1467

43. Maguen S, Hebenstreit C, Li Y, et al. Screen for disordered eating: Improving the accuracy of eating disorder screening in primary care. *Gen Hosp Psychiatry.* 2018;50:20–25. doi:10.1016/j.genhosppsych.2017.09.004

44. Cotton MA, Ball C, Robinson P. Four simple questions can help screen for eating disorders. *J Gen Intern Med.* 2003;18(1):53–56. doi:10.1046/j.1525-1497.2003.20374.x

45. Sorensen CJ, DeSanto K, Borgelt L, Phillips KT, Monte AA. Cannabinoid hyperemesis syndrome: Diagnosis, pathophysiology, and treatment—A systematic review. *J Med Toxicol.* 2017;13(1):71–87. doi:10.1007/s13181-016-0595-z

46. Arnulf I, Rico TJ, Mignot E. Diagnosis, disease course, and management of patients with Kleine–Levin syndrome. *Lancet Neurol.* 2012;11(10):918–928. doi:10.1016/S1474-4422(12)70187-4

47. Voderholzer U, Haas V, Correll CU, Körner T. Medical management of eating disorders: An update. *Curr Opin Psychiatry.* 2020;33(6):542–553. doi:10.1097/YCO.0000000000000653

48. Harrington BC, Jimerson M, Haxton C, Jimerson DC. Initial evaluation, diagnosis, and treatment of anorexia nervosa and bulimia nervosa. *Am Fam Physician.* 2015;91(1):46–52.

49. Boyle S. How should the law determine capacity to refuse treatment for anorexia? *Int J Law Psychiatry.* 2019;64:250–259. doi:10.1016/j.ijlp.2019.05.001

50. Dyer C. Woman with anorexia is discharged after doctors say that she is untreatable. *BMJ*. 2016;353:i2038. doi:10.1136/bmj.i2038

51. Gans M, Gunn WB. End stage anorexia: Criteria for competence to refuse treatment. *Int J Law Psychiatry*. 2003;26(6):677–695.

52. Appelbaum PS, Rumpf T. Civil commitment of the anorexic patient. *Gen Hosp Psychiatry*. 1998;20(4):225–230. doi:10.1016/S0163-8343(98)00027-9

53. Douzenis A, Michopoulos I. Involuntary admission: The case of anorexia nervosa. *Int J Law Psychiatry*. 2015;39:31–35. doi:10.1016/j.ijlp.2015.01.018

SECTION III

SPECIFIC POPULATIONS FREQUENTLY ENCOUNTERED AS PSYCHIATRIC EMERGENCIES

15

Children and Adolescents

Heidi Burns, Bernard Biermann, and Nasuh Malas

Introduction

One in five youth in the United States have a diagnosed mental health condition at any given time.[1] Due to the dearth of child and adolescent psychiatrists and limited access to child psychiatric services, emergency departments (EDs) have increasingly become the setting for managing mental health crises involving children and adolescents. ED mental health visits increased by 21% between 2006 and 2011, with a corresponding 34% increase in visits for substance use disorders and 71% increase in impulse control disorders.[2] More recent data revealed an increase in pediatric mental health visits from 50.4/100,000 children to 78.5/100,000 between 2012 and 2016.[3] The COVID-19 pandemic has resulted in acute increases in children's mental health concerns while limiting access to community-based mental health resources, resulting in increased ED visits for psychiatric and behavioral concerns.[4]

Pediatric behavioral emergencies are recognized as a public health crisis by the American Academy of Pediatrics and the American College of Emergency Physicians.[5] Reasons for increased rates for mental health-related ED visits among youth include the following:[4]

1. Increased incidence of mental health conditions and symptomatology
2. Increased awareness by families, schools, and primary care providers (PCPs) of the impact of mental health and mental health diagnoses
3. Lack of timely accessible care to meet the needs of youth in local communities
4. Lack of training and education to frontline providers and families as to what is appropriate treatment of pediatric mental health concerns
5. The rise of social media as an added means of distress and potential route of bullying

Emergency departments throughout the United States have become the default setting for managing mental health crises involving youth. This is particularly true in rural areas, urban centers, or large areas of the country in the Midwest, Southwest, and Southeast, where access to child psychiatric care is particularly limited. Unfortunately, many communities have limited access to emergency psychiatrists, let alone psychiatric providers with expertise in child and adolescent psychiatry and emergency psychiatry. Of youth seeking mental health services in the ED, nearly 20% of these youth were medically admitted, twice the rate of youth without a mental health diagnosis.[6] Among youth requiring inpatient psychiatric care, up to 58% may have extended waits in the ED, known as "boarding," that on average can last from 5 to 41 hours in the ED setting, with some cases taking weeks.[7]

Furthermore, ED recidivism rates approach 21% in youth.[8] Because many communities are faced with a lack of child and adolescent mental health providers, the same factors that contribute to an overreliance on emergency rooms for managing psychiatric conditions pose barriers to timely and appropriate disposition options. Outpatient clinics often have long wait times for appointments, and inpatient beds are often unavailable. There is variable accessibility to intermediate services, such as crisis respite services, mobile crisis teams, intensive outpatient programming, or partial hospitalization services, with many areas of the country lacking access to intermediate mental health services altogether. This all contributes to a bottleneck resulting in the gradual rise of the number of youth presenting to the ED for mental health needs, the proportion of youth presenting with psychiatric emergencies compared to the general population of youth seeking emergent care, as well as ED boarding, as youth await more intensive psychiatric care or inpatient psychiatric hospitalization of patients.

Care Settings and Models of Care

Various models of care exist to address psychiatric emergencies in youth, ranging in specificity of expertise and setting. Settings designed specifically with pediatric psychiatric patients in mind are associated with increased support staff to enhance developmentally informed comfort and reduce traumatic stress, provide environmental modifications, and allow for engagement with providers and staff with training and expertise in the care of youth. The goal is to deliver trauma- and developmentally informed care with a focus on reduced use of security, seclusion and restraint, and length of stay.

PCPs are often expected to recognize and respond to mental health emergencies; however, training programs often lack education on addressing these crises and are limited in education on pediatric mental health evaluation and management. Whereas patients present to PCPs with psychiatric emergencies, often such settings only allow referral to the local ED or rely on emergent consultation from specialty providers. These settings may be highly stimulating, have significant ligature risk, offer little space for private information sharing, and provide limited space for seclusion or other intensified intervention for youth with significant agitation or aggression. Some EDs may have access to mental health consultants with variable expertise in child psychiatric care, have designated "safe space" sections for psychiatric patients, or may have "flexible" areas that can be utilized for medical or psychiatric purposes.

Youth may have access to psychiatric emergency services (PES), which are typically staffed 24 hours a day, 7 days a week with a multidisciplinary team, including nursing, social work, and psychiatry. The PES setting is much less common, and many communities may not have a PES available. Although PES have the capacity to provide psychiatric assessment, nonpharmacologic and pharmacologic intervention, as well as utilize restraint/seclusion when necessary, they may have other limitations that make care of youth challenging. Many PES sites do not have private rooms, despite long lengths of stay for some youth; may have adult and youth congregate in the same milieu; and often have limited or no child- and adolescent-specific staff.

An ideal model for managing psychiatric emergencies in youth includes 24-hour access to care, staff with specific training and expertise in the assessment and evaluation of youth, an environment designed to minimize safety hazards and promote comfort in a developmentally informed way, the capacity to safely keep patients until an appropriate disposition can be determined (including crisis beds for extended observations), provision of nonpharmacologic and pharmacologic intervention, as well as the capability of utilizing seclusion or restraint when indicated and only when necessary. This model is embodied in the Comprehensive Psychiatric Emergency Program (CPEP), which provides high-quality, timely, and comprehensive care for youth in psychiatric crisis. However, it is resource-intensive and only provided in a few sites in the world. CPEP also includes crisis outreach, which is a mobile crisis intervention program offering outreach to the community, including homes, residential programs or schools; and "crisis beds."

Other innovative, yet less commonly available, services exist to meet the gap for youth in psychiatric emergency. Psychiatric urgent care allows youth to be seen for non-emergent crisis counseling, conflict resolution, simple medication adjustments, and supportive care not rising to the level of needing a locked unit with 24-hour observation. Urgent care can aid in diffusing crises and interpersonal conflict commonly seen among youth, decrease symptom severity, and increase patient satisfaction, while obviating the need for youth and families to seek care in the busy ED environment. Furthermore, youth may benefit from accessing mobile crisis support in which care is delivered to the home or another setting, such as school or a residential setting for crisis management or in situ stabilization. In this way, mobile crisis teams are often able to divert patients from the ED setting by maintaining safety outside of the hospital and decrease utilization of hospital emergency services.

Telepsychiatry further expands outreach for either initial evaluation or consultative care by using remote audiovisual capability for assessment, diagnosis, and disposition. Recently, given capacity to reach remote areas, these services are gaining increased use in the emergency room setting. The COVID-19 pandemic has spurred the use of technology to extend the reach of the ED to aid local EDs and PCPs in the support of youth with psychiatric emergencies in their locality or to provide direct care to youth who require more acute psychiatric care. Telepsychiatry has been shown to be cost-effective, and data suggest that families are accepting of telepsychiatry with similar outcomes to in-person care.[9] This care can be particularly beneficial for youth who struggle outside the home environment, including youth with medical comorbidities, developmental delay, or autism.[9]

Psychopathology

Neuroanatomy and Neurophysiology of Acute Affective and Behavioral Dysregulation

Acute affective and behavioral dysregulation in the ED is a common initial presentation, with multiple etiologies influencing presentation. Although multifactorial, there are common pathways impacted in youth that result in the phenotypic manifestations of behavioral and affective dysregulation. The prefrontal cortex and the limbic structures, which are underdeveloped in youth, are integral to emotion regulation and processing, stimuli processing, and mediation of cognitive processes through emotional modulation.[10] Behavioral and emotional regulation requires higher order processes, including working memory, inhibitory control, abstract thought, decision-making, executive functioning, and cognitive skills. There is a relative limitation among youth in the ability to regulate emotion, as well as associated cognition, behavior, and impulse control. With adolescence, hormonal changes can have downstream effects on the still developing pathways involved in emotion regulation, resulting in more reactive and dysregulated behaviors in response to the still immature ability to manage emotional impulses.

Important Disease Considerations in the Pediatric Population

Suicide and Self-Injury

- It is the second leading cause of death for youth in the United States[11]
- Suicide rates steadily climbing, with a nearly 100% increase in annual ED visits for suicidal ideation and behavior without a statistically significant increase in overall ED visits.[12]
- Child psychopathology and child-reported family conflict are highly correlated to risk of suicidality.[13]
- Caregivers may often have poor awareness of suicidal ideation or behavior in youth, with poor inter-informant agreement with self-report by youth.[13]
- Interpersonal conflict, particularly with peers or romantic relationships, fractured sense of self or identity, past traumatic experiences, and significant familial distress are all important antecedents to suicidal ideation or behavior in youth.
- Suicidality also correlated with increased screen time use and was reduced with greater parental supervision or positive school involvement.[13]

Depression

- Presents to ED as worsening neurovegetative symptoms, suicidal ideation or behavior, severe interpersonal conflict, academic decline, or behavioral dysregulation.[14]
- Be careful to distinguish adjustment disorders and subclinical depression related to maladaptive coping from progression to clinical depression.
- Average age of onset is between ages 11 and 14 years and often increases as youth progress through early adulthood.[15]
- May have less insight and more irritability compared to adults.
- Other common symptoms include poor frustration tolerance, somatic manifestation of emotional distress, and social withdrawal.
- Monitor externalizing behaviors and interpersonal conflict as clue to presentation of depression.
- Providers should inquire about decline in social and academic function as a proxy for depression severity.

Anxiety

- Most common psychiatric condition of childhood, with a prevalence of up to 13% and presenting at an average age of 11 years.[16]
- Can be transient along a spectrum of adaptation to incident stress or may be entrenched as part of the individual's temperament or emerging personality.
- Can present with school refusal, worsening interpersonal conflict, aggression, behavioral outbursts, or somatic complaints.[16]
- Highly comorbid with mood, attention, or behavioral disturbances.
- May first manifest with entry into school or progression through school where separation from attachment figures, interpersonal stressors, or academic pressures may elicit significant fear and worry.

- Associated with school avoidance or absenteeism and also declining academic performance.
- When untreated, it can influence development of chronic irritability and increase risk of depression. It can also lead to an increase in high-risk behaviors, declining physical and academic functioning, and substance use and suicidal behaviors.[17]
- Youth may present more undifferentiated symptoms for a shorter time and with less insight into those symptoms compared to adults.[17]

Substance Use

- Rising use of cannabis, opioids, and vaping of tobacco.
- Nearly three-fourths who develop substance use disorders in adulthood indicate substance use began before age 17 years; 1 in 10 indicate substance use prior to puberty.[18]
- Can manifest with sudden changes in behavior, increased risk-taking behaviors, or a decline in function at school, home, or socially.
- Adolescence characterized by increased risk-taking, peer pressure, and impulsivity.
  - Individuals endorsing cannabis use in adolescents are at six times higher risk for developing a substance use disorder in adulthood compared to those who started use after age 18 years.[19]
- Earlier onset of substance use is predictive of chronic psychosocial and functional impairments, including increase risk of substance use disorders, conduct disorders (CDs), difficulties with school, legal concerns, interpersonal challenges, and high-risk sexual behaviors.[18]
- Often comorbid with CDs, anxiety, depression, post-traumatic stress disorder (PTSD), and attention-deficit/hyperactivity disorder (ADHD).
- Suicide attempts strongly associated with substance use in youth, even when controlling for the presence of mood disorders.[20]
- Important to screen for substance use disorders and address as part of core pediatric care in the emergency psychiatry setting.[15]

Psychosis

- Often overreported and symptoms more often manifestations of dissociation, severe anxiety, traumatic stress, or youth with autism or intellectual disability who may struggle describing experience or internal states.
- Normal childhood experiences of magical thinking, illusions, and imaginary play can be misinterpreted as psychotic.
- Seventeen percent of youth aged 9–12 years and 8% of adolescents describe psychotic-like experiences, most without psychotic disease.[21]
- Important to rule out underlying medical disease impacting perception and mentation.
- Rarely, may suggest a primary psychotic disorder when there is considerable prodromal decline with preceding negative symptoms and progressive thought disorganization.
  - Abrupt decline in mentation or fluctuating change, particularly at younger ages, is more suggestive of a primary organic cause.

Delirium and Altered Mental Status

- Deficit in awareness and attention with associated cognitive disturbances; abrupt change from baseline function; fluctuating course; and due to physical disease, substance use or withdrawal, or both, not better explained by another developmental or neurocognitive process.[22]

- Prevalence of up to 40% in medically ill youth in the ED setting.[22]
- Risk factors include preexisting developmental delay or physical disease, younger age, ongoing pain, polypharmacy, sleep–wake changes, and environmental overstimulation.
- Common etiologies resulting in pediatric delirium include infection, respiratory illness, seizure, dehydration, drug intoxication or withdrawal, or central nervous system disease.
- Delirium diagnosis may be confounded by the presence of developmental delay, whereas youth with developmental delay are at 3.5 times higher risk of developing delirium.[22]
- Youth present with more nonspecific symptoms, such as intense anxiety, sleep disturbance, irritability, aggression, withdrawal, or disturbances in executive functioning, with less evidence of psychosis or severe cognitive disturbance that may be more apparent in adults with delirium.
- Imperative to obtain a thorough history of premorbid function, review symptom timeline and development from collaterals, and conduct a thoughtful medical assessment.

Mania

- Can be overdiagnosed and conflated with mood lability, emotional reactivity, chronic irritability, risk-taking behaviors, or regressed emotional modulation.
  - Common nonspecific findings seen in anxiety, mood, and trauma-related disorders in youth.
  - Chronic psychosocial distress and high expressed emotion in the home can shape this emotional and behavioral dysregulation.
  - Can be further modeled based on familial responses to distress.
- Transient manifestations of mood lability and affective dysregulation can be seen in maladaptive coping in normally developing youth without psychopathology.
- Discrete evidence of mania or hypomania is much less common in youth.
  - Obtaining collateral information, exploring more specific symptoms for mania (decreased need for sleep or grandiosity), and asking for concrete examples of episodes can aid in diagnostic assessment.
  - More commonly, may present with subthreshold or atypical symptoms, including significant mood lability, impulsivity, irritability, recklessness, outbursts, or aggression.
  - Assessment should search for other explanatory models for symptom development when more classic manifestations of mania are not described.

Trauma and Acute Stress

- Common, pervasive factor in presentation of psychiatric emergency.
- Highly heterogeneous with diverse presentations.
- Always considered as part of the diagnostic formulation.
- Youth with past trauma can react violently due to perceived threat, at times appearing innocuous to others, which can result in severe behavioral dysregulation, agitation, and aggression.
- Behavioral escalation can be rapid with little insight into antecedent stressors.
- Factors suggestive of traumatic stress influencing psychiatric emergency:
  - History of behavioral escalation with re-traumatization

- History of significant trauma (particularly physical and sexual abuse)
- History of chronic irritability or poor interpersonal effectiveness
- Poorly controlled symptoms of post-traumatic stress or traumatic grief
- Chronic avoidance
- Worsening hypervigilance

Aggression

- Often multifactorial with a wide breadth of potential etiologies.
- Important to first rule out any potential underlying medical conditions and sources of pain (constipation, otitis media, headache, fracture, or dental disease).
  - Autoimmune, endocrine, and neurologic conditions may initially manifest with behavioral changes in the setting of personality or cognitive disturbance.
  - Often, youth with nonverbal autism or intellectual disability may manifest agitation in the setting of constipation, pain, seizures, infection, self-inflicted injuries, or other medical problems.
- Other common psychiatric conditions in youth that may influence aggression include sensory overstimulation or chronic distress in youth with
  - Autism or intellectual disability
  - Trauma or attachment difficulties experiencing acute distress
  - An acute manic or psychotic episode
  - Substance intoxication or withdrawal
  - Severe anxiety with associated behavioral dysregulation

Autism and Developmental Delay

- Increasing prevalence with increasing utilization of emergency services.
- Presenting concerns include aggression, stereotypic behavior, repetitive or ritualistic behavior, obsessional or inflexible thinking, or self-injury.
- Evaluation complicated by communication limitations, restricted and repetitive interests and behaviors, and social deficits.
  - Compounded by a stimulating ED environment and frequent transitions and change in ED characteristics.
  - Functional and cognitive limitations can further complicate evaluation and management.

Attachment Disorders

- Reactive attachment disorder (RAD) presents with children who appear distant, rarely seek comfort, and have difficulty regulating emotions.
- Disinhibited social engagement disorder (DSED) presents with an overly familiar child who often approaches strangers, has loose boundaries, and can present as disinhibited or behaviorally dysregulated.
- Severe neglect, deprivation, or institutionalization are risk factors for the development of RAD and DSED.
- Although less common, RAD and DSED are underrecognized.
- Present due to significant emotional dysregulation, regressed tantrum behaviors, self-injury, or demonstration of provocative or disinhibited behavior.
  - Differential includes autism spectrum disorder, developmental delay, ADHD, and depression; common comorbidities may include ADHD, PTSD, and quasi-autism.

Disruptive Behavior Disorders

- Oppositional defiant disorder (ODD) presents in 12.6% of youth, with CD presenting in 6.8%.[15]
- ODD presents with irritability, frequent argumentation, and vindictiveness toward authority figures for at least 6 months.
- CD must be present for 12 months and characterized by antisocial behavior, including violence toward people or animals, destruction of property, theft, and deceitfulness.
- ODD starts in school-age children and is observed more in males than females.
- Risk is increased with low socioeconomic status; inconsistent, permissive, or overly punitive parenting; and exposure to violence.
- Common comorbidities include CD, mood disorders, substance use, aggressive behavior, and ADHD.
- Family- and community-based therapeutic approaches are recommended for management.

Eating Disorders

- The National Comorbidity Survey Replication–Adolescent Supplement found that 2.7% of adolescents reported having an eating disorder, with a much higher prevalence in females.[15]
- Influenced by identity formation; increased valuation of peer perception resulting in significant social pressures; body image concerns; as well as significant individual, familial, and societal pressures related to physical appearance.
- Inherent to eating disorders is a lack of patient insight into disease development with limitations in verbalizing symptomatology.
- Familial report and involvement are crucial to the diagnosis and management.
- Often develop in the context of wanting to "eat healthier" or a change in dietary habits with a gradual loss of control and escalating restrictive eating.
  - Other behaviors seen include excessive exercise, binging, purging, fixation on a goal weight, black-and-white valuation of food as "good" or "bad," excessive activity related to food, or avoidance of eating in front of others.
  - Youth are less likely to have binging and purging behaviors, and when they occur, they are typically later in the disease course.[23]
- High level of comorbid psychopathology, including depression, anxiety, OCD, and borderline personality disorder.
- May present acutely for bradycardia, hypotension, severe weight loss, electrolyte abnormalities, dehydration, or other physical sequelae of chronic malnutrition.
  - Close multidisciplinary evaluation and management, development of a structured refeeding and monitoring protocol, family engagement, clear expectations for activity and feeding, as well as close supervision of refeeding process are all necessary ingredients for management.
- Less commonly, may present with restrictive eating and weight loss related to aversive experiences associated with eating rather than distorted body image, known as avoidant restrictive food intake disorder.
  - Less distress about body image or the nutritional content of food.
  - More distress about physical or other sensory experiences related to eating.
  - Management involves more behavioral interventions to decouple the conditioned negative physical experience of eating with food and nutrition.

Somatic Symptom and Related Disorders
- Characterized by subjective report of physical symptoms incongruous with the medical evaluation and influenced by psychological distress.
- Prevalence in pediatric primary care settings can be as high as 50% of visits and is responsible for 15–20% of U.S. health care costs each year.[24]
- Frequently visit the ED and often have high rates of recidivism.
- Often present as gastrointestinal, neurological, and pain-related complaints.
- Evaluation built on concurrent mental health and physical health evaluation, unified and consistent evidence-based language use, and communication with the family regarding the multifactorial nature of the presentation of somatic symptom and related disorders.
- Management is an iterative process that is founded on setting clear goals and expectations, education, and brief cognitive–behavioral therapy.
  - Focus on improving functioning in small, achievable steps, while shifting the focus away from impairment.
  - The goal is to deliver diagnosis and conceptualization in a multidisciplinary fashion after a thoughtful biopsychosocial assessment and translate the template of a treatment plan to the outpatient setting, or maintain it in the inpatient setting if inpatient care is warranted.[24]

Development

Youth who develop psychiatric illness can be affected in drastically different ways based on the impacts on functioning, self-perception, interpersonal and familial interactions, understanding of illness, and each child's notion of the impact of psychiatric illness on their future. In the setting of a psychiatric emergency, typically less impairing coping strategies and personality traits can become heightened and pervasive. Delivery of information related to diagnosis, management, or disposition, at times, may result in a mix of emotions, including disbelief, anger, sadness, distress, and detachment, depending on the perception of the child or the child's recognition of familial reaction. Understanding these developmental factors aids in differentiating pathology from normal development, as well as provides a deeper understanding of the patient experience from a developmentally informed perspective.

Preschool youth are quickly expanding their cognitive, emotional, and social understanding of the world while building more physical independence. They are heavily reliant on their caregivers for comfort, support of activities of daily living, and modeling. However, they are also growing their interactions with and reactions to the world around them. Having secure attachments, routine, and a supportive environment without high expressed emotion is important for the child to develop a sense of stability and security. Language abilities rapidly grow at this age, where children have more capacity for imaginative play and symbolism. This can often be a time in which the social–emotional aspects of autism spectrum disorder become evident to families and community providers. During this time, youth are able to exhibit theory of mind and understand both internal states and how others may be perceiving or experiencing them. Youth are also starting to problem-solve more and understand societal expectations and morality. This is also a time when youth begin to attend day care and preschool, where their social interactions start expanding outside the household and they must learn to take turns, follow instructions, maintain a routine, and regulate their behaviors. Common challenges at this age include aggression and behavioral regulation, attachment, separation anxiety, attentional difficulties, impulsivity, social reciprocity, interpersonal interaction, and emotional expression.

School-aged youth have some insight into the antecedents of their behavior, are more aware of their internalizing symptoms, and have an improved sense of behavioral norms. Challenges meeting behavioral norms or conforming to expectations from family and school can result in increased demoralization and distress from the child. Furthermore, peer relationships take on a more important role for youth at this age. Therefore, struggles interpersonally with other youth may be more evident or result in more psychological distress, predisposing the child to risk of psychiatric illness. Specifically, bullying becomes an increasing consideration to be mindful of in this age group and can significantly impact self-esteem and self-perception. Chronic anxieties can progress to depression. Furthermore, greater academic demands are placed on youth, which may compound risk related to interpersonal interactions. School-age children can often be reasoned with, provided concrete explanation of care, and offered a modicum of control in their environment to stem further worries. Youth at this age can take a more active role in their care and provide input on care decisions.

By adolescence, the individual can have a more abstract and nuanced understanding of their condition, the interactions between different organ systems, and the relationship between their physical and emotional health. Adolescence is also a time that the individual is forming their identity, their relationships to their peers and the world, and assuming more autonomy of their care. Functionality, appearance, academics, peer relationships, and sexuality take on an even more important place in the mind of an adolescent. The adolescent may be more cognizant of how psychiatric illness can impact interactions with peers, perception by others, and their future. There can be considerable variability in the ability to adaptively cope with distress at this age. Maladaptive personality traits and a more entrenched unhelpful coping style can appear more prominently at this age. Adolescents are often active participants in their care, or if avoidant, they should be encouraged to be engaged in care and provide assent when feasible.

Family Considerations

Psychiatric illness can have dramatic effects on familial interactions. An understanding of the family's history with psychiatric illness, structural composition, interactional style, and resiliency is critical early in evaluation and management. Disruptions in familial functioning can result in poor limit setting, limited empathy, child resentment of the family, disorganized interactions, and fracturing of relationships within the family. The emotional health of the caregiver can have significant impacts on the child and places the child at considerable risk of psychopathology.

Primary caregivers can be particularly vulnerable to the distress of observing their child impaired, distressed, or in discomfort. A sense of helplessness, lack of control, and worry can engender a variety of responses from the primary caregiver. These responses can include avoidance and detachment or overinvolvement with a desire to control aspects of care that they may have little or no control over. These strong emotions, along with the physical toll of supporting a child with psychiatric illness and the difficulty of juggling multiple competing roles and tasks, can result in significant caregiver burden.

In addition, parental separation, divorce, and poor adjustment to their child's psychiatric illness can result in considerable distress and maladjustment for the child.

Sibling interactions and response to psychiatric illness in their brother or sister are an often-missed aspect of care, with little attention dedicated to sibling health and its impacts on the child. Siblings may take on an overly parental role and engage in communications or responsibilities that result in a fractured sense of structure and hierarchy in the family. The sibling may then be taxed with responsibilities that can result in traumatic experience, distress, chronic worries, irritability, or burnout.

Systems of Care

Outside of the immediate family system, there are unique systems of care that youth interface with that require consideration when youth present to the ED. These systems may offer collateral information on the individual's symptom evolution, may be a source of support or additional resource, may be an ongoing stressor for the patient or family, or may be intimately involved in the delivery of treatment or supervision of the patient's care needs longitudinally.

School

Often, youth may spend most of their waking day at school, and therefore it serves as an important source of information and perspective into the child's presentation. Schools are also one of the most common referral sources to the ED, either due to screening for suicide or other psychopathology or due to observations of concern relating to the child's conduct, interpersonal interactions, or emotional well-being. Understanding the child's academic performance, ability to attend to tasks and instruction, interactions with authority figures such as teachers, and interactions with peers provides valuable information to assist in the diagnostic assessment. School serves as a source of social connectedness and an opportunity for youth to shape their identities and self-worth, whether in a way that is nurturing or a means that feels invalidating to the child. School also provides academic, developmental, and, occasionally, mental health services that can provide tremendous support for youth and intervene early to mitigate progression of psychopathology. In this way, schools can provide valuable resources in a feasible and natural way to youth and families to address emotional, cognitive, and developmental needs in an environment that is more familiar and often closer to the family's residence.

Developmental Services

Youth with learning disabilities, autism spectrum disorder, physical disabilities, or intellectual disability may have access to developmental resources in the community or school. These services can range from physical therapy, occupational therapy, and speech therapy to applied behavioral analysis or other intensive behavioral services. Awareness of these services and communication with developmental support staff can be crucial in identifying patient baseline functionality and progress with treatment, as well as deviation from the patient's normative functioning. Antecedents to behavioral health emergency, triggers for distress, strategies to ameliorate behavioral escalation, and important insights into the child's development and behavior can often be gleaned by interfacing with these developmental services. Furthermore, identifying developmental needs and establishing engagement with appropriate developmental services can be tremendously helpful in reducing visits to the ED and use of unnecessary psychopharmacology and also may have more lasting benefit in the patient's treatment.

Pediatric Medical Care

As mentioned previously, primary care pediatrics is often at the front lines of the evaluation and management of childhood psychopathology. Developing a strong relationship with primary care practices may aid in early identification of youth mental illness but also may aid in empowering pediatricians to manage youth in their practices while reducing visits to the ED. Engagement in mental health care in the primary care setting results in more regular adherence to treatment, engagement in visits, and more willingness to accept mental health care among youth and families.

Child Protective Services

As mandated reporters of suspected abuse or neglect, the ED unfortunately may be a setting in which the maltreatment of youth is detected and reported to Child Protective Services (CPS). CPS can be helpful in investigating matters of abuse, neglect, or significant familial negative influence on the perpetuation of child psychopathology. Because CPS workers are often not clinicians, it is important to provide clear, succinct, and detailed accounts of the concerns and why the concerns raised could jeopardize the well-being and safety of the child. Occasionally, this may be more nuanced, and it is critical to relay the gravity of the concerns, the impact on the child, and be objective in doing so. General concern or suspicion of maltreatment can be relayed to CPS because it is not the obligation of the ED provider to substantiate or prove the concerns. Rather, it is the obligation of the ED to report concerns that may put the child at considerable harm due to abuse or neglect, and CPS is then to investigate those concerns to determine if they carry substance. Other common reasons for contacting CPS in the ED setting include the following:

- Child abandonment
- Repeated inability to ensure patient safety and lethal means restriction in the home, despite repeated education and counseling, for youth with a high risk of suicide
- In some states, when the primary caregiver is refusing more intensive or a higher level of psychiatric care when an alternative level of care is clearly unsafe and jeopardizes the well-being of the child

Foster Care or Other Congregate Living

Nearly one in two youth in the foster care system exhibit a psychiatric or behavioral concern.[25] These youth are less likely to receive intensive psychological or behavioral services and more likely to be overmedicated with psychopharmacology. Common psychiatric conditions seen in this population include attachment disorders, PTSD, depression, anxiety, learning difficulties, and ADHD. However, it is fairly common that these youths may accumulate diagnostic labels to suggest more severe psychopathology, such as bipolar disorder or schizophrenia, due to misdiagnosis related to more maladaptive forms of distress management, including dissociation, mood lability, aggression, and regressed behavior. It is very important to be aware of the potential pitfalls and epidemiology associated with this population, as well as the chronic traumatic stress experienced, to accurately diagnose and treat youth who may present from foster care or group homes, as well as to advocate for their best longitudinal care.

Law Enforcement/Legal System

Youth may also present from juvenile detention or be escorted by law enforcement for psychiatric evaluation in the ED setting. The context of their presentation and the implications on future legal proceedings may have a significant influence on the individual's presentation and evolution of symptoms over time. It is important to screen for development and cognitive deficits, past adverse life events or trauma, and comorbid substance use in this population to obtain a broader understanding of the individual's experience so as to help formulate the case conceptualization. Furthermore, evaluation and treatment may be impacted by guardianship status, court order, or future implications related to the potential legal action being taken. In these circumstances, it is important to have close communication with your health system's legal team, social work, as well as local and state agencies involved in the legal matters influencing the child's presentation to the ED.

Assessment

General Principles

The evaluation and management of psychiatric emergencies begin at triage. With rare exceptions, children present with an adult, which may be a parent or guardian, law enforcement, emergency medical service personnel, school staff, or social worker. The evaluation begins by observing the interaction between caregivers and the patient, including level of cooperation, interaction, attachment, and fear of both parties. In some instances, separating the parent and child becomes necessary, either to diffuse a crisis or to help establish rapport with a potentially uncooperative youth. The evaluation is iterative and reflective with incorporation of new observations, interactions, and collateral information as the course of the ED stay progresses and as symptoms evolve.

Unique Aspects of History Gathering and Examination

Gathering a comprehensive history usually involves interviewing children and their caregivers, together and separately (Box 15.1). This should be coupled with a focused physical examination and mental status examination (Box 15.2). The age and developmental status of the child can determine whether the patient should be interviewed separately from a parent and in which order or whether interviews should be conducted with both parties together. With younger children, it often makes sense to begin interviews with the child and parent present. This helps the child feel comfortable and allows for more extensive initial symptom history to be gathered. This is also a good opportunity to witness parent–child interactions and get a glimpse of parenting style. Adolescents may be given the choice of meeting with the clinician first if possible, which may help establish rapport and trust while validating adolescent autonomy. If more than one clinician is involved in the adolescent's care, it may be meaningful to separate the parent and the adolescent and conduct concurrent interviews to gather independent reports that can then be reviewed in totality later. In addition, a brief period of separation may be necessary if families present in conflict.

Whenever possible, obtaining collateral information can help clarify or validate the history. Valuable information and perspective may be gleaned from school personnel, a psychiatrist or therapist, a case manager, a probation officer, the PCP, and/or the other parent or another family member. Birth history, developmental history, family history, and early childhood history can be highly informative and may not be ascertained directly from the child. Effective questioning of a child typically involves understanding of the child's development and cognitive status. Young children might have a different concept of time, so using life events, such as birthdays, holidays, or grade in school, as anchors might be helpful. Also, some matters, such as sexual behaviors, substance use, and even suicidality, are clearly more pertinent to adolescents or preteens than to younger elementary-age children and, as such, need to be explored in a developmentally appropriate manner. Youth and caregiver report may also be discordant, and it is important to be aware that youth tend to be more accurate in reporting internalizing symptoms, whereas caregivers often provide more valid report of externalizing symptoms and behaviors.[26]

Patients with developmental disability or cognitive impairment may not be able to participate in an interview, and history must be gathered primarily from caregivers. Caregiver bias may influence interpretation of symptoms, perception of child functionality, and factors driving presentation; therefore, the clinician must be as objective as possible and parse through caregiver subjectivity. Symptoms often include aggressive or other dangerous behaviors; self-injury; property destruction; and functional decline, including decreased intake of food. Other considerations include catatonic states—either classic catatonia, with negativism, mutism, or unusual posturing, or agitated catatonia, with purposeless movements or unprovoked outbursts. History should include information about behaviors, antecedents, calming strategies including effective PRN medication, or other nonpharmacologic coping strategies.

Lethality assessment in youth should account for the seriousness of the attempt; past history of suicidal ideation and behavior; family history of suicide; the extent of psychiatric and psychological comorbidity exhibited by the patient; past exposures to adverse childhood experiences or traumatic experiences; comorbid chronic physical illness; and factors that may impact sense of identity, hopefulness, connectedness, and self-worth. It is common for youth to exhibit more impulsivity and reduced insight into suicidal ideation or behavior, yet this does not obviate the need to conduct a thorough and thoughtful risk assessment and identify level of risk and how to best ensure patient safety given the unique factors influencing pediatric suicide.

Box 15.1 Child and Adolescent Psychiatric History Gathering in the Emergency Setting

- **Identifying information**: age, gender identity and pronouns, family status (household members, grade in school, living with biological family, adoptive parents, or in foster care)
- **Chief complaint**: reason for coming to the ED (elicit patient and caregiver rationale)
  - Is there an emergency? Why now?
  - Who has concerns: Patient? Parents? School?
- **History of presenting illness**: symptoms with time frame and course, recent changes, associated stressors, treatment adherence
  - How is this impacting the patient and family?
  - Include psychiatric review of systems with a focus on mood and anxiety disorders, learning difficulties, developmental disorders, trauma, eating and feeding disorders, behavioral disturbance and suicidal ideation or behavior.
- **Psychiatric history**: previous diagnoses, hospitalizations, others levels of care, history of ambulatory psychiatric care and psychotherapy (including types of therapies and medications)
  - Medications: doses, time frames, beneficial effects and side effects
- **Medical history**: any acute or chronic medical issues, medications, history of hospitalizations, surgeries, head injuries, seizures, allergies, immunization status
- **Family history**: relevant psychiatric or medical issues (including suicide, developmental disorders, and substance use) and associated treatment in first-degree biologic relatives
- **Developmental history**: pregnancy and delivery history including any intrauterine exposures, review of prenatal care
  - Review developmental milestones (gross and fine motor, language, social) and if on time
- **Social history**: review living arrangements (who is there, biological or adoptive vs. foster parents), parental status and custody arrangements, relationships with family members, family stressors (financial, legal), friendships, extracurricular or other activities
  - History of significant poverty or deprivation? Food insecurity?
  - Safety issues: gun in home, how are medications stored?
  - Social media and internet use
  - Sexual activity and contraceptive use with safety questions: Similar age? Consensual?
- **Substance use history**: tobacco, nicotine, vaping, cannabis, alcohol, prescription drugs (opiates and amphetamines/stimulants), other street drugs (cocaine, opiates, hallucinogens, synthetics), and over-the-counter medications
  - Characterize age of first use, frequency and duration, and attempts to reduce or quit use
- **Trauma history**: any history of experiencing or witnessing abuse—physical, emotional, sexual
  - Ask about bullying (either victim or perpetrator)
  - Ask about intimate partner violence
  - Identify evidence of neglect
- **Educational history**: grade in school, performance, history of any special education services (504 plan or IEP), behavioral issues at school (suspensions or detentions), attendance history, past neuropsychological testing
- **Legal history**: any history of legal problems or criminal activities, any CPS involvement

---

Box 15.2 Considerations in the Emergency Department Pediatric Mental Status Examination

---

- **Physical appearance**: Observe hygiene, posture, age-appropriate clothing, distinguishing hair styles, piercings or tattoos.
  - Look for areas of superficial injury on the forearms and other exposed areas.
  - Observe for dysmorphic facial features, neurocutaneous findings.
  - Monitor level of apparent physical comfort, including evidence of physical distress, tachypnea, diaphoresis, or pupillary changes.
- **Interaction with examiner and other adults**: Level of cooperation and social reciprocity, eye contact, use of hand gestures.
  - Observe interactions when parents are present and how this may change when alone with the examiner.
- **Mood and affect**
  - Watch for irritability, which may be a sign of depression in children.
  - Ask about separation anxiety (common in younger children) and social anxiety (common in preteens and teens).
  - Incongruent affect and mood lability may be signs of past attachment difficulties, social–developmental difficulties, or a history of trauma.
- **Psychomotor behavior**: Observe for tics or other movements, level of coordination, gross motor or fine motor abnormalities.
  - Monitor for evidence of hyperactivity and ability to sustain engagement in an activity as a marker for possible ADHD or a marker of high psychosocial distress and related behavioral dysregulation.
- **Orientation**: Target to developmental age and cognitive status.
  - What type of place is this? Is it morning, afternoon, or night?
  - Sometimes may provide choices for younger youth.
- **Form and content of thinking**: Broader differential for hallucinations, "Do the voices seem like they are inside your head, or from outside of you?"
  - Magical thinking or imaginary friends may be developmentally appropriate.
- **Cognitive**: Developmentally appropriate vocabulary and fund of knowledge?
- **Attention and concentration**: Observe for hyperactivity, impulsivity, and obvious distractibility, which may be signs of ADHD.
- **Judgment and insight**: Do they appreciate the seriousness of their symptoms? Are they aware of how preceding factors led to future events or current presentation? Can they understand relationships between events or interacting aspects of the patient's experience? Can they make reasonable decisions based on facts and guidance?
  - Keep in mind that adolescents may have unrealistic standards for risk-taking behaviors, which may be age appropriate if not impairing and/or persistent.

Laboratory and Diagnostic Examination

An important part of psychiatric ED evaluation is considering a broad differential for symptom presentation and thoughtful evaluation of potential physical health factors influencing the child's symptoms. However, there are no specific standards to guide this medical evaluation in the pediatric population receiving psychiatric evaluation in the ED. Laboratory assessment may be driven by exam findings, clinical history, hospital policy, or as part of "medical clearance" prior to transfer. Many EDs still obtain basic laboratory studies in the assessment of pediatric patients, which is partly driven by many inpatient psychiatric units requiring medical clearance prior to acceptance for admission.

Diagnostic testing that may be particularly useful in youth is obtaining a complete blood count to assess for anemia, which can factor in presentations of fatigue (particularly adolescent females with heavy menses) or in youth who may have lead toxicity or anemia of chronic illness. Youth with eating disorders, dehydration, or poor nutrition may have electrolyte abnormalities that are important to assess and monitor. Certain medications can also impact renal and hepatic function and may warrant laboratory assessment. Worsening anxiety or mood can sometimes be the initial harbinger for the presentation of endocrine disorders; therefore, glucose monitoring, urinalysis, and thyroid studies can be helpful in this regard. Acute infectious processes are also common irritants in youth, particularly youth with neurodevelopmental disorders, or may be a cause of delirium. Obtaining a urinalysis and complete blood count can be helpful in this regard as well, particularly in female youth. Pregnancy screens should be routinely obtained for females. If overdose is suspected, salicylate, acetaminophen, or ethanol levels may be obtained, or gas chromatography–mass spectrometry may be performed. Head imaging may be indicated in the setting of head trauma with loss of consciousness or other concerning features, first-episode psychosis, or acute mental status changes. Further diagnostic studies are often guided by specific exam findings or collaboration with pediatric providers and subspecialists.

Formulation and Differential Diagnosis

It is important to have a clear framework to develop a conceptualization of the child's presentation and incorporate the evident and potential etiologies influencing patient presentation. Establishing a comprehensive formulation requires asking the question, "Why now?" and understanding the "how" of the patient's current manifestations of acute decompensation. This also incorporates static factors that predispose youth to risk of psychiatric emergency, precipitating factors that escalate that risk, perpetuating factors that maintain risk, as well as potential protective factors that may be fostered to mitigate risk and aid in de-escalation.[27,28] The formulation must be reviewed dynamically across the patient's clinical course and be flexible to the changes in the patient's presentation and response to interventions. Several confounding factors can influence the diagnostic formulation in youth and should be considered when the treatment response does not align with the formulation or when diagnostic clarity appears elusive. Common confounding factors include psychological trauma, attachment disorders, anxiety, neurodevelopmental disorder, substance use, and medical illness.

Nonpharmacologic Management

Strategies for prevention, identification, and management of etiologic factors, acute treatment and surveillance, and risk attenuation for pediatric behavioral emergencies are closely intertwined and overlapping processes. The presentation is often evolving; sometimes rapidly, and thus the evaluation and management interventions must change iteratively and remain flexible throughout the care process. Management of any pediatric behavioral emergency is founded on early nonpharmacologic and environmental modification, adjusted based on ongoing assessment of antecedents to the patient's presentation and response to these interventions. Early and frequent use of these interventions can mitigate the use of psychopharmacology and can significantly improve care outcomes for the patient and family[27] (Box 15.3).

Prevention

Prevention in the emergency room setting starts with identifying the unique risks a pediatric patient may have and incorporating those risks into the evaluation and management plan to reduce risk of escalating psychopathology while reinforcing strengths, resiliency, and previously identified calming strategies. This includes three principle components:

- Standardized care practices to ensure evidence-based approaches are routinely and consistently applied to care
- Advanced screening for patient risk through formal screening practices or through information gathered from caregivers about the child
- Universal precautions and environmental practices provided for all youth to provide care that is developmentally informed and ensures a care environment oriented to the pediatric patient

Common prevention practices address several factors related to the pediatric care experience, including the following:

- Regular psychoeducation and communication, both with caregivers and the child
- Close engagement with supportive caregivers and other family members
- Awareness of developmental needs, including sensory needs, physical mobility, toileting, nutritional needs, and communication style
- Monitoring and addressing sleep deprivation, hunger, and pain
- Addressing environmental factors that may hinder or support patient comfort

Psychoeducation and Communication

Education directed toward the child should be developmentally informed and collaborative to ensure consistent delivery of information to the child. Discussion should be provided at a time and in a setting in which the child feels safe and can listen to the information to aid in comprehension. Using pictures, models, play, and toys can help the child understand their emotional and physical needs and how they may interact.

Language is key in providing education because children may be receptive to certain analogies, phrasing, word use, or images. For example, explaining different emotions using superheroes may resonate for one child, whereas using emotional "temperature" as a framework for communication of emotion may work better for another child. Using language that is concrete, simple, succinct, familiar, and nonthreatening can be the

Box 15.3 Nonpharmacologic Interventions for Youth in Psychiatric Emergency

- Environment
  - Reducing noise pollution
  - Providing comfort measures such as blankets or pillows
  - Providing a consistent care team
  - Clustering care to promote privacy and sleep
  - Removing excessively bright or fluorescent lights
  - Offering white noise or soothing music
  - Adequate temperature control
  - Providing food and drink
  - Posting schedules and information in the room
  - Allowing for familiar objects, toys, and comfort items to be present with the patient
- Individual
  - Utilization of distraction techniques and incorporating useful soothing strategies
  - Provision of education
  - Providing anticipatory guidance and preparation for change
  - Offering models, pictures, and dolls to explain care
  - Understanding triggers for distress
  - Supporting communication and functioning, including understanding developmental needs
  - Utilization of physical therapy, occupational therapy, or speech therapy when necessary
  - Providing technology such as a tablet, television
- Familial
  - Engagement of supportive family and caregivers
  - Separation of unsupportive family
  - Modeling ways that the family successfully aids in de-escalation of the child
  - Understanding familial experience, culture, and values
  - Including family in providing reassurance, explaining care, and in the de-escalation process
- System
  - Standardization of protocols for common psychiatric emergencies in youth
  - Implementing screening
  - Training and education
  - Use of developmentally and trauma-informed care and language practices
  - Inclusion of key caregivers and family members in care
  - Incorporating age-appropriate themes in the child's care experience
  - Involvement of social work in child's life early and routinely in care

difference between education that is well received and that which may generate further anxieties and exacerbate underlying depression.

Educational interventions geared toward caregivers and family should focus first on decreasing their own distress and enhancing their understanding of what is happening to their child. It should be geared to the education, literacy level, language, and baseline understanding of the caregiver. Equally important is empowering family with the necessary information and tools to be integral to treatment of their child. It can be helpful to ask, in advance, the caregiver's understanding of the child's psychiatric illness and current needs. This includes reviewing the impact of disease on the child's physical, social, and emotional functioning, as well as gauging any concerns that the caregiver may have. Checking for understanding after sharing communications can ensure that the family and the providers have a shared understanding of the factors influencing the child's presentation and management.

Awareness of Developmental Needs

Early recognition of unique patient developmental needs is key in the successful prevention and management of pediatric behavioral emergencies. Although this should be a routine part of nursing and physician assessment of the pediatric patient, key components of the assessment can often be missed, resulting in lost opportunities to understand the patient and intervene proactively. Therefore, embedding a standardized assessment of patient developmental needs and functioning, including their ability to communicate and receive information, can be highly informative to the patient's care.

Youth, in particular, may have a variety of visual, auditory, olfactory, tactile, and oral sensory needs that can be valuable to the care in the ED setting. Although youth with ASD or DD may routinely need assessment for sensory needs, all youth should be at least asked about sensory sensitivities because these needs occur along a spectrum and may antagonize or perpetuate distress in a child with limited awareness or insight. This assessment should focus both on sensory deprivation and on stimulation needs. Youth may have needs related to their activities of daily functioning, including physical mobility, toileting, and nutritional needs. As children age, they increasingly value their autonomy and independence; therefore, understanding these limitations early, how they impact function, and what supports are needed and/or preferred by the patient and family, in addition to addressing these needs in a proactive and normalizing way, can significantly impact the pediatric patient experience in the ED setting. Use of adaptive devices, access to appropriate toileting and hygiene post-toileting, and use of gastrostomy, nasogastric, or nasojejunal tubes are all considerations in the care of youth that can influence presentation, reduce symptoms, and enhance the care experience for patients and families.

Communication needs, as described previously, afford emergency room staff and providers a window into how the child perceives their environment and relates their experiences to others. Determining expressive and receptive language skills and how communication is conveyed provides greater insight into the patient experience. This may involve understanding whether the patient uses a communication board, tablet, sign language, or certain vocalizations and/or gestures to relay information. Each patient and family may have unique communication styles that are used within that family structure to aid with effective communication and garner confidence from the patient and family that the care team will attempt to understand and interact with the patient in the most meaningful way possible.

Environment

The environment is a powerful medium to aid in ameliorating symptoms, and robust environmental adjustments can result in significant symptomatic improvement. Modifications include room temperature control, reduction of bright or fluorescent lighting, reduced noise contamination, allowance of physical space for mobility, and reduction of use of physical restraints. Facilitating the creation of a familiar environment by having recognizable objects and family members as well as stability in caretakers and daily routines has been shown to be beneficial. Any items that may be distressing to the patient or potentially used as a weapon should be removed to reduce the risk of escalation of patient behavior or distress. In addition, items that may be soothing to the patient, such as a tablet, a television, or a favorite toy or item, should be provided to reinforce the patient's ability to self-soothe and stay occupied in more adaptive activities.

Psychotherapy

In addition to effective communication, environmental adjustments, risk mitigation, and psychoeducation, brief behavioral and psychotherapeutic intervention can be a powerful management strategy for youth and families. Specific modalities utilized more commonly for the pediatric population include cognitive–behavioral therapy, dialectical behavioral therapy, brief exposure and response prevention, biofeedback, functional behavioral analysis, applied behavioral therapy, and family therapy. Considerations in utilizing these therapies in youth in psychiatric emergency include the following:

- Variable attention span requiring regular reinforcement, use of models and pictorials, and use of play to maintain engagement.
- Limited insight with increased focus on behavioral intervention, conditioning, and reinforcing adaptive coping strategies.
- Therapy must be catered to the developmental stage of the patient.
- Being mindful of language use with avoidance of jargon and utilizing language that is familiar to the patient.
- Familial or dyadic therapies can be invaluable, particularly when interpersonal or familial conflict is influencing patient presentation.

In addition, children can easily become overwhelmed by the environment, frequent transitions, and change, as well as misunderstand or overly internalize events in the emergency room. Using a "here and now" focus with therapy and focusing on discrete, concrete tasks or coping strategies can be more easily incorporated for children than more complex or future-oriented approaches.

Pharmacologic Management

The guiding principle for management of pediatric behavioral emergencies is the use of effective prevention strategies, de-escalation techniques, and the least restrictive interventions possible. Aligned with recently published national consensus guidelines on the management of psychiatric emergencies in youth, the primary goal for pharmacologic management should be treating the underlying cause or causes of symptom presentation while calming the child to allow for ongoing evaluation and treatment.[28] According to recent literature, benzodiazepines, antihistamines, and antipsychotics are the most common agents used for agitation in the emergency setting for pediatric patients.[29] Due to the varying etiologies of agitation in the emergency situation, there is no "one-size-fits-all" medication recommendation for all patients. Given these limitations, it is important to keep the considerations discussed next in mind.

Among youth, the therapeutic window for psychopharmacology is narrower, response may be more variable, side effect risk is higher, and metabolism may require more frequent yet smaller doses. Collaboration with pharmacy and utilization of pharmacologic guides can aid with weight-based dosing in youth, which is much more common than seen in adults. The patient's age, route of medication delivery, weight, and medication naivety should all be considered when dosing medications in youth. Given that many medication trials have not been performed on the pediatric population, providers should keep in mind that factors such as liver size, body fat percentage, gastrointestinal absorption, and glomerular filtration rate could all differ in the pediatric patient and result in differing pharmacokinetic effect.[29] When possible, oral administration should be offered prior to intramuscular injection, primarily to minimize risk to the patient. It can be helpful from a patient alignment standpoint to offer a choice between oral or injection. If intravenous administration is possible, this is considered superior to intramuscular administration given that it is often less distressing to the pediatric population than an injection, unless intravenous access is already available.[29]

Awareness of Side Effect Profiles in Youth

Youth commonly have more heterogeneous responses to psychopharmacology and may commonly experience neuroexcitation and paradoxical responses due to narrow therapeutic thresholds and significant central nervous system sensitivity to psychotropic medications. Common agents that may elicit these paradoxical responses include antihistamines (i.e., diphenhydramine), benzodiazepines, anticholinergics (including some antiemetics), antibiotics, and stimulants. These paradoxical responses can result in mood dysregulation, disinhibition, rage, confusion, and severe sleep disturbance. Youth with intellectual disability, developmental disorders, or underlying neurologic disorders may have higher risk of these negative responses to psychopharmacology. Reviewing past medication trials with parents to confirm any abnormal responses or allergic reactions and using low doses with close observation for response are important steps to avoid these potential paradoxical reactions.[28]

The use of antipsychotic medication in pediatric patients who may be naive to these agents may result in extrapyramidal syndromes in the emergency setting. Acute dystonic reactions may present as torticollis, fixed gaze, muscle stiffening, involuntary spasms, or paralysis. Examples include oculogyric crisis, which specifically affects the extraocular muscles, and laryngeal dystonia, which can cause breathing difficulty, stridor, and choking. Akathisia is also a common acute syndrome following the administration of antipsychotics and is characterized by a feeling of restlessness. Consider adding an anticholinergic agent, such as benztropine or diphenhydramine, if these symptoms occur, while stopping or reducing the use of the offending agent. Tardive dyskinesia is very unlikely to occur with the acute use of antipsychotics but may be seen with chronic or excessive use, which may be evident on presentation to the ED as a primary or secondary concern. Youth are also more susceptible to the development of neuroleptic malignant syndrome; early awareness and rapid management are crucial, with many youth requiring critical care to manage this presentation.

A particular challenge has been increasing and excessive use of antipsychotic medications for wider indications and with reduced metabolic monitoring in youth. This is compounded by an obesity epidemic and a bidirectional relationship between obesity, poor nutrition, and sedentary dietary habits with the development of psychopathology in youth.[13] With use of antipsychotics, youth are at higher risk for poor glycemic control, dyslipidemia, weight gain, and metabolic syndrome. The metabolic effects of these agents may persist even 1 year after discontinuation, making antipsychotic use and monitoring paramount in the psychiatric emergency care of the pediatric population.[30] With the use of antipsychotics, the underlying etiology being managed, intended duration and frequency of use, metabolic monitoring, and appropriate counseling and education should be a routine aspect of care of youth in the ED setting.

Longitudinal Care

Disposition

Disposition planning for any child should start at the beginning of an encounter and be routinely reflected upon within the interdisciplinary team and with the family. A clear sense of criteria for progressing to a higher level of care should be established and either overtly discussed or at least routinely reviewed. This should be communicated clearly with the patient and family to ensure transparency because escalation or de-escalation of care can carry strong emotional responses and significantly disrupt the daily activities of a child or family or both. Every opportunity should be made to have the child seen by mental health providers who can offer psychiatric and psychological support that matches the severity and frequency of need. Care should be taken to obviate potential barriers to seeking outpatient psychiatric care, including insurance coverage, transportation, accommodations for physical health needs at the mental health facility, and coordination of medical and mental health visits so as to consolidate care when feasible. Close communication between mental health and physical health providers is essential and can reduce iatrogenic injury, improve rapport with the patient and family, and result in improved clinical outcomes.

The criteria for inpatient psychiatric care for youth are similar to those for adults. Other criteria that may warrant consideration for inpatient psychiatric admission include the following:

1. Significant familial distress, psychosocial challenges, or caregiver difficulty to support ongoing patient psychiatric needs such that the patient is at high risk for severe decompensation or dysfunction without inpatient psychiatric stabilization and engagement with the family around these care needs
2. Severe treatment non-adherence in the setting of worsening depression, self-injurious behavior, or suicidal ideation that has not been stemmed by less restrictive interventions and is resulting in risk of imminent harm to the patient or others

3. Complex development, psychiatric, physical, and psychological factors influencing significant patient dysfunction and clinical decompensation warranting inpatient psychiatric assessment, particularly for youth with eating disorders, autism, intellectual disability, or medical comorbidities where subspecialty psychiatric services may be limited in less restrictive environments

Key Takeaways

- Increasingly, youth are seeking emergency psychiatric care at higher rates and are comprising a higher proportion of visits in ED settings.
- The increase in pediatric behavioral emergencies is influenced by increasing psychopathology in youth with diminishing access to care.
- Presentations in youth can be highly variable with, at times, atypical manifestations.
- Care is informed by a developmentally and trauma-informed assessment and management approach.
- Early awareness of risk, engagement with family, regular education, and nonpharmacologic intervention can be critical in minimizing progression of pathology and reducing use of medications, restraint, and seclusion in youth.
- Close and regular involvement with the caregiver and family is crucial.
- Medication management often involves use of low doses of psychotropic medications that is etiologically informed, with close monitoring for side effects or paradoxical response.
- Further research should focus on strategies to mitigate ED use, enhance collaboration with primary care, and reduce recidivism.

References

1. Nasir A, Watanabe-Galloway S, DiRenzo-Coffey G. Health services for behavioral problems in pediatric primary care. *J Behav Health Serv Res*. 2016;43:396–401.

2. Torio CE, Encinosa W, Berdahl T, et al. Annual report on health care for children and youth in the United States: National estimates of cost, utilization and expenditures for children with mental health conditions. *Acad Pediatr*. 2015;15:19–35.

3. Abrams A, Badolato G, Pastor W, et al. Racial disparities in pediatric mental health-related emergency department vistis: A five-year, multi-institutional study. American Academy of Pediatrics National Conference and Exhibition, November 2018.

4. Leeb RT, Bitsko RH, Radhakrishnan L, et al. Mental health-related emergency department visits among children aged <18 years during the COVID-19 pandemic—United States, January 1–October 17, 2020. *MMWR Morb Mortal Wkly Rep*. 2020;69:1675–1680.

5. American Academy of Pediatrics, Committee on Pediatric Emergency Medicine, American College of Emergency Physicians and Pediatric Emergency Medicine Committee. Pediatric mental health emergencies in the emergency medical services system. *Pediatrics*. 2006;118(4):1764–1767.

6. Sheridan D, Spiro DM, Fu R, et al. Mental health utilization in a pediatric emergency department. *Pediatr Emerg Care*. 2016;31(8):555–559.

7. McEnany FB, Ojugbele O, Doherty JR, et al. Pediatric mental health boarding. *Pediatrics*. 2020;146(4):e20201174.

8. Goldstein AB, Frosch E, Davarya S, Leaf PJ. Factors associated with a six-month return to emergency services among child and adolescent psychiatric patients. *Psychiat Serv.* 2007;58:1489–1492.

9. Malas N, Klein E, Tengelitsch E, et al. Exploring the telepsychiatry experience: Primary care provider perception of the Michigan Child Collaborative Care (MC3) program. *Psychosomatics.* 2019;60(2):179–189.

10. Ahmed SP, Bittencourt-Hewitt A, Sebastian CL. Neurocognitive bases of emotion regulation development in adolescence. *Dev Cogn Neurosci.* 2015;15:11–25.

11. Burstein B, Agostino H, Greenfield B. Suicidal attempts and ideation among children and adolescents in US emergency departments, 2007–2015. *JAMA Pediatr.* 2019;173(6):598–600.

12. Janiri D, Doucet GE, Pompili M, et al. Risk and protective factors for childhood suicidality: A US population-based study. *Lancet Psychiatry.* 2020;7(4):317–326.

13. Malas N, Plioplys S, Pao M. Depression in medically ill children and adolescents. *Child Adolesc Psychiatr Clin N Am.* 2019;28(3):421–445.

14. Merikangas KR, He JP, Burstein M, et al. Lifetime prevalence of mental disorders in U.S. adolescents: Results from the National Comorbidity Survey Replication–Adolescent Supplement (NCS-A). *J Am Acad Child Adolesc Psychiatry.* 2010;49(10):980–989.

15. Bardach NS, Neel C, Kleinman LC, et al. Depression, anxiety and emergency department use for asthma. *Pediatrics.* 2019;144(4):e20190856.

16. Beesdo K, Knappe S, Pine DS. Anxiety and anxiety disorders in children and adolescents: Developmental issues and implications for DSM-V. *Psychiatr Clin North Am.* 2009;32(3):483–524.

17. Poudel A, Gautam S. Age of onset of substance use and psychosocial problems among individuals with substance use disorders. *BMC Psychiatry.* 2017;17:10.

18. Substance Abuse and Mental Health Services Administration. *Results from the 2012 National Survey on Drug Use and Health: Summary of National Findings.* NSDUH Series H-46, HHS Publication No. (SMA) 13-4795. Substance Abuse and Mental Health Services Administration; 2013.

19. Wu P, Hoven CW, Liu X, et al. Substance use, suicidal ideation and attempts in children and adolescent. *Suicide Life Threat Behav.* 2004;34(3):408–420.

20. Kelleher I, Connor D, Clarke MC, et al. Prevalence of psychotic symptoms in childhood and adolescence: A systematic review and meta-analysis of population-based studies. *Psychol Med.* 2012;42(9):1857–1863.

21. Malas N, Brahmbhatt K, McDermott C, et al. Pediatric delirium: Evaluation, management, and special considerations. *Curr Psychiatry Rep.* 2017;19(9):65.

22. Gerson R, Malas N, Feuer V, et al. Best Practices for Evaluation and Treatment of Agitated Children and Adolescents (BETA) in the emergency department: Consensus statement of the American Association for Emergency Psychiatry. *West J Emerg Med.* 2019;20(2):409–418.

23. Gerson R, Malas N, Mroczkowski MM. Crisis in the emergency department: The evaluation and management of acute agitation in children and adolescents. *Child Adolesc Psychiatr Clin N Am.* 2018;27(3):367–386.

24. Lock J, La Via MC, American Academy of Child and Adolescent Psychiatry (AACAP) Committee on Quality Issues (CQI). Practice parameter for the assessment and treatment of children and adolescents with eating disorders. *J Am Acad Child Adolesc Psychiatry.* 2015;54(5):412–425.

25. Malas N, Ortiz-Aguayo R, Giles L, et al. Pediatric somatic symptom disorders. *Curr Psychiatry Rep.* 2017;19(2):11.

26. Jacobsen H, Bergsund HB, Wentzel-Larsen T, et al. *Children Youth Services Rev.* 2020;108.

27. De Los Reyes A, Augenstein TM, Wang M, et al. The validity of the multi-informant approach to assessing child and adolescent mental health. *Psychol Bull.* 2015;141(4):858–900.

28. Baker M, Carlson GA. What do we really know about PRN use in agitated children with mental health conditions: A clinical review. *Evid Based Ment Health.* 2018;21:166–170.

29. Chun TH, Mace SE, Katz ER, et al. Executive summary: Evaluation and management of children with acute mental health or behavioral problems: Part II. Recognition of clinically challenging mental health related conditions presenting with medical or uncertain symptoms. *Pediatrics.* 2016;138(3):e20161574.

30. Dayabandara M, Hanwella R, Ratnatunga S, et al. Antipsychotic-associated weight gain: Management strategies and impact on treatment adherence. *Neuropsychiatr Dis Treat.* 2017;13:2231–2241.

16

Geriatrics

*Daniel Cho, Junji Takeshita, Victor Huynh, Ishmael Gomes,
and Earl Hishinuma*

Introduction

An Aging Problem

The oldest of the baby boomers turned age 65 years in 2011, and the number of U.S. geriatric-aged adults is expected to exceed 70 million by 2030, which would account for an estimated 20% of the overall population.[1] The prevalence of geriatric patients with psychiatric disorders is 20–25%.[2] Despite these numbers, outpatient mental health resources are often underutilized by this population; approximately half of geriatric patients who acknowledge a psychiatric disorder receive treatment from any outpatient provider, whereas only 3% see a psychiatrist.[3]

Data have shown that in recent years, older adults have presented to emergency departments (EDs) for psychiatric reasons at increasing rates. Furthermore, for overall ED use, this cohort has higher visit rates; has increased duration of ED stays; is more likely to be repeat users; and, when admitted, has longer hospitalizations.[4]

These factors likely suggest an increase in ED utilization by geriatric patients for emergency psychiatric services in the upcoming decades. This chapter provides a practical approach to the evaluation and management of common geriatric psychiatry emergencies, while serving as both a reference and introductory text for clinicians working in the ED or emergency consult setting.

Special Considerations for the Geriatric Psychiatry Patient

Numerous biopsychosocial factors contribute to geriatric psychiatry emergencies, which makes evaluation and management especially challenging.

Biologic Factors
Medical Comorbidities
In the United States, 80% of people aged 65 years or older have at least one chronic medical condition.[5] The high rates of comorbid medical and psychiatric illnesses in this population can be challenging because psychiatric complaints are often vague and can be caused or exacerbated by medical issues.

Prescription Medications

Although geriatric patients account for only 12% of the U.S. population, this age group contributes to 34% of all prescription and 30% of all over-the-counter medications. Among elderly patients taking five or more medications, 35% experienced an adverse drug reaction.[6] Polypharmacy is the leading cause of delirium among geriatric patients, and it can also result in other serious reactions, including falls, depression, confusion, hallucinations, and malnutrition.[7] In the emergency setting, medication reconciliation is paramount. Efforts should be made to use the lowest effective dose or safely discontinue any medications that could potentially be contributing to a psychiatric emergency. Common medications of concern can be found in the American Geriatrics Society Beers Criteria.

Age-Associated Changes in Physiology and Pharmacokinetics

In a normal-aging brain, there are substantial changes in neurotransmitter substrate, enzyme, and receptor activity within the dopaminergic, cholinergic, and adrenergic pathways. Reductions in dopamine activity through progressive loss of striatum D_2 receptors can increase the risk of parkinsonism and extrapyramidal effects associated with antipsychotics and other dopamine antagonists. In addition, due to cholinergic cell loss and decreased choline acetyltransferase, cholinergic function declines with age. Thus, the elderly individual may be more susceptible to anticholinergic toxicity and experience impairments in cognition, memory, and coordination. Physical manifestations of anticholinergic toxicity, including reduced secretions, constipation, and falls, can also contribute to potential medical emergencies. Finally, decreased adrenergic function may lead to increased risk of orthostatic hypotension, cardiac abnormalities, sexual dysfunction, and altered response to medications.[7–9]

The bodies of aging individuals undergo physiologic changes that alter pharmacokinetics. During the aging process, increasing body fat stores lead to a larger volume of distribution and reduced elimination of lipid-soluble drugs. Lower water volume and serum albumin levels increase free plasma concentrations of medications, resulting in increased susceptibility to drug toxicity.[10] Hepatic metabolism and clearance of drugs are dependent on hepatic blood flow, hepatic volume, and enzymatic activity in hepatocytes, which have all been found to decline with age. Hepatically cleared medications may have a delayed clearance, and medications with active metabolites may have a delayed onset of action. Renal function as measured by glomerular filtration rate also declines with age, which may impair clearance of medications.[10] For example, elderly individuals are more susceptible to lithium toxicity.

Table 16.1 summarizes age-related changes in distribution, metabolism, and elimination of drugs, as well as their clinical implications. As a general rule, current medications must be evaluated extensively and new therapies monitored closely. When starting medications, it is prudent to abide by the adage "start low and go slow."

Drugs of Abuse

Although illicit drug use typically declines after young adulthood, nearly 1 million adults aged 65 years or older carry a substance use disorder diagnosis.[11] Illicit substance or alcohol intoxication can precipitate mood, anxiety, and psychotic or manic episodes and

Table 16.1 Physiologic, Pharmacokinetic, and Pharmacodynamic Changes with Aging

Age-Related Changes	Clinical Implications
↓ Dopaminergic function	↑ Risk of extrapyramidal symptoms
↓ Cholinergic function	↑ Risk of anticholinergic toxicity
↓ Adrenergic function	↑ Risk of hypotension, cardiac abnormalities, sexual dysfunction
↓ Plasma albumin	↑ Free drug serum concentrations, ↑ risk of toxicity
↓ Total body water volume	
↑ Body fat	↓ Lipid-soluble drug clearance, ↑ risk of toxicity
↓ Hepatic function	↓ Hepatic metabolism and clearance, ↑ risk of toxicity
↓ Renal function	↓ Renal excretion, ↑ risk of toxicity

Adapted from Mulsant and Pollack[7] and Catterson et al.[8]

can lead to increased risk for suicide. Withdrawal syndromes can precipitate delirious or agitated states.

Psychosocial Factors
Transition Periods
Many geriatric psychiatric crises arise in the setting of acute stressors, particularly during significant life transitions. Erickson's seventh stage, generativity versus stagnation (ages 40–65 years), describes a period in which adults exhibit work productivity, raise families, and are involved in larger scale community activities. For example, facing retirement can lead to significant loss of identity and purpose, and in times of a crisis (e.g., a pandemic), an abrupt transition may even trigger a psychiatric emergency. Major life events, including the loss of parents, spouses, or children, divorce, and decline in physical functioning also lead to forced transitions.

Elder Abuse
Current evidence suggests approximately one in six older individuals experience elder abuse, which includes physical, verbal, psychological, financial, and sexual abuse.[12] Elder abuse can lead to significant psychological distress and precipitate mood disorders, anxiety, and substance abuse.

Family Dynamics
Changes in family dynamics play a major role in geriatric mental health. In the midst of the COVID-19 pandemic, abrupt changes in family health have brought these caregiver issues to the forefront. Geriatric patients are losing loved ones unexpectedly with resultant grief and suffering or may rapidly have to adjust to becoming a caregiver for an acutely ill family member, which may lead to burnout or guilt over their inability to provide the necessary care. Patients themselves may have to abruptly transition from the provider role to becoming a perceived burden on the family when illness arises. These changes in family dynamics can precipitate psychiatric emergencies.

Approach to the Geriatric Psychiatric Emergency

Initial Safety Assessment and Triage

When an elderly patient presents to the ED, the psychiatrist's priority is to assess for danger to self or others and to establish safety. Compared to younger individuals, geriatric patients have increased rates of depression and completed suicide. Furthermore, violent and aggressive behaviors associated with medical conditions such as dementia and delirium are more prevalent in the elderly.[10,13] Despite these elevated risks, achieving safety may be difficult in the elderly individual who may be physically frail, disabled, and with significant medical comorbidities.

When a patient requires evaluation due to concerns of suicidality or homicidality, the patient should be placed under adequate supervision and prevented from leaving the ED until the evaluation is completed. Safety precautions must be pursued and may include placement in a private room, removal of potentially dangerous objects, and one-to-one supervision by trained staff.[14] In the case of an acutely agitated patient, the etiology of agitation should be determined and addressed if associated with reversible causes, such as akathisia, intoxication, or withdrawal. Underlying disease states that may be contributing to risk should be targeted, as in the case of delirium. Pain should be appropriately assessed and managed. Because sensory deficits may contribute to agitation, corrective eyeglasses or hearing aids should be provided where appropriate. Environmental risk factors should be addressed, such as removal from excessive stimuli, loud noises, or potential perceived threats. Nonpharmacologic approaches to agitation should be attempted, including verbal de-escalation, distraction, and reassurance.[15]

Chemical restraints may be a necessary strategy for management of severe agitation by means of sedation. Older patients, however, may be more susceptible to side effects with these medications due to age-related physiologic, pharmacokinetic, and pharmacodynamic changes, placing them at elevated risk for adverse effects, including worsening confusion, oversedation, falls, paradoxical agitation, and extrapyramidal symptoms.[20] Medications considered for chemical restraint must be carefully selected and depend on specific disease states to minimize adverse effects.

Observational studies have suggested that physical restraints may be associated with increased fall risk, direct injury, increased agitation, and psychological distress.[16] Due to these concerns, physical restraints should be avoided when possible. However, such restraints may be necessary for severely agitated patients at risk of harming themselves or others; to allow delivery of appropriate medical care; or to prevent removal of medical devices, such as lines or catheters. As a general rule, when physical restraints are necessary, the least restrictive approach should be utilized and the need for continuing restraints should be evaluated frequently.

History and Physical

As with all patients, when an elderly adult presents to the ED, it is critical to obtain an accurate history of the presenting complaint. This may be a challenge because older patients frequently present with complaints that may not be overtly psychiatric in nature. Described symptoms may be diffuse, nonspecific, and often somatic, such as fatigue, weakness, poor appetite, or insomnia. This clinical picture may be further complicated because the geriatric population may be more vulnerable to acute and chronic medical conditions that may mask or enhance symptom presentation.

In some cases, patients may not be able to provide any reliable history at all, with information that may be absent, inaccurate, or confabulated. This may be the case with cognitive impairment in dementia, thought disorganization in psychosis, confusional and altered consciousness states such as delirium or coma, and neurologic complications such as aphasia or dysarthria. Due to the limited accuracy of the history obtained from the older patient, valuable information can be gleaned from physical signs and auxiliary informants.

It is crucial to utilize collateral sources of history, including families, caregivers, and other treating providers. These informants may have more familiarity with the patient and may be able to identify subtle changes that emergency providers may overlook. They may report changes in cognition, personality, or behavior, including agitation, aggression, violence, self-harm, social withdrawal, declining memory, changes in activities of daily living, decreased oral intake, and insomnia. Informants may be able to provide a baseline level of functioning, a timeline, and the character and frequency of presenting symptoms. However, objectivity and cautious skepticism are necessary in evaluating collateral historians because the geriatric population is highly vulnerable to abuse, neglect, and exploitation. It is for this reason that the patient history should be gathered separate from collateral to limit intimidation and coercion. If abuse is suspected or confirmed, state-dependent procedures for reporting should be followed in collaboration with local law enforcement and adult protective services.

In addition to history taking, an accurate and complete physical and neurological examination can help elucidate any underlying medical conditions that may be contributing to current presentation. There is considerable symptom overlap and complex interplay of medical, neurologic, and psychiatric disorders that require careful attention for accurate diagnosis and subsequent treatment. Although difficult to perform on an acutely agitated patient, a complete and targeted physical exam is recommended, which may provide valuable clues. The physical exam may help reveal an indwelling catheter that is identified as the nidus for the deliriogenic urinary tract infection, healed lacerations to a forearm from a previously undisclosed history of depression and suicidality, multiple ecchymoses in varying stages of healing inflicted by a frustrated caretaker, a distended abdomen found to be a potential cause for discomfort, or fecal smearing in the demented and constipated patient. Vital signs may reveal a fever and hypoxia, evidence of a pneumonia, and a cause for acute mental status changes. A neurologic exam may equally prove its utility, identifying focal neurologic changes that may suggest a left temporal stroke, which is highly associated with depression. Common medical comorbidities and psychiatric manifestations are listed in Box 16.1.

Laboratory and Imaging Studies

Due to the elevated risk of comorbid medical conditions and increased vulnerability in the geriatric population, routine laboratory tests and imaging studies are recommended to identify or exclude medical causes for neurobehavioral symptoms. At minimum, labs obtained should include complete blood count, metabolic profile, urinalysis, and urine toxicology to evaluate for any intoxicants and hematologic, metabolic, or infectious processes. Additional tests, when clinically relevant and guided by clinical suspicion, may

---

Box 16.1 Common Emergency Room Geriatric Psychiatric Presentations

---

Altered mental status
Confusion and disorientation
Memory disturbance
Perceptual disturbance
Personality changes
Risk of self-harm and suicide
Risk to others and property
Severe agitation and aggression
Failure to thrive
Insomnia
Deterioration in activities of daily living
Catatonia
Substance intoxication and withdrawal
Adverse drug reactions

---

be performed for thyroid function, hepatic function, ammonia, drug levels, vitamin B_{12}/folate, heavy metals, and autoimmune markers. Although not necessary unless clinically indicated, selective use of imaging studies may be of utility in evaluating underlying causes of presentation. For example, chest radiography may reveal a subtle pneumonia or fractured ribs from an unwitnessed fall at home. Neuroimaging studies should also be guided by a concerning history or findings on neurologic examination. Computed tomography may reveal a new stroke and foci for seizure activity and associated hallucinations, or magnetic resonance imaging findings of diffuse white matter hyperintensities may be suggestive of subcortical ischemia and vascular dementia. With advancing age and increasing polypharmacy, there is an elevated risk of cardiac abnormalities, arrhythmias, and especially QT prolongation associated with psychotropics, and thus an electrocardiogram is recommended. Additional studies, such as an electroencephalogram (EEG), although rarely used in the emergency setting, may be utilized to identify a seizure or to confirm delirium states.

Cognition and Capacity

Informed consent is an integral facet of medical care, and a patient must have medical decision-making "capacity" to provide consent and receive (or refuse) recommended treatment. When a patient lacks capacity, this decision may rely on surrogate decision-makers and advance directives. As many as 25% of psychiatric consults in the hospital are sought for capacity determination, with up to 48% of these patients found to lack decisional capacity.[17] The elderly population is particularly vulnerable, facing end-of-life decisions with increasing risk of impaired cognition, while simultaneously at elevated risk of experiencing emergencies requiring emergent medical intervention. The emergency provider may be faced with the ethical dilemma of balancing patient autonomy and protecting the patient from consequences of cognitive

Table 16.2 Medical Decision-Making Capacity Assessment Criteria

Component	Requirement
Choice	Patient must be able to consistently indicate a preferred treatment choice.
Understanding	Patient must be able to grasp fundamental understanding of conditions, risks, and benefits of specific treatment options communicated by physician.
Appreciation	Patient must be able to acknowledge medical condition and likely consequences of treatment options if accepted or refused.
Reasoning	Patient must be able to engage in rational process of manipulating relevant information, comparing treatment options and consequences, and offer reasoning for selection of choice.

Adapted from Appelbaum.[17]

impairment. Although the intricacies of this process are beyond the scope of this chapter, a provider should be prepared to perform a capacity assessment. Four criteria must be met for a patient to be deemed to have medical decision-making capacity: choice, understanding, appreciation, and reasoning.[17,18] The details are listed in Table 16.2.

Disposition

When delirium is suspected in the elderly patient who presents in the ED, medical hospitalization often follows to allow for adequate diagnostic workup and treatment of underlying causes. Identification of underlying causes may be difficult to ascertain in the emergency setting, and additional time and provider coordination are often required for therapeutic interventions. Although appropriate for management of neurobehavioral symptoms associated with delirium, psychiatric units may be ill-equipped to manage medically fragile patients and may be without resources for a complete medical workup. In some cases, delirium associated with acute intoxication may clear during emergency observation, and patients may be subsequently discharged to prior arrangements.

Management of Specific Geriatric Psychiatry Emergencies

Delirium, Dementia, and Depression/Decompensated Psychiatric Illness

Background
Delirium
Delirium is a neurocognitive syndrome characterized by disturbances in attention and cognition that develop over a short period of time, and it tends to have a waxing and waning course. It is considered a reversible form of brain dysfunction that is a direct consequence of another medical condition, substance intoxication/withdrawal, or exposure to a toxin. Delirium often occurs in the context of acute illness,

hospitalization, and postoperative status and is associated with a multitude of adverse consequences, including prolonged hospitalizations, institutionalization, cognitive and functional decline, mortality, and increased cost of medical care. Delirium may progress to stupor, coma, and death, particularly with untreated progression of the underlying disease process. Disturbance of the sleep–wake cycle is also common in delirium. Individuals may exhibit a wide array of neuropsychiatric symptoms, including hallucinations, thought disorganization, mood lability, agitation, anxiety, depression, irritability, euphoria, and apathy.[19-21]

There are three classifications of delirium that are separated by psychomotor phenotypes: hyperactive, hypoactive, and mixed. In hyperactive delirium, an individual may experience a heightened level of psychomotor activity accompanied by mood lability, agitation, and combative behavior. This subtype is generally more readily identified in the ED and hospital setting due to the typically disruptive behaviors associated with the condition. Hypoactive delirium, however, is characterized by decreased activity; patients appear sluggish, lethargic, and approaching stuporous. Although more common in the elderly, it is underrecognized and often mistaken for other psychiatric and neurologic diagnoses, frequently misdiagnosed as dementia or depression. Mixed-type delirium generally presents as rapidly fluctuating levels of psychomotor activity; however, this type of delirium may also present as normal levels of psychomotor activity.[20]

Delirium remains one of the most underrecognized disorders and is often underdiagnosed in both the hospital and the emergency setting. In the general population, prevalence of delirium is low, estimated at 1% or 2%, with risk increasing with age. In hospitalized patients, prevalence increases dramatically, and delirium is the most common psychiatric syndrome observed, with occurrence rates estimated to be 29–64%. In the ED, it is estimated that 10–30% of elderly patients will present with delirium, with only 24–35% of these patients correctly diagnosed.[19,22]

Dementia

Dementia is a chronic, steadily progressive neurocognitive process leading to impairments in memory, thinking, and behavior beyond what would be expected in normal aging. Although there are numerous subtypes of dementia, the most common by far is Alzheimer's disease (AD), accounting for 60–70% of all cases.[23]

There are various stages to AD, starting with mild cognitive impairment (MCI). In MCI, signs and symptoms are subtle and there is no impact on daily functioning. Patients may have insight into their mild deficits and can compensate for them. In early stages of dementia, symptoms begin to interfere with daily activities and become noticeable to others. There are typically problems with short-term memory, word-finding, and executive function. In the middle stages of Alzheimer's dementia, almost all new information is lost, and there are significant deficits in problem-solving, social judgment, and basic self-care. Patients may be able to complete simple chores or tasks, but they require assistance with most everything.[24] In late stages, patients typically lose all of their activities of daily living and instrumental activities of daily living and require 24-hour care to ensure safety. Patients with dementia typically utilize emergency psychiatric services for acute neuropsychiatric symptoms, including agitation, depression, apathy, delusions, hallucinations, and sleep impairment. It has been estimated that 50–80% of patients with dementia experience neuropsychiatric symptoms at some point in the course of illness.[23]

Depression

The geriatric population is not immune to primary psychiatric disorders, with specific prevalence estimates at 6% with a diagnosable depressive disorder, 0.6% with schizophrenia, and 0.6–3.7% with alcohol use disorders.[2] Geriatric patients with underlying psychiatric illnesses often present to the ED for acute decompensation, such as active suicidal ideations, worsening psychosis, or agitation. Depression in the elderly is often heterogeneous, and it is associated with dementia, delusions, and/or anxiety in more than 45% of cases.[25]

Etiology and Risk Factors

Delirium

The etiology of delirium is poorly understood and has been conceptualized as multifactorial with complex interplay between patient vulnerability and precipitating factors resulting in brain dysfunction. With increasing age, comorbidities, and decreased homeostatic function, the elderly are more vulnerable to noxious stimuli and acute illness. Predisposing risk factors that may identify vulnerable patients include history of delirium, dementia, cognitive impairment, disorientation, sensory impairments, use of physical restraints, comorbid illness, history of strokes, depression, and substance abuse.[21,26,27]

There are a wide range of precipitating factors for delirium, including physiologic stressors, metabolic and electrolyte derangements, infection (sepsis, urinary tract infections, and pneumonia), intoxication, withdrawal, and other central nervous system (CNS) insults. Potential precipitants are listed in Table 16.3, utilizing the mnemonic "I WATCH DEATH." These physiologic changes have been proposed to induce delirium through multiple mechanisms, such as neuroinflammation, hypoxia, and oxidative stress. These can cause changes

Table 16.3 I WATCH DEATH Mnemonic for Potential Precipitants for Delirium

Infection	HIV, sepsis, pneumonia, urinary tract infection
Withdrawal	Alcohol, benzodiazepine, opiate
Acute metabolic	Acidosis, alkalosis, electrolyte derangement, hepatic failure, renal failure
Trauma	Head trauma, burns, postoperative status, use of restraints
CNS pathology	Diffuse axonal injury, encephalitis, hemorrhage, hydrocephalus, penetrating injury, stroke
Hypoxia	Anemia, respiratory failure, shock
Deficiencies	Vitamin B_{12}, folate, niacin, thiamine
Endocrinopathies	Derangements of cortisol, glucose, thyroid, parathyroid
Acute vascular/Autoimmune	Arrhythmias, encephalopathy, hemorrhage, hypertensive emergency, shock, stroke, autoimmune disease
Toxins	Illicit drugs, pesticides, prescription drugs, solvents
Heavy metals	Lead, mercury

CNS, central nervous system.
Adapted from Gower et al.[30]

in blood–brain barrier permeability, neurotransmitter substrate and receptor activity, and dysregulation of the reticular activating system. Relative neurotransmitter deficiencies of acetylcholine, γ-aminobutyric acid (GABA), and melatonin along with excess dopamine, epinephrine, and N-methyl-D-aspartate (NMDA) have all been implicated in the etiology of delirium and have guided potential treatment modalities.[21,28,29]

Dementia

Individuals affected by AD have loss of synapses and neurons in the cerebral cortex, leading to atrophy of the affected regions. Microscopically, there are buildup of plaques (insoluble β-amyloid peptide and cellular material) and neurofibrillary tangles (hyperphosphorylated collections of microtubule-associated protein τ inside cells).[31] Environmental and lifestyle risk factors are listed in Table 16.4.

Depression

The diathesis–stress model postulates that genetic predisposition to depression is activated by stressful psychosocial life events.[33] On a micro-level, there are deficiencies in the neurotransmitters serotonin, norepinephrine, and dopamine. Temperament, including low self-esteem, poor coping, and negative attitudes, can contribute to depression. Stressful childhood events, such as violence, neglect, abuse, or low socioeconomic status, also increase risk for depression.

It is important to be aware of risk factors for suicide because risk is higher in the geriatric population. Specific risk factors for suicide are listed in Box 16.2.

Differential Diagnosis

Distinguishing between delirium, dementia, and depression can be difficult due to overlapping symptomology. The delirious patient is commonly misdiagnosed with

Table 16.4 Risk Factors for Alzheimer's Dementia

Age	10% of patients older than age 65 years, 30–40% of patients older than 85 years
Gender	Women > men
Family history	Increased risk for AD
Genetics	40–65% of people with AD have apolipoprotein E4 gene
Down syndrome	Typically early onset AD in 30s and 40s
Head injury	Traumatic brain injury with loss of consciousness and amnesia can increase AD risk in later ages
Low education	Increase risk for AD
Alcohol	Dependence may increase risk
Diet	Healthier, vegetarian diets may be protective
Maternal age	Increased maternal age
Estrogen deficiency	Increased risk in postmenopausal women
Other factors	High cholesterol, hypertension, cardiovascular accident, diabetes mellitus

AD, Alzheimer's dementia.
Adapted from Khouzam.[32]

> ## Box 16.2 Risk Factors for Suicide
>
> Family history of suicide
> Family history of child maltreatment
> Previous suicide attempts
> Psychiatric illness, particularly major depressive disorder
> History of alcohol and substance use
> Hopelessness
> Impulsive or aggressive tendencies
> Cultural and religious beliefs
> Local epidemics of suicides
> Isolation
> Barriers to accessing mental health treatment
> Physical illness
> Easy access to lethal methods
> Unwillingness to seek help due to stigma
>
> From Centers for Disease Control and Prevention.[34]

depression due to the cognitive impairments associated with "pseudodementia." Dementia and its subtypes may also mimic delirium, with similar behavioral disturbances associated with "sundowning" or perceptual disturbances present with Lewy body dementia. These syndromes may be distinguished by the onset and course of symptom development as well as characteristic inattention and fluctuating consciousness of delirium.[35] Additional distinguishing characteristics are described in Table 16.5.

Assessment

There are multiple challenges in establishing an accurate diagnosis in the ED, including the acuity of symptoms, fluctuating course, and confused and potentially agitated patients. A comprehensive history may help identify any precipitating factors of delirium, especially trauma, recent surgery, hospitalizations, changes in medications, and recent substance use.[20,27] Several diagnostic and screening instruments with high sensitivity can be used to rapidly identify delirious patients. The Delirium Triage Scale can be performed in less than 20 seconds and guide additional delirium evaluation. The Confusion Assessment Method (CAM) has become the most widely accepted diagnostic and screening tool for delirium. It can be performed in less than 5 minutes with a sensitivity of 94–100% and specificity of 90–95%. The CAM evaluates for acute mental status changes and fluctuating course, inattention, disorganized thinking, and altered levels of consciousness.[36]

For patients with suspected dementia, cognitive testing should be performed, such as the Mini-Cog, Folstein Mini-Mental Status Examination, or the St. Louis University Mental Status Examination. Many hospitals have implemented brief suicide screening tools that are administered to every ED patient. These screening tools can range from a few direct questions about hopelessness and suicidality to more comprehensive questionnaires, such as the Columbia-Suicide Severity Rating Scale, which is considered the gold standard and differentiates between interrupted,

Table 16.5 Characteristics of Delirium, Dementia, and Depression

	Delirium	Dementia	Depression
Onset	Rapid, abrupt	Slow, insidious	Variable, cyclical
Course	Fluctuating, reversible with treatment	Chronic, progressive	Variable, reversible with treatment
Consciousness	Impaired, fluctuates	Intact, may be impaired late stage	Intact
Attention	Impaired, fluctuates	Intact, may be impaired late stage	Variable
Orientation	Impaired, fluctuates	Intact, may be impaired late stage	Generally intact
Memory	Recent impaired, remote may be intact	Recent and remote impaired	Generally intact, may be selectively impaired
Thought process	Often disorganized, incoherent	Linear to impoverished, may be disorganized late stage	Linear to impoverished
Perceptions	Hallucinations and delusions common	Intact, delusions may be present late stage	Generally intact, may have mood-congruent hallucinations and delusions
Behavior	Psychomotor agitation or retardation	Intact, agitation may present late stage and occur in the evening	Generally intact
Insight	Variable, fluctuates	Poor	Generally intact, may focus on memory impairment

Adapted from Downing et al.[35] and Gower et al.[30]

aborted, and actual suicide attempts. Utilizing other standardized tools, such as the Geriatric Depression Scale or Patient Health Questionnaire–9, can further assist in the diagnosis of depression.

A complete and thorough workup is suggested for all patients who present with psychiatric symptoms, but it is of utmost importance in the geriatric population. Delirium may be a harbinger for serious medical illness and mortality, emphasizing the need for appropriate workup. Vital signs and physical and neurological exam should be performed routinely. Basic laboratory tests should also be obtained, including complete blood count, basic metabolic panel, thyroid studies, urinalysis, and urine toxicology. Additional tests, when clinically relevant, may include hepatic function, ammonia, drug levels, vitamin B_{12}/folate, heavy metals, and autoimmune markers. Neuroimaging may be guided by neurological evaluation and should be considered in acute mental status changes. If there is suspicion for CNS infection, lumbar puncture may be necessary.[27] Although rarely performed in the emergency setting, EEG may be used to identify seizure activity or differentiate between underlying neuropsychiatric conditions. Although with limited sensitivity and specificity, EEG studies typically reveal generalized slowing in delirium, and the presence of specific patterns, such as triphasic waves, may predict etiology and severity.[37] The general approach to assessment of altered mental status is described in Table 16.6.

Table 16.6 Assessment of Altered Mental Status

History	Baseline cognition
	Acuity and character of mental status changes
	Medical history, including recent surgeries, hospitalizations, diagnoses, medications
	All current medications, supplements, interactions
	Substance use history
	Psychiatric history
	Social history
Physical examination	Vital signs
	Sensory evaluation
	Signs of infection, dehydration, acute illness
Neurological examination	Focal neurologic signs, tremor, clonus, asterixis
Laboratory evaluation	Complete blood count, basic metabolic panel, urinalysis, urine toxicology
Additional considerations	Vitamin B_{12}, folate, hepatic function tests, ammonia, HIV, rapid plasma regain, erythrocyte sedimentation rate, heavy metals, urine porphyrins, cortisol, anti-nuclear antibody, serum drug levels
	Arterial blood gas
	Electrocardiography
	Chest radiography
	Lumbar puncture
Neuroimaging	Identify signs of head trauma, hemorrhage, hematoma
	Identify stroke, structural lesions, encephalitis
Electroencephalography	Identify seizure activity
	Generalized slowing common in delirium

Adapted from Inouye SK, et al.[27]

Treatment

Delirium

In the delirious patient, preventing, identifying, and treating the underlying cause are the cornerstones of treatment. This may present a challenge because delirious patients, especially hyperactive and mixed types, may be confused, combative, and uncooperative. Therefore, symptomatic management is the primary target in the ED setting to minimize morbidity and mortality, including neurobehavioral symptoms of agitation, impaired cognition, and perceptual disturbances. Although a risk factor for prolonging delirium, cautious use of physical and/or chemical restraints may be required to maintain safety for the patient and staff, in addition to facilitating adequate workup and delivery of necessary care.

Nonpharmacologic Approaches

Nonpharmacologic strategies include sleep–wake regulation, reorientation, sensory optimization, early mobilization, and examination of nutritional status. Environmental precipitants should be addressed, such as removing the patient from loud noises and bright lights. Because untreated pain may precipitate and prolong delirium, pain should be assessed and managed appropriately. Maintenance of daily routines and familiar activities have also been effective in reducing neurobehavioral symptoms. Familiar faces and objects may provide comfort and assist with prevention and recovery of delirium.[21,28]

Pharmacologic Approaches

As a general principle, goals of pharmacologic interventions for delirium in the ED are to rapidly manage severe agitation and psychotic symptoms, if present, while avoiding exacerbation of delirium. Medications should be carefully selected and minimized due to the risk of interactions and toxicity in the elderly and vulnerable populations. Although anticholinergic medications have been effective for sedation and management of agitation in the general population, they should be avoided in the elderly patient. Anticholinergic medications are deliriogenic, and the risk of toxicity is elevated with increasing polypharmacy and anticholinergic burden. Treatment of toxicity may require metabolization of offending agents or use of antidotes, such as physostigmine.[38] Narcotic medications should be provided for acute management of pain at the minimum dose possible because pain is a risk factor for delirium. However, narcotics have been implicated to prolong delirium due to CNS effects, although data are inconsistent.[39] Benzodiazepines have been shown to exacerbate delirium and should be avoided in the delirious patient under most circumstances. Special cases include alcohol, barbiturate, or benzodiazepine withdrawal, in which benzodiazepines remain the mainstay of treatment to limit progression of the withdrawal syndrome to seizures, autonomic dysregulation, hallucinations, and potentially death.[40]

Antipsychotics

Use of antipsychotics in the treatment of delirium has been controversial. There are no U.S. Food and Drug Administration (FDA) indications for the use of antipsychotics in delirium, and the literature has been inconclusive. There is conflicting evidence regarding the use of antipsychotics, demonstrating inconsistent findings in reducing delirium incidence, duration, disease burden, length of stay, and mortality.[41] Nevertheless, antipsychotics have been commonly used as a first-line pharmacologic approach to manage neurobehavioral symptoms of delirium. Antipsychotics can improve symptoms of psychosis, including hallucinations, delusions, and paranoia, by addressing proposed dopamine excess.[28] To ensure the safety of an aggressive patient and treating clinicians, antipsychotics can be used judiciously as a chemical restraint. Furthermore, sedating properties may confer benefit in establishing a consistent sleep–wake cycle. Haloperidol has been studied most extensively and has been widely used due to its versatile routes of administration, especially intramuscular and intravenous formulations for extreme agitation. However, risk of QT prolongation, potentially fatal arrhythmias (Torsades de pointes), and elevated risk of extrapyramidal symptoms remain concerns. Second-generation antipsychotics risperidone, quetiapine, olanzapine, ziprasidone, and aripiprazole have also been widely used.[28,41] For the elderly patient in the ED, selection of first- or second-generation antipsychotics for management of neurobehavioral symptoms of delirium should be guided by target symptoms, cardiac status, available route of administration, and associated side effects. Table 16.7 lists specific antipsychotic medications and properties.

Non-antipsychotics

Valproic acid (VPA) may be an effective treatment option for severe agitation in the delirious elderly patient when antipsychotics are contraindicated. In the general population,

Table 16.7 Antipsychotics Used for Neurobehavioral Symptoms of Delirium

Antipsychotic	Route of Administration	Anticholinergic/Sedation	QT Prolongation
Haloperidol	PO, IM, IV, (LAI)	+	+, +++ (IV)
Risperidone	PO, rapid dissolve, (LAI)	+	+++
Quetiapine	PO	+++	++
Olanzapine	PO, rapid dissolve, (LAI)	+++	++
Ziprasidone	PO, IM	+	+++
Aripiprazole	PO, (LAI)	–	+/–

IM, intramuscular; IV, intravenous; LAI, long-acting injectable; PO, oral.
Data from Huhn et al.[42]

VPA has been used to decrease agitation through chemical sedation and can be administered orally and intravenously with rapid onset. VPA may be particularly beneficial in delirium due to proposed deliriolytic effects mediated by action on GABA, glutamate, dopamine, and acetylcholine pathways. Although rare, VPA is associated with hyperammonemic encephalopathy, and this must be considered when it is used as a primary or adjunct management of agitation in delirium. Other adverse effects include hepatotoxicity, pancreatitis, and blood dyscrasias.[43]

Several medications are effective in preventing and treating delirium, although these have limited use in the ED setting because acute behavioral and psychotic symptoms remain the primary targets. Melatonin is commonly prescribed in the delirious hospitalized patient, addressing proposed melatonin deficiency and dysregulation of the sleep–wake cycle.[28] Alpha-2 agonists have been used extensively in intensive care unit patients for sedation, analgesia, and sympatholysis while avoiding deliriogenic GABAergic agents, demonstrating reduced incidences of delirium. Cardiovascular effects of bradycardia and hypotension have limited its regular use in the emergency room.[28]

Dementia

Treatment of neuropsychiatric symptoms of dementia begins with nonpharmacologic management, similar to that of delirium. Caregiver training is also an important aspect of nonpharmacologic management.

Meta-analyses have shown no clear evidence for the use of typical antipsychotics, aside from low-dose haloperidol for reducing aggression.[44] However, the risk for extrapyramidal side effects and sedation may outweigh the benefits. Atypical antipsychotics, primarily olanzapine and risperidone, have moderate evidence in reducing neuropsychiatric symptoms of dementia and display limited side effects at low doses. However, they have also shown statistical significance for cardiovascular and cerebrovascular accidents, prompting a black box warning for a 1.6–1.7 times risk for all-cause mortality. The antidepressant citalopram was found to improve agitation and lability in demented patients. It may best be suited for anxious behaviors, such as repetitive vocalizations or pacing. However, citalopram can prolong the QT interval and should be used cautiously, especially in patients who are also taking antipsychotics. VPA has not been shown to be efficacious in treating this population, and carbamazepine has shown mixed results. However, if patients have underlying bipolar disorder or present primarily with manic

Table 16.8 Medications for the Neuropsychiatric Symptoms of Dementia

Medications	Target Symptoms	Adverse Effects
Haloperidol	Aggression	EPS, sedation
Risperidone	Agitation	EPS, increase in CVA, MI
Olanzapine	Agitation	Sedation, increase in CVA, MI
Citalopram	Agitation, anxiety	Prolonged QTc
Rivastigmine, galantamine	Cognition, function	Gastrointestinal SE, headache
Memantine	Cognition, function	Agitation

CVA, cardiovascular accident; EPS, extrapyramidal symptoms; MI, myocardial infarction.

symptoms, VPA, lithium, and carbamazepine should be considered. Cholinesterase inhibitors show a small but consistent benefit for cognition and function but not for neuropsychiatric symptoms. The NMDA antagonist memantine shows similar results for function but not for neurocognitive symptoms.[44] Table 16.8 summarizes medications for the neuropsychiatric symptoms of AD.

Depression

Acute management of depression involves ensuring a safe, supportive, and protective environment for patients. Determining the appropriate care setting can be challenging due to the high rates of comorbid delirium and dementia. It has been shown that delirious patients admitted to psychiatric units are less likely to undergo complete diagnostic assessments.[45] If there is a high suspicion for delirium, it is recommended that patients be admitted to the medical floor, with psychiatry assisting for the management of depression. Collaboration between psychiatric, medical, and even geriatric teams allows for better overall management of this particularly challenging cohort.

Due to the delayed onset of action of antidepressants, it is not recommended they be started in the ED. The patient's medication list should be reviewed prior to starting new medications to prevent interactions. Fluoxetine is FDA approved for geriatric depression.[46] However, citalopram may be a good choice in patients with comorbid dementia. Somatic treatments, such as electroconvulsive therapy, should be considered early in treatment course for severe symptoms or acute suicidality.

Education and Training

There is great importance in educating and training the future health care workforce in serving ED geriatric patients with psychiatric needs.[47] Although there are no specific Liaison Committee on Medical Education requirements for medical student exposure, they may experience educational opportunities in the ED that may entail working with geriatric psychiatry patients. In addition to these experiences providing specific learning opportunities for medical students (e.g., delirium, dementia, depression, and suicidality), they may also inspire medical students toward careers in related fields, such as emergency medicine, geriatric medicine, or psychiatry.

There are more specific guidelines for psychiatry residents based on the Accreditation Council for Graduate Medical Education (ACGME):[48]

Residents must demonstrate competence in the evaluation and treatment of patients of different *ages* and genders from diverse backgrounds, and from a variety of ethnic, racial, sociocultural, and economic backgrounds.

Resident experience in geriatric psychiatry must include one month full-time equivalency (FTE) of organized experience focused on areas unique to the care of the elderly. Each resident's geriatric psychiatry experience must include: (a) diagnosis and management of mental disorders in geriatric patients with coexistent medical disorders; (b) diagnosis and management, including management of the cognitive component, of degenerative disorders; (c) basic neuropsychological testing of cognitive functioning in the elderly; and (d) management of drug interactions. Resident experience in emergency psychiatry must be conducted in an organized, supervised psychiatry emergency service. This experience must not be counted as part of the 12-month outpatient requirement. Resident experiences must include crisis evaluation and management, and triage of psychiatric patients. On-call experiences alone must not fulfill the requirement for resident experience in emergency psychiatry.[48]

The ACGME also has specific competencies for geriatric psychiatry fellows:

Fellows must demonstrate competence in diagnosis and treatment of all major psychiatric disorders seen in elderly patients, including adjustment disorders, affective disorders, anxiety disorders, delirium, dementias/neurocognitive disorders, iatrogenesis, late-onset psychoses, medical presentations of psychiatric disorders, personality disorders, sexual disorders, sleep disorders, substance-related disorders, and continuation of psychiatric illnesses that began earlier in life.

Fellows must demonstrate proficiency competence in recognizing and managing psychiatric co-morbid disorders, including dementia/neurocognitive disorders, and depression, as well as agitation, wandering, changes in sleep patterns, and aggressiveness.

Experience should include consultation to inpatient, outpatient, and emergency services, as well as consultative experience in chronic care facilities.[49]

Allied health care providers who work in the ED can also benefit from education and training in serving geriatric psychiatry patients. These include other physician attendings, nurses, social workers, and ED technicians.

Education and teaching can occur in various forums and environments, but they all address critical appraisal of the literature and understanding of the research process.[48] Bedside learning and supervision through technology are more direct methods of active and applied learning. Didactic instruction can entail lectures (e.g., grand rounds), seminars, problem-based learning, and assigned readings coordinated with concurrent clinical experiences. These teaching methods can be further enhanced through case conferences, in which the focus is on specific patient cases that have generalizable knowledge and principles in patient safety and care, and journal clubs, in which the focus is on specific research studies or reviews that have generalizable knowledge and principles in clinical psychiatric content and research methodologies. Finally, local, regional, national, and international conferences, including annual meetings of the American Association of Geriatric Psychiatry and the American Association of Emergency Psychiatry, focus on a wide variety of contemporary topics.

Telepsychiatry

There have been growing issues in providing the necessary services in the ED for psychiatry patients, geriatric patients included.[50] One primary concern is the ability to provide on-site coverage by a psychiatrist given the issues of limited workforce and cost,[52] especially in rural areas or emergency disaster situations.[50]

One increasingly utilized solution has been coverage through telepsychiatry—that is, mental health services through "real-time" long-distance audiovisual technology (e.g., WebEx, Jabber, and Zoom). Although variations of telehealth began in the 1950s, telehealth and telepsychiatry use have increased only relatively recently due to lower costs, faster electronic processing, Health Insurance Portability and Accountability Act (HIPAA)-compliant technology, increased agency approval for reimbursement, and greater public acceptance of technology in general and telehealth in particular.[50] Of particular relevance, SARS-CoV-2/COVID-19 has accelerated the use of telehealth and telepsychiatry as an effective means of exposure prevention, and greater accommodations have been made to reimburse such services.

Telepsychiatry in the ED with geriatric psychiatry patients may need to include camera control (e.g., physical examination, psychomotor symptoms, and extrapyramidal side effects) and staff assistance for patients who are delirious, combative, agitated, aphasic, hearing or vision impaired, homicidal, or suicidal.[52] Particular attention should be given to technology equipment that could pose patient safety issues (e.g., electrical cords for suicide).[50] Other technical issues include identifying and implementing technology that works given the unique circumstances for a given ED (e.g., ability for wireless communication to work in the ED), providing technological support (e.g., to fix glitches), training personnel (e.g., on how to use the new technology), redefining personnel roles (e.g., person responsible for setting up the technology to interface with the patient), and so on. In addition to HIPAA, legal issues include capacity and consent, duty to warn, access to firearms, licensure in different states (e.g., medical license, state-controlled substance license, and the Drug Enforcement Agency), malpractice insurance, and reimbursement regulations.[50]

Although more research is needed on the effectiveness of telepsychiatry in general, the literature suggests that telepsychiatry can be comparable to in-person services and may even have advantages for certain psychiatric disorders (e.g., anxiety) and locations (e.g., corrections and rural areas).[50] In particular, for the ED, telepsychiatry can increase efficiency by decreasing wait times and lengths of stay. However, more research is needed on telepsychiatry services for geriatric psychiatry patients in the ED, given the types of disorders encountered (e.g., delirium, dementia, depression, and suicidality) and accompanying issues that are addressed (e.g., decisional capacity and caregiver burden). Further details on the field of telepsychiatry in emergency services are presented in Chapter 5.

SARS-CoV-2/COVID-19

The coronavirus SARS-CoV-2/COVID 2019 (COVID-19) was discovered in Wuhan, China, in December 2019 and has yet to be fully understood by scientists.[53] What is known is that the virus is part of the coronavirus family, which is common in people, along with many other animals such as cattle, camels, cats, and bats. However, the COVID-19 virus is a novel (or new) coronavirus that was yet to be seen in humans.[53] COVID-19 spreads through person-to-person contact through airborne transmission and less commonly through contaminated surfaces, and it very rarely spreads from animal-to-person contact.[54]

Age is one of the most robust risk factors for both morbidity (e.g., hospitalization) and mortality (i.e., death) due to COVID-19 (Table 16.9).[55] Tragically, 95% of Americans who were killed by COVID-19 were aged 50 years or older.[56] For many individuals in the 50+ years age range, a mixture of chronic conditions, such as diabetes or cancer, along with an aging immune system creates conditions that allow for the virus to wreak havoc on this vulnerable population.[56]

Given the risk factors of age and medical condition comorbidity, higher rate of infection than that for the flu, and consequent morbidity and mortality, COVID-19 has major ramifications for serving geriatric psychiatry patients residing in such environments as nursing homes,[57] corrections, inpatient units, and the ED. The spread of COVID-19 can be prevented through distancing socially (keeping space of at least 6 feet from others), using face coverings when indoors, washing hands when possible, cleaning and disinfecting surfaces, and isolating and staying home when sick.[54]

In the case of the ED and providing psychiatric assessment and treatment services, prevention of COVID-19 is the first course of action. There must be clear procedures for screening, isolating, and treating COVID-19-positive patients in the ED. These procedures should include the use of personal protective equipment (gloves, medical masks, respirators, eye protection, gowns, aprons, and boots or closed-toe work shoes) and consideration of telepsychiatry as an option.

However, providing services to geriatric psychiatry patients in the emergency room within the context of COVID-19 is further complicated by the symptoms of delirium, dementia, and depression (e.g., confusion, agitation, and aggression), the common need for information from family members and caregivers despite social distancing, and the consideration of the negative impact of social isolation of the elderly.[58]

Table 16.9 Morbidity and Mortality of COVID-19 by Age Range

Age Range (Years)	Hospitalization	Death
18–29	Comparison group	Comparison group
30–39	2× higher	4× higher
40–49	3× higher	10× higher
50–64	4× higher	30× higher
65–74	5× higher	90× higher
75–84	8× higher	220× higher
85+	13× higher	630× higher

It is recommended that any COVID-19-positive patient requiring psychiatric admission be admitted to a COVID-19-specific medical unit and be kept in isolation for the appropriate quarantine time. Collaborative care between medical and psychiatric providers is essential in managing the sequelae of the virus and mental health symptoms. Telepsychiatry should be utilized, if available, to limit the chance of transmission. After the necessary quarantine time, if a patient still requires psychiatric stabilization, they may be transferred to an inpatient psychiatry unit.

Very encouraging has been the development of multiple vaccines (i.e., by Pfizer-BioNTech and Moderna) that appear to be highly effective and, currently, the prioritization of vaccination for high-risk individuals, including long-term care facility residents and the elderly, especially those with underlying medical conditions.[59]

References

1. The state of aging and health in America 2013. Centers for Disease Control and Prevention. Published 2013. https://stacks.cdc.gov/view/cdc/19146

2. Jeste DV, Alexopoulos GS, Bartels SJ, et al. Consensus statement on the upcoming crisis in geriatric mental health: Research agenda for the next 2 decades. *Arch Gen Psychiatry*. 1999;56(9):848–853.

3. Lebowitz BD, Pearson JL, Schneider LS, et al. Diagnosis and treatment of depression in late life: Consensus statement update. *JAMA*. 1997;278(14):1186–1190.

4. Aminzadeh F, Dalziel WB. Older adults in the emergency department: A systematic review of patterns of use, adverse outcomes, and effectiveness of interventions. *Ann Emerg Med*. 2002;39(3):238–247.

5. He W, Sengupta M, Velkoff VA, et al. 65+ in the United States: 2005. Current Population Reports No. P23-209, U.S. Census Bureau. U.S. Government Printing Office; 2005.

6. Hanlon JT, Schmader KE, Koronkowski MJ, et al. Adverse drug events in high risk older outpatients. *J Am Geriatr Soc*. 1997;45(8):945–948.

7. Mulsant BH, Pollack BG. Psychopharmacology. In: Blazer DF, Steffans DC, eds. *The American Psychiatric Publishing Textbook of Geriatric Psychiatry*. 4th ed. American Psychiatric Publishing; 2009:387–411.

8. Catterson ML, Preskorn SH, Martin RL. Pharmacodynamic and pharmacokinetic considerations in geriatric psychopharmacology. *Psychiatr Clin North Am*. 1997;20(1):205–218.

9. Sera LC, McPherson ML. Pharmacokinetics and pharmacodynamic changes associated with aging and implications for drug therapy. *Clin Geriatr Med*. 2012;28(2):273–286.

10. Centers for Disease Control and Prevention and National Association of Chronic Disease Directors. The state of mental health and aging in America Issue Brief 1: What do the data tell us? National Association of Chronic Disease Directors; 2008.

11. National Institute on Drug Abuse. Substance use in older adults DrugFacts. Published July 9, 2020. Accessed December 4, 2020. https://www.drugabuse.gov/publications/substance-use-in-older-adults-drugfacts

12. Elder abuse. World Health Organization. Published December 12, 2017. https://www.who.int/news-room/fact-sheets/detail/mental-health-of-older-adults

13. Walsh PG, Currier G, Shah MN, Lyness JM, Friedman B. Psychiatric emergency services for the U.S. elderly: 2008 and beyond. *Am J Geriatr Psychiatry*. 2008;16(9):706–717.

14. Betz ME, Boudreaux ED. Managing suicidal patients in the emergency department. *Ann Emerg Med.* 2016;67(2):276–282.

15. Kennedy M, Koehl J, Shenvi CL, et al. The agitated older adult in the emergency department: A narrative review of common causes and management strategies. *J Am Coll Emerg Physicians Open.* 2020;1(5):812–823.

16. Frank C, Hodgetts G, Puxty J. Safety and efficacy of physical restraints for the elderly: Review of the evidence. *Can Fam Physician.* 1996;42:2402–2409.

17. Appelbaum PS. Assessment of patients' competence to consent to treatment. *N Engl J Med.* 2007;357(18):1834–1840.

18. Marco CA, Derse AR. Refusal of life-saving therapy. In: Jesus J, Rosen P, Adams J, et al., eds. *Ethical Problems in Emergency Medicine: A Discussion-Based Review.* Wiley-Blackwell; 2012:89–97.

19. American Psychiatric Association. *Diagnostic and Statistical Manual of Mental Disorders.* American Psychiatric Publishing; 2013.

20. Oh ES, Fong TG, Hshieh TT, Inouye SK. Delirium in older persons. *JAMA.* 2017;318(12):1161–1174.

21. Thom RP, Levy-Carrick NC, Bui M, Silbersweig D. Delirium. *Am J Psychiatry.* 2019;176(10):785–793.

22. Inouye SK. Delirium in hospitalized older patients: Recognition and risk factors. *J Geriatr Psychiatry Neurol.* 1998;11:118–125, 157–158.

23. Dementia. World Health Organization. Retrieved December 15, 2020. https://www.who.int/news-room/fact-sheets/detail/dementia

24. Budson A, Solomon P. *Memory Loss: A Practical Guide for Clinicians.* Elsevier; 2011.

25. Meyers BS, Klimstra SA, Gabriele M, et al. Continuation treatment of delusional depression in older adults. *Am J Geriatr Psychiatry.* 2001;9(4):415–422.

26. Ahmed S, Leurent B, Sampson EL. Risk factors for incident delirium among older people in acute hospital medical units: A systematic review and meta-analysis. *Age Ageing.* 2014;43(3):326–333.

27. Inouye SK, Westendorp RG, Saczynski JS. Delirium in elderly people. *Lancet.* 2014;383(9920):911–922. doi:10.1016/S0140-6736(13)60688-1

28. Maldonado JR. Acute brain failure: Pathophysiology, diagnosis, management, and sequelae of delirium. *Crit Care Clin.* 2017;33(3):461–519.

29. Maldonado JR. Delirium pathophysiology: An updated hypothesis of the etiology of acute brain failure. *Int J Geriatr Psychiatry.* 2018;33(11):1428–1457.

30. Gower LE, Gatewood MO, Kang CS. Emergency department management of delirium in the elderly. *West J Emerg Med.* 2012;13(2):194–201.

31. Bouras C, Hof PR, Giannakopoulos P, Michel JP, Morrison JH. Regional distribution of neurofibrillary tangles and senile plaques in the cerebral cortex of elderly patients: A quantitative evaluation of a one-year autopsy population from a geriatric hospital. *Cerebral Cortex.* 1994;4(2):138–150.

32. Khouzam HR. The geriatric patient. In: *Handbook of Emergency Psychiatry.* Mosby Elsevier; 2007:307–399.

33. Caspi A, Sugden K, Moffitt TE, et al. Influence of life stress on depression: Moderation by a polymorphism in the 5-HTT gene. *Science.* 2003;301(5631):386–389.

34. Risk and protective factors. Centers for Disease Control and Prevention. n.d. https://www.cdc.gov/violenceprevention/suicide/riskprotectivefactors.html, 2021.

35. Downing LJ, Caprio TV, Lyness JM. Geriatric psychiatry review: Differential diagnosis and treatment of the 3 D's—delirium, dementia, and depression. *Curr Psychiatry Rep.* 2013;15(6):365.

36. Mariz J, Costa Castanho T, Teixeira J, Sousa N, Correia Santos N. Delirium diagnostic and screening instruments in the emergency department: An up-to-date systematic review. *Geriatrics.* 2016;1(3):22.

37. Kimchi EY, Neelagiri A, Whitt W, et al. Clinical EEG slowing correlates with delirium severity and predicts poor clinical outcomes. *Neurology.* 2019;93(13):e1260–e1271.

38. Dawson AH, Buckley NA. Pharmacological management of anticholinergic delirium—Theory, evidence and practice. *Br J Clin Pharmacol.* 2016;81(3):516–524.

39. Swart LM, van der Zanden V, Spies PE, de Rooij SE, van Munster BC. The comparative risk of delirium with different opioids: A systematic review. *Drugs Aging.* 2017;34(6):437–443.

40. Lonergan E, Luxenberg J, Areosa Sastre A. Benzodiazepines for delirium. *Cochrane Database Syst Rev.* 2009;2009(4):CD006379.

41. Neufeld KJ, Yue J, Robinson TN, et al: Antipsychotic medication for prevention and treatment of delirium in hospitalized adults: A systematic review and meta-analysis. *J Am Geriatr Soc.* 2016;64:705–714.

42. Huhn M, Nikolakopoulou A, Schneider-Thoma J, et al. Comparative efficacy and tolerability of 32 oral antipsychotics for the acute treatment of adults with multi-episode schizophrenia: A systematic review and network meta-analysis. *Lancet.* 2019;394(10202):939–951.

43. Sher Y, Miller Cramer AC, Ament A, Lolak S, Maldonado JR. Valproic acid for treatment of hyperactive or mixed delirium: Rationale and literature review. *Psychosomatics.* 2015;56(6):615–625.

44. Tariot, PN. Pharmacological treatment of neuropsychiatric symptoms of dementia. *JAMA.* 2005;293(18):2211–2212.

45. Han JH, Shintani A, Eden S, et al. Delirium in the emergency department: An independent predictor of death within 6 months. *Ann Emerg Med.* 2010;56(3):244–252.e1.

46. Tollefson GD, Bosomworth JC, Heiligenstein JH, Potcin JH, Holman S. A double-blind, placebo-controlled clinical trial of fluoxetine in geriatric patients with major depression: The Fluoxetine Collaborative Study Group. *Int Psychogeriatr.* 1995;7(1):89–104.

47. Robichaux GT Jr, Fitz-Gerald CM, Fitz-Gerald MJ. Special populations in psychiatric emergency services: The geriatric patient. In: Fitz-Gerald MJ, Takeshita J, eds. *Models of Emergency Psychiatric Services That Work.* Springer; 2020:189–199.

48. ACGME program requirements for graduate medical education in psychiatry. Accreditation Council for Graduate Medical Education. Published 2020. https://www.acgme.org/globalassets/pfassets/programrequirements/400_psychiatry_2022v2.pdf

49. ACGME program requirements for graduate medical education in geriatric psychiatry. Published 2020. Accreditation Council for Graduate Medical Education. https://www.acgme.org/globalassets/pfassets/programrequirements/407_geriatricpsychiatry_2022v2.pdf

50. Fitz-Gerald P, Park T. Telepsychiatry. In: Fitz-Gerald MJ, Takeshita J., eds. *Models of Emergency Psychiatric Services That Work.* Springer; 2020:153–164.

51. Gray NA, Takeshita J. Financial considerations for emergency psychiatry services. In: Fitz-Gerald MJ, Takeshita J, eds. *Models of Emergency Psychiatric Services That Work*. Springer; 2020:143–151.

52. Parekh R. Geriatric telepsychiatry. Published 2020. https://www.psychiatry.org/psychiatrists/practice/telepsychiatry/toolkit/geriatric-telepsychiatry

53. About COVID-19. Centers for Disease Control and Prevention. Published September 1, 2020. https://www.cdc.gov/aging/covid19/index.html

54. How COVID-19 spreads. Centers for Disease Control and Prevention. Published October 28, 2020. https://www.cdc.gov/coronavirus/2019-ncov/prevent-getting-sick/how-covid-spreads.html?CDC_AA_refVal=https%3A%2F%2Fwww.cdc.gov%2Fcoronavirus%2F2019-ncov%2Fprepare%2Ftransmission.html

55. Older adults. Centers for Disease Control and Prevention. Published December 13, 2020. https://www.cdc.gov/coronavirus/2019-ncov/your-health/about-covid-19.html

56. Nania R. 95 percent of Americans killed by COVID-19 were 50 or older. American Association of Retired Persons. Published October 30, 2020. https://www.aarp.org/health/conditions-treatments/info-2020/coronavirus-deaths-older-adults.html

57. Paulin E. Is extended isolation killing older adults in long-term care? American Association of Retired Persons. Published September 3, 2020. https://www.retirementresourceguide.com/2020/09/15/is-extended-isolation-killing-older-adults-in-long-term-care

58. National Academies of Sciences, Engineering, and Medicine. *Social isolation and loneliness in older adults: Opportunities for the health care system*. National Academies Press; 2020.

59. Vaccines for COVID-19. Centers for Disease Control and Prevention. Published December 13, 2020. https://www.cdc.gov/coronavirus/2019-ncov/vaccines/index.html

17

Developmental Disabilities

Justin Kuehl

Introduction

Individuals with developmental disabilities may present with genuine psychiatric emergencies within the context of a behavioral disturbance. Often, the emergency situation occurs secondary to an acute manifestation of threatening or dangerous behaviors. This can include verbal aggression, physical agitation, self-injurious behavior, or even suicidal behaviors. Whereas it is easy to recognize the emergency situation, it is far more difficult to determine the etiology of the disturbance, much less an effective intervention. In part, this can be attributed to a lack of formal instruction and clinical exposure to this population.

In many countries, there is little or no training offered during undergraduate preparation for medical school nor during the years of psychiatric specialization.[1] According to survey results from child and adolescent psychiatry fellowship programs, trainees will only see one to five patients per year with a diagnosis of either autism spectrum disorder (ASD) or intellectual disability (ID).[2] The same trainees will receive an average of 4 hours per year of lectures regarding ASD and 3 hours per year concerning ID. These findings clearly demonstrate the need for more education regarding the unique needs of this population. As such, this chapter provides information and recommendations for best practice.

In beginning to consider the complexities of working with individuals with developmental disabilities, it is important to note that the term "development disability" has a very broad definition. According to the Centers for Disease Control and Prevention,[3] developmental disabilities encompass "a group of conditions due to an impairment in physical, learning, language, or behavior areas." The condition must begin during the developmental period and persist throughout an individual's entire life. The disability also tends to have a direct impact on an individual's daily functioning. Based on these parameters, developmental disabilities include ID, ASD, cerebral palsy, attention-deficit/hyperactivity disorder (ADHD), learning disability, vision impairment, and hearing loss. In the United States, it is estimated that approximately one in six children aged 3–17 years have one or more developmental disabilities.

The fifth edition of the *Diagnostic and Statistical Manual of Mental Disorders* (DSM-5)[4] groups developmental disabilities in a section titled "Neurodevelopmental Disorders." This section includes three of the aforementioned developmental disabilities—ID, ASD, and ADHD—in addition to specific learning disorder.

It also encompasses several types of communication disorders, motor disorders, and other neurodevelopmental disorders. Given the sheer number of disorders that are included under this heading, it is necessary to narrow the scope of the discussion in this chapter. Most of the review and commentary pertain specifically to ID and/or ASD, so it is beneficial to provide a brief review of the DSM criteria for these two diagnoses.

Intellectual Disability

Within the diagnostic nomenclature, the term "intellectual disability" is still relatively new. The DSM-IV-TR[5] still utilized the term "mental retardation" as the correct descriptive label. There were three diagnostic criteria necessary to establish the diagnosis. First, the individual must present with deficits in intellectual functioning as confirmed by an IQ score of approximately 70 or less. Second, there must be deficits in adaptive functioning. These deficits have to occur in at least two of the following areas: communication, self-care, home living, social/interpersonal skills, use of community resources, self-direction, functional academic skills, work, leisure, health, and safety. Third, these deficits must be evident prior to the age of 18 years. The relative severity of the disability was further described using the specifiers mild, moderate, severe, and profound. These four specifiers were defined by corresponding 15- to 20-point decreases in an individual's IQ score.

With the introduction of the DSM-5, the three essential criteria remained intact, although the descriptions were modified. First, it is still necessary to identify deficits in intellectual functioning as confirmed by clinical evaluation and individualized standard IQ testing; however, the current criterion does not include the clear demarcation of an IQ score less than 70. This change was supported by the desire to shift the focus to deficits in adaptive functioning rather than the estimate of intellectual functioning. The change also acknowledges the fact that IQ scores become increasingly unreliable when testing an individual in the severe or profound range. Second, it remains necessary to identify deficits in adaptive functioning that significantly impact conceptual, social, and practical skills. Depending on the severity of the deficits in adaptive functioning, the individual will require progressively more support from others. As such, the four specifiers (mild, moderate, severe, and profound) are now associated with the deficits in adaptive functioning rather than the individual's IQ score. Table 17.1 offers a succinct comparison regarding this fundamental change between the two most recent versions of the DSM. Last, the onset of both intellectual and adaptive deficits still must occur during the

Table 17.1 DSM Criteria for Intellectual Disability

Diagnostic Specifier	Approximate Percentage Distribution by Specifier	DSM-IV-TR Criteria (Specifier Based on IQ Ranges)	DSM-5 Criteria (Specifier Based on Adaptive Functioning Deficits)
Mild	85	IQ range = 50–55 to approximately 70	Intermittent support needed
Moderate	10	IQ range = 35–40 to 50–55	Limited support needed
Severe	3–4	IQ range = 20–25 to 35–40	Extensive support needed
Profound	1–2	IQ range = <20 or 25	Pervasive support needed

From the American Psychiatric Association.[4,5]

developmental period. It is noteworthy that the DSM-5 avoids a firm cutoff (e.g., before age 18 years) and instead suggests that onset must occur in childhood or adolescence.

Autism Spectrum Disorder

In the DSM-IV-TR, there was a section titled "Pervasive Developmental Disorders." There were several disorders included in this section: autistic disorder, Asperger's disorder, pervasive developmental disorder, not otherwise specified (PDD-NOS), Rett's disorder, and childhood disintegrative disorder. As research continued to accumulate, the evidence suggested that these diagnoses were not easy to differentiate. It was also noted that autism presents across a spectrum ranging from mild types to increasingly severe. As a result, modifications to this diagnostic category were recommended.

The DSM-5 collapsed the aforementioned disorders into a single diagnosis, "autism spectrum disorder." This diagnosis requires three essential criteria. First, the individual must display persistent deficits in social communication and interaction. These deficits can manifest in several ways, such as poor social–emotional reciprocity, difficulty comprehending nonverbal communications, and challenges establishing and maintaining relationships with others. Second, the individual will display repetitive patterns of behaviors, interests, or activities. This must include at least two behavioral concerns, such as repetitive motor movements, inflexible routine or behaviors, fixated and extremely intense interests, and abnormal reactions to sensory input. Third, the symptoms must occur in the early developmental period. Table 17.2 offers a visual perspective of the three essential diagnostic criteria and a few behavioral examples.

Comorbidity with Mental Illness

Challenges in Identifying Co-Occurring Mental Illness

There is a general lack of research regarding the co-occurrence of intellectual and developmental disability (IDD) and mental illness.[6] Numerous factors have contributed to this issue. The heterogeneity of the term "developmental disability" presents a fundamental challenge for researchers because they must choose what specific disorders should be included or excluded in a study. Researchers also struggle with changes in the categorization of developmental disabilities over the course of time. For example, the DSM-IV-TR categorized ASD as an "Axis I" disorder, which presents the conundrum of whether it should be considered as a co-occurring "psychiatric" disorder or as a developmental disability. There are also other diagnostic systems besides the DSM. For example, the various editions of the *International Classification of Diseases* (ICD) use diagnostic criteria that are quite similar to the DSM; however, this still presents a dilemma when trying to conduct comparable research.

In the available research literature, there is little consistency regarding what diagnoses should be included as examples of co-occurring mental illness. It is common to include various types of serious and persistent mental illness, such as all psychotic disorders and major mood disorders. There is less consideration for other types of mental illness, such as adjustment disorders or substance use disorders. There is also variability in the research literature regarding whether "challenging behaviors" should be identified as a

Table 17.2 DSM-5 Criteria for Autism Spectrum Disorder

Diagnostic Criteria	Behavioral Examples
A. Persistent deficits in social communication and social interaction (must present with all 3)	
1. Deficits in social–emotional reciprocity	Abnormal social approach and failure of normal back-and-forth conversation Reduced sharing of interests, emotions, or affect Failure to initiate or respond to social interactions
2. Deficits in nonverbal communicative behaviors	Poorly integrated verbal and nonverbal communication Abnormalities in eye contact and body language Deficits in understanding the use of gestures Total lack of facial expression and nonverbal communication
3. Deficits in developing, maintaining, and understanding relationships	Difficulty adjusting behavior to suit various social contexts Difficulty sharing in imaginative play or in making friends Absence of interests in peers
B. Restricted, repetitive patterns of behavior, interests, or activities (at least 2 of 4)	
1. Stereotyped or repetitive motor movements, use of objects, or speech	Simple motor stereotypies Lining up toys Flipping objects Echolalia Idiosyncratic phrases
2. Insistence on sameness, inflexible adherence to routines, or ritualized patterns of verbal or nonverbal behavior	Extreme distress at small changes Difficulties with transitions Rigid thinking patterns Greeting rituals Need to take same route Need to eat same food every day
3. Highly restricted, fixated interests that are abnormal in intensity or focus	Strong attachment to or preoccupation with unusual objects Excessively circumscribed or perseverative interests
4. Hyper- or hyporeactivity to sensory input or unusual interest in sensory aspects of the environment	Apparent indifference to pain/temperature Adverse response to specific sounds or textures Excessive smelling or touching of objects Visual fascination with lights or movement
C. Symptoms must be present in the early developmental period	

From the American Psychiatric Association.[4]

co-occurring issue. Severe behavioral disturbances are not part of the diagnostic criteria for ID; however, they should not necessarily be categorized as a uniquely separate co-occurring issue.[6]

There are also inconsistencies regarding the methods of data collection and the selection of appropriate subjects.[7] Given that individuals with IDD present with variable levels of comprehension and expressive verbal abilities, there is a frequent need to rely on caregivers to provide the data. Some research studies rely on questionnaires or checklists that gather self-reported measures completed by parents, legal guardians, or direct support professionals. This raises inherent concerns regarding the accuracy of diagnostic impressions. In other studies, trained professionals utilize professional interviews and structured tools to reach diagnostic conclusions. These studies may produce more reliable and valid diagnoses, yet even these more rigorous methods fail to address the most significant limitation.

Until the second half of the 20th century, it was generally believed that individuals with ID could not also experience mental health problems.[8] It was thought that deficits in cognitive functioning precluded individuals from subjectively experiencing distress (e.g., feelings of depression or anxiety). These beliefs perpetuated the notion of "diagnostic overshadowing," a term first used in the research literature in 1982.[9] This refers to the tendency for clinicians to attribute symptoms or behaviors to an IDD and underdiagnose the presence of comorbid psychopathology. For example, an individual with IDD likely will experience problems with executive functioning that can result in behavioral disinhibition. Although diminished self-control could be appropriately attributed to the IDD, this does not preclude the possibility of other plausible explanations. Disinhibition is a common symptom associated with a manic episode. Likewise, an individual with a psychotic disorder may exhibit disorganized behavior as a primary symptom. It is also possible that a substance use disorder may be a contributing factor. The sheer number of plausible explanations highlights the challenges in identifying co-occurring disorders.

There have been efforts to help facilitate accurate identification of mental illness in individuals with IDD. The National Association for the Dually Diagnosed developed the *Diagnostic Manual—Intellectual Disability: A Clinical Guide for Diagnosis of Mental Disorders in Persons with Intellectual Disability* (DM-ID). The original edition was published in 2007, which correlated with DSM-IV-TR diagnoses. A subsequent edition was published in 2017 to align with the DSM-5. The text serves as an excellent reference for practitioners and researchers. For many disorders, the DSM diagnostic criteria are carefully modified such that they are increasingly applicable for individuals with ID. It also highlights the need for practitioners to adapt their methods of eliciting certain clinical information (e.g., relying on behavioral observations more than verbal self-report). The DM-ID is not the only effort to adapt diagnostic criteria for individuals with IDD and co-occurring psychiatric disorders. The DC-LD is another example of a system developed in England, which serves to compliment ICD-10 and DSM-IV-TR criteria.[10]

Estimated Prevalence of Co-Occurring Mental Illness

Although individuals with IDD can experience the same mental disorders as the general population, estimates of prevalence have varied substantially. In the United States, some of the best data derive from the National Core Indicators (NCI). This project aims to gather annual data from state-level agencies that provide services to individuals with ID. Respondents are considered to be dually diagnosed when they report at least one of the following categories of mental health conditions in addition to ID: mood disorder, anxiety disorder, psychotic disorder, or other mental health diagnosis. Based on survey data that were collected in 2017 and 2018 in 35 states and the District of Columbia, approximately 48% out of 22,513 respondents met the criteria for a dual diagnosis.[11] At the individual state level, the percentages ranged from 34% to 64%.

Some the best prevalence data derive from Europe and particularly the United Kingdom. One of the more rigorous studies to assess prevalence rates was conducted by Cooper et al.[12] They completed a large-scale population-based study in England that included 1,023 participants. The results varied depending on which diagnostic system was applied. The point prevalence rate of co-occurring mental illness was 40.9% using clinical diagnostic criteria, 32.5% with the DC-LD, 16.6% with the ICD-10-DCR, and 15.7% with the DSM-IV-TR. These rates of comorbidity included a wide range of mental illnesses, but it is worth noting that the most common co-occurring diagnostic category was simply "problem behavior." These results suggest there are elevated rates of mental illness in this population, although they also highlight the difficulty in determining what diagnostic categories should be included in a research study.

Another robust study from Europe utilized Scotland's 2011 census data and assessed the prevalence of mental health conditions among individuals with ID.[13] Of note, the census achieved an estimated 94% response rate, which possibly makes this the largest and most complete population study available. The overall rate of ID in the population was 0.5%. Of those individuals with ID, the rate of mental health conditions was 21.7% compared to a rate of 4.3% in the rest of the general population. This study was not without limitations. The term "mental health conditions" was very broadly defined, and the census data were gathered via self-reports. For many individuals with ID, the responses were likely provided by proxies (e.g., a parent or professional caregiver), and this would also impact the reliability of the data. Nevertheless, these findings strongly suggest that individuals with ID have substantially higher rates of mental health problems than the general population.

Despite a relative dearth of research and associated limitations, it appears clear that there are elevated rates of certain psychiatric disorders within the IDD population. Based on this premise, there will be emergencies related to the exacerbation of psychiatric symptoms. A thorough evaluation would be necessary to determine the best intervention and course of treatment; however, the ability to conduct such an assessment relies on a practitioner's skill in correctly identifying the underlying condition. Subsequent sections of this chapter delineate many important considerations in order to complete a good assessment.

Psychiatric Assessment of Individuals with IDD

Identifying the Presenting Problem

Some individuals with IDD will exhibit challenging behaviors that are difficult to manage in the community setting, which can result in an emergency situation. By definition, a challenging behavior occurs with either "such intensity, frequency or duration that the physical safety of the person or others is placed in serious jeopardy or [that] behavior which is likely to seriously limit or deny access to the use of ordinary community facilities."[14] There are data that illustrate the incidence rate of challenging behaviors. According to NCI survey results collected during 2012 and 2013, 43% of 12,718 respondents required at least some or even extensive support to manage challenging behaviors.[14] Of those requiring any amount of support, 51% needed support for self-injurious behavior, 87% required support for disruptive behavior, and 55% received support for destructive behavior. These individuals were significantly more likely to have been diagnosed with one or more co-occurring mental illnesses. More than three-fourths of respondents requiring support were prescribed at least one kind of medication for a mood disorder, anxiety disorder, behavior challenges, psychotic disorder, or other mental illness. Based on these data, it is no wonder that many individuals with IDD present with psychiatric emergencies.

Additional analysis of NCI data provides a more in-depth look at self-injurious behavior (SIB), which is defined as self-inflicted harmful behavior that can result in injury and cumulative physical damage.[15] Based on the 2015–2016 administration of the Adult Consumer Survey, which included 15,581 responses, 17.8% indicated a need for some support to manage SIB and 5.4% expressed a need for extensive support. Individuals who required any amount of support were significantly more likely to have a co-occurring mental illness, such as a mood disorder, an anxiety disorder, and/or a psychotic disorder. Also of note, individuals exhibiting SIB were less likely to use verbal communications. This compounds the difficult in assessing these individuals and further complicates the ability to ascertain the etiology of the behavior.

In addition to self-injurious behavior, it is also imperative to consider the potential for suicide in this population. In the past, it was believed that low intelligence served as a buffer against suicidal thoughts and behaviors because individuals did not have the cognitive capacity to conceptualize, plan, or act on these thoughts.[16] This misconception may still contribute to the ongoing lack of well-designed research studies on this topic.[17] Contrary to this belief, the available literature does support the notion that suicidality must be evaluated in this population. Many of the same risk factors that are known in the general population apply to this population (e.g., women are more likely to attempt suicide, but men are more likely to succeed). A history of abuse, family instability, and lack of social support are also common risk factors. In summary, the potential for suicide exists in this population and may correlate with the onset of a behavioral crisis.

Gathering Collateral Information

Gathering reliable collateral information should be at the forefront of any emergency situation involving individuals with IDD. Although time is of the essence when conducting an assessment, there are a multitude of reasons why it is essential to thoroughly complete this process. Caregivers can offer some of the most crucial information in order to formulate an accurate diagnosis and develop the best course of treatment. In taking a moment to reflect on the importance of their role, it can be helpful to regard them as the true "experts" concerning the individual with IDD. Whether as a parent, legal guardian, or direct support professional (DSP), caregivers spend many hours with the individual compared to practitioners who have a very time-limited interaction while performing the clinical assessment. As such, it is recommended that practitioners remain keenly aware of the valuable information that caregivers can provide.

According to survey data collected as part of the NCI, individuals with a dual diagnosis of mental illness and intellectual disability are significantly more likely to live in a group residential setting.[11] As such, there is an increased likelihood that a DSP employed by an agency will have access to much of the individual's relevant health information. The DSP should have documentation (e.g., a health log) that summarizes an individual's medical history, relevant diagnoses, prescribed medications, and recent appointments. It is also beneficial to ask if the individual with IDD has a behavioral support plan, which will identify the frequency, intensity, and recommended interventions for any challenging behaviors. A formal plan should provide a comprehensive summary, which can serve to quickly convey salient information to a practitioner.

When gathering self-reported information from a DSP, it can be useful to ask about the duration of their professional relationship with the individual. A DSP who has long-standing rapport may be attuned to even subtle changes in behavior. A practitioner can inquire about the individual's baseline behavior and then ask about any recent changes. This should include questions about changes that may correlate with various psychiatric disorders (e.g., sleep, appetite, and mood). The correct identification of such behavioral changes strongly contributes to an accurate diagnosis.

A caregiver can help identify various psychosocial stressors that may be contributing to a behavioral crisis. It is reasonable to predict a psychiatric emergency within the context of a significant stressor such as moving to a new residence, starting a new job/day program, or the death of a loved one. Other changes that may seem rather minor could in fact serve as significant triggers for an individual with IDD. For example, the cancelation of a scheduled visit with family could lead to a behavioral crisis for a residential provider. Likewise, a change in the regularly assigned DSP could result in issues for other covering staff members. It is particularly important to inquire about changes in routine when evaluating an individual with ASD. "Insistence on sameness" and "inflexible adherence to routines" are explicitly included in the DSM-5 diagnostic criteria, so any changes warrant heightened consideration because they could help explain the cause of a behavioral crisis.

Last, a caregiver should be able to provide some insight regarding an individual's preferred communication style and any relevant deficits. A sign language interpreter may be necessary to conduct the evaluation. Individuals with deficits in expressive language may benefit from the use of visual aids, pictures, or diagrams. Other individuals may present with idiosyncratic methods of communication, which caregivers may understand and be able to assist with interpreting them. Additional considerations regarding communication are discussed in more depth later in this chapter.

Despite all the benefits offered by collateral informants, it is also necessary to maintain a healthy skepticism regarding the veracity of their reports. The provision of care for individuals with IDD can correlate with stress and burnout. The corresponding pressure to alleviate a challenging behavior and resume "normal" functioning becomes a primary goal. As such, caregivers may exaggerate symptoms and ultimately advocate for certain outcomes (e.g., requests for medication changes or admission to an inpatient hospital) even when this level of intervention may not be warranted. In summary, it is important to provide a supportive and empathetic opportunity that allows the caregiver to be heard while still maintaining appropriate objectivity.

Verifying the IDD Diagnosis

Prior to beginning a psychiatric assessment, it is beneficial to try to verify the presence of an IDD. Many psychiatric evaluations begin with the assertion that an individual "seems" to have cognitive limitations or "appears" to have an intellectual disability. Although certain elements of a good clinical interview and mental status exam can help verify the presence of a developmental disability, it can be exceedingly difficult to achieve a valid new diagnosis in the context of an emergency situation. For example, there are simply not enough time and/or resources to complete a standardized test of intelligence. A reliable test such as the Wechsler Adult Intelligence Scale–Fourth Edition can take 60–90 minutes when administered by a trained professional. Likewise, a thorough assessment of adaptive functioning relies on the use of other standardized measures that are very time-consuming. Even if there were an opportunity to conduct a formal and thorough assessment, it would be unreasonable to complete such testing due to the likelihood of invalid results (i.e., an individual likely could not put forth their best effort in the midst of a crisis). Based on these factors, it is preferably to seek a diagnosis provided by a reliable collateral source.

In the absence of a verified diagnosis, it is essential to proceed with caution rather than make a definitive determination. When there is any degree of diagnostic uncertainty, it is preferable to list the IDD as a provisional diagnosis. The use of this specifier will still convey the strong presumption that an IDD exists; however, it also indicates a degree of reluctance due to the absence of essential information. Likewise, a clinician could choose to list the developmental disability as a "rule out" diagnosis as a means to alert future practitioners of the suspected diagnosis.

It is worth noting the significant ramifications of inaccurate diagnostic work. The documentation authored by a practitioner has "staying power" as part of an individual's medical record. Often, a singular diagnosis of an ID serves as the basis for future practitioners to justify their own conclusions. For example, a practitioner may reference "per review of the medical record" and utilize a prior diagnosis in making the current one. To many nonclinicians (e.g., researchers, auditors, quality assurance personnel, and managed care organizations), a diagnosis is frequently viewed as a definitive medical decision. As a result, an initial misdiagnosis can serve to perpetuate itself to the degree that it becomes immutable fact.

It is also important to consider the sources of funding for long-term support services. In the past, the services for individuals with developmental disabilities and mental health needs were integrated into single state departments.[18] Over time, there has been increasing variability regarding how each state finances and monitors publicly funded programs. Due to further budget constraints and a narrowing of eligibility criteria, it has become increasingly difficult for individuals to access the proper services to address their needs. Therefore, a single misdiagnosis can have a long-term impact by relegating an individual into the wrong service delivery system. The individual may not receive optimum care nor will their needs be met in the best way. In summary, there are many reasons to exercise care and caution when making diagnostic decisions.

Communication Issues

A typical diagnostic assessment relies heavily on self-reported symptoms and the ability to provide subjective descriptions of experiences and feelings. Although this is the standard approach for psychiatric evaluations, it is not reasonable for individuals with IDD due to limitations in communication. Most individuals will experience varying degrees of deficits in both expressive and receptive language.[6] Therefore, it is necessary to account for these issues and modify various aspects of the evaluation accordingly.

There are a few general recommendations that can positively influence the entire interview. First, it is important to speak directly to the individual with IDD. Often, there is a tendency to talk about an individual with a disability rather than to them. By maintaining a person-centered approach, there is an increased likelihood for full engagement and cooperation. Second, it is important to be mindful of the vocabulary used during the evaluation. It needs to be appropriate to the developmental level of the individual, and it is beneficial to use simple sentences, speak slowly, and pause frequently. The use of medical jargon should also be avoided. Third, the interview questions should consist of clear and unambiguous language. This will help reduce confusion and the need for further clarification. It is best to use concrete language when formulating questions (e.g., "Do you feel sad?") as opposed to more abstract language (e.g., "How do you feel?"). The need for clarity is further exemplified when assessing for the presence of auditory hallucinations. Presenting the question, "Do you hear voices?" will routinely elicit an affirmative response unless additional clarification is sought. The practitioner should explain that genuine hallucinations are categorically different than "self-talk" or other examples of normal internal dialogue.

For individuals with mild to moderate ID, the limitations in both receptive and expressive language will be minimal. Nevertheless, these individuals may have other barriers to fully expressing themselves. If they do not completely understand a question, it may be easier to simply answer "yes" or "no" rather than asking for clarification. This can be an adaptive way of minimizing or even masking their disability, which often is a learned approach to cope with difficult situations. These individuals may also be aware of the inherent power differential between practitioners and patients. They may strive to appease the practitioner by providing responses that they believe are most favorable. In order to mitigate the potential for these issues to arise, the practitioner should be sure to ask additional clarifying questions as needed.

For individuals with severe and even profound ID, receptive language tends to be better than expressive language. This can lead to frustration given that individuals may understand the questions but will experience an inability to convey adequate responses. As previously noted, the practitioner should consider the use of additional means of communication (e.g., visual aids, pictures, or diagrams) to further support the process of communication. The use of gestures can also be helpful in these situations.

Communication deficits are one of the most apparent characteristics for individuals on the autism spectrum. As such, the clinical interview may present challenges because the usual reciprocity of verbal interactions likely will not occur. Some individuals will present with stilted or overly literal speech. Others may display issues with echolalia (i.e., the tendency to repeat the exact words that were uttered). In addition, these individuals likely will not read the nonverbal cues that typically help convey verbal language. This includes an inability to fully appreciate social cues, facial expressions, and tone of voice. An awareness of these factors can help the practitioner temper the validity of the clinical interview and focus on other available clinical information.

Comprehension Issues

For individuals with IDD, it is reasonable to presume there are associated deficits in comprehension. Their ability to understand will be impaired secondary to difficulties in adequately receiving information, evaluating it, and reaching reasonable conclusions.

Ultimately, this will impact their judgment and overall assessment of a situation. Although these challenges will be present at baseline, they are more than likely exacerbated in the midst of a crisis situation. With these considerations in mind, it is essential for the practitioner to approach the evaluation with a modified perspective.

For example, a risk assessment for suicide would need to be adapted depending on an individual's level of comprehension. As part of any standard risk assessment, the practitioner will routinely inquire about any recent suicidal thoughts or plan. The practitioner will also consider the underlying intent of any suicide attempt. Based on these factors, the practitioner will ascribe a risk level and determine the appropriate interventions and course of treatment. In the case of an individual with ID, the plan and intent should be assessed with consideration of impaired judgment and reasoning. The individual may believe that ingesting a few pills amounts to a lethal overdose. Although the practitioner will have the knowledge of what constitutes a harmful dose, it is essential not to base clinical judgment solely on the factual evidence. In this situation, the intent of the suicide attempt must be considered relative to the individual's cognitive deficits.

Due to impairments in comprehension and judgment, many individuals with IDD will have a substitute decision-maker (e.g., parent or legal guardian). Nevertheless, it remains important to engage them in the decision-making process. A lack of decisionality should not imply a lack of interest, nor does it suggest that the individual does not have an opinion. On the contrary, a person-centered practitioner will continue to fully involve the individual in the assessment process. This is empowering for the individual, and it helps establish and maintain therapeutic rapport, which will likely yield a better overall assessment.

Medical Comorbidities

Individuals with IDD have a greater tendency to either underreport or inaccurately report physical pain and discomfort. Therefore, it is the responsibility of the provider to consider the possibility that underlying medical comorbidities are a contributing factor in a behavioral crisis. It can be beneficial to conduct a good review of systems with a keen awareness of potential sources of pain or distress. Although it is not possible to review all scenarios in this chapter, there are some medical issues that frequently occur within this population.

It can be beneficial to consider whether sensory issues are a contributing factor in behavioral crises. Based on a review of the literature by Owen et al.,[19] vision problems are far more common among individuals with ID. This includes issues such as refractive errors, strabismus, cataracts, and keratoconus. If visual deficits are not adequately identified and addressed, they could contribute to barriers in communication and overall frustration for an individual. Likewise, there could be problems related to any condition that diminishes an individual's ability to hear. A simple ear infection can cause significant irritability, pain, and overall distress. For individuals with limited verbal language, these physical symptoms can be the primary causal factors in a behavioral crisis.

There is a greater tendency for individuals with ID to display poor oral hygiene, which contributes to problems such as dental caries, gingivitis, and periodontal disease.[19] Several factors that may contribute to these findings. Many individuals with IDD experience decreased physical coordination, which can create challenges in completing daily dental care. There also may be an aversion to attending routine dental checkups, which reduces the opportunity for preventative care and further exacerbates any existing issues. As a result, the onset of associated pain may be expressed through maladaptive behaviors leading to a crisis.

Without the benefit of a verbal self-report, it can be exceedingly difficult to determine when someone is suffering from a headache. Furthermore, the etiology of headaches varies widely, which also makes intervention difficult. For example, seasonal allergies can create sinus congestion and serve as the precipitating factor in need of treatment. Individuals with known seizure activity can experience headaches during either the prodromal stage or the postictal phase. The onset of migraine headaches could also clearly correlate with a behavioral response. If migraine headaches are suspected, it may be beneficial to encourage prophylactic treatments.[20]

Gastrointestinal problems are common in individuals with IDD. Disorders such as gastroesophageal reflux disease and irritable bowel syndrome can contribute to several distressing symptoms, including coughing, choking, sore throat, diarrhea, bloating, constipation, and fecal impaction.[21] Any one of these symptoms could be expressed through disruptive behavior. Another disorder that may co-occur in this population is pica, which poses its own concerns such as constipation, blockages, or infections. Food allergies are also a necessary consideration given the associated distress.

As a final consideration, it can be useful to order routine lab work to help to rule out underlying medical concerns. A simple urinalysis can help detect whether a urinary tract infection is contributing to pain and discomfort. Likewise, an individual with a known thyroid disorder would benefit from a thyroid-stimulating hormone test to measure the hormone level. Given that hyperthyroidism can mimic the symptoms of a manic episode and hypothyroidism can look like a depressive episode, it is essential to first consider other courses of treatment.

Psychopharmacology

Any psychiatric evaluation includes a review of the individual's current medication list. For individuals with IDD, there are several unique factors that require additional consideration. Based on the prevalence rates that were previously discussed, it is clear that mental illness co-occurs with IDD. When this is the case, it can be appropriate to treat the symptoms of the mental illness with the usual psychotropic medications; however, very few medications have been specifically tested in individuals with IDD.[22] In part, this is due to the inherent challenges in conducting ethical research with this vulnerable population (issues regarding consent, difficulty assessing outcomes, etc.). Potential research opportunities are further complicated by the fact that psychotropic medications are often prescribed to address challenging behaviors rather than a co-occurring mental illness.

Second-generation antipsychotic medications have been prescribed to address challenging behaviors, and there is evidence to support their use. The U.S. Food and Drug Administration has approved the use of both aripiprazole and risperidone for individuals with ASD, and additional research suggests that one is not better than the other in treating irritability in children and adolescent.[23] On the contrary, Tyrer et al.[24] conducted a large multisite study comparing haloperidol, risperidone, and placebo for aggression in non-psychotic individuals with ID and found no benefit over placebo. In addition to the antipsychotic medications, mood stabilizers (particularly anticonvulsants) have also been used to address behavioral concerns such as aggression. Some antidepressant medications that are known to address symptoms of obsessive–compulsive disorder have been used as treatment for the repetitive behaviors in ASD. Certain benzodiazepines have been prescribed for their calming effects. Although each class of medications offers some benefits, there are additional concerns that must be considered.

Again, it is important to acknowledge that individuals with IDD will likely experience limitations in their ability to self-report symptoms. This makes the identification of medication side effects more difficult. It is incumbent on practitioners to thoroughly consider the known side effects of various medications. For example, a number of psychotropic medications can cause akathisia. For individuals with deficits in expressive language, it is difficult to describe their subjective experience, and the practitioner needs to primarily rely on behavioral observations to identify this side effect. Some of the psychotropic medications can lower the seizure threshold, which is a concern given that 25% of individuals with ID have comorbid epilepsy.[25] In these cases, the individual may be prescribed increasing amounts of anticonvulsant medications although this can lead to an increased risk of drug interactions. Some other medications will have anticholinergic side effects resulting in dry mouth, constipation, or urinary retention that could have a causal relationship with challenging behaviors. Benzodiazepines may provide a desired sedative effect; however, there is also an increased likelihood for behavioral disinhibition that could compound existing problems.[26] By no means should this serve as an exhaustive list of potential side effects, but it highlights the need to carefully consider relevant possibilities. Often, medication side effects are not identified, and they are addressed as additional behavioral problems in need of treatment.

It is important to reflect on the overall utilization of medications in this population. Hellings and Jain[21] note that individuals with ID take an average of 10 medications per day for treatment of physical and psychiatric diagnoses. The NCI survey data suggest similar concerning trends regarding medications specifically for psychiatric conditions and behavior challenges. Hiersteiner and Bradley[14] reported that 15% of 12,718 respondents took medications as treatment for four different reasons (i.e., mood disorder, anxiety disorder, psychotic disorder, and behavior challenges). They also noted that 6% of all respondents reportedly did not need behavioral support nor had they been diagnosed with behavioral challenges, yet they still were prescribed medication for behavioral challenges. These data suggest there is an overreliance on the use of medications. They also highlight the difficulty in determining whether each medication has beneficial or detrimental effects.

Prescribing medications for individuals with IDD involves a great deal of complexity. The difficulty in making accurate diagnoses and the risks of deleterious side effects are great. As such, there are a few reasonable guidelines for consideration. First, the best pharmacological treatments are directly linked to a valid psychiatric diagnosis. Again, this highlights the need for thoughtful and accurate diagnostic work. Second, if possible, polypharmacology should be avoided. The drug interactions make it exceedingly difficult to ascertain which medications are the most effective (or even necessary). Third, it is good practice to start with the minimum recommended dose of a medication and then wait to ascertain the effects. Subsequent increases should also be minimal in order to help provide additional clarity regarding the benefits of the medication.

Trauma

As part of any thorough crisis assessment, it is essential to inquire about any history of trauma. This should begin with consideration for any past significant traumatic experiences. The IDD population has a substantially higher rate of victimization. Serious violent victimization (e.g., rape, sexual assault, robbery, or aggravated assault) has been reported to be three times higher for individuals with disabilities.[27] This statistic does not account for other instances of significant abuse or neglect. The probability of these negative experiences increases for individuals who have resided in congregate settings such as large institutions or group homes. As a result of such events, there is a greater likelihood of developing post-traumatic stress disorder (PTSD); however, it is difficult to accurately make this diagnosis.

As with other psychiatric disorders, the criteria for PTSD are not easily identified or applied to individuals with IDD. The details regarding a traumatic event may be difficult to ascertain given the limitations in self-report for individuals with communication deficits. It is essential for caregivers to provide the information, yet the details may not be known, reported, or recognized.[28] It is also difficult to distinguish the essential symptoms associated with PTSD.[29] The re-experiencing of a traumatic event may be displayed through observable maladaptive behaviors, which sometimes includes self-injurious behavior. Likewise, hyperarousal can present as agitation or acting-out behavior. The avoidance of stimuli associated with the trauma can be misinterpreted as noncompliance. Therefore, the collateral information and any challenging behaviors must be considered within the context of any known history of trauma.

Practitioners tend to agree on serious incidents that constitute significant trauma. It can be far more difficult to gauge the relative severity of other experiences that can be just as traumatic. In her work developing eye movement desensitization and reprocessing as an effective treatment for trauma, Francine Shapiro was the first to introduce the concepts of "big T trauma" and "little t trauma." The big T trauma events are evident: rape, abuse, disasters, etc. The little t traumas occur repeatedly over the course of time and can have a similar disruptive impact. Harvey[30] expanded on these ideas by suggesting that individuals with IDD experience an increased frequency of little t trauma throughout their lives. Seemingly minor events such as name-calling, teasing, and exclusion can have cumulative impacts on individuals. If this is part of their history, then a new event can cause a similar retriggering of these past negative experiences. It may even correlate with the behavioral disturbance that led to the crisis event. Therefore, it is essential to ask caregivers about any social interactions that may have precipitated the psychiatric emergency. Likewise, it is important to ask the individual with IDD whether something had been irritating them and how it may be related to past events.

It is also important to view significant life events through the trauma perspective. Certain stressors may not be perceived as overly significant by a practitioner, yet they are experienced that way by the individual with IDD. Hastings et al.[31] noted an association between recent life events and general psychiatric problems. Some examples of the most frequently occurring life events included moving residence, serious illness or injury to self, serious illness or problems for a close relative or friend, and death of a close family friend or other relative. They found that the presence of one or more of such life stressors was predictive of psychiatric problems. Likewise, Lunsky and Elserafi[32] further correlated the experience of stressful life events and emergency department visits. They noted six specific life events that increased the likelihood of a hospital visit: a move of house or residence; serious problem with family, friend, or caregiver; problems with police or other authority; unemployment for more than 1 month; recent trauma/abuse; and drug or alcohol problems. These studies offer a salient reminder that stressful situations can be predictive of psychiatric crisis, which emphasizes the need to assess for their presence.

Through a person-centered approach, it is important for a practitioner to take the perspective of the individual with IDD and consider whether other stressors may be contributing factors. For individuals who are living in supported settings, such as group homes, many of the freedoms that are taken for granted are not available to them. For example, personal privacy is limited in a congregate setting. Freedom of choice may be quite limited (e.g., bedtimes are established, meal plans are made, and schedules are organized). Although it is hoped that individuals have some input into these decisions, this often is not the case. This can produce conflict with caregivers and/or peers, which results in stress for the individual. Therefore, it is essential to take these into consideration because the resolution of such conflicts may defuse the crisis situation.

As part of this discussion regarding trauma assessment, it is also important to briefly reflect on the potential use of restraints. In the midst of a behavioral crisis, practitioners maintain a duty to keep the individual and others safe from harm. As the threat of physical aggression increases, the use of a brief manual hold or more extensive forms of restraint may be necessary; however, it is important to reflect on the individual's past experiences. If the individual had been a victim of abuse, the restraint can serve as a trigger to those memories. The individual may react with an increased amount of aggression as a "fight or flight" response is initiated. As such, it is highly recommended that the use of restraints remains an absolute last resort for individuals with IDD.

Conclusion

When a behavioral crisis occurs in a community setting, there are only a few available options. Certainly, caregivers can attempt to work though the crisis on their own. If the situation poses a significant threat of danger to the individual or others, caregivers could reach out to law enforcement for assistance. As another option, caregivers may seek emergency psychiatric services. In such situations, it is important for practitioners to provide thoughtful diagnostic services and evidence-based care. This begins by actively listening to the concerns shared by caregivers and demonstrating responsivity to their needs.

Caregivers provide constant care for individuals with IDD, which is an enormous responsibility that is relatively unheralded. Often, the physical, emotional, and mental toll can result in caregiver burnout. This mostly occurs when caregivers do not receive the adequate support that they need. So when challenging behaviors do occur, the caregivers deserve additional help to address the situation. They are seeking professional opinions and guidance from highly educated practitioners. As such, it is incumbent to offer this support rather than hastily turn them away, which fosters a sense of helplessness and generates feelings of isolation.

It is also important to acknowledge that individuals with IDD are chronically underserved by the health care system. Being turned away in the midst of an emergency situation further contributes to this disparity in care. Therefore, it is essential to offer equitable care and to consider the possibility that the individual has a treatable condition. This begins with a thorough assessment and an accurate diagnosis, which will yield the best possible outcome. As noted in this chapter, diagnostic certainty can only be achieved when practitioners account for the uniqueness of this population. Astute practitioners will modify their standard clinical evaluations to account for deficits in communication and comprehension. It is important to remember that observable behavior is a form of communication that can guide the evaluative process. Furthermore, it is imperative to never overlook the potential impacts of co-occurring medical conditions (especially ones that cause pain or discomfort), the effects/side effects of medications, and any history of trauma.

As a core principle of the Hippocratic Oath, there is a duty to "help the sick." Individuals with developmental disabilities are not "sick," but they do deserve the benefit of a thorough assessment that can accurately identify the presence of co-occurring psychiatric or medical conditions which can be managed and/or mitigated. It is our responsibility to rise to this challenge.

References

1. Deb S, Kwok H, Bertelli M, et al. International guide to prescribing psychotropic medication for the management of problem behaviours in adults with intellectual disabilities. *World Psychiatry*. 2009;8(3):181–186. https://doi.org/10.1002/j.2051-5545.2009.tb00248.x

2. Marrus N, Veenstra-Vander Weele J, Hellings J, et al. Training of child and adolescent psychiatry fellows in autism and intellectual disability. *Autism*. 2014;18(4):471–475. https://doi.org/10.1177%2F1362361313477247

3. Facts about developmental disabilities. Centers for Disease Control and Prevention. Published 2020. https://www.cdc.gov/ncbddd/developmentaldisabilities/facts.html#ref

4. American Psychiatric Association. *Diagnostic and Statistical Manual of Mental Disorders*. 5th ed. American Psychiatric Publishing; 2013.

5. American Psychiatric Association. *Diagnostic and Statistical Manual of Mental Disorders*. 4th ed., text revision. American Psychiatric Association; 2000.

6. Fletcher RJ, Barnhill J, Cooper SA, eds. *Diagnostic Manual—Intellectual Disability: A Textbook of Diagnosis of Mental Disorders in Persons with Intellectual Disability*. NADD Press; 2017.

7. Buckles J. The epidemiology of psychiatric disorders in adults with intellectual disabilities. In: Hemmings C, Bouras N, eds. *Psychiatric and Behavioral Disorders in Intellectual and Developmental Disabilities*. 3rd ed. Cambridge University Press; 2016:34–44.

8. Bouras N. Historical and international perspectives of service. In: Hemmings C, Bouras N, eds. *Psychiatric and Behavioral Disorders in Intellectual and Developmental Disabilities*. 3rd ed. Cambridge University Press; 2016:1–14.

9. Reiss S, Levitan GW, Szyszko J. Emotional disturbance and mental retardation: Diagnostic overshadowing. *Am J Ment Defic*. 1982;86(6):567–574.

10. Royal College of Psychiatrists. *DC-LD: Diagnostic Criteria for Psychiatric Disorders for Use with Adults with Learning Disabilities/Mental Retardation*. RCPych Publications; 2001. https://doi.org/10.1046/j.1365-2788.2002.00403.x

11. Bradley V, Hiersteiner D, Maloney J, Vegas L, Bourne ML. What do NCI data reveal about people who are dual diagnosed with ID and mental illness? [Data brief]. National Core Indicators; 2019. https://www.nationalcoreindicators.org/upload/core-indicators/NCI_DualDiagnosisBrief_Oct072019.pdf

12. Cooper SA, Smiley E, Morrison J, Williamson A, Allan L. Mental ill-health in adults with intellectual disabilities: Prevalence and associated factors. *Br J Psychiatry*. 2007;190:27–35. https://doi.org/10.1192/bjp.bp.106.022483

13. Hughes-McCormack LA, Rydzewska E, Henderson A, MacIntyre C, Rintoul J, Cooper SA. Prevalence of mental health conditions and relationship with general health in a whole-country population of people with intellectual disabilities compared with the general population. *Br J Psychiatry*. 2017;3(5):243–248. https://doi.org/10.1192/bjpo.bp.117.005462

14. Hiersteiner D, Bradley V. What do NCI data reveal about individuals with intellectual and developmental disabilities who need behavior support? [Data brief]. National Core Indicators; 2014. https://www.nationalcoreindicators.org/upload/core-indicators/NCI_DataBrief_MAY2014_ADDENDUM_04_20_15.pdf

15. Bradley V, Hiersteiner D, Rotholz D, Maloney J. What do NCI data show about respondents who need support for self-injurious behavior? [Data brief]. National Core Indicators; 2017. https://www.nationalcoreindicators.org/upload/core-indicators/NCI_DataBrief_SelfInjuriousBehavior_May2017.pdf

16. Merrick J, Merrick E, Lunsky Y, Kandel I. A review of suicidality in persons with intellectual disability. *Isr J Psychiatry Relat Sci*. 2006;43(4):258–264. http://doctorsonly.co.il/wp-content/uploads/2011/12/2006_4_5.pdf

17. Dodd P, Doherty A, Guerin S. A systematic review of suicidality in people with intellectual disabilities. *Harv Rev Psychiatry*. 2016;24(3):202–213. https://doi.org/10.1097/hrp.0000000000000095

18. Pinals DA, Hovermale L, Mauch D, Anacker A. The vital role of specialized approaches: Persons with intellectual and developmental disabilities in the mental health system [Policy brief]. National Association of State Mental Health Program Directors; 2017. https://www.nasmhpd.org/sites/default/files/TAC.Paper_.7.IDD_.Final_.pdf

19. Owen PL, Kerker BD, Zigler E, Horwitz SM. Vision and oral health needs of individuals with intellectual disability. *Ment Retard Dev Disabil Res Rev*. 2006;12(1):28–40. https://doi.org/10.1002/mrdd.20096

20. Baldridge KH, Andrasik F. Pain assessment in people with intellectual or developmental disabilities. *Am J Nurs*. 2010;110(12):28–35. https://doi.org/10.1097/01.naj.0000391236.68263.90

21. Hellings JA, Jain S. The interface between medical and psychiatric disorders. In: Hemmings C, Bouras N, eds. *Psychiatric and Behavioral Disorders in Intellectual and Developmental Disabilities*. 3rd ed. Cambridge University Press; 2016:231–241.

22. Ruedrich S. Psychopharmacology. In: Hemmings C, Bouras N, eds. *Psychiatric and Behavioral Disorders in Intellectual and Developmental Disabilities*. 3rd ed. Cambridge University Press; 2016:139–150.

23. Ghanizadeh A, Sahraeizadeh A, Berk M. A head-to-head comparison of aripiprazole and risperidone for safety and treating autistic disorder: A randomized double blind clinical trial. *Child Psychiatry Hum Dev*. 2014;45(2):185–192. https://doi.org/10.1007/s10578-013-0390-x

24. Tyrer P, Oliver-Africano PC, Ahmed Z, et al. Risperidone, haloperidol, and placebo in the treatment of aggressive challenging behavior in patients with intellectual disability: A randomized controlled trial. *Lancet*. 2008;371(9606):57–63. https://doi.org/10.1016/s0140-6736(08)60072-0

25. McGrother CW, Bhaumik S, Thorp CF, Hauck A, Brandford D, Watson JM. Epilepsy in adults with intellectual disabilities: Prevalence, associations and service implications. *Seizure*. 2006;15(6):376–386. https://doi.org/10.1016/j.seizure.2006.04.002

26. Kalachnik JE, Hanzel TE, Sevenich R, Harder SR. Benzodiazepine behavioral side effects: Review and implications for individuals with mental retardation. *Am J Ment Retard.* 2002;107(5):376–410.   https://meridian.allenpress.com/ajidd/article-abstract/107/5/376/ 805/Benzodiazepine-Behavioral-Side-Effects-Review-and?redirectedFrom=fulltext

27. Sick R. Justice and people with IDD [Issue brief]. American Association on Intellectual and Developmental Disabilities; 2015. https://www.aaidd.org/docs/default-source/National-Goals/justice-and-people-with-idd.pdf?sfvrsn=683b7f21_0

28. Dodd P, Kelly F. Stress, traumatic, and bereavement reactions. In: Hemmings C, Bouras N, eds. *Psychiatric and Behavioral Disorders in Intellectual and Developmental Disabilities.* 3rd ed. Cambridge University Press; 2016:99–108.

29. Tomasulo DJ, Razza NJ. Posttraumatic stress disorder. In: Fletcher R, Loschen E, Stavrakaki C, First M., eds. *Diagnostic Manual—Intellectual Disability: A Clinical Guide for Diagnosis of Mental Disorders in Persons with Intellectual Disability.* NADD Press; 2007:215–224.

30. Harvey K. *Trauma-Informed Behavioral Interventions: What Works and What Doesn't.* American Association on Intellectual and Developmental Disabilities; 2012.

31. Hastings RP, Hatton C, Taylor JL, Maddison C. Life events and psychiatric symptoms in adults with intellectual disabilities. *J Intellect Disabil Res.* 2004;48(1):42–46. https://doi.org/ 10.1111/j.1365-2788.2004.00584.x

32. Lunsky Y, Elserafi J. Life events and emergency department visits in response to crisis in individuals with intellectual disabilities. *J Intellect Disabil Res.* 2011;55(7):714–718. https://doi. org/10.1111/j.1365-2788.2011.01417.x

18

Perinatal Patients and Related Illnesses, Symptoms, and Complications Related to Pregnancy

Sarah Slocum

Introduction

Discussion of psychiatric emergencies in pregnancy must also include the current state of pregnancy and sexuality in the United States. Recent studies have shown that 1 in 6 women and 1 in 33 men are victims of sexual assault, 1 in 4 women and 1 in 9 men are victims of domestic violence, and approximately half of pregnancies are "unintended," with 18% being classified as "unwanted." [1-3] Within emergency psychiatry, these are situations of which we must be cognizant to address with patients.

Given that 50% of pregnancies are unplanned, it is likely that half of women do not account for potential pregnancy when discussing medication changes with their physician. It also brings to light that without point-of-care testing, 50% of pregnant women may not know to disclose a pregnancy when being seen in an emergent setting.

There is a nationwide movement to promote asking every reproductive age female whether they plan a pregnancy within the next year, so as to allow for shared decision-making regarding medications.[4] Although an emergency setting may not seem like an ideal location to employ this question, it should be made routine, along with questions regarding suicidal ideation, sex trafficking, and domestic violence.

Any discussion of pregnancy is incomplete without also addressing the topic of contraception. As psychiatrists, we should be aware that many contraceptives (including estrogen and progesterone hormonal contraceptives) are metabolized through CYP3A4 enzymes. These enzymes are induced by psychotropics such as phenobarbital, oxcarbazepine, carbamazepine, topiramate, modafinil, and St. John's wort. Relatedly, hormonal contraceptives inhibit oxidation of some psychotropics through CYP1A2, 2B6, 2C19, and 3A4, which can lead to increased levels of benzodiazepines, tricyclic antidepressants, valproic acid, and lamotrigine. These facets must be considered when prescribing medications to someone taking hormonal contraception, as well as when evaluating for recent changes in a psychiatric patient.

In terms of presentations to the emergency room, particular attention should be paid to the sections regarding management of agitation, psychosis, and restraints. For medications, in particular, clinicians should not automatically stop or taper psychotropic medications in the setting of pregnancy, with few exceptions (namely valproic acid and high-dose daily benzodiazepines). Few other psychotropics cause such harm that a thoughtful risk–benefit analysis cannot proceed before making changes to medication regimens. It is highly desirable for mothers to be psychiatrically stable during pregnancy and the postpartum period, and efforts should be made to maintain medication regimens that promote this stability when reasonable.

Management of Acute Agitation

As with routine management of agitation, verbal de-escalation and offers of comfort items (blankets, food, etc.) should precede use of physical or chemical restraint, when possible. Restraints should be avoided during pregnancy unless absolutely necessary to maintain the safety of the patient and/or staff. It is important to note that should physical restraints be required for treatment of agitation in pregnancy, an effort should be made to position the patient in a left lateral recumbent position, instead of utilizing classic supine positioning, so as to avoid compression of the inferior vena cava by the gravid uterus. This is of increasing concern as pregnancy progresses and the uterus increases in weight. Depending on which type of positioning is possible for the patient, it is reasonable to utilize increased frequency of checks for complications and vital sign assessment. Use of multidisciplinary care teams is extremely important for pregnant patients experiencing psychosis, so as to maximize the potential for risk mitigation and positive outcomes.

Medications should be provided to assist with agitation. As needed atypical or typical antipsychotics or benzodiazepines are quite reasonable treatments for acute agitation, with choice of agent depending on symptomatology. See Chapter 2 for further details regarding management of acute agitation, including Project BETA (Best Practices in the Evaluation and Treatment of Agitation) recommendations. There is no need to deviate from Project BETA recommendations based solely on pregnancy status. During agitated episodes, the risk of using evidence-based medications is less than the risk of either purposeful or inadvertent harm to mother or fetus. As such, chemical treatment of agitation is strongly recommended. Furthermore, this can help avoid or minimize physical restraint time.

Psychotic Disorders

Pregnancy is a high-risk time for exacerbation of psychotic illnesses, whether a primary psychosis such as schizophrenia or affective disorders with psychotic features. It is thought that psychotic illnesses predispose women to many different possible complications, in both the medical and the psychiatric realms. For example, women with schizophrenia have increased risk of obstetric complications, including changes in fetal weight (small or large for gestational age), as well as increased risk of preterm labor and pre-ecclampsia.[5] Psychiatric illness can also result in patient self-harm, which in turn can lead to direct fetal harm: Somatic delusions or beliefs that the fetus is evil can lead to significant self-harm by means such as stabbing self in the abdomen. Alternatively, psychotic denial of a pregnancy can precipitate a lack of antenatal care.

Postpartum psychosis, which is most often observed in patients with a history of bipolar disorder (see below), must be discussed in detail. Diagnostic criteria for postpartum psychosis and a comparison to other postpartum illnesses are displayed in

Table 18.1 Diagnostic Criteria for Postpartum Psychosis and a Comparison to Other Postpartum Illnesses

	Baby Blues	Postpartum Depression	Postpartum Anxiety	Postpartum Psychosis
Incidence	Up to 85%	10–15%	10–20% (studies vary)	0.1–0.2%
Timeline	Onset 2–3 days, resolves within 10–14 days	Onset between 2 weeks and 2 months, can last months to years	Onset between days and 2 months, can last months to year	Onset sudden, typically within 2 weeks, can last weeks to months
Key symptoms	Fatigue, low mood, tearful, irritable	Low mood, fatigue, guilt, poor sleep/ appetite, suicidal thoughts, anhedonia	Excessive worry, feelings of dread, sleep disruption, racing thoughts, intrusive thoughts, palpitations, nausea, sweating	Hallucinations, delusions, disorganized behavior, sleep disturbance, confusion
Treatment and disposition	Supportive; self-limited; encourage help with infant; 20% progress to postpartum depression	Antidepressant medication, psychotherapy	Antidepressant medication, psychotherapy	Antipsychotic medication; strongly consider inpatient hospitalization given 5% suicide and 4% infanticide rate

Table 18.1; symptoms typically begin within 1 or 2 weeks of delivery. Although the disorder has a low prevalence, estimated at 0.2% of pregnancies, it is key to note that this disorder, specifically, has a 5% rate of suicide and a 4.5% rate of infanticide, marking it as a true psychiatric emergency.[6] As such, patients who present postpartum with any symptoms of psychosis (hallucinations, paranoia, and disorganized behaviors or thought processes), hyperreligiosity (belief that patient or child is possessed, demonic, called to be an "angel," etc.), decreased need for sleep, or loss of maternal drive ("my child will be better off without me") should be taken extremely seriously. The provider should pay particular attention to ascertaining the location of the child and ensuring the child's current caretaker is informed of the severity of the disorder as well. Inpatient admission is preferred for mothers struggling with postpartum psychosis, given the high-risk nature of the illness. If that is not feasible, follow-up should be frequent, and a robust, involved support system is essential for the patient, as well as the health and safety of the dependents. A particular emphasis should be placed on sleep patterns. In situations in which breast-feeding the infant is significantly affecting a patient's sleep schedule, it is recommended to transition to a different method of feeding (providing formula or pumped milk overnight) so as to maximize maternal rest.

In addition to postpartum psychosis, there are other psychotic disorders related to pregnancy. In some patients, a psychotic denial of pregnancy can exist. For all clinical purposes, these patients should be treated in line with a delusional disorder. If denial is to the point where it affects prenatal care and maternal health, treatment is certainly indicated. Some patients also display pseudocyesis, a delusional belief in pregnancy that may present with somatic symptoms consistent with pregnancy, although medical workup is negative for such. If causing functional impairment, then psychiatrists should explore treatment options while taking into consideration that antipsychotics may increase the patient's somatic symptoms, including weight gain, abdominal distention, galactorrhea, and breast growth and tenderness.

Affective Disorders

Mood and affective disorders constitute the most common psychiatric illnesses in pregnancy, with varying severity. A large number of women enter pregnancy with a preexisting affective diagnosis, although a significant number also develop initial symptoms during the inter- or postpartum periods. It is important to note that mental health disorders, mostly affective disorders, are the number one complication of pregnancy and that suicide is the second most common cause of death in postpartum women. How clinicians approach women struggling in the pre-, inter-, and postpartum periods is integral in forming a therapeutic alliance and connecting these women to appropriate care. Thoughts of depression, anxiety, or other presentations should be taken seriously, validated, and not underestimated by psychiatrists or other health care staff.

Specifically, major depressive disorder has a prevalence of approximately 10–15% during pregnancy and postpartum.[7] Women are at increased risk if they have had a prior history of depression; endorse a low socioeconomic status; express having poor social supports; or express having major life stressors, including being victims of intimate partner violence (IPV).[7,8] It is also important to note that IPV rates have been reported to increase during pregnancy, with a prevalence of 5–9%.[8]

For all new-onset or worsened affective disorders during pregnancy, some medical workup is indicated. Specifically, it is recommended to rule out anemia and thyroid dysfunction, substance abuse, and to evaluate what other medications a patient is prescribed.

There are multiple depressive-type illnesses associated with pregnancy. According to the U.S. Health Resource and Services Administration, approximately 80% of mothers experience "baby blues," a time-limited, less severe depressive illness, the symptoms of which are delineated in Table 18.1. Given its high prevalence, it is important to distinguish this illness from perinatal depression, anxiety, or bipolar disorder.

Bipolar disorder, whether diagnosed preconception or later, merits close follow-up through the postpartum period due to its association with postpartum psychosis. There is a high risk of relapse during pregnancy, including a 23% chance of experiencing a mood episode (most commonly depression).[9] Specific risk factors for relapse include having experienced a prior postpartum mood episode, abrupt cessation of medications, and discontinuation of medications immediately surrounding pregnancy; these also portend a higher chance of prolonged illness. Again, a particular emphasis should be placed on sleep hygiene in peripartum women with bipolar disorder because disrupted sleep is a risk factor for a mood episode. Sleep shifts in which nocturnal care is split with a partner or other support person and/or utilization of formula/pumped milk overnight should be recommended.

Anxiety and Obsessive–Compulsive Disorders

Anxiety disorders can manifest prior to, during, or after pregnancy. Although some anxiety surrounding pregnancy is common, pathologic anxiety during pregnancy is associated with adverse fetal and developmental outcomes, including increased risk for preterm birth, as well as poorer neurodevelopmental outcomes through "fetal programming."[10] Specifically, there are noted negative impacts on long-term learning, motor development, and behavior.[10]

Intrusive thoughts are a frequent manifestation of anxiety in pregnancy, and they can be extremely distressing to mothers and families. It is important to be able to differentiate intrusive thoughts stemming from anxiety from those related to obsessive–compulsive disorder (OCD) and psychosis. Consider, for instance, a mother's intrusive thought about "putting baby in an oven." When stemming from anxiety, this is ego-dystonic. The mother will often demonstrate significant distress over these thoughts and will even take great pains not to be left alone with the child, cook while watching the child, etc. Because intrusive thoughts are not often discussed, many women will not report them to providers for fear of hospitalization, Child Protective Services involvement, or shame. These thoughts can be so debilitating that the patient may lose sleep or exhibit other functional impairments. Thus, it is important for psychiatrists to normalize these thoughts, even offering examples such as the one above.

Women struggling with OCD can also present with similar intrusive thoughts. Separately, they may have obsessions more typical of OCD, including fear of germs or paranoia. It is important to assess what compulsions these women perform because the time required to do so may significantly impact time with baby or self-care time.

Suicidality

Suicide is not a rare event in the postpartum period. In fact, recent studies have identified overdose and suicide as the two most common causes of death in the first year postpartum.[11] The diagnoses most commonly associated with suicide in this period are postpartum depression and postpartum psychosis. Whereas most hospitals have rigorous, established protocols for obstetric emergencies such as postpartum hemorrhage, such protocols are not readily available for clinicians attempting to treat peripartum mental illness. Thus, it falls on clinicians, especially psychiatrists, to have a low threshold to serve as consultants for colleagues treating women at risk and to develop a thorough understanding of the intricacies of peripartum mental health treatment.

Pregnancy Loss

Spontaneous abortion occurs in 15–20% of pregnancies; women and families who suffer a spontaneous abortion can struggle with psychiatric manifestations of loss, including complicated grief, acute or post-traumatic stress disorder (PTSD), or depression.[12] There can be a significant discrepancy between expected physical recovery time (days) to the grief process. In addition, patients may believe their own actions caused the loss, which can manifest as clinical guilt. There is an increased risk of psychiatric complications in patients who undergo recurrent loss or experience loss at an advanced gestational age, after having reassuring ultrasounds, or after experiencing fetal movement. It is important to recall that fathers and other family members can experience complications as well.

Induced abortion can also have psychiatric manifestations. As previously stated, the Guttmacher Institute reports that approximately half of pregnancies in the United States are unintended; of these, 40% are terminated by induced abortion. Rates of induced abortion have been declining since 1973. Data show that patients can have some time-limited guilt, although most patients report relief as the predominant emotion.[13] Furthermore, in patients who are denied termination, resulting children have poorer outcomes than matched controls or even their own siblings.[14] Although psychiatrists should not provide directive recommendations to women seeking a termination, they should be able to validate a woman's distress in the setting of this decision and be familiar with data on psychiatric outcomes of both mother and children, so as to allow the patient to make an informed decision. In addition, patients who are facing a late-term abortion in the setting of a significant fetal defect or maternal illness should be expected to have psychiatric concerns specifically related to such.

Assisted Reproduction

Another less commonly addressed area of perinatal psychiatry is the treatment of women and couples who are utilizing assisted reproductive technology (ART). Multiple studies have reported psychiatric side effects from the medications necessary for egg retrieval and embryo transfer, including mania and psychosis.[15] Specifically, clomiphene and leuprolide administration during low estrogen states results in increased dopaminergic activity, which can contribute to development of psychosis.[15] In addition, patients undergoing ART treatments can exhibit symptoms consistent with depressive, anxiety, and trauma-based illnesses, as well as somatic symptoms.[16] Depending on the severity of these symptoms, patients may benefit from pharmacologic treatment and would almost certainly benefit from psychotherapy. Routine follow-up is recommended for women who exhibit psychiatric symptoms during ART treatment.

Substance Abuse in Pregnancy

Of concern is that onset of substance use disorders in women tightly corresponds to reproductive age. The most commonly abused substances in pregnancy are tobacco, alcohol, marijuana, and other illicit substances, respectively.[17] Surveys, which likely underrepresent true levels of substance use, indicate that approximately 6% of pregnant women report using illicit substances and 8.5% report alcohol consumption. Many women are reluctant to discuss their substance use with providers, given fear of Child Protective Services involvement and the potential for loss of custody or other legal repercussions. According to the Guttmacher Institute, 23 states consider substance abuse during pregnancy to be child abuse and therefore subject to mandatory reporting laws. Furthermore, 3 states consider such use to be grounds for "civil commitment."

It is imperative that psychiatrists develop a comfort level for routinely asking all pregnant women about their current and former substance use so as to allow for risk mitigation and treatment. In doing so, psychiatrists can also serve as role models to physician colleagues and other members of the health care team.

Although treatment of substance use disorders during pregnancy is similar to treatment of nonpregnant patients, there are a few important caveats. First, alcohol and opioid withdrawal states can be life-threatening to a fetus. Therefore, admission for detoxification and medication management can be justified, even in the absence of other risk factors such as suicidal ideation. In addition, the MOTHER study demonstrated that although buprenorphine and methadone are both effective at aiding maternal abstinence, buprenorphine resulted in less fetal movement abnormalities and a less severe manifestation of neonatal abstinence syndrome compared to methadone.[18] However, depending on a patient's past treatment history, availability of psychiatrists or addiction providers, and need for structure, either treatment could be justified.

Neonatal abstinence syndrome (NAS) is not to be confused with the neonatal adaptation syndrome seen from serotonin withdrawal. Although the term NAS can be utilized to discuss infant withdrawal from multiple substances, it most classically refers to opioid withdrawal. Infant symptoms are not the subject of this chapter, but it is important to be able to discuss this syndrome with mothers during their pregnancy. According to the March of Dimes, most infants develop signs and symptoms of NAS within 3 days of birth, although symptoms may occur later. Depending on the severity, infants may require days to weeks or months to recover. Signs and symptoms of NAS include tremor, hypertonia, poor feeding or weight gain, fussiness, increased crying, fever, yawning, diarrhea, emesis, sneezing, and congestion. It is difficult to precisely predict which infants will develop NAS; much depends on the substance and amount utilized, the mother's and the infant's metabolism, and the infant's gestational age at delivery. Infants with NAS have an increased risk of sudden infant death syndrome, seizures, jaundice, and low birth weight. There are ongoing investigations into the correlation between maternal opioid use, NAS, and developmental delays and other behavior, speech, and sleep problems. Some infants require medication treatment for severe symptoms, including opioid replacement therapies; they may also require additional nutrition support and specialized nursing care. Mothers with opioid use disorder should discuss NAS with their obstetric and pediatric providers prior to delivery so that providers can inform mothers of the possible treatment outcomes as soon as possible. The role of the psychiatrist is to support and validate the mother's decision-making process and to assist in providing information about medication-assisted treatment. Despite the risks of NAS, maintaining the mother on an opioid replacement therapy is standard of care, and it provides mitigation from the risks of using unregulated illicit substances or undergoing opioid withdrawal.

Trauma and Stressor-Related Disorders

Acute trauma and PTSD can begin or flare during or after pregnancy. In addition to preexisting or non-pregnancy-related traumas, not all women experience a smooth perinatal course, and trauma related to pregnancy or birth can occur. Women who have an unexpected outcome, such as postpartum hemorrhage, an infant diagnosed with a serious medical condition soon after birth, or even unanticipated caesarian section delivery, can struggle with these events. It is important to note that a woman's existing ideas of how birth "should" go versus how birth does go, in addition to a patient's existing coping skills and defense mechanisms, can inform the degree of distress. This is further present in the postpartum period regarding lactation. Some women feel "forced" into breast-feeding, whereas others wish to breast-feed but are unable to so for a number of reasons. In these cases, it is our role to be supportive and to provide accurate medical information, without imposing our own choice patterns upon a patient. Clinicians should take care to be nonjudgmental of patients and should make efforts to use language that does not assume every mother is adjusting easily to motherhood.

Providing medication management for PTSD symptoms is indicated during pregnancy if a woman's symptoms are functionally impairing. Standard first-line treatment with a selective serotonin reuptake inhibitor (SSRI) is appropriate, with similar recommendations when initiating treatment for anxiety or depression, as outlined below.

Personality Disorders in Pregnancy

Much like substance use disorders, personality disorders in pregnancy are managed similarly to those in nonpregnant patients. Furthermore, the interplay between personality disorders and complex trauma must be recalled. In every clinical scenario, trauma-informed care should be utilized consistently. For all patients, clear communication, boundaries, and delineated expectations for the physician–patient relationship are integral to successful treatment. However, particular attention should be paid to patients with a history of sexual abuse, abuse during pregnancy, or new traumas resulting from pregnancy or delivery because these conditions can flare with subsequent pregnancies.

As in nonpregnant patients, diagnostic accuracy should be maintained. For instance, if a patient has hallucinations that are trauma-based and not secondary to a primary psychotic illness, it may be in the best interest of both the patient and the fetus to attempt to manage the mother's symptoms with psychotherapy instead of medication during pregnancy. Although it remains standard of care to provide medications to the mother if indicated, physicians should minimize fetal risk by discontinuing or not initiating unnecessary medications during pregnancy.

Psychotropic Medication Use in Pregnancy and Lactation

As previously mentioned, good psychotropic stewardship does not begin when a woman is already pregnant. Instead, it is incumbent on every psychiatrist to acknowledge that any female patient of reproductive age should be counseled on a medication's use in pregnancy, regardless of whether that patient is planning a pregnancy. In addition, it is integral to assess a woman's expectations for pregnancy at least once per year. In this vein, the use of known, significantly teratogenic medications such as valproic acid should be stringently avoided in women of reproductive age, except in rare circumstances such as a history of sterilization. Less reliable methods of birth control, such as oral contraceptives, condoms, and family planning methods, are not sufficient means of contraception to justify use of teratogenic medications.

In general, if a patient is stable on psychotropic medications before or when pregnancy is diagnosed, those medications should be changed only if they present a risk of harm to the fetus that is deemed greater than the risk of destabilizing the mother's mental health. Although medication changes are indeed sometimes necessary, an immediate reaction to discontinue psychotropics in pregnancy is not appropriate and should be avoided. Many states or academic institutions now have dedicated perinatal psychiatrists who are available to act as resources, especially in the area of psychotropic management in pregnancy and lactation.

The most commonly used psychotropics in pregnancy are SSRIs. These medications are generally considered safe and well-tolerated. More recent large studies of these medications do not indicate a significant risk of teratogenicity or poor neurodevelopmental outcomes. For infants, the most common effect is a neonatal adaptation syndrome, which occurs in approximately 30% of infants who were routinely exposed to SSRIs during development. This syndrome is non-dose-dependent and commonly appears as increased infant irritability, poorer sleep, and possibly poorer feeding habits for the first 3–5 days of life. It is managed conservatively with skin-to-skin contact; swaddling; and small, frequent feedings. There are no known long-term adverse effects for infants who experience adaptation symptoms.

Specifically, when starting a new medication for depression or anxiety in pregnancy, escitalopram and sertraline are commonly considered. Escitalopram tends to be well-tolerated but can have a narrow dosing range, given the maximum recommended daily dose of 20 mg. Sertraline, although possessing the lowest transfer rate into breast milk of any of the SSRIs, can cause significant gastroesophageal reflux disease (GERD); it is important to note that sertraline has not been proven *safer* than other SSRIs in pregnancy. All SSRIs transfer into breast milk with a rate <10%, which is the standard acceptable cutoff transfer rate according to the American Academy of Pediatrics.[19,20] As is recognized in adult psychiatry, treatment of pregnant women with paroxetine is not generally considered first-line, given its short half-life and risk of withdrawal phenomenon. Furthermore, initial studies on paroxetine displayed a link with persistent pulmonary hypertension of the newborn, although newer, larger trials have not confirmed a causal relationship.[21]

In addition, it has been well described that untreated maternal mental illness increases morbidity and mortality related to pregnancy and birth. Treatment for psychiatric illness must be standard of care during pregnancy and/or lactation. Recent large studies have demonstrated a small, likely clinically insignificant risk of preterm delivery (mean ½ week earlier delivery) and decreased birth weight (mean decrease of 74 g), as well as lower 1- and 5-minute APGAR scores in neonates who were exposed to SSRIs in utero.[22] Although these differences were statistically significant for both mothers without psychiatric illness and mothers with untreated mental illness, the clinical states were still within normal limits for births, further supporting the idea that clinical significance of the results is questionable.[22] Furthermore, evidence that SSRI use during pregnancy increases the risk of stillbirth, neonatal, or post-neonatal mortality is lacking.[23]

Given the known increase of bleeding potential with SSRIs, there has also been concern about increased rates of postpartum hemorrhage. However, data show that although this risk does exist, the average amount of increased bleeding is <100 mL, again raising the question of whether this difference is clinically significant compared to the risk of untreated maternal mental illness.[24] In terms of cardiac abnormalities, SSRI exposure during the first trimester (while the cardiac system is forming embryologically) was not associated with an increase in abnormalities.[25]

Regarding specific selection of SSRI agent during pregnancy or postpartum, preference should be given to preexisting medication trials. If the patient has been successfully treated with an SSRI previously, it should be resumed and titrated to effective dose. If an agent is already at maximum dosing and is not completely controlling symptoms, it may be reasonable to trial a different agent. When selecting a new agent, patients typically exhibit good tolerance of escitalopram, sertraline, fluoxetine, mirtazapine, and duloxetine.

Specific agent selection should be dependent on desired side effect profile. Note that it is reasonable to breast-feed with each of these medications. Furthermore, it is important to state that some women, especially those with preexisting GERD or frequent loose stools, may not tolerate sertraline, which tends to affect the serotonin receptors located within the gastrointestinal tract at higher frequency.

Regarding atypical antipsychotics, which are the most commonly prescribed antipsychotics in pregnancy, studies indicate that the rate of major malformations remains low at 1.4% of pregnancies (versus 1.1% of control group; odds ratio = 1.25).[26] This data is reassuring and indicates that it is unlikely that the risk of teratogenicity should increase significantly beyond that for the general population, although further studies are ongoing.[26] It is generally believed that there is no one atypical antipsychotic which is safer in pregnancy than another. Treatment should be tailored to the individual patient and favorable side effect profile. As with all patients, monitoring for metabolic syndrome and typical screening requirements, such as evaluating lipid profile, hemoglobin A1C, weight, waist circumference, and possibly electrocardiogram for QTc assessment, should occur as indicated.

Antiepileptic medications (AEDs) are commonly used in women for mood stabilization and bipolar disorder, in addition to their uses in the field of neurology. Given the risk of destabilization and the comorbidity between bipolar disorder and postpartum psychosis, frequent monitoring and continued medication management are often recommended. However, it is vital to ensure diagnostic accuracy before continuing any treatment in pregnancy, so as to minimize unnecessary risks to the mother and fetus. Specifically, valproic acid, lithium, and lamotrigine merit individual discussion.

Lithium has long been the gold standard for treatment of bipolar disorder. Although classically associated with a risk of Ebstein's anomaly, a defect of the right ventricular outflow tract (RVOT) of the fetal heart when exposure occurs in the first trimester during cardiac development, the absolute clinical risk of such remains incredibly low. More recent studies indicate a general population risk for cardiac malformations of 1.15% in patients without lithium exposure; in the setting of lithium, the absolute risk of such increases to 2.41%, with an adjusted risk ratio of 1.65.[27] This risk is somewhat dose-dependent, with a demarcation of increasing risk at ≥900 mg PO total daily dose. For RVOT obstructions, specifically, the risk in an unexposed fetus is 0.18% versus 0.60% in exposed fetuses, with an odds ratio of 2.66.[27] Given the still-low absolute risk of malformations, it is recommended that serious consideration be given to continuing lithium treatment in women with confirmed bipolar disorder who desire to be or become pregnant. Note that the dosing of lithium in pregnancy must increase, given changes in body water distribution. In general, serum lithium levels decrease during the first trimester to a nadir in the second trimester, before increasing slightly. Lithium levels and creatinine should be monitored closely until at least 34 weeks of pregnancy and then at least weekly until 2 weeks postpartum.[28] Consideration should be given to split (twice daily) dosing to minimize extremes in serum lithium levels. Dose may need to increase during pregnancy to maintain therapeutic levels per serum monitoring, and common practice dictates that at the time of delivery, dose should be immediately decreased either down to prepartum dosing or to two-thirds of immediate pre-delivery dosing, to prevent lithium toxicity in the setting of postpartum fluid shifts.[28] It is therefore beneficial to know the patient's baseline lithium dosing prior to pregnancy.

Valproic acid is another commonly utilized AED. However, it carries significant teratogenic risks to the fetus in addition to ongoing neurodevelopmental consequences. Valproic acid should be avoided in all reproductive-aged women regardless of contraceptive status. Among first-trimester exposures, there is an increased incidence of major congenital malformations of 6.1% over the baseline risk of approximately 3%, with a specific focus on the increased risk of neural tube defects.[29] Furthermore, valproic acid has been associated with a significantly increased risk of autism spectrum disorder and childhood autism in children who were exposed to it in utero.[30] These children exhibited an absolute risk of autism spectrum disorder diagnosis of 4.15% when exposed versus 2.24% in unexposed children.[30] Given both the teratogenic and neurodevelopmental effects, alternate treatments should be sought, and valproic acid should be discontinued in any reproductive-aged female or immediately upon diagnosis of pregnancy, with subsequent close monitoring and initiation of an alternate agent if indicated. Discontinuation should occur even if the patient has a well-established pregnancy, past the time frame of neural tube development. If valproic acid must be used in a reproductive-aged female, there must be long-term contraception in place, such as sterilization, intrauterine device, or similar. Family planning, oral contraceptives, or even injections such as medroxyprogesterone acetate are not sufficient.

Possibly the most preferred mood stabilizer in pregnancy, if one is indicated, is lamotrigine. Lamotrigine was previously identified to carry a possible increased association with orofacial cleft abnormalities as well as club foot; however, follow-up studies have not borne this out.[31] In fact, studies indicate the additional orofacial cleft risk to be <2% in exposed children, and researchers were not able to conclude that there is an independently increased risk of club foot in lamotrigine-exposed infants, although further studies are needed to assess this risk.[31] Although there is a theoretical risk of Stevens–Johnson syndrome in an exposed infant, this has not been reported clinically.

Benzodiazepines, which are γ-aminobutyric acid subtype A receptor agonists, are sometimes necessary for treatment of panic disorder or in an emergent setting for treatment of agitation or withdrawal. Furthermore, patients may become pregnant while taking benzodiazepines, and clinicians may need to provide patient education and management. When using benzodiazepines in pregnancy, patients should take the lowest possible effective dose at the lowest frequency to control symptoms; benzodiazepines should be used no more than two or three times per week. Patients who become pregnant while taking higher or more frequent doses should be tapered, although taper must be by a maximum of 25% total daily dose per week to prevent seizures or other physiologic withdrawal. For instance, a patient taking 4 mg total of clonazepam daily should taper to 3 mg total daily dose for 1 week, then to 2 mg total daily dose for 1 week, etc. Among women who regularly use benzodiazepines in pregnancy, there is an association with preterm labor, low birth weight, and caesarian delivery; higher doses in particular are associated with poor muscle tone (hypotonicity and "floppy baby" syndrome), poor feeding, respiratory depression, and drowsiness at delivery.[32] There is the potential for neonatal withdrawal from benzodiazepines after delivery as well, which could manifest with physiologic symptoms including tachycardia and seizures. Similarly, benzodiazepines are also secreted into breast milk, and efforts to maintain infrequent, as-needed use should continue following pregnancy.[32] It is also important to discuss with patients that due to the nocturnal needs of infants, taking sedating medications at bedtime may impact infant care and safety. For mothers who require longer sleep stretches, scheduling sleep shifts with a partner or other caretaker can be effective.

Gender Identity and Sexual Orientation

This chapter would not be complete without mentioning the subject of gender identity and sexual orientation. The Trevor Project has reported that LGBTQ+ teenagers are five times more likely to attempt suicide; furthermore, their attempts are five times more likely to require medical treatment than those of their heterosexual, cis-gendered peers. In addition, children and teens experiencing family rejection on the basis of their identity attempt suicide more than eight times as often. These statistics indicate that routine discussion of gender identity and sexual orientation should be a part of every psychiatric risk assessment.

Psychiatrists should discuss gender identity and sexual orientation openly and routinely with patients as part of their social history. It is important to avoid assumptions regarding either topic and to allow patients to express themselves as desired. One subtle, yet noticeable strategy includes the placement of one's own personal pronouns in email or professional document signature lines in order to help destigmatize pronoun selection for transgender youth and adults. For those desiring more proactive strategies, joining an "Out or Ally List" at one's own institution represents another significant step that can be taken in support of LGBTQ+ patients and their families and also to acknowledge a commitment to treatment of this population without prejudice.

References

1. Tjaden P, Thoennes N. *Prevalence, Incidence, and Consequences of Violence Against Women: Findings from the National Violence Against Women Survey*. U.S. Department of Justice; 1998:16.

2. Truman JL, Morgan R. *Nonfatal Domestic Violence, 2003–2012*. U.S. Department of Justice; 2014:21.

3. Finer LB, Zolna M. Declines in unintended pregnancy in the United States, 2008–2011. *N Engl J Med*. 2016;374(9):843–852.

4. Allen D, Hunter MS, Wood S, Beeson T. One Key Question: First things first in reproductive health. *Matern Child Health J*. 2017;21(3):387–392. doi:10.1007/s10995-017-2283-2

5. Vigod S, Kurdyak P, Dennis C, et al. Maternal and newborn outcomes among women with schizophrenia: A retrospective population-based cohort study. *BJOG*. 2014;121(5):566–574. doi:10.1111/1471-0528.12567

6. Brockington I. Suicide and filicide in postpartum psychosis. *Arch Womens Ment Health*. 2017;20:63–69.

7. Halbreich U, Karkun S. Cross-cultural and social diversity of prevalence of postpartum depression and depressive symptoms. *J Affect Disord*. 2006;91(2–3):97–111. doi:10.1016/j.jad.2005.12.051

8. Saltzman LE, Johnson CH, Gilbert BC, Goodwin MM. Physical abuse around the time of pregnancy: An examination of prevalence and risk factors in 16 states. *Matern Child Health J*. 2003;7(1):31–43.

9. Viguera AC, Tondo L, Koukopoulos AE, Reginaldi D, Lepri B, Baldessarini RJ. Episodes of mood disorders in 2,252 pregnancies and postpartum periods. *Am J Psychiatry*. 2011;168:1179–1185.

10. Dunkel Schetter C, Tanner L. Anxiety, depression and stress in pregnancy: Implications for mothers, children, research, and practice. *Curr Opin Psychiatry*. 2012;25(2):141–148. doi:10.1097/YCO.0b013e3283503680

11. Goldman-Mellor S, Margerison CE. Maternal drug-related death and suicide are leading causes of postpartum death in California. *Am J Obstet*. 2019;221(5):489.e1-489.e9. doi:10.1016/j.ajog.2019.05.045

12. Kersting A, Wagner B. Complicated grief after perinatal loss. *Dialogues Clin Neurosci*. 2012;14(2):187–194.

13. Charles VE, Polis CB, Sridhara SK, Blum RW. Abortion and long-term mental health outcomes: A systematic review of the evidence. *Contraception*. 2008;78(6):436–450. doi:10.1016/j.contraception.2008.07.005

14. Kubicka L, Roth Z, Dytrych Z, Matejcek Z, David H. The mental health of adults born of unwanted pregnancies, their siblings, and matched controls: A 35-year follow-up study from Prague, Czech Republic. *J Nerv Ment Dis*. 2002;190(10):653–662.

15. Seeman MV. Transient psychosis in women on clomiphene, bromocriptine, domperidone and related endocrine drugs. *Gynecol Endocrinol*. 2015;31(10):751–754. doi:10.3109/09513590.2015.1060957

16. Burns LH. Psychiatric aspects of infertility and infertility treatments. *Psychiatr Clin North Am*. 2007;30(4):689–716. doi:10.1016/j.psc.2007.08.001

17. Forray A. Substance use during pregnancy. *F1000Research*. 2016;5(887):1–9. doi:10.12688/f1000research.7645.1

18. Jones HE, Finnegan LP, Kaltenbach K. Methadone and buprenorphine for the management of opioid dependence in pregnancy: *Drugs*. 2012;72(6):747–757. doi:10.2165/11632820-000000000-00000

19. Sachs HC; Committee on Drugs. The transfer of drugs and therapeutics into human breast milk: An update on selected topics. *Pediatrics*. 2013;132(3):e796–e809. doi:10.1542/peds.2013-1985

20. Chad L, Pupco A, Bozzo P. Update on antidepressant use during breastfeeding. *Can Fam Physician*. 2013;59:633–634.

21. 't Jong GW, Einarson T, Koren G, Einarson A. Antidepressant use in pregnancy and persistent pulmonary hypertension of the newborn (PPHN): A systematic review. *Reprod Toxicol*. 2012;34(3):293–297. doi:10.1016/j.reprotox.2012.04.015

22. Ross L, Grigoriadis S, Mamisashvili L, et al. Selected pregnancy and delivery outcomes after exposure to antidepressant medication: A systematic review and meta-analysis. *JAMA Psychiatry*. 2013;70(4):436–443.

23. Stephansson O, Kieler H, Haglund B, et al. Selective serotonin reuptake inhibitors during pregnancy and risk of stillbirth and infant mortality. *JAMA*. 2013;309(1):48–54.

24. Palmsten K, Hernandez-Diaz S, Huybrechts KF, et al. Use of antidepressants near delivery and risk of postpartum hemorrhage: Cohort study of low income women in the United States. *BMJ*. 2013;347:1–15. doi:10.1136/bmj.f4877

25. Huybrechts KF, Cohen LS, Mogun H, Setoguchi S. Antidepressant use in pregnancy and the risk of cardiac defects. *N Engl J Med*. 2014;370(25):2397–2407.

26. Cohen LS, Viguera A, McInerney K, et al. Reproductive safety of second-generation antipsychotics: Current data from the Massachusetts General Hospital National Pregnancy Registry for Atypical Antipsychotics. *Am J Psychiatry*. 2016;173(3):263–270.

27. Patorno E, Huybrechts KF, Bateman BT, et al. Lithium use in pregnancy and the risk of cardiac malformations. *N Engl J Med.* 2017;376(23):2245–2254. doi:10.1056/NEJMoa1612222

28. Wesseloo R, Wierdsma A, van Kamp I, et al. Lithium dosing strategies during pregnancy and the postpartum period. *Br J Psychiatry.* 2017;211:31–36.

29. Angus-Leppan H, Liu RSN. Weighing the risks of valproate in women who could become pregnant. *BMJ.* 2018;361:1–8. doi:10.1136/bmj.k1596

30. Christensen J, Gronborg TK, Sorensen MJ, et al. Prenatal valproate exposure and risk of autism spectrum disorders and childhood autism. *JAMA.* 2013;309(16):1696–1703.

31. Dolk H, Wang H, Loane M, et al. Lamotrigine use in pregnancy and risk of orofacial cleft and other congenital anomalies. *Neurology.* 2016;86(18):1716–1725. doi:10.1212/WNL.0000000000002540

32. Shyken JM, Babbar S, Babbar S, Forinash A. Benzodiazepines in pregnancy. *Clin Obstet Gynecol.* 2019;62(1):156–167. doi:10.1097/GRF.0000000000000417

19

Victims of Physical and Sexual Violence

Kristie Ladegard and Jessica Tse

Introduction

Globally, approximately 470,000 people are victims of homicide every year. Hundreds of millions more men, women, and children suffer nonfatal forms of interpersonal violence, which contributes to lifelong physical, behavioral, and mental health consequences for individuals and families, as well as undermining the social and economic development of whole communities and societies.[1] As experts who understand the biological aspects of violence as well as the societal, environmental, and economic conditions that affect health, psychiatrists are uniquely positioned to help prevent violence.[2] Through definitions, current statistical data, identification, approach recommendations, and reporting considerations, we review interpersonal violence, including homicide, sexual violence, intimate partner violence (IPV), child abuse, human trafficking, and elder abuse.

Homicide and Other Interpersonal Violence

Homicide is defined as the killing of a person by another with intent to cause death or serious injury, by any means including police brutality and mass shootings. In the United States in 2017, 1.1 million nonfatal assault-related injuries occurred among adults aged 25 years or older, and nearly 3.15 million incidents of assault were experienced by victims aged 25 years or older. That is more than 1 in 10 adults involved in violent incidents.[3] The health effects of different forms of violence at different ages can be cumulative. Assault-related injuries are associated with a high risk of recurrent victimization and negative health outcomes. Some victims suffer permanent injuries that limit their ability to work.[3] Psychological effects include anxiety; depression; post-traumatic stress disorder (PTSD); aggression; guilt; and a heightened sense of vulnerability with higher risk of PTSD, depression, and sexually transmitted infections (STIs).[3] In addition, adult perpetrators of violence are also more likely than others to die by suicide.[3] In addition to its direct impact to the physical and mental health of victims and perpetrators, interpersonal violence also has serious negative effects on the psychological health and socioeconomic status of surviving family members.

Homicide is caused by mix of factors at the individual, relationship, community, and societal levels. In communities in which young males make up a greater share of the population, poverty, economic inequality, ethnic fractionalization, and the availability of guns and alcohol are also risk factors for homicide.[1] Involvement with violence is generally lower among adults aged 25 years or older than among youth aged 15–24 years.[3] Access to firearms garners special attention given lethality and notable increased risk for violence and homicide. In 2018, there were 39,740 firearm-related deaths in the United States, or nearly 109 people dying from a firearm-related injury each day; 6 out of every 10 deaths were firearm suicides, and more than 3 out of every 10 were firearm homicides.[4] Current strategies to address firearm-related injury and death include safety education in schools and communities about safe handling, storage, and disposal, in addition to implementing youth-oriented violence prevention programs with a focus on behavioral management, developing conflict resolution skills, and increasing positive interactions with role models.[2]

Police Brutality

Recently, the police have drawn increased attention for injuring or killing citizens in Minneapolis, Minnesota; Ferguson, Missouri; Baltimore, Maryland; New York City; and elsewhere throughout the country. The actual incidence of homicides due to police use of force is unknown. Although the Centers for Disease Control and Prevention (CDC) reported 616 deaths in 2017 (an incidence of 0.20 per 100,000 people), the number determined by other sources is substantially higher.[3] The use of force can have dire implications for communities of color, communities with prior police contact, and family members and friends of people who have been targets of police use of force. This contributes to cycles of disadvantage, diminished community resilience and cohesion, and intergenerational trauma.[3] It is critical to acknowledge how violence experienced by the individual can affect their broader community and how the aggregated experience of violence within a community can impact the health and well-being of the individual.[3]

Child Maltreatment and Youth Violence

Case Example

Cindy, a 14-year-old female, presents to the psychiatric emergency room after her school placed her on a hold due to concerns that she wrote in a class essay that she wanted to kill herself. Her mother is in the waiting room and when interviewed states that Cindy used to be one of the best students in school but now is disruptive in her classes and frequently skips school. Cindy is initially irritable, keeping her eyes downcast, and smells like she may be under the influence of marijuana. She alleges that her stepfather has been drinking alcohol more frequently and has been very explosive toward her and her mother.

Exposure to trauma including violence is a major public health concern that affects a vast number of children in the United States. Childhood trauma encompasses a wide range of experiences that threaten the life, safety, or physical well-being of a child and includes child abuse and neglect, domestic violence, community violence, murder or suicide of a family member, severe accidents, and natural disasters.

Statistics from numerous studies attest to the rampant and long-lasting effects of childhood trauma.[5] Epidemiologic studies estimate that as many as 70% of U.S. children and adolescents experience some form of trauma.[6] Rates of childhood trauma are even higher in low-income urban communities, with studies of high-risk urban youth reporting a prevalence of more than 90%.[7] It has also been reported that 60% of youth aged

0–17 years were victims or witnesses of interpersonal violence in 2012, and 26% of youth experienced violence in their homes.[8] Finally, approximately one in four women and one in seven men report childhood experiences of sexual abuse.[9] Medical providers are often the first line of response to children's exposure to trauma and are in a unique and vital position to prevent or reduce long-term and even lifelong consequences.

Child and adolescent abuse has short- and long-term impacts on both physical and mental health. Any trauma a child experiences in this time frame can significantly impact the composition of their brain indefinitely. Studies show the impact of trauma not only on brain development but also on how a child forms attachment, self-regulates, cognition, and self-concept.[10] Child abuse is one of the leading causes of injury-related mortality in infants and children.[11] An abused child has an approximately 50% chance of being abused again and has an increased risk of dying if the abuse is not caught and stopped after the first presentation.[12,13] When physicians recognize and treat these cases upon examination, they have an opportunity to prevent significant morbidity and mortality.

Types of Abuse

There are four main types of child abuse: neglect, emotional, physical, and sexual abuse.[11] Medically, each is approached differently, but all require that the physician report suspicions to appropriate authorities and involve other members of the health care community.

Neglect is defined as failure to provide for a child's basic physical, emotional, educational/cognitive, or medical needs.[14] If neglect is suspected, the physician should obtain a full medical history (e.g., prenatal and postnatal care, diet, immunizations, major illnesses, growth curve, developmental milestones, hospitalizations, and previous physician visits), psychosocial history (e.g., family composition, IPV, job status, use of drugs and alcohol in the home, and past involvement with Child Protective Services), and a complete physical examination.[11] Management of neglect includes arranging a home visit by a physician, social worker, or home nurse; scheduling frequent medical follow-up; and obtaining a social work consultation. If the caregiver refuses to cooperate with these interventions, then Child Protective Services should be contacted.[5]

The Office on Child Abuse and Neglect defines *emotional abuse* as abuse that results in demonstrable harm (e.g., impaired psychological growth and development) of a child.[15] Patterns of behavior that should raise concern about the possibility of emotional abuse include social withdrawal, excessive anger or aggression, eating disorders, failure to thrive, developmental delay, and emotional disturbances (e.g., depression, anxiety, fearfulness, and history of running away from home).[11] If the episode of suspected emotional abuse is isolated and there is no immediate danger to the child, family therapy, parental training, and other supportive therapy for the child and family are recommended. If emotional abuse is recurrent or there is a possibility of imminent harm, Child Protective Services should be contacted and removal of the child from the home considered.[16]

Physical abuse should be part of the differential diagnosis for all injuries in children.[17] The American Academy of Pediatrics and the American College of Radiology consider a skeletal survey the method of choice for skeletal imaging in suspected child physical abuse cases; therefore, a skeletal survey is mandatory for all children younger than age 3 years with suspicious trauma.[18,19] Once physical abuse of a child is suspected, the physician is required by law to report it to proper authorities. Medical management can range from inpatient care to outpatient treatment with close follow-up by a physician, a social worker, and Child Protective Services. Criteria for considering admission includes medical indications (e.g., severe burns, head injury, and requirement for serial examinations), unsafe home environment, delayed outpatient Child Protective Services evaluation, and inpatient observation of child–parent interactions.[20]

The World Health Organization (WHO) defines *sexual abuse* as an act of involving a child in a sexual engagement without their full comprehension to give informed consent. WHO also views sexual abuse as a situation in which the child has not fully undergone complete development to engage in sexual activities. Less than 10% of substantiated child sexual abuse cases have physical findings on examination;[21] therefore, the history is the most important part of the sexual abuse evaluation. The provider should document carefully the child's history. A thorough physical examination should be performed at the time of initial interview if the reported incident occurred less than 72 hours before and the patient has a history highly suggestive of abuse.[11] For these instances, sexual assault kits (i.e., rape kits) usually are available in emergency departments or child abuse centers.[11] Examinations should be done by health care professionals familiar with forensic examinations (e.g., experienced primary care physicians, emergency department personnel, or sexual assault nurse examiners).[18] Children may feel helpless and ashamed to speak up when they are sexually abused. Although physical examination by physicians will rarely confirm sexual abuse, providers can be powerful advocates for children by reporting concerns to appropriate agencies, thereby allowing for a multidisciplinary investigation to take place while simultaneously offering children and families support.

Regardless of the type of abuse that a child may present with, providers must be knowledgeable of the mandatory reporting guidelines in their state. For detailed information on specific state statutes, visit the website for the National Clearing House on Child Abuse and Neglect.[22] The psychiatric emergency room may frequently be the first place a child or adolescent presents with traumatic experiences such as abuse, and providers must be vigilant in assessing and treating them. By being competent and keeping up to date on this topic, providers have an opportunity to positively impact a youth's life while preventing the devastating long-term consequences of abuse.

Intimate Partner Violence and Sexual Violence

Case Example

A timid-appearing, non-English-speaking young female presents to the emergency department with vague gastrointestinal concerns. She is accompanied by a male companion who insists on translating on the patient's behalf, is resistant to the patient having a physical exam, and is reluctant to leave the patient's side. The emergency department provider expresses concern because the patient struggles to make eye contact, appears subdued and unkempt, and has notable bruises of varying ages and burn marks on her forearm.

The World Health Organization defines IPV as behavior within an intimate relationship that causes physical, sexual, or psychological harm, including acts of physical aggression, sexual coercion, psychological abuse, and controlling behavior by current and former spouses and partners. An intimate partner is defined as "a person with whom one has a close personal relationship that can be characterized as with emotional connectedness, regular contact, ongoing physical contact and/or sexual behavior, identify as a couple or familiarity, and knowledge about each other's lives."[23] IPV affects both men and women, but women are more likely to experience severe victimization that results in injury and the need for medical care.[3] In addition, perpetrators are often victims of IPV as well, and thus they may suffer from the combined effects of being both perpetrator and victim.[3] The most extreme form of IPV is intimate partner homicide; 55.3% of homicides of women are related to IPV, and half of those are due to firearms.[3] Recent estimates of prevalence in the United States from the National Intimate Partner and Sexual Violence Survey "indicate that 1 in 4 women and 1 in 10 men have experienced contact sexual violence, physical violence, and/or stalking by an intimate partner resulting in consequences such as injury, need for medical care, or posttraumatic stress symptoms."[24]

Types of Intimate Partner Violence

1. *Physical violence* is the intentional use of physical force with the potential for causing death, disability, injury, or harm.[23]
2. *Sexual violence* (SV) is further divided into five categories and includes attempted or completed acts. These acts occur without the victim's freely given consent and include situations in which the victim is unable to consent because of being incapacitated (e.g., intoxication, lack of consciousness, or lack of awareness) through their voluntary or involuntary use of alcohol or drugs.[23]
   • Rape or penetration of victim and includes completed or attempted, forced, or unwanted vaginal, oral, or anal insertion
   • Victim was made to penetrate someone else
   • Nonphysically pressured unwanted penetration, including verbal intimidation and misuse of authority to consent or acquiesce to penetration
   • Unwanted sexual contact, including intentional touching of the victim or making the victim touch the perpetrator, either directly or through the clothing without the victim's consent
   • Noncontact unwanted sexual experiences, including unwanted sexual events that are not of a physical nature that occur without the victim's consent.
3. *Stalking* is a pattern of repeated, unwanted attention and contact that causes fear or concern for one's own safety or the safety of someone else, such as a family member or friend.[23] Examples include unwanted communication via phone calls, texts, voice messages, or emails; being watched or followed with nonconsenting invasion of privacy (spying, recording, etc.); and the perpetrator appearing when the victim does not want to see them.[25] The National Intimate Partner and Sexual Violence Survey (NISVS) reports that approximately 1 in 6 women and 1 in 17 men have been stalked at some point in their lives and reported feeling very fearful that they or someone close to them would be harmed or killed as a result.[25] Numerous studies have reported that stalking can lead to psychological distress, such as depression and PTSD.
4. *Psychological aggression* is the use of verbal and nonverbal communication with the intent to harm another person mentally or emotionally and/or to exert control over another person.[23] Examples include expressive aggression (name-calling and

humiliating or degrading behaviors), coercive control (limiting access to money, friends, or transportation, excessive monitoring, and making threats to loved ones or possessions), threats of physical or sexual violence, control of reproductive or sexual health, exploitation of victim's vulnerability or perpetrator's vulnerabilities, and gaslighting.[23] Psychologically aggressive acts are not physical acts of violence and may not be perceived as aggression because they are covert and manipulative in nature. Psychological aggression "frequently co-occurs with other forms of intimate partner violence and research suggests that it often precedes physical and sexual violence in violent relationship."[25] The impact of psychological aggression by an intimate partner is every bit as significant as that of physical violence.

Non-Partner Sexual Violence

The World Health Organization defines sexual violence as any sexual act, attempt to obtain a sexual act, or other act directed against a person's sexuality using coercion, by any person regardless of their relationship to the victim.[1] Although sexual assault is most common among young women, men and older women also are victims of sexual assault. In 2016, WHO reported 7% global lifetime prevalence of women who suffer non-partner sexual violence at some time in their life, with rates for women being 11-fold higher than those for men.[3]

Sexual violence is often a life-altering event associated with numerous physical and mental health consequences, as noted previously. Suicide attempts and completed suicides are four times higher in sexual assault victims than in the general population, and eating disorders are more than two times greater in this population.[3] The psychological consequences of sexual assault are greatly influenced by the response the victim receives from their social network, the medical community, and the criminal justice system, with increased risk for poorer outcomes when their community is unresponsive or unsupportive.[3] Whereas most identified rape victims will be triaged directly to a rape crisis treatment team, unreported victims may first present to a psychiatric emergency room.[3]

The risk factors that increase the likelihood of SV perpetration are similar to those for IPV; however, additional individual risk factors for perpetration include preference for impersonal sex; sexual risk-taking for perpetration; early sexual initiation; hostility toward women or general aggressiveness and acceptance of violence, including coercive sexual fantasies; and prior sexual victimization or perpetration.[26] Additional relationship factors include family environment characterized by physical violence, conflict, lack of emotional support, and poor parent–child relationships (particularly with fathers); association with sexually aggressive, hypermasculine, and delinquent peers; and involvement in a violent or abusive intimate relationship.[26] Protective factors include parental use of reasoning to resolve family conflict, emotional health and connectedness, academic achievement, and empathy or concern for how one's actions can affect others.[27] As for IPV, community and societal factors include poverty, community tolerance of SV, and lack of institutional supports from police and judicial systems. Societal norms that support SV, sexual entitlement, gender inequality, and high levels of crime or other forms of violence also increase risk of SV perpetration.[26]

Screening for rape remains a challenging task, in part because the victim may feel too ashamed or guilty to talk about what happened or may not define the violation as rape, as in many cases of spousal or date rape. Prevention strategies currently being evaluated and implemented include rape awareness education in schools and communication and relationship skills building.

Special Considerations

Pregnant Women

In the United States, suicide and homicide are leading causes of pregnancy-associated mortality.[23] Overall highest prevalence of IPV during pregnancy was reported in non-Hispanic American Indian/Alaskan Native and non-Hispanic Black females.[23] Reproductive coercion is a prominent aspect of IPV and includes behaviors aimed at controlling reproductive or sexual health, such as refusal to use birth control, coerced pregnancy termination or continuation, sabotage of birth control efforts, etc.[23] During pregnancy, IPV also poses a risk to the health and well-being of the fetus or fetuses and has also been associated with adverse pregnancy outcomes such as preterm birth, low birth weight, and small for gestational age contributing to an increased risk of developmental and behavioral issues.[23,28] Maternal adverse health behaviors include late and missed prenatal care appointments, poor weight gain, higher rates of smoking and alcohol use, and substance abuse as a direct result of IPV.[23] Added risk factors for pregnant women include jealousy or anger toward the unborn child, pregnancy-specific conflicts, and whether pregnancy was unwanted or unexpected for one partner. These women may be more than four times more likely to experience violence during pregnancy.[29]

Violence Against Men

Male victimization is a significant public health problem, according to estimates in the NISVS. Throughout the United States, nearly one-fourth of men reported some form of contact SV in their lifetime. Approximately 1 in 10 men experienced contact SV, physical violence, and/or stalking by an intimate partner during their lifetime and reported some form of IPV-related impact. Commonly reported IPV-related impacts among male victims were fear, concern for safety, and symptoms of PTSD, among others.[30]

Special Populations

Intimate partner violence may also be increased in lesbian, gay, bisexual, transgender, queer, or questioning couples, with sexual minority respondents reporting rates of IPV at least as high as those in heterosexual couples. The NISVS reported in 2010 that the risk may be highest in bisexual women (61%) compared with lesbian women (44%) and heterosexual women (35%).[30] IPV prevention programs must reach out to and support victims regardless of sexual orientation and ensure access to culturally sensitive services.[28] Veterans and those in the military are another notable population. Rates of IPV may be affected by unique stressors such as deployments, separations, and relocations, as well as stressors related to combat. A higher lifetime prevalence of IPV exists in military populations than in the civilian population. In addition, increased rates of violence are also found in immigrant populations, the members of which may find it difficult to locate resources or support due to language barriers and fears about deportation. "Women with disabilities and developmental delays are also more at risk owing to reliance on their partners and families for care, as are elderly women, who are often abused by partners or adult children."[28]

Human Trafficking

Human trafficking, also known as "modern slavery," remains a clandestine yet significant public health problem throughout the world, including the United States. It is associated with enduring adverse health and mental health outcomes.[31,32] Trafficking humans does not always indicate the movement of people from one location to another but, rather, equates to commerce in humans for their subsequent exploitation.[33] Most health care providers are unaware of the scope and complexities of human trafficking, making identification difficult.

In the United States, populations vulnerable to trafficking include children in the child welfare and juvenile justice systems, runaway and homeless youth, and children working in agriculture.[34] "Children are perhaps the most vulnerable population to human trafficking and are frequently targeted not only because of the ease of kidnapping but also because of their long-term value."[32] In addition, American Indians and Alaska Natives, migrant laborers, foreign national domestic workers in diplomatic households, employees of businesses in ethnic communities, populations with limited English proficiency, persons with disabilities, rural populations, and LGBTQ individuals are all vulnerable, with risk factors for trafficking identified as previous abuse, poverty, limited education, and substance misuse."[35] The most widely recognized form of human trafficking is sexual exploitation, but trafficking exploitation occurs in many different forms in the United States ("commercial sex, hospitality, sales crews, agriculture, manufacturing, janitorial services, construction, shipyards, healthcare, salon services, fairs and carnivals, peddling and begging, and domestic service"[35]). Anyone can become a victim of trafficking, and some victims will not display any obvious indicators of abuse.

The mental health consequences of human trafficking are extensive, and many human trafficking victims may require extensive and long-term mental health treatment.[36] The most commonly reported mental health problems in this population include depression, anxiety, PTSD, and attempted suicide. Addiction has a complex relationship with human trafficking: It can exacerbate a trafficked person's vulnerability; be part of a captor's means of coercing a captive person to submit, incentivizing a captive person to remain captive; and be used by the captive person as a mechanism of coping with the physical and mental traumas of being trafficked.[37] Although alcohol, marijuana, and cocaine have been reported as being utilized, opioids are an especially effective coercion tool for traffickers because they numb both emotional and physical pain.

Evaluation of possible trafficking victims is challenging because patients who have been exploited rarely self-identify.[35] As with IPV, not all trafficked persons are ready to leave their exploitative situation or even acknowledge that they are being exploited.[36] It is critical to approach all patients with a culturally sensitive trauma-informed care perspective, which prioritizes a safe environment for the clinical encounter and helps the patient regain a sense of agency and autonomy during the clinical encounter.[31,37] Involving social workers, case managers, and advocates early in suspected cases of human trafficking is highly recommended given their training in handling diverse and culturally sensitive situations.[35]

In addition to medical care, a trafficked patient's identified needs may include shelter, substance abuse treatment, legal services, and law enforcement.[36] Clinicians should respectfully and honestly discuss the possibility of or need for law enforcement involvement.[35] Many trafficked persons have a poor relationship with law enforcement because it may lead to unintended consequences, such as arrest of the patient for outstanding warrants or loss of patient trust. Law enforcement should be involved in state-specific mandated reporting scenarios, by patient request, or when clinicians appreciate imminent danger to staff or the patient.[35,36] If law enforcement is deemed necessary, connecting with the National Human Trafficking Resource Center Hotline may help in identifying which law enforcement officials would be most appropriate for the case at hand.

COVID-19 Considerations

Data suggest that violence, including IPV, increases during humanitarian crises and emergencies such as the COVID-19 pandemic. Managing the fear of the disease, restructuring of the household routine, increasing isolation with an abusive partner, and coping with financial hardship may exacerbate an already tenuous relationship, which may precipitate IPV episodes.[34] Enforcement of recommendations for self-isolation, lockdown, and closing of nonessential businesses puts victims in constant danger by the imposed and continuous proximity with the perpetrator and removes important protective factors, such as moments of relative freedom when the perpetrator or victim goes to work or access to support by additional people. Isolation and control have been critical tactics applied by violent partners; COVID-19 provides new opportunities of perpetration, including threats linked to the fear of infection, limiting or denial of necessary items, controlling transmission of reliable information about the pandemic, or spreading misinformation to further manipulate the victims.[34] Many victims may experience greater risk for economic abuse and may abandon or delay plans to seek independence from their abuser. In addition, calling hotlines or seeking safe spaces became much more challenging, limiting opportunities for victims to seek refuge or assistance.

Risk Factors

The CDC reports that certain individual, relational, community, and societal factors are linked to a greater likelihood of IPV perpetration but might not be direct causes, and not everyone who is identified as "at risk" becomes involved in violence.[23,26,38] Individual risk factors include past history of child maltreatment; psychological or personality disorders; violent behaviors; alcohol or substance abuse; physical, mental, or intellectual disability; youth and old age; limited education; low income; medical illness; recent migration; sexual or visual minority; and Indigenous status.[39] Relationship risk factors include marital discord, friends who engage in violence, need for overcontrol, jealousy, negative attitude toward women, and having other sexual partners;[39] however, having high friendship quality and tangible support from neighbors can be protective. Community factors that increase risk include poverty and associated factors, limited neighborhood support and cohesion, weak community sanctions against IPV, and high density of businesses that sell alcohol. Neighborhood cohesiveness, willingness to intervene for the common good, and having coordination of resources available among community agencies may be considered protective factors.[38] Societal factors such as gender inequality, cultural norms that support aggression toward others, societal income inequality, weak health, and educational, economic, and social policies increase overall risk for IPV.[39]

Health Implications of Intimate Partner Violence and Sexual Violence

Victims of IPV experience acute physical and mental health effects such as those sustained directly from injury and physical violence and intimidation, as well as indirect consequences such as chronic health problems related to prolonged stress, with adverse effects potentially persisting for years even after IPV stops.[23,38] Health consequences may also be related to

> the health damaging behaviors that victims use to cope with the abuse, such as smoking and substance use. Furthermore, such violence reduces victims' ability to be economically independent and can lead to lost productivity, missed work or school, unemployment, and housing instability.[3]

Physical health consequences frequently documented include direct injuries to the head, neck, or face;[3] fractures; lacerations; burns; urinary tract infections; STIs; HIV; unintended pregnancies; various gynecological syndromes; and numerous reproductive health consequences as a result of SV.[23] Functional disorders (conditions for which there is no identifiable medical cause) are common and include irritable bowel syndrome, other gastrointestinal symptoms, fibromyalgia, various chronic pain syndromes, and overall poor health.[23]

Mental health consequences include increased risk for depression, anxiety, PTSD, suicidality, and chronic mental illness. Women are 2.5 times more likely to experience depressive symptoms, suicidal ideation and behaviors, and have poor psychological adjustment than women who are not exposed to IPV.[1,3,23] IPV is also associated with alcohol and drug abuse, eating and sleep disorders, physical inactivity, poor self-esteem, PTSD, self-harm, and unsafe sexual practices.[23]

Specific to intimate partner sexual violence (IPSV), a unique pattern of adverse outcomes includes shame and elevated risk for PTSD, depression, problematic substance use, and suicidality compared with exposure to other forms of IPV. Multiple studies have found that victims of IPSV experienced higher levels of trauma-related symptoms of intrusion, avoidance, hyperarousal, and dissociative symptoms compared to those with nonsexual IPV.[40] "Adverse sexual health consequences of IPSV are

> more severe than in other forms of interpersonal violence given the mechanism, repetition, and frequency of abuse. Unlike sexual assault by a stranger or acquaintance, IPSV victims are often subject to repeated sexual assaults by their partner, which can predispose to a higher risk for adverse sexual health effects such as physical trauma to genitals during sexual assault, or pregnancy and STIs from lack of birth control or barrier protection.[40]

Children who witness IPSV in a parent are at a higher risk of internalizing behaviors than children who witness physical violence alone.[40]

Evaluation and Identification

Approaching patients of suspected IPV or SV in a trauma-informed manner allows the health care provider to support patients, rather than seeking disclosure of IPV as the ultimate goal. Trauma-informed care is a patient-centered approach in which the health care team realizes the widespread impact of trauma and understands potential paths for recovery; recognizes the signs and symptoms of trauma in clients, families, staff, and others involved with the system; responds by fully integrating knowledge about trauma into policies, procedures, and practices; and seeks to actively resist re-traumatization on the part of the patient.[23,26,38,41]

Creating an environment in which patients feel comfortable discussing IPV is imperative. Making resources (brochures and posters) available in waiting rooms and more discrete locations (bathrooms) gives the message that IPV is an important health issue and one that providers are willing to discuss.[39] Patients are more likely to disclose their experience of violence when practitioners listen and use open-ended questioning and when questioning is done in privacy. Others present should be asked to leave for the interview and examination; resistance to leaving may provide important diagnostic information about perpetration. The relational aspect of the questioning (e.g., concern and eye contact), rather than the particular words used, may be the most important factor when evaluating. Providers may want to avoid using terms such as "victim," "abused," or "battered" and instead mirror the patient's own word choices or use words such as "hurt," "frightened," or "treated badly."[42]

During the clinical encounter, observations such as inconsistent explanation of injuries, delay in seeking treatment, frequent emergency department or urgent visits, medication nonadherence, and missed appointments should heighten the clinician's suspicion of IPV.[43] Additional observations include apparent social isolation, inappropriate or incongruent affect, and avoidance of eye contact. Victims may appear jumpy, fearful, evasive, hostile, or cry readily. Typically, abusers do not want their victims to form an allegiance with one clinician and may believe the victim will be less likely to find an ally in an emergency department where care may be more fragmented. Victims may be accompanied by an overly attentive partner who may frequently answer most or all questions for the patient or by a verbally abusive partner who may also be reluctant to leave the patient alone in the examination room, which should raise flags for concern.

The psychiatric provider may not be the first clinician to evaluate the patient and will more likely work as part of the health care team. The provider should also learn the victim's common presenting complaints, which may include gynecologic conditions (premenstrual syndrome, STIs, unintended pregnancy, and chronic pelvic pain), somatic complaints (chronic pain, irritable bowel syndrome, headaches, and musculoskeletal pain), and mental health complaints (depression, suicidality, anxiety, and eating disorders).[42]

Typically, victims of IPV present with injuries on the central part of the body, such as the breasts, abdomen, and genitals; wounds on the head and neck; injuries on the forearms, suggesting possible defensive positioning; and bruises of different ages, which may suggest repeated abuse.[42] Evidence of sexual assault, including STIs (including HIV infection) or unintended pregnancy, may be present. The health care team should treat acute injuries, and the patient will likely require additional laboratory work, imaging, or official forensic examination by a sexual assault nurse examiner (SANE) if sexual assault is suspected or confirmed;[44] a SANE examination requires patient consent and cooperation.

Recommendations

Providers should be aware that leaving the relationship is not the only path to safety; other options may exist. "Providing a safe, respectable, compassionate place where a patient can reveal IPV is an important first step and providing education and support in a non-judgmental and caring manner empowers patients to make healthy change."[39] Coordination with the medical team and early involvement of social workers are recommended not only to support the patient by providing counseling, safety planning, and provisions for legal, financial, and housing resources but also to assist the medical team in navigating potential reporting, medicolegal, and ethical concerns.[38,47]

In the acute presentation and immediate management, the provider should reassure that the patient is in a safe and confidential environment. The provider should treat acute injuries, make inquiries regarding whether or not the patient feels safe to return home, help mobilize social supports, assist with providing referrals to appropriate services, and set up a follow-up care provider (primary care physician or mental health provider) to monitor for emergence of depression, PTSD, and substance abuse. Psychiatric providers are in the unique position to provide psychoeducation about the effects of trauma, including anxiety, hyperarousal, irritability, sleep disturbance, and re-experiencing phenomenon, in addition to providing therapeutic strategies such as grounding techniques. Helping the patient create a safety plan with an "escape" or emergency kit may help the patient feel more empowered, yet not force the patient to make the difficult decision to leave their perpetrator. Depending on the presentations, providers may also consider psychopharmacologic interventions with anxiolytics such as short-term use of benzodiazepine (lorazepam and clonazepam) or hydrocortisone.[38] Regarding long-term management and follow-up care, data from meta-analyses and random control trials support eye movement desensitization and reprocessing and trauma-focused cognitive–behavioral therapy and indicate greater efficacy in addressing PTSD and comorbid substance use disorders.[41] When appropriate, psychopharmacologic interventions such as selective serotonin reuptake inhibitors are useful in targeting reduction of depression, anxiety, and PTSD symptoms, with moderate strength of evidence for fluoxetine, paroxetine, and venlafaxine.[41]

Screening

The U.S. Preventive Services Task Force (USPSTF) recently updated recommendations to promote screening as a method for detection of IPV and also emphasized that intervention and referral to support services for IPV are necessary to reduce violence and abuse, as well as associated physical or mental harm in women of reproductive age.[45] Perceived barriers to evaluation and intervention of suspected IPV cases include personal discomfort; concern for personal safety; resource constraints including limited time; lack of knowledge, education, or training regarding screening; and perception of inadequate follow-up resources and support staff available to support victims. Psychiatric providers, who are charged with caring and treating all patients, must make a significant effort to overcome the fears and biases of members of this vulnerable and mistreated population in order to support and care for them. There is no "gold standard" tool, but short clinician surveys such as HITS (Hurt, Insult, Threaten, Scream), STaT (Slapped, Threatened, and Throw), and WAST (Woman Abuse Screening Tool) have demonstrated high sensitivity and specificity in multiple comparative analysis.[42]

Reporting Requirements

Because requirements for reporting vary, the clinician needs to be familiar with state or country law regarding situations in which reporting is mandated. Mandatory reporting of IPV is controversial, and laws requiring reporting of IPV are aimed at identifying and protecting victims; however, this may place victims in danger of retaliation or increased abuse, supersede women's autonomy, and could negatively affect the patient–physician relationship and decrease disclosure of abuse by patients.[39] Domestic violence programs, either community- or hospital-based, can often aid with reporting and/or guidance about whether reporting is indicated. Generally, state laws provide immunity from civil or criminal liability for filing reports of abuse if completed in good faith.[28]

The following commonly require reporting:

- Abuse of disabled persons: Harm to disabled persons must be reported to the Disabled Persons Protection Commission.
- Weapon use: In most states, injury resulting from assault with a firearm or knife or causing "grave bodily harm" mandates reporting.
- Elder abuse
- Child abuse: Within the United States, domestic violence involving a child must be reported if the child is younger than age 18 years and if sexual and physical abuse, or neglect of a child is suspected.

Social workers and the hospital team can assist patients in initiating a domestic violence protective order, legally preventing perpetrators from contact with patients if patients believe they are in danger. In general, a community advocate or legal advisor will assist the patient with obtaining this document. Evidence of the effectiveness of protection orders is inconsistent, but they may be one of the many options that may help victims of IPV feel empowered.

Elder Abuse

Case Example

An older male with multiple medical comorbidities presents to the emergency department in a wheelchair accompanied by his caretaker with chief complaints of difficulty sleeping and increased irritability. He is dressed in multiple layers of clothing despite the warm weather, with food stains on his face and long untrimmed nails. The patient initially sits quietly while the caretaker answers most questions for the patient until the patient abruptly shouts that his caretaker knows nothing and "doesn't care about me at all" while glaring angrily. The caretaker does not appear phased by this outburst and continues to outline their concerns, while also expressing increased frustration with the patient.

Elder abuse, including neglect and exploitation, is a serious problem in the United States that is frequently underreported yet common, affecting 5–10% of community-dwelling older adults annually,[46] with 50% of older victims of violent crime being assaulted by a family member or caregiver.[44] From 2002 to 2016, more than 19,000 homicides occurred, and more than 643,000 older adults were treated in the emergency department for nonfatal assaults. Studies have indicated that these estimates grossly underestimate the incidence of elder abuse and that for every incident reported or detected case of elder abuse, approximately 23 cases remain unreported and undetected.[3] In addition, individuals of ethnic minority (African American, Hispanic, and non-White) were 2.1 times more likely to experience elder abuse.[3]

Elder abuse and neglect are complex phenomena with multiple underlying etiologies, with research describing familial or learned behaviors, preexisting IPV (later termed elder abuse due to patient age), as well as increased victimization as the older adult develops more functional and/or cognitive disabilities leading to stressed caregivers becoming abusive or neglectful.[44] Often, the older individual may be afraid or unable to speak of the abuse because they may depend on or deeply care for the perpetrator, and thus the older individual frequently suffers in secrecy.[46] Providers are often faced with other challenges, specifically balancing autonomy and the well-being of vulnerable adults when treating or seeking to prevent elder abuse.[46]

Forms of Violence

Violence experienced by older adults can be categorized into three main forms: violence directed toward older adults, including IPV; self-directed violence (suicide or nonfatal self-harm); and violence perpetrated by older adults against others.[46]

Violence directed toward older adults is typically identified as elder abuse, which is defined as an intentional act or failure to act that causes or creates a risk of harm to an adult aged 60 years or older. Older adults may be targets of perpetration because of their perceived vulnerability and lower likelihood of reporting. Violence can be perpetrated by strangers or by someone who is known to the victim and in a position of trust.[46] Many older adult victims of IPV may have suffered for decades in an abusive relationship but given their current age, it is now termed elder abuse.[46] Late-onset IPV describes a pattern of IPV that begins in later adulthood and is thought to be related to retirement, new roles in partnership, disability, cognitive impairment, and sexual changes related to the aging process.[43]

The most common types of abuse or violence identified by the CDC include physical abuse, sexual abuse, emotional or psychological abuse, neglect, and financial abuse. Financial abuse is a concerning phenomenon described as the illegal, unauthorized, or improper use of an elder's money, benefits, belongings, property, or assets for the benefit of someone other than the older adult, and it can be difficult to identify for the physician; however, it is not the focus of this chapter.[47] The other common types of abuse are defined as follows:[46]

> *Physical abuse* is the intentional use of physical force (hitting, kicking, pushing, slapping, or burning) to cause the older adult illness, pain, injury, functional impairment, distress, or death.
>
> *Sexual abuse* is the forced or unwanted sexual interaction of any kind with an older adult, including unwanted sexual contact or penetration or noncontact acts such as sexual harassment.
>
> *Emotional or psychological abuse* refers to verbal or nonverbal behaviors that inflict anguish, mental pain, fear, or distress on an older adult, including humiliation or disrespect, verbal and nonverbal threats, harassment, and geographic or interpersonal isolation.
>
> *Neglect* is the failure to meet an older adult's basic needs (food, water, shelter, clothing, hygiene, and essential medical care).

Regarding self-directed violence, self-harming behaviors and suicide attempts are of particular concern, with suicide rates higher among older adults. Women's suicide rates peak in midlife, and men's suicide rates continue to a peak into old age at a rate that is 3.6 times greater than the age-adjusted overall rate for men and women combined.[44] Older adults are also more likely than younger adults to use firearms rather than other methods in suicide attempts and are more likely to live alone and therefore less likely to be found in sufficient time to be rescued after suicide attempts. "These characteristics, combined with reduced physical resilience to survive an attempt, lead to higher fatality rates in suicide attempts in later life."[44]

Although older adults are more often the victims rather than the perpetrators of violence, it is necessary to recognize the two main scenarios wherein older adults might inflict harm onto others: IPV that continues into later life and violence perpetrated toward relatives or others with dementia or other progressive chronic brain diseases. Alzheimer's disease is the most common type of dementia, and the long-term gradual decreases in cognition and memory, accompanied with anxiety, delusions, and paranoia, can all contribute to behavioral changes and potentially violent outbursts.[44] "Approximately 20 percent of home-based dementia caregivers experience violence or aggression, which may be associated with subsequent placement of the person with dementia in a long-term care facility."[44]

Risk Factors

A complex constellation of risk factors at the levels of the victim, perpetrator, relationship, community, and society can increase the likelihood of elder abuse.[3] Notable risk factors include cognitive impairment, medical illness, functional disability or dependence, psychiatric illness, substance misuse, low socioeconomic status, and social isolation or low social support.[44]

Firearm access requires special consideration because there is an increased risk for violence perpetration and also increased mortality. Although potentially controversial, it has also been a focus of many prevention efforts, with increased attention to education in firearm safety, storage, and removal. Firearm access can increase the risk of serious injury or death, with higher rates of firearm access in the older population contributing to higher completed suicide rates in the context of other risk factors for violence, such as depression, PTSD, or heavy alcohol use.[44] Yet, firearm ownership can also be a source of identity and pride, which highlights the challenge of balancing safety with autonomy. Veterans in particular may be at elevated risk because of the high rate of firearm ownership and multiple risk factors for experiencing elder abuse, including poor physical health, functional dependence, social isolation, and a high prevalence of past trauma and subsequent elevated rates of PTSD.[44] Providers should make efforts to review how to store guns safely in the home, such as ensuring ammunition and firearms are separated and in a locked safe, and possibly ask patients to consider removing firearms from the home.

Health Implications of Elder Abuse

Multiple studies have shown that victims of elder abuse have increased mortality, poorer general health, chronic pain, sleep disturbance, and metabolic syndrome compared to those who have not been abused.[3] Immediate and short-term consequences include increased presentation to the emergency department or hospitalizations for minor to major injuries, unaddressed or worsening chronic illnesses likely related to neglect, as well as poorer quality of life.[44] Psychological consequences that have been studied more extensively include higher levels of stress and depression, increased risk for developing fear and other anxiety reactions, and increased suicidal thinking and attempts in the abused population. Any type of mistreatment can leave victims feeling fearful, depressed, and isolated, with self-blame further exacerbating psychological impact.[44]

Evaluation

Studies have shown that physical abuse and neglect are consistently unrecognized in the emergency setting as well as outpatient office setting in comparison to the reported prevalence in the community,[48] with victims often presenting with somatic complaints rather than the outright complaint of abuse.[44,49] One challenge to elder abuse identification is obtaining a reliable history because many older adults who are at increased risk for mistreatment may suffer from cognitive impairment, affecting their ability to accurately report. Paranoia may pose an additional complication because it is often a common feature with certain types of dementia versus increasing fear and distrust resulting from prolonged abuse or neglect.[44] Language and cultural considerations may also pose additional barriers. In addition, many victims may be reluctant to report abuse or neglect because of guilt, same, or fear of reprisal; however, obtaining a complete and accurate medical history is critical to evaluate for abuse or neglect.[44]

During a patient evaluation, indications from medical history that may suggest possible elder abuse or neglect include unexplained injuries; past history of frequent injuries or patient referred to as "accident prone"; delay between onset of medical illness and seeking medical attention; recurrent visits to the emergency department for similar injuries; using multiple physicians and emergency departments ("doctor shopping") for care rather than their primary care provider; and noncompliance with medications, appointments, or physician directions.[44] Patients may present with signs of neglect, including dirty clothing, poor dental hygiene, and untrimmed or dirty fingernails.[44]

Ideally, providers should attempt to interview the patient separately when possible, given the limitations noted above. Providers should observe behavioral signs which may offer clues that suggest elder abuse and neglect, including fear, poor eye contact, anxiety, low self-esteem, and helplessness. When the caregiver is the suspected perpetrator, providers should also observe patient–caregiver interaction for signs of strain and seek collateral evidence from other sources, such as other providers or family members.[48] Conflicting accounts, caregiver frequently interrupting or answering for the older adult, and observed fearful or hostile behaviors toward the caregiver may also be concerning signs that may suggest elder mistreatment.

Interviewing caregivers separately may reveal discrepancies in the patient's history and provide the opportunity to explore whether changes or stressors have occurred in the patient's residence and whether the caregiver believes the patient is a burden. Providers should approach this interview as an opportunity to learn more about the patient, and it allows the clinical team the opportunity to provide a potentially overburdened caregiver supportive resources such as respite services. Potential indications that a caregiver may be overwhelmed or burdened include a caregiver's inattentive or disengaged manner or appearing frustrated, angry, or expressing frustration. Neglect may be related to the caregiver's lack of knowledge or understanding of the patient's care needs, in which case the clinical team should provide education and re-evaluate the level of care services.[44]

Screening Tools

The Centers for Medicare and Medicaid Services' Physician Quality Reporting System, Measure No. 181, focuses exclusively on elder mistreatment and gives examples of screening tools for elder maltreatment, including the Elder Abuse Suspicion Index, the Vulnerability to Abuse Screening Scale, and the Hwalek–Sengstock Elder Abuse Screening Test, which it notes are psychometrically sound instruments with demonstrated reliability and validity indices.[44] Providers are encouraged to become familiar with their facilities' screening tools and utilize them to evaluate cases of suspected elder mistreatment.

Recommendations

During a psychiatric evaluation, if there are notable signs of physical injury requiring urgent attention, including reported or suspected sexual abuse, an official forensic examination such as SANE may be necessary in addition to laboratory work, imaging, thorough physical examination, and medical treatment of acute injuries. Coordination with the medical team and early involvement of social workers are recommended because they are uniquely qualified to assist in reporting and provide counseling, safety planning, and appropriate resources to patients and caregivers.[44] Resources such as home health services (e.g., Meals on Wheels), medical transportation services, adult day care, senior centers, substance use treatment options, and respite care may provide much needed support for an overwhelmed caregiver.[44]

If the suspected abuser is present, the clinical team should ensure that the patient does not have contact with the suspected abuser during the evaluation This may be challenging, particularly if the suspected perpetrator is a health care proxy, caregiver, or power of attorney. It may require involving the hospital administration and legal department to assist with issues regarding health care, decision-making, and guardianship.[44]

Intervention and prevention efforts must be balanced with the competing goals of autonomy and protection. If a patient experiencing abuse or neglect declines intervention or services, assessment of capacity to refuse may be needed in this vulnerable population. This is similar to the management of IPV: When a victim has the capacity to refuse care, their choice to return to an unsafe environment must be respected. Attempts to provide psychoeducation about violence, abuse, safety planning, and appropriate community services should be made even when the patient refuses intervention.[44]

Prevention strategies currently being evaluated/implemented include educational intervention and caregiver support programs, as well as increased efforts for educating health care workers to recognize potential signs of neglect or abuse. Current campaigns focus on the prevalence and prevention of suicide in older adults and firearm safety, specifically raising awareness among professionals and the public.[44] Interventions should not be based exclusively in health care systems, and a cornerstone of healthy aging is enabling older adults to remain independent, active, and involved in their communities.[44]

In 2018, the USPSTF updated its recommendations on elder mistreatment screening, concluding that current evidence is insufficient to assess the balance of benefits and harms of routine screening of all older adults for abuse and neglect in health care settings.[45] However, given the enormous potential impact on an individual patient and their health, commentators have strongly advocated that clinicians evaluate for elder mistreatment as part of routine care.[24,44,45]

Reporting Requirements

Suspected or confirmed elder abuse or neglect should be reported; the provider does not need to prove what is occurring because reporting allows for the investigatory process to begin. Adult Protective Services is the agency that investigates these cases, but it functions differently from Child Protective Services, and requirements may vary by state.[50] All health care providers (physicians, nurses, social workers, etc.) and administrators are mandated by law to report suspected elder mistreatment and can be found to be negligent if they fail to do so.[43,44,50] Additional information can be obtained from any state's Department of Health website and the National Adult Protective Services website; any Area Agency on Aging is able to aid in reporting suspected mistreatment.

If the older adult is a resident of a long-term care facility, a separate process often exists for investigating suspected mistreatment through the state agency that surveys these facilities. Identifying the appropriate avenue for investigation can be done through the available Adult Protective Services agency or the state department of child and family services. Contacting the police is always an option, especially in an urgent situation.[49]

Violence Resources National Domestic Violence Hotline 800-799-7233 (toll-free, 24/7) 800-787-3224 (TTY/toll-free) http://www.thehotline.org/get-help National Victims of Crimes Hotline 1-855-4-VICTIM (855-484-2846)
Child Abuse National Clearinghouse on Child Abuse and Neglect *Specific state statutes* http://www.childwelfare.gov/systemwide/laws_policies/search/index.cfm Child Abuse Evaluation & Treatment for Medical Providers http://www.ChildAbuseMD.com Childhelp National Child Abuse Hotline USA *Crisis counseling* http://childhelpusa.org 1-800-4-A-Child (1-800-422-4453) National Child and Traumatic Stress Network *Trauma-informed care while doing trauma assessments* https://www.nctsn.org National Children's Advocacy Center https://www.nationalcac.org American Professional Society on the Abuse of Children Covid Resources https://www.apsac.org/covid-19
Elder Abuse Eldercare Locator 800-677-1116 (toll-free) https://eldercare.acl.gov

National Adult Protective Services Association
202-370-6292
https://www.napsa-now.org
National Center on Elder Abuse
855-500-3537
https://ncea.acl.gov

Community-Based Supports
- Area Agencies on Aging, which are funded by State Units on Aging using federal funds, should be key players in such efforts.
- Senior Corps volunteers (55 years or older) provide peer companionship in which individuals are linked with vulnerable elders to reduce social isolation and help with everyday tasks.

Intimate Partner Violence and Sexual Violence
CDC
Dating Matters Strategies to Promote Healthy Teen Relationships https://www.cdc.gov/violenceprevention/intimatepartnerviolence/datingmatters/index.html

Futures Without Violence
Contains brochures, posters, and safety planning cards
https://www.futureswithoutviolence.org
Mandatory reporting compendium
http://www.futureswithoutviolence.org/userfiles/file/HealthCare/Compendium%20Final.pdf

National Coalition Against Domestic Violence
Online tool to crease safety plan
http://www.ncadv.org

National Sexual Assault Hotline
1.800.656.HOPE (4673)
https://www.rainn.org/resources

National Teen Dating Abuse Helpline
1.866.331.9474
1.866.331.8453 (TTY)

Human Trafficking
National Human Trafficking Resource Center
Hotline: 1-888-373-7888 (available 24/7)
BeFree text: 233733 (available 3–11 p.m. Eastern Standard Time)
https://traffickingresourcecenter.org

Administration for Children & Families, Office on Trafficking in Persons
https://www.acf.hhs.gov

HEAL Trafficking and Hope for Justice
http://healtrafficking.org

International Organization for Migration
Trafficked Persons Guidance for Healthcare Providers
http://publications.iom.int/system/files/pdf/ct_handbook.pdf

National Health Collaborative on Violence and Abuse
http://nhcva.org/2014/04/15/webinar-human-trafficking

References

1. The Violence Prevention Information System (Violence Info). World Health Organization. Accessed December 31, 2020. https://apps.who.int/violence-info

2. Hargarten SW, Christiansen A. Violence prevention and control: A public health approach. In: Glick RL, ed., *Emergency Psychiatry: Principles and Practice*. Lippincott Williams & Wilkins; 2008.

3. Rivara F, Adhia A, Lyons V, et al. The effects of violence on health. *Health Aff.* 2019;38(10):1622–1629. doi:10.1377/hlthaff.2019.00480

4. Firearm violence prevention. Centers for Disease Control and Prevention. Accessed January 4, 2020. https://www.cdc.gov/violenceprevention/firearms/fastfact.html

5. Effects of complex trauma. National Child Traumatic Stress Network. Accessed January 28, 2021. https://www.nctsn.org/what-is-child-trauma/trauma-types/complex-trauma/effects

6. Fairbanks JA. The epidemiology of trauma and trauma related disorders in children and youth. *PTSD Res Q.* 2008;19(1):1–3.

7. Wilson HW, Woods BA, Emerson E, Donenberg GR. Patterns of violence exposure and sexual risk in low-income, urban African American girls. *Psychol Violence.* 2012;2(2):194–207.

8. Finkelhor D, Ormrod R, Turner H, Hamby S. School, police, and medical authority involvement with children who have experienced victimization. *Arch Pediatr Adolesc Med.* 2011;165(1):9–15.

9. Feiguine RJ, Ross-Dolen MM, Havens J. The New York Presbyterian Pediatric Crisis Service. *Psychiatric Q.* 2000;71(2):139–152.

10. Lieberman AF, Ghosh Ippen C, van Horn P. Child–parent psychotherapy: 6-month follow-up of a randomized controlled trial. *J Am Acad Child Adolesc Psychiatry.* 2006;45(8):913–918.

11. McDonald KC. Child abuse: Approach and management. *Am Fam Physician.* 2007;75(2): 221–228.

12. Saade DN, Simon HK, Greenwald M. Abused children: Missed opportunities for recognition in the ED. *Acad Emerg Med.* 2002;9:524.

13. Rosenberg LA. Effects of maltreatment on the child. In: Wissow LS, ed. *Child Advocacy for the Clinician: An Approach to Child Abuse and Neglect*. Williams & Wilkins, 1990:12.

14. Ludwig S. Child abuse. In: Fleisher GR, Ludwig S, Henretig FM, Ruddy RM, Silverman BK, eds. *Textbook of Pediatric Emergency Medicine*. 4th ed. Lippincott Williams & Wilkins; 2000.

15. Goldman J, Salus M, Wolcott D, Kennedy K. *A Coordinated Response to Child Abuse and Neglect: The Foundation for Practice*. National Clearinghouse on Child Abuse and Neglect Information; 2003. http://www.childwelfare.gov/pubs/usermanuals/foundation/index.cfm

16. Hamarman S, Bernet W. Evaluating and reporting emotional abuse in children: Parent-based, action-based focus aids in clinical decision-making. *J Am Acad Child Adolesc Psychiatry.* 2000;39:928–930.

17. Committee on Child Abuse and Neglect, American Academy of Pediatrics. When inflicted skin injuries constitute child abuse. *Pediatrics.* 2002;110:644–645.

18. American College of Radiology. ACR practice guideline for skeletal surveys in children. Resolution 22. Accessed January 26, 2021. http://www.acr.org/s_acr/bin.asp?CID= 543&DID=12286&DOC=FILE.PDF

19. American Academy of Pediatrics, Section on Radiology. Diagnostic imaging of child abuse. *Pediatrics.* 2000;105:1345–1348.

20. American Academy of Pediatrics, Committee on Hospital Care and Committee on Child Abuse and Neglect. Medical necessity for the hospitalization of the abused and neglected child. *Pediatrics.* 1998;101(4 Pt 1):715–716.

21. Heger A, Ticson L, Velasquez O, Bernier R. Children referred for possible sexual abuse: Medical findings in 2384 children. *Child Abuse Negl.* 2002;26:645–659.

22. Child Welfare Information Gateway. Child abuse & neglect. Accessed January 27, 2021. http://www.childwelfare.gov/can/index.cfm

23. Chisholm CA, Bullock L, Ferguson JEJ 2nd. Intimate partner violence and pregnancy: Epidemiology and impact. *Am J Obstet Gynecol.* 2017;217(2):141–144. doi:10.1016/j.ajog.2017.05.042

24. Miller E, Beach SR, Thurston RC. Addressing intimate partner violence and abuse of older or vulnerable adults in the health care setting—Beyond screening. *JAMA Intern Med.* 2018;178(12):1583–1585. doi:10.1001/jamainternmed.2018.6523

25. Breiding MJ, Basile KC, Smith SG, Black MC, Mahendra RR. *Intimate Partner Violence Surveillance: Uniform Definitions and Recommended Data Elements. Version 2.0.* National Center for Injury Prevention and Control, Centers for Disease Control and Prevention; 2015.

26. Niolon, PH, Kearns M, Dills J, et al. *Preventing Intimate Partner Violence Across the Lifespan: A Technical Package of Programs, Policies, and Practices.* National Center for Injury Prevention and Control, Centers for Disease Control and Prevention; 2017.

27. Basile KC, Smith SG, Breiding MJ, Black MC, Mahendra RR. *Sexual Violence Surveillance: Uniform Definitions and Recommended Data Elements. Version 2.0.* National Center for Injury Prevention and Control, Centers for Disease Control and Prevention; 2014.

28. Lutgendorf MA. Intimate partner violence and women's health. *Obstet Gynecol.* 2019;134(3):470–480. doi:10.1097/AOG.0000000000003326

29. Henshaw E, Marcus S. Psychiatric emergencies during pregnancy and postpartum and review of gender issues in psychiatric emergency medicine. In: Glick RL. *Emergency Psychiatry: Principles and Practice.* Lippincott Williams & Wilkins; 2008.

30. Smith SG, Zhang X, Basile KC, et al. *The National Intimate Partner and Sexual Violence Survey (NISVS): 2015 Data Brief–Updated Release.* National Center for Injury Prevention and Control, Centers for Disease Control and Prevention; 2018.

31. Recknor F, Gordon M, Coverdale J, Gardezi M, Nguyen PT. A descriptive study of United States-based human trafficking specialty clinics. *Psychiatr Q.* 2020;91(1):1–10. doi:10.1007/s11126-019-09691-8

32. Costa CB, McCoy KT, Early GJ, Deckers CM. Evidence-based care of the human trafficking patient. *Nurs Clin North Am.* 2019;54(4):569–584. doi:10.1016/j.cnur.2019.08.007

33. Myths and facts about human trafficking. Administration for Children and Families, Office on Trafficking in Persons. Published 2017. https://www.acf.hhs.gov/otip/about/myths-facts-human-trafficking

34. Moreira DN, Pinto da Costa M. The impact of the Covid-19 pandemic in the precipitation of intimate partner violence. *Int J Law Psychiatry.* 2020;71:101606. doi:10.1016/j.ijlp.2020.101606

35. Shandro J, Chisolm-Straker M, Duber HC, et al. Human trafficking: A guide to identification and approach for the emergency physician. *Ann Emerg Med.* 2016;68(4):501–508.e1. doi:10.1016/j.annemergmed.2016.03.049

36. Gibbons P, Stoklosa H. Identification and treatment of human trafficking victims in the emergency department: A case report. *J Emerg Med.* 2016;50(5):715–719. doi:10.1016/j.jemermed.2016.01.004

37. Stoklosa H, MacGibbon M, Stoklosa J. Human trafficking, mental illness, and addiction: Avoiding diagnostic overshadowing. *AMA J Ethics.* 2017;19(1):23–34.

38. Stewart DE, Vigod S, Riazantseva E. New developments in intimate partner violence and management of its mental health sequelae. *Curr Psychiatry Rep.* 2016;18(1):4. doi:10.1007/s11920-015-0644-3

39. Sugg N. Intimate partner violence: Prevalence, health consequences, and intervention. *Med Clin North Am.* 2015;99(3):629–649. doi:10.1016/j.mcna.2015.01.012

40. Barker LC, Stewart DE, Vigod SN. Intimate partner sexual violence: An often overlooked problem. *J Womens Health.* 2019;28(3):363–374. doi:10.1089/jwh.2017.6811

41. Stewart DE, Vigod SN. Update on mental health aspects of intimate partner violence. *Med Clin North Am.* 2019;103(4):735–749. doi:10.1016/j.mcna.2019.02.010

42. Weil A. Intimate partner violence: Intervention and patient management. UpToDate; 2020.

43. Beach SR, Carpenter CR, Rosen T, Sharps P, Gelles R. Screening and detection of elder abuse: Research opportunities and lessons learned from emergency geriatric care, intimate partner violence, and child abuse. *J Elder Abuse Negl.* 2016;28(4–5):185–216. doi:10.1080/08946566.2016.1229241

44. Rosen T, Platts-Mills TF, Fulmer T. Screening for elder mistreatment in emergency departments: Current progress and recommendations for next steps. *J Elder Abuse Negl.* 2020;32(3):295–315. doi:10.1080/08946566.2020.1768997

45. US Preventive Services Task Force. Screening for intimate partner violence, elder abuse, and abuse of vulnerable adults: US Preventive Services Task Force final recommendation statement. *JAMA.* 2018;320(16):1678–1687. doi:10.1001/jama.2018.14741

46. Violence prevention. Centers for Disease Control and Prevention. Accessed December 31, 2020. http://cdc.gov/violenceprevention/elderabuse/fastfact.html

47. Elder abuse. National Institutes of Health, National Institute on Aging. Published 2020. Accessed December 31, 2020. https://www.nia.nih.gov/health/elder-abuse

48. Mercier É, Nadeau A, Brousseau AA, et al. Elder abuse in the out-of-hospital and emergency department settings: A scoping review. *Ann Emerg Med.* 2020;75(2):181–191. doi:10.1016/j.annemergmed.2019.12.011

49. Swagerty DL Jr, Takahashi PY, Evans JM. Elder mistreatment. *Am Fam Physician.* 1999;59(10):2804–2808.

50. 2013 Nationwide survey of mandatory reporting requirements for elderly and/or vulnerable persons. National Adult Protective Services Association. Updated December 2015. Retrieved January 2, 2021. http://www.napsa-now.org/wp-content/uploads/2016/05/Mandatory-Reporting-Chart-Updated-December-2015-FINAL.pdf

SECTION IV

DISPOSITION, AFTERCARE, LEGAL ISSUES, AND FUTURE DIRECTIONS

20

Tool, Constraint, Liability, Context

Law and Emergency Psychiatry

John S. Rozel and Layla Soliman

With great power comes great responsibility.

—Apocryphal

I fought the law and the law won.

—The Clash

Introduction and General Considerations

Few areas of clinical medicine are as entwined with the law as emergency psychiatry. The legal concepts underpinning our craft include patient rights, duties to third parties, and commitment laws, to name a few. Balancing these elements is complex yet critical to the successful practice of the discipline. And the intersection is not accidental: More than any other aspect of clinical medicine, emergency psychiatry routinely involves the modification or disruption of patients' fundamental legal rights. Proper practice of emergency psychiatry requires proper and frequent application of legal tools, as it does with medical science. Such responsibility must not be taken lightly, nor used capriciously.

Although at times the concept of interacting with legal systems seems daunting, note that understanding defeats fear. The legal context of emergency psychiatry is not just about rules and consequences but also about finding tools and pathways to effective intervention, collaboration, and protection of patient rights, patient and community safety, and physician decision-making. This chapter guides the reader through essential elements of ethical and legal concepts as they apply to the practice of emergency psychiatry.

Importantly, the legal rules—which derive from statutes enacted by legislatures and common law standards arising from appellate and supreme court decisions—can vary substantially across legal jurisdictions and over time. Some legal standards arise from federal sources, such as the Health Insurance Portability and Accountability Act (HIPAA) regulations for privacy or the *Jaffee v. Redmond* standard for psychotherapist privilege arising from the Supreme Court. Many standards evolve from state-level legislatures or courts (e.g., commitment laws or duties to third party standards). Although this chapter discusses many general precepts, the reader is urged to explore and understand the nuances of their own jurisdiction's rules and customs.

Law plays a variety of roles in emergency psychiatry. The legal standards and procedures encompassing voluntary and involuntary commitment and consent for psychiatric evaluation are the foundation on which emergency psychiatry exists: These laws provide opportunities for intervention and protections of patients' rights. These standards are generally more stringent and specific than the laws guiding other types of medical treatment and, while adhering to national minimal standards, vary substantially between states. Furthermore, the looming specter of malpractice risk hangs over all areas of health care. Although psychiatry and emergency medicine are not expressly high risk,[1] there are many features of emergency psychiatry that may be concerning, including brevity of engagement, lack of access to collateral information, and the challenges of working with patients and supports who may be deeply vested in outcomes that are clinically contraindicated. Emergency psychiatry interacts with law enforcement routinely, and an understanding their duties, limitations, and culture is essential to successful outcomes. Finally, emergency psychiatry exists in the same environment as the rest of health care—heavily regulated and bounded by laws and rules covering billing, employment, facility design, and other factors.

Even the most skilled emergency psychiatrists, including those with forensic training, cannot be expected to master all the intricacies of law as applied to their work. Cultivating a network of skilled, accessible, and collaborative advisors is essential. Hospital attorneys who understand the work and the mission of emergency psychiatry are invaluable, as are experienced risk management professionals who can guide the psychiatric emergency services (PES) team through complex cases. Finding useful resources for nuanced information, such as guides for understanding duties to third parties, laws for treatment of minors, and other areas of the law, can be invaluable.

Finally, even with these resources, humility is warranted. The cases seen in PES are routinely complex and extraordinarily complicated. Outlier cases—such as those involving minors, people with intellectual disability or progressive dementia, people with active criminal justice issues, among other factors—may defy even the most scrupulous attempts to apply available law. At times, imperfect solutions will need to be accepted while care is handed off to other providers for definitive management.

Ethical Considerations

The practice of emergency psychiatry comes with unique rewards and challenges. Ethical issues account for a variety of challenges that one may encounter. Often, we are called upon to balance our role as advocates for patients, our obligation to act in a patient's best interest even if that is at odds with what the patient wants, and our duty to third parties. In this section, we explore some common categories of ethical issues and possible approaches to resolving potential conflicts.

Agency and Duty

Psychiatrists in an emergency setting may be confronted by dual agency in a variety of scenarios.[2] Their roles as hospital employees, learners, team members, and supervisors can occasionally create tension within the physician–patient relationship. For example, a resident physician may feel comfortable discharging the patient but their supervisor may not, or the reverse. Furthermore, a resident or other trainee must balance their obligation to the patient with deference to their supervisor's experience, and even with their duty to learn from each patient.[3] There are risks to different team members presenting mixed messages, as well as the inherent risk of the decision sometimes needing to be made even without team consensus. Of course, every effort should be made to reach such consensus, but there may be some areas in which that cannot be achieved.

Confidentiality and Collateral Information

Another potential for conflicting duties arises when the patient and their family have markedly different perspectives on symptom severity and need for treatment. Yet another conflict may arise when balancing duty to third parties against the patient's right of confidentiality. Similarly, when evaluating and treating children and adolescents, the perceived interests of the minor and their parents may not align. The need to involve family/supports in the patient's treatment whenever possible further complicates the navigation of such conflicts.

Broadly, the following interventions can be utilized:

1. Supervisors, learners, and other team members should discuss cases prior to communicating recommendations to patients whenever possible, particularly when differing viewpoints are foreseeable (e.g., when there may be more than one reasonable course of action).
2. Upfront communication with patients regarding the need to involve a third party such as family or law enforcement should be undertaken at the beginning of the evaluation. Basically, this amounts to a discussion of the limits of confidentiality.
3. Utilization of group discussions with the patient and their supports can be very helpful in resolving conflict.

However, physicians should be prepared for times when conflicts between parties cannot be resolved and we must make the best judgment we can with the available data. Depending on jurisdictional limitations on confining the patient while more data are gathered, one may be frequently faced with making a judgment with an incomplete data set. In such cases, documentation of the limitations on the physician's ability to gather relevant data is essential. Although legal limitations on the ability to hold the patient or gather information can be frustrating, at times they can simplify the decision-making process by default. Some of the more difficult decisions arise when we find ourselves in a gray area—when we may be able to override the patient's wishes and contact a source of collateral information—but we must decide whether the benefit outweighs the risk.

Medicine, and psychiatry in particular, relies heavily on building a relationship with the patient and their supports. Ideally, patients will be able to identify at least one reliable source of collateral information whom they are willing to have staff contact. However, when they cannot, psychiatrists must consider the risks and benefits of breaching patient preferences by using permitted disclosures under HIPAA and related jurisdictional standards.[4] Although these communications may be legally permissible, they may seem like a violation to the patient. Simply stated, just because one can does not mean one should.

There may be a variety of reasons to decide to forego collateral information. For example, a person may be in a high-conflict divorce from their spouse and releasing even a minimum of information could have adverse impact on custody issues. Revealing information such as a relapse of a substance use disorder may impact existing relationships. Domestic violence situations could mean that a person has been cut off from most other supports and that their spouse is not a safe person for them to rely on in recovery.

A common conflict with collateral informants involves patients and supports having conflicting perspectives on the events that led to the patient's presentation. At times, the clinician can reconcile such conflict relatively easily—for example, based on the patient's history and/or current clinical presentation. Nevertheless, the conflicts can place the clinician in the difficult situation of trying to build rapport with the patient while also taking opposing viewpoints into account. Rarely, one encounters collateral sources that are not operating in good faith or whose views are clouded by unhealthy relationship dynamics.

To be clear, for most cases, collateral information should be sought and obtained whenever possible. However, the cases that tend to cause the most consternation are not those in the vast majority. Ultimately, in those cases, rationale for obtaining or foregoing collateral contact should be carefully documented. When collateral contact is made despite the patient's objection, the nature of the information revealed and the basis for revealing it, as well as steps taken to protect the patient's privacy, should be part of the record.

Building Relationships with Families and Their Support Network

Once the decision has been made to include the patient's natural supports, an assessment of their supports' knowledge of the mental health system and their loved one's illness/crisis should be made. Often, such information can be found in the record. Prior documentation might include who was involved in the patient's care previously and the extent to which they were supportive of recommendations. Prior records may not always be available, such as when someone is presenting for psychiatric care for the first time or is presenting to your system for the first time. In these cases, the patient may be able to give some insight into the mindset of their family/support systems toward mental health.

Psychoeducation for families and patients about their illness is a key component in building relationships. Such education should also include signs of decompensation to monitor for and steps to ensure safety and maximize the chances of successful treatment. For example, families may be surprised to learn that the time of highest risk for patients is immediately after they are discharged from the hospital, particularly the first 3 months. In a sense, having just been discharged from the hospital may give loved ones a false sense of security because they intuitively believe that the patient is "well" and therefore at a low risk, if even temporarily. If the patient presents in the early phase of a psychotic or bipolar illness, families may not realize that insight can be a double-edged sword. On the one hand, it can increase the chances of treatment adherence. On the other hand, it can increase suicidal ideation as a person comes to terms with a life-changing diagnosis.

When appropriate, linking the family or natural supports of a patient to an appropriate advocacy and support group may be useful. The National Alliance for Mental Illness has broad national and local accessibility and can provide an array of resources and supports for family members. Family members may find it invaluable to seek their own understanding of the legal and ethical issues related to supporting a loved one with chronic mental illness.[5]

Family members can be essential allies in supporting the health and safety of patients. They play a critical role in helping identify when a patient is decompensating or when the patient needs to return for further assessment and management. They can provide invaluable information about how a current presentation differs from baseline. The skilled emergency psychiatrist build relationships with and engages families to aid in the evaluation and care of patients and their loved ones.

Cultural Competence

Psychiatrists and other members of the clinical team must also consider the cultural aspects of how a person and their supports respond to a mental health crisis or psychiatric diagnosis. Often, when we think of cultural competence, we focus solely on cultures other than our own. We must realize that although we often think of culture and ethnicity as synonymous, this puts us at risk of oversimplifying the concept of cultural competence and missing an opportunity to reduce health care disparities. Failing to recognize medicine as its own culture furthers that risk.[6]

Although an understanding of other cultures is essential, we must also note the challenges of the dominant culture in which we practice. Cultural identity is multifactorial, and pertinent elements will differ by patient. Common elements include race, ethnicity, gender, sexual orientation, disability, language, religion, and age. Many people find that because of their identification with one or more of these categories, they have had experiences in their life in general or interacting with health/mental health systems that shape how they are able to interact now. This can impact how people understand the causes or symptoms of illnesses, what treatments may be appropriate, whether systems are fair, and how systems respond to perceived unfairness. For example, prior poor experiences with law enforcement can have a significant impact on a family, patient, or physician being willing to contact police for a "wellness check."[7]

Putting aside our own goals for the patient and hearing the patient's and family's priorities represent the first major step in finding common ground. Simply stated, clinicians are experts in biomedicine; patients are experts in their own experience of distress.[6] Although it is beyond the scope of this chapter to delve deeply into the significant literature of cross-cultural clinical work, systemic racism, and implicit bias, these factors can have significant impact on the experience of patients across the spectrum of emergency psychiatric services, and efforts to proactively address these issues may reduce the risk for clinical errors, unnecessary aggravation of patients and families, and risk for malpractice litigation driven by poor experiences.

To Admit or Not to Admit? Risks and Benefits of Inpatient Psychiatric Admission

The assessment in the emergency setting comes down to one overarching decision: What is the correct level of care given the patient's needs? In many cases, this will be obvious. For example, a patient who is severely depressed and unable to complete activities of daily living would be best served by an inpatient admission. However, many cases are not so clear-cut.

Although patients may verbalize suicidal, homicidal, or aggressive ideation or other distress, it does not mean that inpatient admission is the best intervention. For example, patients who have failed to benefit from multiple admissions and have failed to engage in care while admitted may not benefit from readmission. Similarly, a patient displaying hallmarks of seeking secondary gain (or known from prior, similar, and well-documented presentations as seeking secondary gain) may not benefit. However, it would not be advisable for the clinician to make that determination absent a review of prior records or a track record of encountering the same individual multiple times.

Conditional threats of suicide or violence often cloud the clinical picture. Of course, factors such as homelessness, substance use, conflict at home, and maladaptive personality traits increase the risk of suicide. It is important to consider the desperation a person might feel under such circumstances, as well as their historical interaction with the mental health system.

Threats that one will harm themself or someone else if discharged should be assessed systematically, while monitoring one's own countertransference. When discharging such a patient, consider the six steps in Box 20.1.[8] There is significant overlap between the steps and standard procedure for assessing and documenting a patient's risk and the plan to mitigate that risk.

Chronic risk for suicide is not the same as acute risk for suicide. Similar to considerations of violence risk management, suicide risk management must focus on identifying and disrupting dynamic risk factors.[9] Inpatient psychiatric settings are not always the best environment for this. Although it may satisfy a clinician's short-term liability concerns, there are patients for whom it can reinforce a pattern of maladaptive coping skills and prevent them from participating in longer term psychotherapy and other interventions that will improve their prognosis over time. In such cases, it is very important to realize that there is no decision-making pathway that will eliminate the risk of suicide. Some of these patients will die by suicide, and we must be able to extricate concerns over

---

Box 20.1 Steps for Discharge of Contingently Suicidal Patients

1. Define and document the clinical situation.
2. Assess and document current suicide risk. It is important to document stressors that may be increasing the patient's risk above the baseline, even if they are at chronic risk.
3. Document modified dynamic or protective factors, especially those that have been modified by treatment thus far, and the recommended plan.
4. Document the reasons continued care in the acute setting is not indicated—for example, patterns of not participating in treatment, not following recommendations, or worsening in a given treatment setting.
5. Document your discussion of discharge, including efforts to solve identified or presenting problems, reconcile with, or explanations of the decision with the patient.
6. Consult with a colleague and document consultation, even if informal discussion only.

Adapted from Bundy et al.[8]

liability or anxiety related to losing a patient from what will ultimately benefit the patient the most. Certainly, there are acute stressors that can increase chronically at-risk patients' level of risk. In such cases, hospitalization may be indicated.[10]

Legal Considerations for Admission

Involuntary commitment laws exist in some form in every state. At a minimum, there are "emergency hold" laws to allow for further assessment that are broadly used throughout the United States.[11] These laws are typically reserved for people who are either unwilling to voluntarily participate or lack the capacity to make such a decision. In addition to requiring evidence that a patient has a mental illness, such laws typically require evidence that because of the mental illness, the patient poses a danger to themself or someone else. In some instances, this might include posing a danger to oneself through inability to care for oneself.[12] The vast majority of states also have a mechanism for civil commitment to participate in outpatient treatment, sometimes referred to as "assisted outpatient treatment."

States very widely in the specifics of their involuntary commitment laws: the threshold for initiation, who can initiate, how an emergency hold is initiated and reviewed, how people of different ages are handled, how outpatient commitment modifies emergency evaluation or involuntary inpatient admission, the impact of psychiatric advanced directives or guardianship orders on commitment processes, what disorders are or are not included, how subsequent reviews are handled, among many others. It is incumbent on every emergency psychiatrist to have a rigorous understanding of the laws and procedures for voluntary and involuntary commitment in their jurisdiction. Involuntary commitments can have far-reaching implications for patients, including disqualifying them from owning a weapon, joining the military, etc. Such implications should be taken into consideration when weighing the risks and benefits of an involuntary commitment. At the same time, the risk of allowing a person who meets involuntary commitment criteria to leave the emergency room often outweighs the risks noted above.

Legal Interventions and Firearm Access

When formulating a patient's risk of suicide or violence, access to lethal means (firearms) should be taken into consideration. Voluntary hospitalizations generally do not adversely impact a person's Second Amendment rights; depending on jurisdiction, involuntary commitment may limit such rights. Regardless, there is generally no automatic removal of firearms with involuntary admission—so a successful involuntary admission, hospitalization, and discharge may still lead to a person at elevated risk returning to a home with firearms. Recent discharge, as has often been noted, may be a risk factor for suicide.[13]

Extreme Risk Protection Orders (ERPOs; also known as red flag laws, gun violence restraining orders, among other terms) are another potential tool to reduce risk. ERPOs can be a useful tool for emergency psychiatrists, especially when there is concern for violence or suicide risk and commitment criteria are not met. Depending on jurisdiction, ERPOs allow a person—for example, a family member, law enforcement, or a clinician—to petition the court for emergency temporary removal of firearms from a person at risk. Just as with involuntary commitment, it is crucial that clinicians understand the laws in their jurisdiction.[14]

For example, in California, immediate and emergent interventions require initiation by law enforcement, whereas longer term restrictions can be initiated by family members and may require court review.[15] The New York SAFE act, passed after the tragic school shooting at Sandy Hook Elementary School in Newtown, Connecticut, includes a provision for mental health professionals to report patients whom they identify as being at risk of harming themselves or someone else.[16]

Different studies have identified potential benefits of ERPO laws in reducing suicide, crime, and possibly mass shootings.[17,18] Further research is needed to be able to definitively point to broad, population-level benefits—but in fairness, the same can be said for involuntary commitment.[19] As with all interventions, they should be individually tailored to the needs of the specific patient.

Managing and Assessing Risk: Beyond "Denies SI/HI"

Suicide and violence are two of the most dreaded, and publicized, outcomes in psychiatry. Fortunately, they are also low base rate events, making prediction difficult. Regulatory groups have advocated for universal screening in all clinical settings. The Joint Commission requires standardized processes across institutions to screen for suicide risk using validated screening and assessment tools, detailed assessment for people who screen positive, determination of a "level of risk," and documentation of an appropriate plan to reduce risk.[20] These standards are not without controversy, especially in psychiatric emergency settings, in which the standard of care is routinely substantially higher than simple screening and the nuances of risk management may fit poorly into a simple high–medium–low stratification.[21,22]

Furthermore, the PES is a unique setting in which suicidality is frequent and the patients at highest risk may be those who most ardently deny suicidality.[23] Nonetheless, the importance of routine and detailed evaluation of suicide risk—including careful evaluation of suicide risk in those who deny suicidality—is the sine qua non of good emergency psychiatry.[24]

Consider instead that our goal should be delivering the highest quality of care possible and focusing on prevention rather than prediction.[9,25] Interventions aimed at disrupting modifiable risk factors and reinforcing or introducing protective factors help patients achieve better quality of life and reduced risk of suicide. Assessing non-modifiable risk factors assists with identifying patients' enduring vulnerabilities, providing valuable information for clinicians.

Given the time pressure in emergency settings, it is important to do an assessment that goes beyond simply asking about suicidal or homicidal ideation and writing down "denies SI/HI." Although the demonstration that the question was asked may be somewhat protective in the event of adversarial review, it does not by itself constitute adequate assessment. For example, if somebody is going through a contentious divorce, it may behoove you to specifically ask about violent thoughts toward their spouse. Regarding suicide risk, the Chronological Assessment of Suicide Events approach describes an equation to uncover "real" intent: stated intent + reflected intent (plans, preparation, time spent thinking about suicide, etc.) + withheld intent = real intent.[26]

Although developed for the purposes of suicide risk assessment, a parallel approach could be applied to violence risk. For example, for a patient who denies violent thoughts or dismisses a prior statement of violent intent as "fleeting," the answer may lay in the "reflected intent." Perhaps they have been driving past the intended target's workplace or thinking about ways to isolate the person. A call to a collateral source of information may reveal that the patient has been talking frequently about getting revenge for a perceived slight, spending time looking at firearms for sale online, etc.

Risk factors for suicide and violence overlap significantly, and in the PES, where both are issues of great concern, it makes sense to screen and assess for both. To the extent possible, we can use the modifiable (dynamic) risk factors as a "to-do" list, while recognizing that not all modifiable risk factors can be addressed within a single treatment encounter. Rather, they should form the basis of interventions during the treatment encounter as well as recommendations for the next level of care.

Examples of modifiable risk factors include current or recent suicidal/aggressive/ homicidal ideation, substance use, psychotic symptoms, mood instability, treatment nonadherence, and readily available lethal means. Examples of non-modifiable risk factors include maladaptive personality traits, severe and persistent mental illness, past suicide attempts, past violence, and traumatic brain injury.

Certain risk factors may be more applicable to diagnostic groups. For example, in bipolar disorder, rapid cycling increases the risk of suicide attempts,[27] whereas irritability and paranoia increase the risk of violence.[28] In post-traumatic stress disorder, a clinical picture with predominantly arousal symptoms, as opposed to avoidance symptoms, can increase the risk of suicide and violence. In schizophrenia, positive symptoms including hallucinations and persecutory delusions increase the risk of violence.[29] Newfound insight can serve as a double-edged sword because it can increase treatment adherence and overall functioning but may also increase the risk of suicide.[30] Note that there are risk factors that fall somewhere between the "modifiable" and "non-modifiable" categories. For example, some maladaptive personality traits or patterns may respond to psychotherapy, depending on the patient's motivation and engagement.

Finally, protective factors can be leveraged to help the patient through a crisis and therefore deserve a clinician's attention as well. For example, a patient with strong family support would likely benefit from a meeting with their supports. Their supports may be able to help problem-solve and can learn to identify warning signs of an impending mood or psychotic episode. Furthermore, they may be able to educate the clinician about warning signs unique to that patient, as well as signs that they have noticed when the patient is beginning to improve.

A patient's risk for suicide and violence changes over time, as does their willingness to share information with a clinician. As such, risk assessment must be a process rather than an event. At best, it is a point-in-time assessment and should be updated periodically to account for changes in risk and protective factors.

Although we focus on prevention rather than prediction, both improve with a conditional or dynamic approach to risk management. This involves examining a particular patient's situation and patterns to describe the set of circumstances under which their risk of violence or suicidal behavior would be increased. Simply stated, risk does not exist in a vacuum and is impacted by the patient's changing environment. Adequate documentation of a risk assessment serves many purposes, including improving patient care, communicating with the next level of care, and mitigating risk of liability in the event of an adverse outcome. For both suicide and violence risk, this dynamic approach to identifying and modifying risk and protective factors as a pathway to management has become the gold standard in clinical risk management.[9,25]

Privacy, Confidentiality, and Duties to Third Parties

Patient privacy in psychiatry is a series of exceptions nested within exceptions. In general, if two people are having a conversation and one discloses potentially sensitive information such as involvement in a crime, there is no expectation of privacy and the other person can share that information as they see fit. Indeed, that second person may be lawfully compelled to share that information with law enforcement or in a court of law. Some relationships are considered special, or privileged, because there is great value to society in protecting such relationships and communication is viewed as an essential and functional part of such relationships. Client communications with attorneys are the archetypal example, and many regions also recognize spousal privilege or priest–penitent privilege. Communications with physicians are viewed as privileged within many jurisdictions, and in the United States, psychotherapeutic communications are also viewed as privileged.[31] Hence the complex array of rules, laws, and regulations governing the confidentiality of medical records and therapeutic communication.

There are areas of medical information that may have heightened protection, including information occurring in the context of treatment in an authorized substance use program, among others.[32] There are also numerous exceptions to these rules, including mandated reporting of child or elder abuse, certain infectious diseases, certain types of violent injuries (e.g., those from apparent felonious assault or firearms), and disclosures to protect third parties from certain types of harm. The definitions and rules relating to such exceptions vary substantially by jurisdiction, and the ethics will vary substantially by clinical context.[33]

Health Insurance Portability and Accountability Act

The Health Insurance Portability and Accountability Act required the U.S. Department of Health and Human Services to enact regulations governing the protection and release of protected health information by organizations using electronic health records and billing Medicare or Medicaid for services. The HIPAA privacy regulations are focused on large-scale breaches of information—that is, handling the data of large groups of patients. It is an imperfect (but, nonetheless, binding) tool for managing the care of an individual patient. Although HIPAA enforcement is generally focused on large-scale breaches of information, allegations of a single breach can be problematic, especially if they reveal an overall pattern of lackadaisical adherence to HIPAA standards.

In terms of managing acute emergencies, HIPAA is relatively permissive in sharing information between directly involved health providers. Psychotherapy notes—documentation of talk therapy intervention and process maintained in separate health records—have higher protections, but basic clinical information including diagnosis, medications, allergies, and medical concerns does not. Unless a patient objects, information can also be shared with family members. Although HIPAA is a complex regulatory schema, the U.S. Department of Health and Human Services maintains a number of useful explainers on clinical applications that serve as useful references.[34]

Note that more restrictive state laws or regulations on privacy may preempt (or be enforced in place of) the federal HIPAA standard. Careful review of federal and local standards is an essential process for any PES.

HIPAA permits a variety of information sharing with law enforcement. This includes information about crimes committed in a health care setting, service of warrants to patients, location of fugitives, and reporting of certain types of crimes such as child abuse or elder abuse.[35,36] Note that for analysis of duty to third-party scenarios, HIPAA provides for permission to warn as long as doing so is in accordance with professional ethics or local jurisdictional standards.[37] Again, be mindful that more stringent state rules may supersede the HIPAA privacy standards.

Note that HIPAA always permits providers to listen to collateral from friends and family of a patient, even if they are limited in the information they can share with providers.

Patient Access to Medical Records

The 21st Century Cures Act was created to expand the ability to share clinical records between health systems and electronic medical records as a way to improve the quality of care. Embedded within the statute is broadly expanded access to medical records by patients.[38] Understandably, some mental health practitioners have concerns that permitting psychiatric patients access to their own records may be particularly problematic or even pose safety concerns to the providers.[39] This same concern has been present for decades and, largely, seems unfounded.[40,41]

Within the PES, records may be considered sensitive for a variety of clinical reasons. Information that clinicians may wish to consider sensitive includes formulation, sources of collateral information, and speculation about motivation or malingering. Within the Cures Act, there are several possible categories that may legitimately overlap and allow restriction of information from the patient. Any hospital policy addressing sequestration of potentially sensitive health records should address legitimate operational needs, the legal boundaries and limits emplaced by the Cures Act, and ethical implications.[42,43]

Duties to Third Parties

Duties to third parties vary substantially by jurisdiction. Although the Tarasoff case may be the most infamous, every state and country has approached the issue of the rights of third parties differently. Indeed, even California—the state where Tarasoff was decided—ultimately did not follow the court's rule of a duty to protect, with the legislature subsequently enacting a statutory duty to warn.[44] As a starting point, a state-by-state summary of relevant duty to third party statutes or court rulings can be found at https://www.ncsl.org/research/health/mental-health-professionals-duty-to-warn.aspx. Note that most countries—with the possible exception of Austria—also have some similar duty to third party standard.[45]

Some states focus on the affirmative duty of a clinician to warn or protect. Others speak only of permission to warn. Some states expressly state that clinicians who take certain actions to warn or protect are immune from civil claims related to violent acts or claims for breach of confidentiality. Some states protect property, although most are

---

Box 20.2 Questions to Consider in Analyzing a Jurisdiction's Duty to Third Party Standard

---

Do I have a duty to warn, protect, or something else?

How imminent does the risk need to be?

Are there alternatives to warning?

Does the threat have to be communicated and explicit?

Do I have a duty for indirect information?

How specific or plausible does the threat need to be?

Did the patient communicate a threat or does the patient pose a threat?

Did the clinician directly hear the threat? (Who else heard the threat?)

Is the target an identified or readily identifiable individual?

Is the target a member of a specific group of people?

Is the target property?

Are their alternatives to warning that may effectively reduce risk?

Is informing law enforcement permitted or required?

---

only concerned with human life or injury. HIPAA provides permission to warn insofar as it is congruent with jurisdictional standards.[37] Questions a clinician may consider in analyzing their jurisdiction's duty to third party standard are summarized in Box 20.2.

Emergency Medical Treatment and Active Labor Act

The Emergency Medical Treatment and Active Labor Act (EMTALA), enacted in 1986, serves as a vital protection to ensure that patients in need of treatment receive appropriate evaluation and—at least—initial stabilizing care of emergency medical conditions without regard to their insurance or ability to pay for services. This serves as a vital protection for patients, especially those with severe mental illness who are often underinsured and at greater risk for psychiatric and medical emergencies. EMTALA also compels hospitals to provide unreimbursed care at great expense, thus creating a significant financial burden on emergency departments that is displaced onto other services and patients.[46,47] It is complicated. It is, nonetheless, the binding legal standard for any hospital that receives Medicare.

EMTALA requires any licensed hospital that participates in Medicare to provide certain essential services to any person who presents for care or who is on the campus appearing to need treatment.[48] A medical screening examination (MSE) must be performed by an appropriately qualified medical professional to rule out an emergency medical condition (EMC). (Note that "MSE" in the context of EMTALA is quite different from the common usage of "MSE" in psychiatry.) Any EMCs must be stabilized prior to discharge or transfer to an appropriate medical facility, and specialized hospitals may not refuse patients appropriate for transfer.[48] Services cannot be delayed or different based on ability to pay or due to discrimination. Failure to comply can result in a complaint, investigation, and fines by the Center for Medicare Services (CMS). EMTALA violations are not a "federalization" of medical malpractice liability, but there are rare (and generally unsuccessful) cases in which EMTALA violations are a focus of civil litigation.[49]

In terms of psychiatric emergencies, EMCs include suicidality, aggression, intoxication, or significant psychiatric symptoms.[50] Stabilization of medical conditions that may be difficult to manage in a psychiatric setting are also a concern, as is identification of medical causes of psychiatric symptoms. Adherence to best practice guidelines for such processes is prudent.[51,52]

Failure to comply with EMTALA can be costly. EMTALA allows CMS to impose fines on hospitals for failure to comply. Although psychiatric EMTALA cases account for just under 20% of EMTALA violations, fines are two to three times greater than those for non-psychiatric cases; typical violations include failure to provide an appropriate medical screening examination, stabilization, or appropriate transfer.[53] Alleged EMTALA violations are addressed through investigation by CMS and may lead to substantial fines.

Strange Bedfellows: Law Enforcement as Partner

Police officers play a frequent, complex, and often essential role in emergency psychiatry. Police are routinely involved in initiating involuntary commitments on people in the community and transporting involuntary patients between hospitals.[54] In some jurisdictions, police are used as sitters for involuntary psychiatric patients being evaluated or boarded in emergency departments. The relationship can be strained because law enforcement is increasingly uncomfortable in this role and subsidizing the health system.[55] Furthermore, just as emergency psychiatry has a legacy of systemic racism and bias, these same factors can play a role in law enforcement involvement in involuntary commitments.[56]

Recent calls for having behavioral health professionals take the lead in managing psychiatric emergencies in the community are not new. Alternative models such as mobile crisis teams using behavioral health professionals alone or co-responding with law enforcement have existed for at least 30 years.[57] Similarly, efforts to divert people with primarily behavioral health concerns out of the criminal justice system, as a practice and as a policy, are well established and effective—even if inconsistently applied.[58]

Fully exploring the complex topic of improved response to psychiatric emergencies in the community with partnerships or partitions between law enforcement and behavioral health warrants a chapter, if not a book, in and of itself.[59] The role of law enforcement as employed staff within an emergency department or PES is equally complex.[60] The essential step is for PES clinicians and their leaders to recognize this as a sensitive and important relationship—a relationship that requires intentional and regular attention to ensure open lines of communication, collaborative review of problematic events, and proactive planning and cross-training.[61]

Finally, threat management is increasingly being recognized as a critical tool for the evaluation of people at risk for engaging in targeted or mass violence, and psychiatric services in general and the PES in particular play an essential role in that effort.[62] Threat management is a systematic and multidisciplinary approach to identifying and intervening with people who have made threats or inchoate acts of violence.[63] Although psychiatric illness may play a limited role in violence, psychiatric professionals can play a critical role in identifying modifiable risk factors and reducing violence risk. Psychiatrists and PES leadership need to be prepared to collaborate with law enforcement and other partners in managing violence risk in high-risk individuals.[64]

Risk Management: Reducing Litigation Exposure

Documentation and consultation are the twin pillars of liability management.[65] Indeed, documentation may be the most essential measure to ensure that treatment which meets or exceeds the standard of care can be defended in a malpractice case should an untoward outcome occur. Malpractice litigation is like high school math: Even if the final answer is wrong, partial credit will be given by the jury to the physician if they show their work.[66] Although psychiatry and emergency medicine are—surprisingly—not viewed as high-risk specialties, any prudent physician should be mindful of mitigating potential risk.[1] Even among lower risk specialties, most physicians accrue at least one lawsuit over the course of their career. The strategy is not to avoid litigation but, rather, to provide care that meets or exceeds the standard of care and to contemporaneously document the care and decision-making to make it easy to defend in the event of adversarial review. To wit: Do not practice defensive medicine. Instead, practice excellent medicine—or at least meet the standard of care—and document defensively.

The PES has many elements that make it higher risk for litigation exposure, including acuity, the possibility of deception by patients (and family members), brevity of contact limiting the ability to nurture positive relationships with patients and families, and, often, a mismatch between resources and clinical needs. And, put bluntly, if an emergency medicine physician mismanages an airway or a resuscitation, a patient may die. If an emergency psychiatrist mismanages a potentially violent patient, many people may die. And none of these concerns alter the fact that a physician can undertake every step of evaluation and management perfectly, exceeding the standard of care, and still be faced with an unavoidable or unpredictable bad outcome. Our work, despite its joys and rewards, can be daunting.

Similarly, psychiatrists need to recognize that admission to inpatient units may or may not be the safest disposition. Fifteen-minute checks, admission, involuntary admission, 1-week follow-up windows, and many other common myths of psychiatric practice are not supported by available evidence.[67] All decisions are risk versus risk, and any prudent physician should acknowledge this fact and document their reasoning accordingly. In the event of litigation, the medical record serves as a critical tool to demonstrate the judgment applied by the clinician; juries expect the application of judgment, not perfect decisions.

When possible, consultation in ambiguous or high-risk cases can be essential. It may yield novel perspectives or recommendations that the psychiatrist at an impasse may apply. It may simply confirm the dilemma that the primary psychiatrist already recognized. Nonetheless, the engagement of a second psychiatrist and the integration of their views into the final plan can provide added resilience to potential litigation—in addition to, it is hoped, improving the care and outcome. As a fallback, there is no shame in admission, especially for high-risk cases with ambiguous formulations.

Reason, Respond, and Record (Don't React)

Although it is unclear if shared decision-making approaches reduce malpractice risk, there is a clear ethical preference for this practice when possible.[68] Well-documented informed consent discussions with patients and families, including explaining the risk of admission for chronic personality driven suicide risk, can be valuable tools.[10] Engaging with family and primary supports in the emergent care of a patient at risk for suicide or aggression is essential: Families are the people most likely to recognize when a patient is at risk, families are the people most likely to assist when a patient is at risk, and families are the most likely people to sue if there is an adverse outcome and they were not engaged collaboratively.

Conclusion

It has been said, likely inaccurately, that the Chinese symbol for "crisis" is a combination of danger and opportunity.[69] The metaphor is apt even if linguistically flawed. At the time of this writing, emergency psychiatry is at just such a juncture: There is a new, broad expansion of crisis and emergency mental health services imminent and driven by multiple factors, including the implementation of a national 988 system for accessing crisis support and broad social efforts to more effectively divert people in the community experiencing behavioral emergencies toward crisis and emergency psychiatric services and away from law enforcement intervention, use of force, and criminal justice outcomes. Although some of this is driven by politicized rhetoric around law enforcement, the strategic shift to and expansion of emergency mental health services out of the hospitals and into the community has been building for years. As policymakers and stakeholders rediscover the valuable role of mobile crisis and co-responding programs (which have existed for at least 40 years[70]), reconsideration of the boundaries and rules of engagement between emergency psychiatry and law enforcement for behavioral emergencies will benefit from fresh appraisal.

It will be critical for PES clinicians and leadership to understand and lead these efforts, to ensure that patients with serious illnesses are cared for and that new systems are designed with safety, recovery, efficiency, and civil rights equally in mind. It is an exciting time to work in emergency psychiatry and an exciting time to explore, expand, and improve the legal and structural tools to help our patients, our discipline, and our communities.

References

1. Jena AB, Seabury S, Lakdawalla D, Chandra A. Malpractice risk according to physician specialty. *N Engl J Med*. 2011;365(7):629–636. doi:10.1056/NEJMsa1012370

2. Robertson MD, Walter G. Many faces of the dual-role dilemma in psychiatric ethics. *Aust N Z J Psychiatry*. 2008;42(3):228–235. doi:10.1080/00048670701827291

3. Hoop JG. Hidden ethical dilemmas in psychiatric residency training: The psychiatry resident as dual agent. *Acad Psychiatry*. 2004;28(3):183–189. doi:10.1176/appi.ap.28.3.183

4. Petrik ML, Billera M, Kaplan Y, Matarazzo B, Wortzel H. Balancing patient care and confidentiality: Considerations in obtaining collateral information. *J Psychiatr Pract*. 2015;21(3):220–224. doi:10.1097/PRA.0000000000000072

5. Tashbook L. *Family Guide to Mental Illness and the Law: A Practical Handbook*. Oxford University Press; 2018.

6. Carpenter-Song EA, Schwallie MN, Longhofer J. Cultural competence reexamined: Critique and directions for the future. *PS*. 2007;58(10):1362–1365. doi:10.1176/ps.2007.58.10.1362

7. Rafla-Yuan E, Chhabra DK, Mensah MO. Decoupling crisis response from policing—A step toward equitable psychiatric emergency services. *N Engl J Med*. 2021;384(18):1769–1773. doi:10.1056/NEJMms2035710

8. Bundy C, Schreiber M, Pascualy M. Discharging your patients who display contingency-based suicidality: 6 steps. *Curr Psychiatry*. 2014;13(1):e1–e3.

9. Pisani AR, Murrie DC, Silverman MM. Reformulating suicide risk formulation: From prediction to prevention. *Acad Psychiatry*. 2016;40(4):623–629. doi:10.1007/s40596-015-0434-6

10. Mammen O, Tew J, Painter T, Bettinelli E, Beckjord J. Communicating suicide risk to families of chronically suicidal borderline personality disorder patients to mitigate malpractice risk. *Gen Hosp Psychiatry*. 2020;67:51–57. doi:10.1016/j.genhosppsych.2020.08.014

11. Morris NP. Reasonable or random: 72-hour limits to psychiatric holds. *PS*. 2021;72(2):210–212. doi:10.1176/appi.ps.202000284

12. Pinals DA, Mossman D. Evaluation for Civil Commitment. Oxford University Press; 2012.

13. Olfson M, Wall M, Wang S, et al. Short-term suicide risk after psychiatric hospital discharge. *JAMA Psychiatry*. 2016;73(11):1119–1126. doi:10.1001/jamapsychiatry.2016.2035

14. Barsotti C. Standing affirm: Firearms, red flag laws, and at-risk patients. *Emerg Med News*. 2021;43(5):14. doi:10.1097/01.EEM.0000751872.54634.b6

15. Pallin R, Schleimer JP, Pear VA, Wintemute GJ. Assessment of extreme risk protection order use in California from 2016 to 2019. *JAMA Netw Open*. 2020;3(6):e207735. doi:10.1001/jamanetworkopen.2020.7735

16. Jacobs J, Fuhr Z. Universal background checking—New York state's SAFE Act. *Albany Law Rev*. 2015;79(4):1327–1354.

17. Swanson JW, Easter MM, Alanis-Hirsch K, et al. Criminal justice and suicide outcomes with Indiana's risk-based gun seizure law. *J Am Acad Psychiatry Law Online*. 2019;47(2):188–197. doi:10.29158/JAAPL.003835-19

18. Wintemute GJ, Pear VA, Schleimer JP, et al. Extreme risk protection orders intended to prevent mass shootings: A case series. *Ann Intern Med*. 2019;171(9):655–658. doi:10.7326/M19-2162

19. Swanson JW. Understanding the research on extreme risk protection orders: Varying results, same message. *PS*. 2019;70(10):953–954. doi:10.1176/appi.ps.201900291

20. National Patient Safety Goal for suicide prevention. The Joint Commission. Published 2019. Accessed May 24, 2021. https://www.jointcommission.org/-/media/tjc/documents/resources/patient-safety-topics/suicide-prevention/r3_18_suicide_prevention_hap_bhc_5_6_19_rev5.pdf?db=web&hash=887186D9530F7BB8E30C28FE352B5B8C

21. Nestadt PS, Triplett P, Mojtabai R, Berman AL. Universal screening may not prevent suicide. *Gen Hosp Psychiatry*. 2020;63(1):14–15. doi:10.1016/j.genhosppsych.2018.06.006

22. Rozel JS. Broken promise: Challenges in achieving effective universal suicide screening. *Acad Emerg Med*. 2022;28(6):705–706. doi:10.1111/acem.14199

23. Simpson S, Goans C, Loh R, Ryall K, Middleton MCA, Dalton A. Suicidal ideation is insensitive to suicide risk after ED discharge: Performance characteristics of the Columbia-Suicide Severity Rating Scale Screener. *Acad Emerg Med*. 2021;28(6):621–629. doi:10.1111/acem.14198

24. Berman AL. Risk factors proximate to suicide and suicide risk assessment in the context of denied suicide ideation. *Suicide Life Threat Behav*. 2018;48(3):340–352. doi:10.1111/sltb.12351

25. Mulvey EP, Lidz CW. Conditional prediction: A model for research on dangerousness to others in a new era. *Int J Law Psychiatry.* 1995;18(2):129–143. doi:10.1016/0160-2527(95)00002-Y

26. Shea SC. *The Practical Art of Suicide Assessment: A Guide for Mental Health Professionals and Substance Abuse Counselors.* Wiley; 1999.

27. Coryell W, Solomon D, Turvey C, et al. The long-term course of rapid-cycling bipolar disorder. *Arch Gen Psychiatry.* 2003;60(9):914–920. doi:10.1001/archpsyc.60.9.914

28. Volavka J. Violence in schizophrenia and bipolar disorder. *Psychiatr Danubina.* 2013;25(1):24–33.

29. Swanson JW, Swartz MS, Van Dorn RA, et al. A national study of violent behavior in persons with schizophrenia. *Arch Gen Psychiatry.* 2006;63(5):490–499.

30. Melle I, Barrett EA. Insight and suicidal behavior in first-episode schizophrenia. *Expert Rev Neurother.* 2012;12(3):353–359. doi:10.1586/ern.11.191

31. Appel JM. Trends in confidentiality and disclosure. *Focus.* 2019;17(4):360–364. doi:10.1176/appi.focus.20190021

32. Bossenbroek MD. Thirty years in the making: 42 C.F.R. Part 2 revisited and revised. *The Health Lawyer.* 2017;29(6):1–11.

33. Fisher MA. *The Ethics of Conditional Confidentiality: A Practice Model for Mental Health Professionals.* Oxford University Press; 2013.

34. Office of Civil Rights. HIPAA privacy rule and sharing information related to mental health. U.S. Department of Health and Human Services. Published 2017. https://www.hhs.gov/sites/default/files/hipaa-privacy-rule-and-sharing-info-related-to-mental-health.pdf

35. Petrila J. Dispelling the myths about information sharing between the mental health and criminal justice systems. CMHS National Gains Center. Published 2007. Accessed March 23, 2015. https://www.usf.edu/cbcs/mhlp/tac/documents/behavioral-healthcare/hipaa/dispelling-myths-of-information-sharing.pdf

36. Petrila J, Fader-Towe H. Information sharing in criminal justice–mental health collaborations: Working with HIPAA and other privacy laws. Council of State Governments Justice Center. Published 2010. Accessed June 4, 2017. https://www.bja.gov/Publications/CSG_CJMH_Info_Sharing.pdf

37. Rodriguez L. Message to our nation's health care providers. Published January 15, 2013. https://www.hhs.gov/sites/default/files/ocr/office/lettertonationhcp.pdf

38. Lye CT, Forman HP, Daniel JG, Krumholz HM. The 21st Century Cures Act and electronic health records one year later: Will patients see the benefits? *J Am Med Inform Assoc.* 2018;25(9):1218–1220. doi:10.1093/jamia/ocy065

39. Chimowitz H, O'Neill S, Leveille S, Welch K, Walker J. Sharing psychotherapy notes with patients: Therapists' attitudes and experiences. *Social Work.* 2020;65(2):159–168. doi:10.1093/sw/swaa010

40. Roth LH, Wolford J, Meisel A. Patient access to records: Tonic or toxin? *Am J Psychiatry.* 1980;137(5):592–596. doi:10.1176/ajp.137.5.592

41. Åkerstedt US, Cajander Å, Moll J, Ålander T. On threats and violence for staff and patient accessible electronic health records. *Cogent Psychology.* 2018;5(1):1518967. doi:10.1080/23311908.2018.1518967

42. Genes N, Appel J. Ethics of data sequestration in electronic health records. *Cambridge Q Healthcare Ethics.* 2013;22(4):365–372. doi:10.1017/S0963180113000212

43. Thom RP, Farrell HM. When and how should clinicians share details from a health record with patients with mental illness? *AMA J Ethics*. 2017;19(3):253–259. doi:10.1001/journalofethics.2017.19.3.ecas3-1703.

44. Buckner F, Firestone M. "Where the public peril begins": 25 years after Tarasoff. *J Legal Med*. 2000;21(2):187–222.

45. Gutiérrez-Lobos K, Wagner E, Schmidl-Mohl B, Schmid-Siegel B. Wrapped in silence: Psychotherapists and confidentiality in the courtroom. *Int J Offender Ther Comp Criminol*. 2000;44(1):33–45. doi:10.1177/0306624X00441004

46. Morreim EH. EMTALA turns 30: Unconstitutional from birth. *The Health Lawyer*. 2015;28(2):32–42.

47. Katz MH, Wei EK. EMTALA—A noble policy that needs improvement. *JAMA Internal Med*. 2019;179(5):693–694. doi:10.1001/jamainternmed.2019.0026

48. Centers for Medicare & Medicaid Services. 42 CFR Parts 413, 482, and 489. Medicare program; Clarifying policies related to the responsibilities of Medicare-participating hospitals in treating individuals with emergency medical conditions. U.S. Department of Health and Human Services. Published 2003. Accessed October 1, 2017. https://www.cms.gov/Regulations-and-Guidance/Legislation/EMTALA/Downloads/CMS-1063-F.pdf

49. Lindor RA, Campbell RL, Pines JM, et al. EMTALA and patients with psychiatric emergencies: A review of relevant case law. *Ann Emerg Med*. 2014;64(5):439–444. doi:10.1016/j.annemergmed.2014.01.005

50. West JC. EMTALA obligations for psychiatric patients. *J Healthc Risk Manag*. 2014;34(2):5–12. doi:10.1002/jhrm.21153

51. Anderson E, Nordstrom K, Wilson M, et al. American Association for Emergency Psychiatry Task Force on Medical Clearance of Adults: Part I. Introduction, review and evidence-based guidelines. *West J Emerg Med*. 2017;18(2):235–242. doi:10.5811/westjem.2016.10.32258

52. Wilson MP, Nordstrom K, Anderson EL, et al. American Association for Emergency Psychiatry Task Force on Medical Clearance of Adult Psychiatric Patients: Part II. Controversies over medical assessment, and consensus recommendations. *West J Emerg Med*. 2017;18(4):640–646. doi:10.5811/westjem.2017.3.32259

53. Terp S, Wang B, Burner E, Connor D, Seabury SA, Menchine M. Civil monetary penalties resulting from violations of the Emergency Medical Treatment and Labor Act (EMTALA) involving psychiatric emergencies, 2002 to 2018. *Acad Emerg Med*. 2019;26(5):470–478. doi:10.1111/acem.13710

54. Redondo RM, Currier GW. Emergency psychiatry: Characteristics of patients referred by police to a psychiatric emergency service. *Psychiatr Serv*. 2003;54(6):804–806. doi:10.1176/appi.ps.54.6.804

55. Meier M. Road runners. Treatment Advocacy Center. Published 2019. Accessed October 7, 2020. https://www.treatmentadvocacycenter.org/road-runners

56. Swartz MS. The urgency of racial justice and reducing law enforcement involvement in involuntary civil commitment. *PS*. 2020;71(12):1211–1211. doi:10.1176/appi.ps.711202

57. Zealberg JJ, Christie SD, Puckett JA, McAlhany D, Durban M. A mobile crisis program: Collaboration between emergency psychiatric services and police. *PS*. 1992;43(6):612–615. doi:10.1176/ps.43.6.612

58. Griffin PA, Heilbrun K, Mulvey EP, DeMatteo D, Schubert CA, eds. *The Sequential Intercept Model and Criminal Justice: Promoting Community Alternatives for Individuals with Serious Mental Illness*. Oxford University Press; 2015.

59. Group for the Advancement of Psychiatry, American Psychiatric Association, eds. *People with Mental Illness in the Criminal Justice System: Answering a Cry for Help: A Practice Manual for Psychiatrists and Other Practitioner*. American Psychiatric Publishing; 2016.

60. Stiebel VG. Safety and security in emergency psychiatry. In: Fitz-Gerald MJ, Takeshita J, eds. *Models of Emergency Psychiatric Services That Work: Integrating Psychiatry and Primary Care*. Springer; 2020:125–134. doi:10.1007/978-3-030-50808-1_12

61. Rozel JS. Armed law enforcement in the emergency department: Risk management considerations. *J Am Assoc Emerg Psychiatry*. 2016;13(3).

62. Medical Directors' Institute. Mass violence in America: Causes, impacts & solutions. National Council for Behavioral Health. Published 2019. Accessed September 21, 2019. https://www.thenationalcouncil.org/wp-content/uploads/2019/08/Mass-Violence-in-America_8-6-19.pdf

63. Rozel JS. Violence: Managing major threats. In: Glick RL, Zeller SL, Berlin JS, eds. *Emergency Psychiatry: Principles & Practice*. 2nd ed. Wolters Kluwer; 2020:345–357.

64. Rozel JS. Targeting targeted violence from the psychiatric emergency service. J Am Assoc Emerg Psychiatry. 2018:4–6. https://www.researchgate.net/publication/330026429_Targeting_Targeted_Violence_from_the_Psychiatric_Emergency_Service

65. Appelbaum PS, Gutheil TG. *Clinical Handbook of Psychiatry & the Law*. 5th ed. Wolters Kluwer; 2020.

66. Rozel JS, Zacharia MZ. Risk management in the emergency department: Liabilities, duties, and EMTALA. In: Zun LS, Nordstrom K, Wilson MP, eds. *Behavioral Emergencies for Healthcare Providers*. Springer; 2021:441–450. doi:10.1007/978-3-030-52520-0_44

67. Berman AL, Silverman MM. Hospital-based suicides: Challenging existing myths. *Psychiatr Q*. 2022;93(1):1–13. doi:10.1007/s11126-020-09856-w

68. Durand M-A, Moulton B, Cockle E, Mann M, Elwyn G. Can shared decision-making reduce medical malpractice litigation? A systematic review. *BMC Health Serv Res*. 2015;15(1):167. doi:10.1186/s12913-015-0823-2

69. Chinese word for "crisis." Wikipedia. Published 2021. Accessed April 25, 2021. https://en.wikipedia.org/w/index.php?title=Chinese_word_for_%22crisis%22&oldid=999807682

70. West DA, Litwok E, Oberlander K, Martin DA. Emergency psychiatric home visiting: Report of four years experience. *J Clin Psychiatry*. 1980;41(4):113–118.

21

Documenting Risk Assessments and High-Acuity Discharge Presentations

Shafi Lodhi

Introduction

All psychiatrists receive substantial training in the assessment of suicidal and homicidal ideation. Throughout residency, psychiatry trainees hone their skills in the assessment and management of patients presenting with a complaint of suicidal or homicidal thoughts. Over the course of one shift, a psychiatrist working in an emergency setting will invariably perform multiple risk assessments and will make disposition decisions for many suicidal and/or homicidal patients.

However, although the assessment of these two chief concerns is an area that all psychiatrists receive extensive training in, the documentation of such assessments is an area in which very few psychiatrists have had formal education. For most practicing psychiatrists, education about risk assessment documentation may have consisted only of a handful of slides during an intern year lecture, followed by informal feedback on their notes from different attendings through the course of their training. As a result of this, documentation of risk assessment varies widely from psychiatrist to psychiatrist and from institution to institution. There is little standardization of what constitutes a "proper" documentation of risk. Even most textbooks and reference works in psychiatry focus primarily on discussing the actual assessment of risk, relegating any discussion on documentation of said assessment to a few sparse pages at the end of a chapter. There is often very little in the way of concrete guidelines or practical advice that can help a psychiatrist learn how to document risk assessment in a proper manner.

Documentation of risk assessment is particularly important in high-acuity discharge presentations, where negative outcomes can place the clinician under the legal spotlight. The law plays a more prominent role in psychiatry than in any other field of medicine.[1] Whereas many physicians in other specialties may go entire careers without coming into contact with the law, it is an almost near-certainty that a psychiatrist will have at least one patient case that is reviewed by a lawyer. In instances in which this proceeds to the level of a psychiatric malpractice lawsuit, documentation will often become the centerpiece of evidence.

This chapter comprehensively discusses the documentation of risk assessments in the emergency psychiatry setting, with particular emphasis placed on high-acuity discharge presentations. The chapter is divided into three sections. The first section presents a brief discussion of the relevant legal background, the importance of documentation, and the purpose of a risk assessment. The second section focuses on the practical aspects of documentation. The necessary elements of a risk assessment, general guidelines, and specific examples of "do's and do not's" of documentation are discussed. Finally, the third section consists of a practical guide to quickly documenting a risk assessment. A step-by-step guide is provided, as well as boilerplate text that can serve to help the reader create their own "dot phrase" in order to aid in documentation. An example of a well-documented risk assessment quickly generated from the guide is also provided.

Legal Background, the Importance of Documentation, and the Purpose of a Risk Assessment

Legal Background

A malpractice lawsuit falls under the legal category of tort. "Tort" derives from the Old French word for wrong and is generally defined as a civil (i.e., noncriminal) wrong, other than a breach of contract. This civil wrong has caused an injury for which a victim may seek damages, typically in the form of money damages, against the alleged wrong-doer. Malpractice, also known as professional negligence, is a tort committed by a medical, financial, legal, or other type of professional that has led to damage to their patient or client.[2]

Psychiatrists are the least likely of all medical specialists to be sued, with only approximately 2.5% of psychiatrists facing a malpractice claim every year.[3] When sued, however, the most common context in which a psychiatrist faces a malpractice claim is the aftermath of a patient suicide.[4]

In order for a physician to be found liable for malpractice, the plaintiff (the party who initiates the lawsuit) must demonstrate the presence of four elements: *dereliction* of *duty* that has *directly* resulted in *damage* to the patient.[4] Known informally as the "four D's of malpractice," the plaintiff must prove all four elements by a preponderance of evidence in order to sustain a successful lawsuit. "Preponderance of evidence" is defined as the likelihood of being "more probably than not" or, in other words, greater than a 50% chance.

Duty
"Duty" begins whenever a doctor–patient relationship is established. Once such a relationship is established, the physician must treat the patient or appropriately terminate the doctor–patient relationship. Of particular importance, under the legal doctrine of *respondeat superior* ("let the master answer"), psychiatrists may also have a duty toward patients who are harmed through the actions of any trainees or nonphysician practitioners that they supervise.[4]

Dereliction
Dereliction does not mean that the plaintiff must simply establish that the physician made any type of error. In cases of psychiatric malpractice, there are two broad types of errors that are considered: errors of fact and errors of judgment.[5] Errors of fact are mistakes that pertain directly to the facts at hand. For example, if a psychiatrist makes a decision that a patient endorsing suicidal thoughts is safe to discharge because the psychiatrist neglected to ask about immediate access to firearms, that psychiatrist has committed an error of fact. If an error of fact results in an adverse outcome for the patient, the physician is more likely to be found negligent.

On the other hand, an error of judgment occurs when the physician properly evaluates and treats the patient according to the standard of care but makes a reasonable clinical decision that happens to be a mistake. In this case, even if that error results in an adverse outcome for the patient, the physician is less likely to be found negligent. Courts have stated,

> For a psychiatrist to be held liable for malpractice based upon a decision . . . it must be shown that the treatment decisions represented something less than a professional medical determination . . . or that the psychiatrist's decisions were not the product of a careful evaluation." (*Ballek v. Aldana-Bernier*, cited in Knoll)[5]

In other words, a psychiatrist is not penalized for making the "wrong" decision per se but, rather, for making a rash decision, or at least a decision that was undertaken without due consideration and thought.

Damage

In order for a malpractice suit to be successful, the plaintiff must also demonstrate that the psychiatrist's action resulted in damage to the patient. Even if a patient is discharged inappropriately without receiving the standard of care, a malpractice lawsuit can only move forward if the patient was damaged by that decision.

Direct Cause

The plaintiff must prove that not only was the patient damaged but also the damages occurred directly due to the substandard level of care the patient received.

Importance of Documentation

Being named in a lawsuit is undoubtedly one of the most stressful experiences that any physician can go through.[6] After the actual providing of empathetic and evidence-based medical care, proper documentation is the strongest defense in a potential malpractice case. The importance of good documentation cannot be overstated. The quality of documentation in the medical record may well be the basis by which a malpractice lawyer accepts or declines a case. "Nothing will stop a malpractice lawyer dead in his or her tracks quicker than a well-documented chart reflecting careful and thoughtful suicide assessments. A well-documented case reflecting good care means a plaintiff's lawyer is likely to lose the case."[7]

Emergency psychiatry is particularly prone to the danger of deficient documentation. Emergency room settings are, by their very nature and design, fast-paced environments. There is constant patient turnover and triaging of multiple acute patients. Given the atmosphere of an emergency room setting, documentation may seem especially burdensome and even frivolous, resulting in the high likelihood of failing to document an adequate risk assessment.

A chart review of all psychiatric evaluations in a busy academic medical center's psychiatric emergency room over 1 year found that documentation was deficient in multiple areas.[8] Startlingly, almost 10% of emergency psychiatry charts failed to even document whether or not suicidal ideation was assessed at all. From a medicolegal perspective, an adverse outcome in any of these 10% of charts could result in the physician being placed in a very precarious position. The physician would need to defend their clinical decision as being careful and reasonable care while also having to justify documentation suggesting that they did not even ask about suicidal thoughts.

Knowing that certain risk factors are important to consider when evaluating a patient does not always translate into these factors being documented in the chart. A Canadian study surveyed both psychiatrists and emergency medicine physicians on which factors they considered important when conducting a risk assessment.[9] This was followed by a chart review of emergency psychiatry patients, evaluating whether these factors were documented in the written risk assessment. The study demonstrated that both psychiatrists and emergency medicine physicians had low documentation rates of the very risk factors that they themselves had deemed important in a proper risk assessment. As the study concluded, "Therefore, a large discrepancy exists, as physicians are aware of the importance of several suicide predictors but are not applying this knowledge by documenting these predictors."[9] Although physicians are undoubtedly incorporating knowledge of these risk factors into their assessment and clinical decision-making, the lack of documentation in the medical record leaves them vulnerable to allegations of substandard care. It is vital that the documented risk assessment accurately reflect the thought that has gone into clinical decision-making.

Although well-written notes do not, in and of themselves, guarantee that good care was provided, a well-documented assessment of risk suggests that thought and care were put into the clinical risk assessment of the patient. Conversely, a sparsely documented assessment of risk may indicate to third parties that the clinical care and risk assessment of the patient were performed without appropriate attention to detail and without considering all relevant factors and angles. It is not uncommon during malpractice trials for medical notes to be put, quite literally, on display—enlarged and printed out on poster boards for juries to view.[5] Careless and haphazard documentation reflects poorly on the physician and may suggest to third parties that standard of care was not provided, even in cases in which the patient received exceptional care.

It is also important to note that good documentation of risk assessment is important regardless of the disposition. Although post-suicide lawsuits are the most common cause of malpractice claims against psychiatrists, lawsuits can also be, and have been, filed when the psychiatrist has decided to admit a patient.[10] The allegation in these lawsuits is that the patient did not meet criteria for involuntary hospitalization, and thus the psychiatrist's decision to admit them against their will constituted false imprisonment and deprivation of civil rights. It is therefore just as important for a psychiatrist to properly document their risk assessment when admitting a patient as when discharging a patient.

A common rationalization for failing to comprehensively document a risk assessment is that it is impossible or impractical for a physician to document everything that transpired during the evaluation.[11] Although this is true, the reality is that vital and relevant information must always be documented. There are few things more vital and relevant when discharging a high-acuity psychiatric patient than risk for harm. Although the phrase "If it wasn't documented, it didn't happen" is inaccurate both legally and medically, it is a prudent sentiment to keep in mind for high-acuity discharges.[12] The fact of the matter is that a physician chooses pertinent information to enter into the medical record. Because suicide and homicide are perhaps the two worst possible outcomes for a psychiatric patient, it is reasonable for a third party such as a jury or lawyer to conclude that if either of those were adequately assessed by the physician, the assessment would have been documented in the medical chart.

Another argument against detailed documentation is that physician liability increases with the amount of information that is documented in the chart. This is a myth—one that is unfortunately still propagated in some training seminars. The reality is that the opposite is true. A lack of documentation opens up the physician to claims that they did not consider certain factors when making the discharge decision.

Good documentation is important for more than just legal protection against malpractice lawsuits. Nobel laureate and psychologist, Daniel Kahneman, describes dichotomous modes of thinking that he refers to as "System 1" and "System 2."[13] System 1 is fast, automatic, and unconscious, and thus more prone to error and cognitive biases. System 2 is slow, logical, and deliberate. This dual-process theory of cognition has gained attention in the emergency medicine literature, in studying how physicians approach patients in an emergency setting.[14] Although the research in this area is still preliminary, it is true to say that the very process of documenting a proper risk assessment results in the physician performing a systematic and structured review of their assessment. In other words, good documentation forces the physician into the deliberative System 2 thinking rather than the intuitive System 1 thinking. By its very nature, good documentation results in more thorough risk assessments and may well play its own role in preventing suicides.

Expectations of a Risk Assessment

In order to know what information to include in a note when documenting a risk assessment, it is important to know what the actual expectations of a risk assessment are. If the expectations are not known, the physician may be susceptible to including extraneous information or to neglecting to include pertinent information when documenting the assessment. One of the most common misconceptions that many psychiatrists believe with regard to risk assessment is that the task ahead of them is one of prediction—that is, predicting the specific likelihood of suicide in the patient they are evaluating. Although tempting to frame risk assessment in this manner, this is neither an accurate description nor a reasonable expectation of a risk assessment. Rather than a task of prediction, risk assessment is a task of stratification, stratifying a heterogeneous set of patients into categories of risk so that groups that deserve important attention can be further evaluated and appropriate steps can be taken to reasonably ensure safety.[15]

From a purely statistical standpoint, most individuals with suicidal thoughts, or even with a history of suicide attempts, do not die by suicide.[16] In the United States, the yearly incident of suicide in the general population is approximately 15 suicides for every 100,000 people, or 0.015% of the total population per year.[17] It has long been known that paradoxically, although suicide is a leading cause of death on a population level, its infrequency on the individual level makes it very difficult to predict the likelihood of suicide in any one person.[18] Even cutting-edge prediction models utilizing advanced statistical tools fail to accurately predict suicide attempts at the individual level.[19] There is no combination of risk factors that guarantees an individual will attempt suicide. Likewise, there is no combination of protective factors that will indubitably protect an individual from ever attempting suicide. An individual with few risk factors and many protective factors may attempt suicide, and an individual with many risk factors and few protective factors may never attempt suicide.[20]

This does not mean that risk assessment is an exercise in futility, done only as a means of practicing medicine defensively to protect against legal repercussions. Risk assessments should not be approached as a predictive task, with the goal of providing a numerical or categorical likelihood of negative outcome. Rather, the goal of a risk assessment is to stratify patients into level of risk so that appropriate steps can be taken for safety.[15] The true purpose of a risk assessment is to provide a structured means to systematically assess both static and dynamic factors of risk and protection. The aim of this systematic assessment is to identify protective factors that can be augmented, identify risk factors that can be ameliorated, and then act on this information in such a way that the likelihood of a negative outcome for the patient is reduced.[21]

The key legal term relevant to risk assessment is "foreseeability." Despite the apparent implication of the term, in the legal context, foreseeability does not refer to predicting a specific act. Rather, foreseeability is generally defined as the reasonable expectation that some damage is likely to arise from certain acts or omission. In other words, it refers to whether or not a doctor reasonably recognized, and adequately dealt with, a particular level of danger.[15]

With this in mind, documentation of a risk assessment should reflect that the physician's decision to discharge or admit was made after synthesizing the patient's current statements, the physician's observations, the patient's previous history, collateral information, and known risk factors. It should also reflect that adequate steps were taken to formulate an appropriate safety plan in order to address any modifiable risk factors.

Numerous risk assessment scales and instruments have been developed to standardize risk assessment. These scales vary in their reliability, and there is no consensus regarding which instruments, if any, are considered validated in an emergency psychiatry population. The use of specific instruments is governed predominantly by local and institutional preference rather than evidence.[22] The use of such scales and instruments can be incorporated into the risk assessment but is neither necessary nor sufficient to document that a proper risk assessment was performed.

Key Elements and General Guidelines

Anatomy of a Risk Assessment

Key Elements
There is no consensus on what constitutes a minimum level of appropriate documentation for a risk assessment. The amount of information documented in a risk assessment will vary from patient to patient. A rule of thumb, albeit with many exceptions, is that patients being discharged who appear to be high acuity and patients being involuntarily admitted who appear to be low acuity merit a higher amount of documentation of risk. The following elements should be considered when documenting a risk assessment and, ideally, would be touched upon, however briefly, in every documentation of risk:[23]

- Facts on which the risk assessment is based, including a mention of
  - Static risk factors
  - Static protective factors
  - Dynamic risk factors
  - Dynamic protective factors

- An overall assessment of level of proximal risk
- An overall assessment of level of chronic risk
- A specific comment on firearms. If there is no access to firearms, this should be documented as a pertinent negative. If there is access to firearms, further documentation about steps taken to address their risk is needed.
- Steps taken to restrict means of committing suicide
- The rationale for the disposition decision made as well as the rationale for not pursuing the alternative option
- Duty to warn/duty to protect, if applicable
- Collateral information or, if unable to obtain, documentation that an attempt was made to obtain collateral
- In the case of admission, documentation of dangerousness or inability to care for self
- In the case of discharge, documentation of lack of imminent danger as well as a safety plan
- Regardless of decision to discharge or admit based on immediate risk, mention of steps taken for chronic risk management

The use of dot phrases and templated text can help with parts of the documentation to increase efficiency when documenting in a busy emergency room setting. However, boilerplate text can never, and should never, completely automate documentation.

Safety Contract

It is important to note that a "safety contract" is not an element of risk assessment documentation. The practice of "contracting for safety" dates back to the mid-1970s and was originally studied in outpatient therapy practices.[24] Even at publication, the study describing contracting for safety faced many criticisms. The decades following publication of that study have failed to produce any evidence that safety contracts are a protective factor against suicide or that refusing to enter into such a contract is a risk factor for suicide.[25] As top psychiatric experts have written, "Under no circumstances should a patient's willingness or reluctance to enter into a verbal or written suicide contract be used as an indicator for discharge planning, especially from an emergency department setting."[26]

It is also important to not confuse a safety contract with a safety plan. A safety contract is a written contract signed by a patient, promising to the physician that the patient will not harm themself. Safety planning, on the other hand, is an intervention in which the physician and the patient will collaboratively identify warning signs, discuss coping strategies that have worked in the past or may work in the future, identify people who can be a source of support when an acute stressor arises, and plan out safety steps that can be taken to mitigate the risk of suicide after discharge. Research has shown that safety planning can help prevent suicide attempts, resolve suicidal ideation, and reduce inpatient hospitalization in certain high-risk patient populations .[27] Part of a safety plan would include how means of suicide can be removed from the environment. Documenting this on paper for a patient to take home is wholly appropriate and is completely distinct from having the patient sign a safety contract.

Assessment and Plan

Although the entire note, including the history of present illness and mental status exam, should support the decision to discharge, it is of utmost importance to pay particular attention to the "Assessment and Plan" portion of the note.[12] It is here that the various data points obtained by the psychiatrist are synthesized and distilled into a cohesive narrative. It is this portion of the note that is most likely to be brought up in any legal proceedings. It is critical that the assessment accurately and comprehensively captures the thought process behind discharge as well as documents whatever plan has been formulated to mitigate risk after discharge. The risk assessment should be worked into the assessment and plan and be more than just one line or a checkbox of factors. A checkbox list or one-sentence assessment gives the appearance that very little thought was given to the decision. Conversely, a well-written and thorough assessment demonstrates that whatever the outcome may have been, the physician who made the decision to discharge did so only after careful clinical consideration.

Guidelines

Ten tips

1. Document the main facts on which the risk assessment is based.

Risk assessment can be broadly conceptualized as a synthesis of four main domains: static risk factors, static protective factors, dynamic risk factors, and dynamic protective factors. Although it is not possible to exhaustively document every single one of these factors, it is important to document the major risk and protective factors that were assessed. See Table 21.1 for a non-exhaustive list of factors to consider when documenting a risk assessment. Do not make the fallacy of only documenting risk factors if admitting or only documenting protective factors if discharging. Documentation should reflect the fact that all pertinent facts were assessed and that the disposition decision was made through a synthesis of all relevant factors. This does not have to be an in-depth narrative of each factor; simply mentioning the factors that were taken into account to make the decision is sufficient.

Do not write:
Patient is safe for discharge, no history of suicide attempts and has plans to go to work on Monday.

Instead, write:
The patient does have several risk factors. Notably, he is an older White male, lives alone, and has decreased social support. However, he also has a significant number of protective factors including the fact he reports no history of suicide attempts, is currently in a stable relationship, reports strong social supports, is currently employed, denies current suicidal ideation, has close outpatient follow-up, and is future-oriented with plans to work on a new project in the office on Monday.

---

2. Document both immediate and long-term risk.

Risk is a dynamic entity and is always assessed as such. Psychiatrists simultaneously assess both the immediate risk that the patient is currently presenting with and the chronic

Table 21.1 Risk Factors and Protective Factors to Consider When Documenting a Risk Assessment

Risk factors	Family history of suicide
	History of physical or sexual abuse as a child
	Previous suicide attempts
	All psychiatric disorders with the exception of intellectual disability and dementia
	History of alcohol and substance abuse
	Feelings of hopelessness
	Impulsive or aggressive tendencies
	Cultural and religious beliefs (e.g., belief that suicide is noble resolution of a personal dilemma)
	Local epidemics of suicide
	Isolation, a feeling of being cut off from other people
	Barriers to accessing mental health treatment
	Relational, social, work, or financial loss
	Physical illness
	Easy access to lethal methods
	Unwillingness to seek help because of the stigma attached to mental health, substance use disorders, and suicidal thoughts
	Suicidal ideation
	Purposelessness
	Unemployment
	Advanced age
	Male gender
	Single
	Being a physician or veteran
	Anticipated or actual losses or life stresses (e.g., romantic breakups, legal problems, academic failures)
	Chronic pain
Protective factors	Effective clinical care for mental, physical, and substance use disorders
	Access to a variety of clinical interventions and support for help-seeking
	Family and community support (connectedness)
	Female gender
	Marriage
	Caregiver for a child (except in postpartum mood and psychotic disorders, teen pregnancy, and extreme economic hardships)
	Ongoing medical and mental health care relationships
	Skills in problem-solving, conflict resolution, and nonviolent ways of handling disputes
	Cultural and religious beliefs that discourage suicide
	Life satisfaction
	Positive coping skills

Information synthesized from Franklin et al.[28] and Weber et al.[29]

risk that the patient will have weeks, months, or even years from presentation. Both of these should be documented in the note in order to reflect that both of them were considered when evaluating the patient. A patient may present with lower imminent risk of suicide while still having an elevated long-term risk of harm to self or others. A proper risk assessment documentation will touch upon not just the patient's immediate risk at the time of evaluation in the emergency room but also the patient's long-term risk after discharge.

> Do not write:
> *The patient's risk is low and therefore the patient is safe for discharge.*
>
> Instead, write:
> *Given the aforementioned risk factors, the patient's overall lifetime risk for future danger to himself or others is moderate. However, given both his protective and risk factors, the imminent risk of harm is low, especially since he is currently future- and goal-oriented, has outpatient psychiatric follow-up established, and is denying suicidal ideation.*

3. Write clearly and do not leave room for inferences.

The goal when documenting risk assessment is to capture the thought process and rationale that went into the disposition decision. When the risk assessment is read afterwards, it should be readily understandable and easy to follow. It is crucial when documenting high-acuity discharges that the documentation clearly and directly explain the thought process behind the decision to discharge.[30] The reader should never need to "read between the lines" or make inferences in order to understand the rationale behind the discharge decision.[12] Expecting the reader to draw their own conclusion opens up the very real possibility that the conclusion the reader takes away from the note will be different than the conclusion intended by the writer.

As a corollary to writing clearly, dispense with the stilted practice of forcing a third-person point of view when writing notes. Many psychiatrists were taught during training that writing medical notes in the third-person point of view is important because it shows that the physician is objective and impartial. The reality, however, is that notes are a record of the physician's thought process and medical reasoning. By their very nature, they are personal and serve to capture one person's thought process at one specific point in time. When documenting a risk assessment and high-acuity discharge, terminology such as "this writer" or "this physician" serves only to confuse the reader and detracts from the actual purpose of the note. An assessment and plan in a medical note is far closer to an op-ed than it is to a news article.[12]

> Do not write:
> *This writer observed several incongruencies between stated suicidal ideation and patient's behavior while in the psychiatric emergency room.*
>
> Instead, write:
> *Although Mr. Smith stated that he felt despondent and could not imagine ever smiling again in his life due to his deep depression and imminent suicidality, I observed Mr. Smith laughing and socializing well with peers in the milieu shortly after we finished the interview. Furthermore, although he reported that he had no appetite at all due to his depression, he repeatedly asked nursing staff for more turkey sandwiches and snacks. These discrepancies suggested to me that Mr. Smith was not being completely forthright about his symptoms and that there was some level of secondary gain to his presentation. Since Mr. Smith is not currently suffering from an acute, decompensated mental illness, a psychiatric hospitalization will not modify his chronic risk of suicide. The best way to help this patient and decrease his suicide risk is not by hospitalization but rather by establishing with an outpatient mental health professional that he can have long-term follow-up to manage symptoms and stressors.*

4. Explain why the disposition is the most appropriate treatment.

In a sense, the risk assessment is an argument justifying why the disposition the physician has chosen is the most appropriate one. In cases in which a patient is endorsing suicidal ideation but the physician still decides to discharge, the documentation should explain why this decision is the most appropriate one. In other words, the treatment rationale should be clearly spelled out in the note. There are two parts to this rationale. One consists of explaining why, despite endorsing suicidality, the physician believes the patient is not imminently at harm to self. The other part consists of explaining why a hospitalization will not be of benefit to the patient. Although a patient may have a long-term risk of harm to self, there is not always a clinical indication for inpatient treatment. If there are no clear factors for inpatient treatment to modify or if an inpatient hospitalization will reinforce maladaptive coping skills, this should be documented in the note to explain the rationale for not admitting a patient endorsing suicidal ideation. Discharging a patient who is endorsing suicidal ideation should only be done when it is clear that the patient is not at imminent risk of harm to self and that hospitalization will not have an impact on suicidality.

Do not write:
The patient does not require inpatient psychiatric hospitalization. Although he is endorsing suicidal thoughts, he is not at harm to himself.

Instead, write:
Mr. Smith has a long history of many hospitalizations and psychiatric emergency room visits. These visits are characterized by endorsements of suicidal ideation but when discharged, the patient does not attempt suicide. Given the patient's presentation and history, I do not believe that the patient has a primary desire to harm himself. Rather, it appears that he uses threats of suicide as a means to communicate his level of distress. Admitting him at this time would only serve to reinforce a maladaptive coping skill, i.e. endorsing suicidal ideation when stressed. We have worked together to devise a safety plan, discussed coping techniques, and given a few hours in the emergency room to decompress. Undoubtedly, given his history of impulsivity and poor distress tolerance, I do have a high concern that he will eventually attempt suicide again in the future. Although this is likely, I cannot predict when it will happen. It occurs in the context of environmental stressors that are unpredictable and the best way to change this would be long- term therapy where he gradually solidifies coping techniques to deal with stressors. A hospitalization will not modify his chronic risk for suicide, and he is no longer imminently suicidal. He will benefit most from long-term outpatient treatment so will be discharged and will follow up outpatient.

---

5. Document the harms of the alternative.

Just like discharging a patient comes with potential negative repercussions for the patient, so too does admission. This is something that, by virtue of their years of training, psychiatrists automatically assess and incorporate into their decision-making when deciding disposition for a patient. However, it is a powerful piece of the risk assessment that is rarely documented. Simply stating that a patient does not require inpatient hospitalization is less cogent of an argument than stating that the harms of an inpatient hospitalization outweigh its benefits. Put into writing the risks and harms of the alternative disposition decision so that the risk assessment demonstrates that not only was the alternative considered but also it was not a benign option that was devoid of any risks. In cases of nonsuicidal self-injury, admitting the patient may be countertherapeutic by reinforcing the belief that self-harm is a way to sustain other's attention and obtain support when distressed.[31]

Do not write:

The patient does not require inpatient hospitalization and is low imminent risk.

Instead, write:

The risks of a psychiatric hospitalization (including loss of freedom, demoralization from institutionalization, removal from community supports, potential of regression in inpatient hospital setting, and impact on financial stability) have been carefully considered and weighed against risks to self or others if discharged. Since he is not currently suicidal, feels hopeful about the future, and has made specific plans in the future such as attending church on Sunday and going for dinner with friends, he would be better served by discharge and outpatient follow-up than inpatient hospitalization.

---

6. Document mitigation of risk.

A risk assessment is not just an assessment of risk. It serves to help inform the larger treatment plan being developed in an emergency room. Part of the purpose in performing a risk assessment is to help identify what concrete steps can be taken to mitigate risk, both immediate and chronic. Once identified, those steps should be carried out and also documented in the note.[12] Short- and intermediate-term mitigation of risk will often involve creation of a crisis plan. Long-term mitigation of risk will often involve referral to outpatient services, including medication management, evidence-based psychotherapy, or both. Because many high-acuity discharge cases involve moderate to high chronic risk, special care should be taken to address what steps were taken to mitigate the chronic risk. If a safety plan was developed with the patient, it should be documented alongside the risk assessment. If the patient refuses to engage in safety planning, document this in the chart, highlighting the attempts made to engage in adaptive problem-solving.[32]

Do not write:

The patient is at elevated chronic risk but as her imminent risk is low, she is safe for discharge at this time.

Instead, write:

As per the risk assessment documented above, the patient's imminent risk for harm to self is low. However, she has many risk factors which elevate her chronic risk. An inpatient psychiatric hospitalization will not modify these risk factors. The best treatment to modify her chronic risk is engagement in dialectical behavioral therapy (DBT). I have referred her to local DBT therapists with whom she can establish care. In addition, I have refilled her SSRI prescription (she has been out for three weeks) and communicated this emergency room visit to her primary psychiatrist so that she can be seen for an appointment as soon as possible.

7. Document collateral.

Collateral information is a key component obtained during the psychiatric evaluation whereby clinicians gather information provided about the patient from the patient's known contacts.[33] Standard of care dictates that proper risk assessment of any high-acuity discharge includes a serious attempt at obtaining collateral information. This can be from a spouse, another close family member, a roommate, or a close friend. Collateral information provides yet another data point that can buttress the physician's decision to discharge. When collateral is obtained, it should always be documented in the chart. A line-by-line transcription is not needed; it is sufficient to mention the name of the person who provided the collateral information, their relationship with the patient, and a general summary of the information they provided.

At times, attempts at obtaining collateral information are unsuccessful. If this is the case, it is vital to document that the attempt was made and that it was unsuccessful. Document not just that an attempt was made but also specifically which family members and friends the attempts were made to reach.

Collateral is so important in a high-acuity discharge that in the case in which collateral cannot be obtained, it is prudent to have a second team member perform an evaluation of the patient. This is typically done by a social worker but, in the absence of one, can be performed by an emergency department (ED) physician or a nurse. If the second clinician is in agreement with the decision to discharge, this should be documented in the note.

Do not write:
Attempts were made to obtain collateral but were unsuccessful.

Instead, write:
We attempted to obtain collateral prior to discharge. Mr. Smith provided us the phone numbers of his mother and father but both numbers were out of service. He was unable to provide us with any other collateral contacts. I discussed this case with the ED psychiatric social worker and asked her to evaluate the patient as well. She did so and agreed that an inpatient psychiatric hospitalization would not be beneficial or therapeutic to the patient at this time.

---

8. Document duty to warn.

If there is an explicit threat toward an identifiable individual, it is important to carry out the duty to warn. Most states either require or permit a psychiatrist to take reasonable steps to inform such a person about threats that have been made against them by the patient. Once law enforcement and the person the threat has been made against have been notified, the patient's chart should reflect that the physician has carried out the duty to warn.[34] This should be explicitly mentioned as part of the risk assessment.

Do not write:
The patient made a threat to hurt his girlfriend if discharged, but given his previous history of threats that he does not act upon, he is at low risk of harm to others.

Instead, write:
Patient was brought into the ED by police after a verbal altercation with his girlfriend during which he stated he wanted to kill himself. On triage, he had stated, "I'm going to

> *mess her up for sending me here." After he had a chance to calm down, he recanted this threat and stated, "I just say stuff like that when angry." As described in the risk assessment, patient does not require, nor would he benefit from, a psychiatric hospitalization. We informed his girlfriend as well as local law enforcement about his threat towards her in order to discharge our duty to warn.*

9. Specifically comment on firearms.

Although firearms are the most common method by which suicide is completed in the United States, they are not the most common method by which people attempt suicide. The reason for this discrepancy is that they are, by a very large margin, the most lethal method with which to attempt suicide. To understand just how lethal a suicide attempt by firearms is, consider that the most common method by which people attempt suicide is by drug overdose. Of these suicide attempts, approximately 3% result in a completed suicide. In a suicide attempt with a firearm, however, approximately 85% of the attempts result in completed suicide.[35] Given that high-acuity discharges are often characterized by impulsive suicidality that waxes and wanes in response to an environmental stressor, it is imperative that access to firearms be addressed and that this be documented in the chart.

If the patient does not have access to firearms, this should be documented in the risk assessment so that it is clear that it was asked about. If the patient does have access to firearms, this should be documented in the risk assessment and incorporated into the disposition decision. If a patient does have access to firearms, steps should be taken, and documented, to mitigate risk of harm. This may include providing education about the lethality of a suicide attempt by firearm, asking a family member or friend to take temporary possession of the firearms, ensuring that the firearms are locked in a safe, utilizing firearm locks, and other means to limit firearms accessibility.[36]

> Do not write:
> *Patient's risk factors include access to firearms.*
>
> Instead, write:
> *Of note, the patient reports that he has access to handguns. I provided education about the lethality of a suicide attempt by firearm (that 85% of suicide attempts by firearm result in fatality). We spoke about steps that could be taken to mitigate risk of harm from his handguns. Although he was reluctant to sell them or dispose of them completely, he agreed to have his mother take temporary possession of them in her house until he felt that he was in a better state of mind. I spoke with his mother who agreed with this plan and will have the firearms removed from his house prior to coming here to pick him up from the hospital.*

10. Avoid pejorative language and instead focus on the underlying motivation.

When writing a risk assessment, care should be taken to use objective, nonjudgmental language. Using phrases such as "frequent flyer," "gamey," "manipulative," "shelter seeking," and "playing the system" suggests that the psychiatrist was diminishing the severity of the patient's presentation. It also suggests, and may even reflect, that the psychiatrist was suffering from an anchoring bias and did not give the patient a fair and balanced evaluation.

As mentioned previously, however, this does not mean that the risk assessment should be written in a manner that the reader needs to make inferences in order to understand the writer's intent. Clearly document the objective findings that were observed and why these findings suggest that the patient is not imminently suicidal. Rather than "cry for help" or "attention seeking," accurately note what was seen and why it suggests that the patient is not at imminent risk of harm to self. This is more beneficial than using pejorative language because it switches the tone of the entire encounter from being adversarial to one in which there is collaboration to address the underlying motivation behind the observed behavior. An individual endorsing suicidal ideation due to an attempt at obtaining shelter from subzero temperatures has a very real unmet need that can be addressed in a more effective way than psychiatric hospitalization. Similarly, a person who chronically endorses suicidal ideation as a way of dealing with any negative relationship stressors still has very real unmet needs that can be addressed in a more effective way than psychiatric hospitalization. Refocusing the assessment to the underlying need is more productive and beneficial for patient care.[37] "Contingent suicidality" is an appropriate term to use and, when relevant, can be worked into the risk assessment to convey the fact that the suicidality is not due to a purely psychiatric disorder.

Do not write:
The patient is malingering and claims he is suicidal in order to game the system to get a place to spend the night. Will discharge as he is not truly suicidal.

Instead, write:
I shared with the patient that despite stating he is suicidal, I observed him laughing with other patients in the milieu and eagerly asking for food. I suggested to him that perhaps his statements of wanting to kill himself stemmed less from a primary desire to harm himself and more as a way to deal with the environmental stressors he is undergoing. He acknowledged that if he was in a more stable environment (it is currently below freezing outside and he is homeless), he would not feel suicidal. We have agreed to keep patient in observation tonight and discharge to a cold shelter tomorrow morning. The patient is agreeable with this plan.

Practical Examples of Risk Assessment Documentation

Quickly Writing a Risk Assessment

Although documenting a thorough risk assessment may seem like a laborious task at first, it is possible to make the process efficient so that no more than 5 minutes are spent documenting the risk assessment. The following guide and boilerplate text can be used to help create dot phrases that will allow a psychiatrist to quickly document a thorough risk assessment.

In the first paragraph, mention risk factors for harm to self:

I performed a thorough risk assessment to evaluate safety for discharge. [Name] has several risk factors for violence towards [him]self and others. Notably, [he] is <25 or >50 years old, male, lives alone, is divorced, has at least one prior suicide attempt or self-harm behavior, has a history of dangerousness to others, is unemployed, has a mood disorder, reports symptoms of psychosis, has comorbid anxiety, reports an impulse control disorder, reports hopelessness, has a personality disorder, endorses a history of trauma, has a cognitive disorder, endorses ongoing substance use, reports a family history of completed suicide, has decreased social support, reports a current plan, suffers from a chronic medical illness, reports chronic pain, has access to guns or weapons.

If there is access to guns or weapons, follow this with an additional paragraph specifically addressing firearms:

Given the elevated risk of completed suicide when there is access to firearms, I spoke to the patient in depth about this. I provided education about the lethality of a suicide attempt by firearm (that 85% of suicide attempts by firearm results in fatality). We spoke about steps that could be taken to mitigate risk of harm from his handguns. [Write final plan about firearm risk mitigation here].

In the next paragraph, document protective factors:

[He] also has a number of protective factors. Notably, [he] is female, denies any previous suicide attempts, denies previous self-harm behaviors or aggression, is currently in a stable relationship, is religious and believes suicide is a sin, reports being satisfied with [his] life, reports strong social supports, denies feeling hopeless, has no history of trauma, is not psychotic, is not endorsing any auditory or visual hallucinations, is not observed to be responding to internal stimuli, has no cognitive dysfunction, is currently employed, denies current suicidal ideation, denies current homicidal ideation, has no ongoing substance abuse problem, has close outpatient follow-up, pattern of help seeking behavior when in crisis, has established relationship with medical professionals, has no access to guns or weapons, and is future-oriented with plans to [mention specific future plans here].

Then, mention collateral:

Collateral information was obtained from [his] [family member] and is reassuring, with [his] [family member] stating that they have a low concern that patient will harm [him]self.

Mention specific observations in the emergency room that contributed to your discharge decision:

During my evaluation of the patient today, [fill in specifics].

Move on to describing chronic and immediate risk stratification:

> Taking into account all of the above information, the overall chronic risk for future dangerousness to self is [low/moderate/high]. [His] **imminent** risk is [low/moderate/high] as [he] now denies SI/HI, has no intent or plan, is clinically sober, future-oriented and goal-oriented, adherent with medication, has good social support, and has outpatient psychiatric follow-up established.

Mention harms of alternative:

> At this time, the risk factors for psychiatric hospitalization (including loss of freedom, demoralization from institutionalization, removal from community supports, potential of regression in inpatient hospital setting, and impact on financial stability) have been carefully considered and weighed against risks to self or others if discharged.

Describe what steps have been taken to mitigate risk, including any safety plan if one was developed:

> As per the risk assessment documented above, the patient has a [high/medium/low] chronic risk for harm to self is low. An inpatient psychiatric hospitalization will not modify these risk factors. The best treatment to modify [his] chronic risk is [therapy/IOP/substance use treatment/other]. I have [what was done to modify the chronic risk.]

Conclude with a summary and follow-up:

> At this time, as [name] is not imminently at risk for suicide, the least restrictive means of reasonably ensuring [his] safety is discharge to the community with follow-up as indicated in [his] discharge instructions. [He] has been given a sheet of information regarding local resources as well as the suicide hotline number (800-273-8255) and instructed that if [he] becomes suicidal in the future to call 911, 800-273-8255, or return to emergency room.

With this guide, the following risk assessment can be generated within 5 minutes:
I performed a thorough risk assessment to evaluate safety for discharge. Mr. Smith has several risk factors for violence towards himself and others. Notably, he is male, lives alone, is divorced, has a mood disorder, has a personality disorder, endorses a history of trauma, and has access to guns or weapons.

Given the elevated risk of completed suicide when there is access to firearms, I spoke to the patient in depth about this. I provided education about the lethality of a suicide attempt by firearm (that 85% of suicide attempts by firearm results in fatality). We spoke about steps that could be taken to mitigate risk of harm from his handguns. I strongly recommended that the patient sell his firearms, but he stated that this was not an option he would consider. We agreed that for the time being, it would be best if his mother took temporary possession of his firearms and kept them in her house until he felt that he was in a better state of mind. I spoke with his mother, who agreed with this plan and will have the firearms removed from his house prior to coming here to pick him up from the hospital.

Mr. Smith also has a number of protective factors. Notably, he denies any previous suicide attempts, denies previous self-harm behaviors or aggression, is religious and believes suicide is a sin, is not psychotic, is not endorsing any auditory or visual hallucinations, is not observed to be responding to internal stimuli, has no cognitive dysfunction, is currently employed, has no ongoing substance abuse problem, has a pattern of help-seeking behavior when in crisis, and is future-oriented with plans to go fishing with his best friend on Sunday. Collateral information was obtained from his mother and is reassuring, with his mother stating that she has a low concern that patient will harm himself.

During my evaluation of the patient today, I noticed that despite stating he was depressed to the point of being suicidal, he had a reactive affect and frequently smiled and joked with staff. On chart review, he has a long history of presenting with suicidal ideation after getting into verbal altercations with his ex-wife on the phone. I shared with the patient my concern that he uses suicidal ideation as a way to express his frustration and that this has become a maladaptive coping mechanism. He agrees with this. At the same time, I am not dismissing the seriousness of his distress, as he is clearly in great psychological and emotional pain when making these statements and it is possible that one day the pain will reach a level where he will act upon his suicidal thoughts. An inpatient psychiatric hospitalization will not be of any benefit in modifying this risk. Rather, long-term engagement with a DBT therapist will have the most effect on modifying his suicidal behavior. I have talked about this at length with him and he has agreed to follow up on a referral that we have made to a DBT therapist.

*Taking into account all of the above information, the overall chronic risk for future dangerousness to self is moderate. His **imminent** risk is low as he now denies SI/HI, has no intent or plan, is clinically sober, future-oriented and goal-oriented, adherent with medication, has good social support, and has outpatient psychiatric follow-up established.*

At this time, the risk factors for psychiatric hospitalization (including loss of freedom, demoralization from institutionalization, removal from community supports, potential of regression in inpatient hospital setting, and impact on financial stability) have been carefully considered and weighed against risks to self or others if discharged.

As Mr. Smith is not imminently at risk for suicide, the least restrictive means of reasonably ensuring his safety is discharge to the community with follow-up as indicated in his discharge instructions. He has been given a sheet of information regarding local resources as well as the suicide hotline number (800-273-8255) and instructed that if he becomes suicidal in the future to call 911, 800-273-8255, or return to emergency room.

Conclusion

Thorough, comprehensive, yet efficient documentation of risk assessment is an important skill that an emergency psychiatrist must master. A few minutes spent properly documenting a risk assessment can pay dividends many times over when it results in better patient care or protection from a malpractice lawsuit.

References

1. Sederer LI. The tragedy of mental health law. *Missouri Med*. 2013;110(2):104–105.

2. Bal BS. An introduction to medical malpractice in the United States. *Clin Orthop Relat Res*. 2009;467(2):339–347.

3. Jena AB, Seabury S, Lakdawalla D, Chandra A. Malpractice risk according to physician specialty. *N Engl J Med*. 2011;365(7):629–636.

4. Frierson RL, Joshi KG. Malpractice law and psychiatry: An overview. *Focus.* 2019;17(4): 332–336.

5. Knoll JL. Lessons from litigation. *Psychiatric Times.* 2015;32(5).

6. Paterick Z, Patel N, Chandrasekaran K, Tajik J, Paterick T. Medical malpractice stress syndrome: A "forme fruste" of posttraumatic stress disorder. *J Med Pract Manag.* 2017;32(4):283–287.

7. Simpson S, Stacy M. Avoiding the malpractice snare: Documenting suicide risk assessment. *J Psychiatr Pract.* 2004;10(3):185–189.

8. Tanguturi Y, Bodic M, Taub A, Homel P, Jacob T. Suicide risk assessment by residents: Deficiencies of documentation. *Acad Psychiatry.* 2017;41(4):513–519.

9. Alavi N, Reshetukha T, Prost E, Antoniak K, Groll D. Assessing suicide risk: What is commonly missed in the emergency room? *J Psychiatr Pract.* 2017;23(2):82–91.

10. Marett CP, Mossman D. What is your liability for involuntary commitment based on faulty information? *Curr Psychiatry.* 2017;16(3):21–25, 33.

11. Sher L. Suicide medical malpractice: An educational overview. *Int J Adolesc Med Health.* 2015;27(2):203–206.

12. Ballas 2017.

13. Kahneman D. *Thinking Fast and Slow.* Farrar, Straus & Giroux; 2013.

14. Cabrera D, Thomas JF, Wiswell JL, et al. Accuracy of "my gut feeling": Comparing System 1 to System 2 decision-making for acuity prediction, disposition and diagnosis in an academic emergency department. *West J Emerg Med.* 2015;16(5):653–657.

15. Reid WH. Risk assessment, prediction, and foreseeability. *J Psychiatr Pract.* 2003;9(1):82–86.

16. Sher L. Preventing suicide. *QJM.* 2004;97(10):677–680.

17. Centers for Disease Control and Prevention. Mortality in the United States, 2018. Data Brief No. 355. Published 2020. https://www.cdc.gov/nchs/products/databriefs/db355.htm

18. Pokorny AD. Prediction of suicide in psychiatric patients: Report of a prospective study. *Arch Gen Psychiatry.* 1983;40(3):249–257.

19. Belsher et al., 2019.

20. Pinals, 2019.

21. Wortzel et al., 2017.

22. Quinlivan L, Cooper J, Steeg S, et al. Scales for predicting risk following self-harm: An observational study in 32 hospitals in England. *BMJ Open.* 2014;4(5):e004732.

23. Sadek J. Documentation requirements of SRA; Documentation and communication. In: *A Clinicians Guide to Suicide Risk Assessment and Management.* Springer; 2019:56.

24. Drye RC, Goulding RL, Goulding ME. No-suicide decisions: Patient monitoring of suicidal risk. *Am J Psychiatry.* 1973;130(2):171–174.

25. Keelin AG, Penn JV, Campbell AL, Esposito-Smythers C, Spirito A. Contracting for safety with patients: Clinical practice and forensic implications. *J Am Acad Psychiatry Law.* 2009;37(3):363–370.

26. Riba MB, Ravindranath D. *Clinical Manual of Emergency Psychiatry.* American Psychiatric Publishing; 2006.

27. Bryan et al., 2017.

28. Franklin JC, Ribeiro JD, Fox KR, et al. Risk factors for suicidal thoughts and behaviors: A meta-analysis of 50 years of research. *Psychol Bull.* 2017;143(2):187–232. doi:10.1037/bul0000084

29. Weber AN, Michail M, Thompson A, Fiedorowicz JG. Psychiatric emergencies: Assessing and managing suicidal ideation. *Med Clin North Am.* 2017;101(3):553–571. doi:10.1016/j.mcna.2016.12.006

30. Francois, Madva, and Goodman, 2014.

31. Joshi, 2021.

32. Bundy, Schreiber, and Pasualy, 2014.

33. Witkin, M. The effect of collateral information on involuntary psychiatric commitment. *Curr Psychiatry.* 2019;18(2):e1–e2.

34. Saxton, Resnick, and Noffsinger, 2018.

35. Drexler, M. Guns and suicide: The hidden toll. Harvard Public Health. Published 2013. https://cdn1.sph.harvard.edu/wp-content/uploads/sites/21/2013/05/HPHSPRING2013gunviolence.pdf

36. Dempsey C, Bendek D, Ursano R. Association of firearm ownership, use, accessibility, and storage practices with suicide risk among US Army soldiers. *JAMA Netw Open.* 2019;2(6):e195383.

37. Lambert and Bonner, 1996.

22

Trauma-Informed Care, Psychological First Aid, and Recovery-Oriented Approaches in the Emergency Room

Benjamin Merotto and Scott A. Simpson

Introduction

Most individuals experience a traumatic event in their life.[1] This trauma may relate to surviving an injury or accident, medical illness, or interpersonal violence. The impact of trauma on survivors can be varied, complex, and insidious. Although most trauma survivors fully recover, as many as one-third will experience consequent psychiatric symptoms, including post-traumatic stress disorder (PTSD).[2] Childhood exposure to trauma is particularly problematic and correlates with the later development of depressive symptoms, substance abuse, and antisocial behaviors;[3] this correlation is stronger for more severe and prolonged trauma. Because trauma is more common among racial and ethnic minority communities, trauma's lifelong consequences disproportionately impact historically underserved persons and thereby fuel other health disparities.[4]

All emergency mental health clinicians will treat patients who have survived trauma. Emergency department (ED) patients may have survived a life-threatening episode just moments before. Families may be learning of the death or disability of loved ones. New and life-changing diagnoses are made with regularity. Life-changing traumatic events occur with regularity in emergency settings, and the environment challenges the resilience of patients and clinicians who have already survived trauma once in their past.

Emergency medical providers are adept at treating severe and unpredictable medical illness. Similarly, managing the aftermath of trauma is an indispensable skill for emergency clinicians, psychiatrists, and service leaders. In this chapter, we describe approaches to reducing the risk of psychological trauma and its consequences in emergency and crisis care settings. First, the recovery model and its application to emergency psychiatry are presented. Then, we describe in greater detail two approaches to fostering a recovery environment in the ED: trauma-informed care (TIC) and psychological first aid (PFA).

The Recovery Model

In a single encounter, emergency clinicians may provide a patient's or family's first impression with mental health care, a healing and reassuring presence at a moment of crisis, or an option of last resort for patients who have had prior adverse experiences with health care. Succeeding in these different roles requires crisis clinicians to be cognizant of the patient's perspectives and their goals for a clinical encounter. Recovery models provide a framework for clinicians to acknowledge patients' perspectives and autonomy in seeking care and for administrators to design systems that cultivate compassionate practice. Understanding the recovery model is elemental to the safe, effective practice of emergency psychiatry.

The recovery model is a treatment philosophy that emphasizes the patient's individual treatment and life goals. These goals may be at odds with traditional aims of conventional medical care. From the recovery perspective, traditional psychiatry overvalues diagnostic assessment and symptom control. These long-standing values are rooted in the history of psychiatry. Historically, mental health care failed to treat psychiatric illness as successfully as other physicians have treated somatic illness. Psychiatric symptom severity was significant even among patients in treatment. To this day, contemporary treatments that achieve substantial reductions in morbidity and mortality related to mental illness may be associated with distressing side effects (e.g., tardive dyskinesia or metabolic syndrome) or frequent episodes of involuntary treatment. Thus, there is often ambiguity as to the best treatment options for many patients. In the past, psychiatric professionals held themselves to be arbiter of these treatment decisions; these paternalistic attitudes led to frequent abuses, including human rights violations.[5]

The recovery movement arose in response to these limitations—and occasional malpractice—of psychiatric medicine. The recovery model reframes the role of psychiatry as a tool for helping patients achieve their personal life goals. Treatment should accommodate the patient's choices and preserve autonomy to the fullest extent possible. For instance, perhaps psychotic symptoms that are not impairing and do not preclude the patient from functioning do not require treatment. Treatment should occur in as least restrictive a manner as possible. Barring imminent risk of harm, patients are permitted to make their own decisions regardless of divergence from prevailing cultural norms. Helping patients achieve recovery requires clinicians to understand their patient's life in a holistic way, in which medical treatment or mental illness may be of relatively little significance.

The notion of minimally restrictive treatment options and a focus on patient-defined recovery seem less revolutionary now than they once were. There has been substantial progress toward including patients' perspectives in treatment planning. For instance, the current *Diagnostic and Statistical Manual of Mental Disorders* often requires significant impairment to be present for making a diagnosis.[6] And the role of the clinician–patient relationship has evolved to appreciate the centrality of the patient's life narrative in treatment.[7] These advances can obscure the ongoing need to promote recovery principles in clinical practice. For instance, patients who present to EDs with suicidal thoughts overwhelmingly experience psychiatric hospitalization rather than less restrictive crisis treatments.[8] Mental health patients remain more likely to experience adverse ED stays than medical patients.[9]

Recovery in Practice

Advancing a recovery model in emergency psychiatry sometimes comes into conflict with traditional medical practices. For example, some hospitals require behavioral

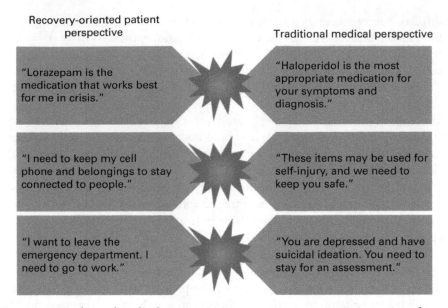

Figure 22.1 Traditional medical perspective versus contemporary recovery-oriented perspective.

health patients to wear certain colored gowns for safety, even when patients may prefer to appear similar to all other patients. Patients may prefer a different medication than that of the clinician. Staff may feel unsafe with patients not receiving injectable medications or with efforts to reduce use of physical restraint. Figure 22.1 illustrates how the traditional clinical and contemporary recovery mindsets can stand in conflict over the course of a clinical encounter.

Patients have described the failings of emergency psychiatry. Survivors of psychiatric crisis attest to the importance of being treated respectfully in a clean and comforting physical environment.[10] Food, water, and warm blankets should be freely available.[11] Most patients who experience restraint or seclusion remember their experience well. These patients emphasize the importance of frequent check-ins by staff and ensuring physical needs are met—bathroom visits, food, and water. The opportunity for patients to give feedback on medication selection is an important component of supporting autonomy.[12] Benzodiazepines are often preferred to antipsychotics, and oral medications are typically preferable to injectable medications.

Many interventions common in emergency psychiatry demonstrate the utility of the recovery philosophy. Harm reduction models of substance use disorder treatment emphasize patients' ability to care for themselves and maintain self-defined functioning, even without abstinence. Psychiatric assessments should involve the patient's supportive contacts not only to inform a safety assessment but also to support a discharge plan.[13] Crisis intervention training for law enforcement officers leads to improved officer satisfaction, reductions in the use of force, and likely reduces unnecessary mental health-related bookings.[14] Recovery also aligns with traditional targets of psychiatric treatment—patients realizing self-defined recovery have been observed to experience less intense suicidal ideation.[15]

Even short patient encounters afford an opportunity to provide evidence-based psychotherapeutic treatment.[16] Figure 22.2 exemplifies how a conflict might be resolved

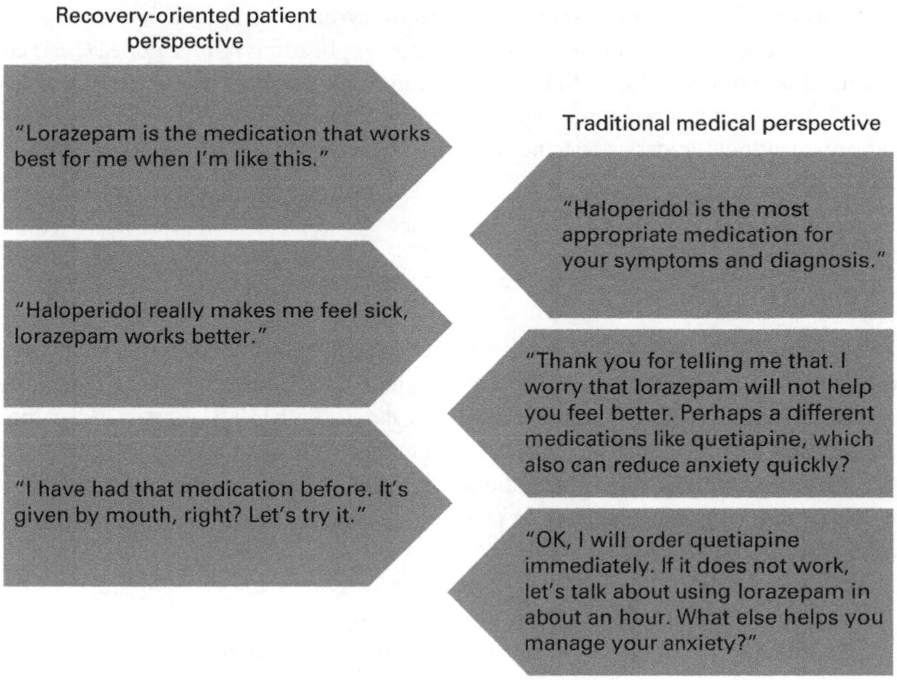

Recovery-oriented patient
perspective

"Lorazepam is the medication that works best for me when I'm like this."

Traditional medical perspective

"Haloperidol is the most appropriate medication for your symptoms and diagnosis."

"Haloperidol really makes me feel sick, lorazepam works better."

"Thank you for telling me that. I worry that lorazepam will not help you feel better. Perhaps a different medications like quetiapine, which also can reduce anxiety quickly?

"I have had that medication before. It's given by mouth, right? Let's try it."

"OK, I will order quetiapine immediately. If it does not work, let's talk about using lorazepam in about an hour. What else helps you manage your anxiety?"

Figure 22.2 Possible conflict resolution in a recovery framework.

in a recovery framework. A recovery approach does not require all decisions to be made by patients. Rather, recovery acknowledges collaborative decision-making and patient autonomy as necessary priorities of treatment, along with maintaining safety. Here, a patient and clinician discuss an appropriate medication treatment for psychotic symptoms. Although the patient prefers a benzodiazepine, the clinician initially believes an antipsychotic is indicated. The patient is given space to share their perspective on this selection, and the clinician offers a different medication choice acceptable to both parties.

A recovery-oriented treatment milieu makes this discussion possible:

- The patient feels empowered to ask for medications.
- The patient's psychiatric symptoms are given prompt attention and credence.
- The clinician believes the patient has a right to provide input into medication selection.
- The patient's request for a benzodiazepine is not presumed to represent addiction or malingering; rather, the clinician affirms a common goal around the patient's well-being in the moment.
- The clinician is willing to compromise on the "ideal" medication to suit the patient's preference.
- There is an effort to provide care by the least restrictive means available through provision of oral medication. The clinician does not threaten to administer an intramuscular injection. (Oral medications are safer for administering staff, too.)
- The clinician ends the exchange by again affirming the ongoing treatment relationship and empowering the patient to give feedback on the effectiveness of treatment.

These examples speak to the benefits of a recovery-oriented approach to emergency psychiatric care and the promise of comprehensive applications of this model. Crisis clinicians must understand how their services may inadvertently risk patients' recovery through retraumatization or inadequate delivery of quality care. TIC offers clinicians and organizational leaders a specific approach to incorporating recovery principles in emergency care.

Trauma-Informed Care

Trauma-informed care is a framework for improving health care delivery in a way that recognizes and responds to the impact of trauma in patients' lives. TIC is not a specific intervention or a therapeutic approach for a specific illness. Rather, TIC is better understood as a philosophy that guides the care of trauma survivors. TIC is a way to broadly apply recovery principles through accommodating an individual's complex reactions to trauma.

The TIC philosophy encompasses a set of tenets intended to support patients' sense of safety and autonomy:[17]

- Ensure patients' physical and psychological safety.
- Conduct organizational operations with trustworthiness and transparency.
- Offer connection to other survivors of trauma.
- Foster collaboration among the clinical team.
- Empower staff and patients to advocate for themselves.
- Recognize and reject biases.

TIC recognizes that patients have experienced trauma, the significance of trauma in a patient's life, and that health care systems have an obligation to reduce the risk of retraumatization.

Reflecting on these principles more deeply reveals how many EDs and crisis environments are not naturally suited to TIC. EDs are chaotic settings with a constant rotation of staff and patients presenting in acute distress. This environment predisposes trauma survivors to experience fear and anxiety. Communication can be challenging and limit patient participation in decision-making. The ED's function to serve complex medically ill patients requires hierarchical teams with rarified expertise, and the clinical culture is susceptible to discounting feedback from less senior team members. In these environments, patients with mental health issues may be prone to be labeled "challenging," "disruptive," or "resource-intensive."[18] One barrier to the use of TIC in emergency settings is staff's concern about the time needed to learn and provide TIC and confusion over how to operationalize TIC principles.[7] Nevertheless, ED staff overwhelmingly advocate for TIC in their practice.[19]

Although providing trauma-informed approaches in the ED may be difficult, perhaps nowhere else can the utility of TIC be more profound. Many ED patients are trauma survivors—survivors of an event in which their autonomy was violated and perhaps their life threatened. A visit to the ED may very well draw vivid parallels to these experiences. Trauma survivors are apt to experience fear, anxiety, and invalidation in unfamiliar and stressful situations.[20]

TIC approaches are heterogeneous in practice. TIC implementation might be imagined from two perspectives: that of the patient and that of the health care team.

From the patient's viewpoint, TIC compels us to imagine how the care environment promotes a sense of safety and reduce the risk of retraumatization. Physical spaces should be clean, welcoming, and navigable. Clinical processes should protect patients' autonomy and offer opportunities for feedback and collaboration. Ideally, organizations should offer peer counseling. In the ED, peer counseling may be accessible via telephone or video modalities, as with an Alcoholics Anonymous or crisis hotlines. Staff should feel knowledgeable answering questions about access to mental health services and comfortable asking sensitive questions about suicidal ideation, substance use, and social history in a nonjudgmental way. Patients should be given high-quality, evidence-based care and allowed to participate in treatment planning to the fullest extent possible.

From the perspective of the care provider, TIC recognizes that the entire treatment team—clinicians, nurses, technicians, and support staff—is at risk of trauma. One study found that one in four emergency responders met criteria for PTSD and described reticence to seek treatment for fear of being unable to work.[21] The physical plant and equipment should be safe. Staff should feel empowered to report dangerous conditions. Staff should receive trainings that describe how trauma impacts the patients they treat and how to treat trauma survivors effectively. Hospital policies should reflect feedback from affected patients and staff. Also, the organization should conduct regular self-reviews of how staff and policies align with trauma-informed approaches.

The Substance Abuse and Mental Health Services Administration describes a multidimensional approach to implementing TIC in health care systems.[17] Table 22.1 describes TIC interventions in emergency psychiatry settings.

The patient, their clinician, and the organization represent a team. This team will thrive or fail together. TIC recognizes that the effects of trauma impact all parties in this team. Patients may be harmed and retraumatized through the care they receive; staff may also be trauma survivors and themselves at risk of retraumatization through their work. Organizational leaders must address these risks, promote a healing environment, and cultivate a healthy clinician–patient relationship.

The experience and sequelae of trauma are not restricted to the hospital. Many emergency care settings, such as prehospital care and disaster response, do not frequently consider the recovery perspective and less easily accommodate the infrastructure of TIC. Techniques such as PFA make the principles of the recovery model universally accessible.

Psychological First Aid

Psychological First Aid, also known as mental health first aid, stress first aid, or community-based psychosocial support, is a specific therapeutic approach that crisis workers can use to aid trauma survivors. PFA is rooted in the recovery model and empowers crisis survivors by ensuring physical and psychological safety, facilitating access to supports, and restoring a sense of agency. It is intended to be compassionate, nonintrusive, and pragmatic. Consistent with the recovery model, PFA allows survivors to lead the level of needed intervention. PFA has been widely adopted as the contemporary disaster response model of choice: Worldwide, aid agencies and humanitarian organizations alike have developed their own versions of PFA programming. Despite their heterogeneity, PFA modules share core foundational themes related to safety, calmness, connectedness, and self-efficacy.[22]

Table 22.1 Examples of Trauma-Informed Care Interventions in Emergency Settings

	Patient-Centered Intervention	Hospital- and Staff-Centered Intervention
Physical environment	Triage medical and mental health patients together, without distinction. Maintain a service with professional appearance that denotes respect for the patient. Orient patients to the availability of food, water, bathrooms, and nursing care on arrival to the ED.	Provide readily accessible and well-trained security staff. Provide personal alarms for staff. Ensure appropriate staff:patient ratios.
Engagement in care	Allow the patient to self-define psychological crisis. Offer appropriate psychiatric treatment immediately, including medications. Offer connection to peer support services (by phone if necessary).	Support staff training in verbal de-escalation and principles of TIC. Allow feedback for policy development.
Treatment	Incorporate peer services into treatment options. Invite patient feedback in treatment planning as much as possible, even if the patient is under an involuntary treatment order. Provide communication on next steps in treatment.	Ensure clinicians have access to appropriate psychiatric consultation when necessary. Provide feedback on quality of care and patient satisfaction.
Operations	Solicit feedback for the patient's experience with crisis services. Provide opportunities for patients to inform hospital policies and procedures. (This may be a standing patient committee to which envisioned changes are proposed.)	Solicit feedback for hospital policies. Allow anonymous reporting of safety concerns. Employ non-retaliation policies. Ensure adequate funding for TIC activities and a safe environment of care.

ED, emergency department; TIC, trauma-informed care.

PFA is often contrasted with another model of early crisis intervention, psychological debriefing, also known as critical incident stress management or critical incident stress debriefing. Debriefing was borne from the experiences of combat veterans returning from military conflict. Its format reflects these martial origins. Debriefings are formal, facilitator-led group exercises in which participants are simultaneously assessed and encouraged to process the facts and fallout of an incident. The goal is to resolve persistent negative emotions and cognitions relating to the event. Debriefing typically follows a prescribed series of steps over a single 1- to 3-hour session.[23] Although debriefings are still used for their relative ease of implementation and low cost, the model lacks efficacy in reducing the risk of PTSD or improving outcomes after exposure to trauma. Moreover, debriefing may worsen reactions to trauma by pathologizing participants' natural responses to an extreme event and overwhelming or retraumatizing survivors with detailed accounts of circumstances.[24] Debriefing is no longer recommended for trauma survivors.[25]

In contrast, PFA delivers pragmatic assistance and bolsters individual adaptive coping skills.[24] The tenets of PFA are highly applicable for emergency settings. By helping providers be culturally sensitive and inclusive, PFA can engage marginalized or disadvantaged persons with significant psychosocial stressors. Many ED patients are suffering from altered perceptions of reality, arriving accompanied by law enforcement, or being held on (or fear being held on) involuntary treatment orders. Persistent stigma surrounding mental illness evokes fear and resistance to seeking help for mental health concerns, and previous negative life experiences can make return visits to hospitals distressing. PFA teaches skills for re-empowering vulnerable patients.

Brief PFA training is accessible through many organizations and online materials, all utilizing similar skills and themes.[26] PFA trains providers on some of the many tools emergency psychiatric clinicians apply to build rapport and foster a good therapeutic alliance. Strategies for starting the session include engaging the patient in a calm, quiet space; introducing oneself by title and role on the treatment team; and addressing the patient in a culturally appropriate and respectful manner. Clinicians are encouraged to communicate in simple, concrete terms; listen actively; and let the patient provide the narrative rather than interrogating with questions. PFA prioritizes attending to the patient's basic needs—food, hydration, sanitation, and contact with loved ones. Table 22.2 describes how specific interventions bring PFA principles to the emergency setting.

Table 22.2 Psychological First Aid and Its Application in the Emergency Department

PFA Actions and Principles	Applications in the ED
Preparing to help	Learn details about disaster (if applicable) and potential risks to patients. Build relationships with community partners who may assist with material needs or ongoing care—food banks, emergency housing, counseling services.
Initiating engagement, establishing and maintaining safety, identifying priority concerns	Engage in verbal de-escalation if necessary.[29] Gather facts regarding provoking incident, only in as much detail as the patient feels comfortable providing. Assess suicide and violence risk. Ascertain emergent medical and social needs that require intervention—decompensated medical illness, unattended children, or pets.
Building alliance and attending to needs and concerns	Introduce yourself by title and role. Address the patient in a manner respectful and appropriate given age, gender, and cultural background. Let the patient speak. Listen actively. Ask the patient, "How can we help?"
Ending your help,[30] planning ahead, empowering, and fostering resilience	Inquire about and reaffirm the importance of healthy social supports. Link the patient with community resources for psychiatric, medical, and social needs. Encourage healthy coping skills—for example, mindfulness and relaxation techniques. Affirm the ED as a safe and supportive place where help can be sought if needed in the future.

ED, emergency department; PFA, psychological first aid.

PFA supports care providers as well. PFA training educates providers on the range of emotional and physical responses individuals experience in response to a traumatic event.[27] Training normalizes these reactions and prepares providers to cultivate an atmosphere of compassion and calming. PFA emphasizes the need for providers to prepare in advance of the patient's arrival. Emergency care organizations should partner with civic organizations and community providers who can assist with patients' material needs. In the event of a specific disaster, clinicians should gather as much information as possible to guide assessment—for example, What medical consequences might result from a chemical exposure? Are commonly accessed shelters and meal sites still open? This information enables responders to assess individuals' needs and problem-solve creatively.

The conclusion of a PFA session reinforces the patient's sense of agency and self-efficacy. Clinicians acknowledge the patient's departure and invite them to return, as necessary. Patients are provided information on accessing community and aftercare resources. Mindfulness interventions help survivors feel better and improve outcomes after trauma.[28]

Conclusion

At its best, emergency psychiatry offers welcoming, compassionate, evidence-based mental health care to all those in need. Doing this successfully, for every patient, is difficult. Nowhere else in mental health care are patients in such acute distress, circumstances more unpredictable, and the challenges of clinical care more complex. Patient relationships may be brief, and the decisions may be life-changing for patients and families. Amid this setting, it is easy to forget that the most effective clinical interventions incorporate the patient's perspective—a perspective that is often fundamentally oriented by a history of social exclusion and trauma. Recovery approaches enable emergency psychiatric teams to deliver better patient care and recognize clinicians' psychological needs in a high-stress clinical environment.

References

1. Felitti VJ, Anda RF, Nordenberg D, et al. Relationship of childhood abuse and household dysfunction to many of the leading causes of death in adults: The Adverse Childhood Experiences (ACE) study. *Am J Prev Med*. 1998;14(4):245–258. doi:10.1016/s0749-3797(98)00017-8

2. Zatzick DF, Kang S-M, Müller H-G, et al. Predicting posttraumatic distress in hospitalized trauma survivors with acute injuries. *Am J Psychiatry*. 2002;159(6):941–946. doi:10.1176/appi.ajp.159.6.941

3. Schilling EA, Aseltine RH, Gore S. Adverse childhood experiences and mental health in young adults: A longitudinal survey. *BMC Public Health*. 2007;7:30. doi:10.1186/1471-2458-7-30

4. Roberts AL, Gilman SE, Breslau J, Breslau N, Koenen KC. Race/ethnic differences in exposure to traumatic events, development of post-traumatic stress disorder, and treatment-seeking for post-traumatic stress disorder in the United States. *Psychol Med*. 2011;41(1):71–83. doi:10.1017/S0033291710000401

5. Buoli M, Giannuli AS. The political use of psychiatry: A comparison between totalitarian regimes. *Int J Soc Psychiatry*. 2017;63(2):169–174. doi:10.1177/0020764016688714

6. American Psychiatric Association. *Diagnostic and Statistical Manual of Mental Disorders.* 5th ed. American Psychiatric Publishing; 2013.

7. Bruce MM, Kassam-Adams N, Rogers M, Anderson KM, Sluys KP, Richmond TS. Trauma providers' knowledge, views, and practice of trauma-informed care. *J Trauma Nurs Off J Soc Trauma Nurses.* 2018;25(2):131–138. doi:10.1097/JTN.0000000000000356

8. Owens PL, Fingar KR, Heslin KC, Mutter R, Booth CL. Emergency department visits related to suicidal ideation, 2006–2013. Statistical Brief No. 220. Agency for Healthcare Research and Quality. Published 2017. Accessed January 31, 2021. http://www.ncbi.nlm.nih.gov/books/NBK442036

9. Kraft CM, Morea P, Teresi B, et al. Characteristics, clinical care, and disposition barriers for mental health patients boarding in the emergency department. *Am J Emerg Med.* 2021;46:550–555. doi:10.1016/j.ajem.2020.11.021

10. Allen MH, Carpenter D, Sheets JL, Miccio S, Ross R. What do consumers say they want and need during a psychiatric emergency? *J Psychiatr Pract.* 2003;9(1):39–58. doi:10.1097/00131746-200301000-00005

11. Thomas KC, Owino H, Ansari S, et al. Patient-centered values and experiences with emergency department and mental health crisis care. *Adm Policy Ment Health.* 2018;45(4):611–622. doi:10.1007/s10488-018-0849-y

12. Lindström V, Sturesson L, Carlborg A. Patients' experiences of the caring encounter with the psychiatric emergency response team in the emergency medical service: A qualitative interview study. *Health Expect Int J Public Particip Health Care Health Policy.* 2020;23(2):442–449. doi:10.1111/hex.13024

13. Simpson SA, Monroe C. Implementing and evaluating a standard of care for clinical evaluations in emergency psychiatry. *J Emerg Med.* 2018;55(4):522–529.e2. doi:10.1016/j.jemermed.2018.07.014

14. Rogers MS, McNiel DE, Binder RL. Effectiveness of police crisis intervention training programs. *J Am Acad Psychiatry Law.* 2019;47(4):414–421. doi:10.29158/JAAPL.003863-19

15. Jahn DR, DeVylder JE, Drapalski AL, Medoff D, Dixon LB. Personal recovery as a protective factor against suicide ideation in individuals with schizophrenia. *J Nerv Ment Dis.* 2016;204(11):827–831. doi:10.1097/NMD.0000000000000521

16. Simpson SA, McDowell AK. *The Clinical Interview: Skills for More Effective Patient Encounters.* Routledge; 2019.

17. SAMHSA's concept of trauma and guidance for a trauma-informed approach. Substance Abuse and Mental Health Services Administration. Published 2014. https://ncsacw.samhsa.gov/userfiles/files/SAMHSA_Trauma.pdf

18. Molloy L, Fields L, Trostian B, Kinghorn G. Trauma-informed care for people presenting to the emergency department with mental health issues. *Emerg Nurse.* 2020;28(2):30–35. doi:10.7748/en.2020.e1990

19. Hoysted C, Babl FE, Kassam-Adams N, et al. Perspectives of hospital emergency department staff on trauma-informed care for injured children: An Australian and New Zealand analysis. *J Paediatr Child Health.* 2017;53(9):862–869. doi:10.1111/jpc.13644

20. Purkey E, Davison C, MacKenzie M, et al. Experience of emergency department use among persons with a history of adverse childhood experiences. *BMC Health Serv Res.* 2020;20(1):455. doi:10.1186/s12913-020-05291-6

21. Tatebe LC, Rajaram Siva N, Pekarek S, et al. Heroes in crisis: Trauma centers should be screening for and intervening on posttraumatic stress in our emergency responders. *J Trauma Acute Care Surg.* 2020;89(1):132–139. doi:10.1097/TA.0000000000002671

22. Schultz JM, Forbes D. Psychological first aid: Rapid proliferation and the search for evidence. *Disaster Health*. 2013;2(1):3–12. http://www.ncbi.nlm.nih.gov/pubmed/28228996

23. Mitchell JT. When disaster strikes . . . the critical incident stress debriefing process. *JEMS*. 1983;8(1):36–39.

24. Kenardy J. The current status of psychological debriefing. *BMJ*. 2000;321(7268):1032–1033. doi:10.1136/bmj.321.7268.1032

25. Rose SC, Bisson J, Churchill R, Wessely S. Psychological debriefing for preventing post traumatic stress disorder (PTSD). Cochrane Database Syst Rev. 2002;2002(2):CD000560. doi:10.1002/14651858.CD000560

26. National Child Traumatic Stress Network and National Center for PTSD. *Psychological First Aid Field Operations Guide*. 2nd ed. U.S. Department of Health and Human Services; 2006. https://www.nctsn.org/sites/default/files/resources//pfa_field_operations_guide.pdf

27. Pollock A, Campbell P, Cheyne J, et al. Interventions to support the resilience and mental health of frontline health and social care professionals during and after a disease outbreak, epidemic or pandemic: A mixed methods systematic review. *Cochrane Database Syst Rev*. 2020;2020(11):CD013779. doi:10.1002/14651858.CD013779

28. Goldberg SB, Riordan KM, Sun S, Kearney DJ, Simpson TL. Efficacy and acceptability of mindfulness-based interventions for military veterans: A systematic review and meta-analysis. *J Psychosom Res*. 2020;138:110232. doi:10.1016/j.jpsychores.2020.110232

29. Simpson SA, Sakai J, Rylander M. A free online video series teaching verbal de-escalation for agitated patients. *Acad Psychiatry*. 2020;44(2):208–211. doi:10.1007/s40596-019-01155-2

30. Snider L, Van Ommeren M, Schafer A. *Psychological First Aid: Guide for Field Workers*. World Health Organization; 2011.

23

Collaborations Within the Emergency Department

Julie Ruth Owen

Introduction

In the United States, the number of hospital emergency department (ED) visits has steadily increased during the past decade; since 2009, ED volumes have increased more than 11%.[1] The proportion of ED visits primarily involving psychiatric concerns (including substance use) has also been on the rise, from 6.6% of all visits in 2007 to 10.9% of all visits in 2016.[2] A retrospective analysis of ED visit data from the National Emergency Department sample examining the years 2010–2014 identified mental health issues (including substance use) as the second-most frequent ED presentation, with abdominal pain ranking as the most frequent.[3]

Utilization of the ED by psychiatric patients has been linked to the mental health resources within the community[4] and impacts ED clinical operations. With increasing volumes of patients presenting to EDs with psychiatric concerns, significant increases in ED length of stay (LOS) have been reported; behavioral health-related ED visits typically have the longest treatment times in comparison to non-mental health visits.[5] In 2017, the average cost per mental and substance use disorders ED visit was 19% higher than the average cost for all ED visits.[6]

Literature on this topic suggests possible barriers to optimal care of psychiatric patients in the ED, including limited space; time constraints; overcrowding; insufficient knowledge and education of staff on the topic of psychiatric illness; negative attitudes and avoidance of psychiatric patients by staff; and complex clinical presentations, including dual diagnoses and acute behavioral disturbances.[7–9] With these challenges in mind, this chapter examines boarding issues and prolonged LOS of psychiatric patients in EDs, various models of care implemented to address these growing concerns, and possible future directions to explore, with the goal of improving ED-based psychiatric patient care delivery and systems-based practices.

Boarding

During the same period of time that the proportion of ED visits primarily involving psychiatric concerns has been on the rise, the availability of crisis and inpatient psychiatric care has been shrinking, without concomitant growth of outpatient care and community-based treatment centers to fill the gap. The arrival of the antipsychotic chlorpromazine to the U.S. market in 1950 signaled that effective treatment of individuals with psychiatric disorders could occur in less restrictive settings.[10] The civil rights movement fueled criticism of psychiatric institutions and amplified calls for more humane psychiatric patient care, and the creation of Medicare and Medicaid in 1960 shifted much of the cost of care for individuals with psychiatric disorders to the American public, who perceived little benefit to institution-based care.[10] President John F. Kennedy signed the Community Mental Health Centers Act in 1963, beginning the "era of deinstitutionalization." In this historic climate, the number of inpatient psychiatric beds declined precipitously, from an all-time high of 559,000 in 1953 to 43,318 in 2010.[11] However, the original funding amount proposed by President Kennedy to create the robust national mental health programming meant to replace state hospitals was gutted by Congress; the Construction Act was passed in 1963, authorizing funds to build community-based treatment centers. The funding amendments needed to staff the centers were not authorized by Congress until 1965.[12] These factors and trends have resulted in an ever-increasing reliance of patients on hospital EDs for psychiatric care and treatment. EDs have manifested the pressure of these demands in a phenomenon referred to as "boarding."

Although there is no established definition of a patient who is boarding in the ED, the situation is generally described as a patient whose ED evaluation is complete and the decision has been made to hospitalize or transfer the patient, but the patient remains in the ED due to deficiencies in staffing or bed availability, patient factors, or other concerns.[13] Although boarding of ED patients generally has been a concern in recent years, with an overall rate of boarding of 11%, the rate of boarding for patients requiring psychiatric treatment has been shown to be nearly double (21.5%) according to data from 2008.[13] In 2014, the American College of Emergency Physicians (ACEP)[14] surveyed ED physicians: 84% of respondents reported ED boarding of their psychiatric patients, with more than half of those reporting daily boarding issues.

Boarding is influenced by a number of patient and systems factors, including the use of restraints and sitters, as well as the insurance status of a patient in need of psychiatric treatment (Table 23.1). In addition, boarding of psychiatric patients presents a steep financial and medical burden to EDs, with an estimated cost of $2,250 per patient and decreased bed turnover.[15,16] Decreased bed turnover negatively impacts overall efficiency of the ED environment, with reduction of ED capacity, prolonged wait times for other ED patients, and more limited availability of ED staff.[17] Moreover, 91% of ED physicians have reported that psychiatric boarding led directly to harm to patients and/or emergency staff.[14]

Patients boarding in EDs awaiting psychiatric treatment are unlikely to receive needed care in the EDs.[13] However, considering the aforementioned description of limited psychiatric treatment resources in the community—particularly inpatient psychiatric beds—it is arguably an antiquated way of thinking to presume that all patients presenting to EDs with psychiatric concerns need to be placed in an inpatient bed and to view "treatment" for these patients as the intervention of a social worker or other ED staff member searching for an inpatient psychiatric bed. Nordstrom et al.[17] published a comprehensive resource document for the American Psychiatric Association that proposes potential solutions and best practice recommendations to the issue of psychiatric patients boarding in the ED, which includes active treatment of psychiatric symptoms (Figure 23.1).

In summary, ED boarding of psychiatric patients is a complex, concerning, and multifactorial issue that has demonstrated significant negative impact on patients, EDs, hospital systems, and the community at large. In order to begin to address this problem, it

Table 23.1 Risk Factors for Emergency Department Boarding of Psychiatric Patients

Patient demographic and social factors	Age >45 years
	Age <18 years
	Male gender
	Homelessness
	± Race (mixed data)
Patient clinical factors	Suicidal ideation
Pediatric population	Diagnosis of autism spectrum disorder
	Diagnosis of intellectual developmental disorder
	Medical illness requiring monitoring
General population	Elevated blood alcohol
	Positive urine drug screen
	History of drug or alcohol abuse
	Use of restraints
	Use of 1:1 observation
	Administration of haloperidol or lorazepam
	Diagnosis of cognitive disorder or dementia
	Diagnosis of personality disorder
	Schizophrenia or other psychotic disorder
Patient insurance status	Government-sponsored insurance
	Lack of insurance
Systems-related factors	Emergency department crowding at any time during day of presentation
	At least three other patients with psychiatric concerns present at the time of patient arrival
	Patient arrival in the evening, overnight, anytime on weekends, or during months without school vacations (pediatric population)
	Patient requiring transfer to another facility
	Patient requiring admission as a psychiatric inpatient

Adapted from Simon et al.[13]

is vital that stakeholders across specialties—particularly, emergency medicine (EM) and psychiatry—collaborate closely to promote patient-centered solutions.

Consult Models

In 2014, ACEP published best practice recommendations for psychiatric patients who present to EDs, which include "psychiatry consultations live or via telemedicine."[18] Specific benefits of psychiatric consultation cited in ACEP's report include a decreased need for inpatient psychiatric admissions and the initiation of pharmacological treatment regimens for psychiatric syndromes.[18] In 2015, the Joint Commission issued a similar directive to "improve access to psychiatrists in the ED" and to "promote improved collaboration between ED providers and psychiatric consultation services to treat and discharge patients, or to reduce ED boarding times."[19] Existing models of psychiatric care delivery in EDs described in the literature universally involve increased collaboration between mental health professionals and ED staff, with notable benefits outlined in Box 23.1. Details of several ED-based psychiatric care delivery models are explored in the following sections.

Role of the Emergency Department

Rapid treatment of agitation
- Prioritize non-coercive de-escalation to calm the patient
- Avoid over-sedation, which is associated with increased ED LOS
- Consider implementation of an objective agitation rating scale
- Identify underlying medical etiologies and treat appropriately
- Train ED staff on techniques to safely and effectively manage agitation
- Consider creation and implementation of specially trained teams to aid in de-escalation of agitation patients

Minimization of restraint and seclusion
- Use physical restraints as a last resort and for the least amount of time necessary

Evaluation of medical comorbidities
- Consider possible medical conditions that could be contributing to patient's psychiatric presentation
- Conduct a medical evaluation specific to the patient's signs and symptoms
- Communicate results of the patient's medical evaluation efficiently and clearly between the ED and any potential receiving facility

Active treatment of psychiatric symptoms
- Initiate treatment of the patient's underlying illness in addition to focusing on agitation mitigation (especially for those patients whose stay in the ED is prolonged)

Implementation of observation units
- Mitigate the need for psychiatric hospitalization

Active treatment for substance-related symptoms
- Treat Intoxication or withdrawal states using a targeted and timely approach
- Consider treatment and monitoring protocols beyond alcohol withdrawal
- Approach the ED evaluation as an opportunity to intervene using motivational interviewing techniques to promote more intensive treatment options for alcohol and other drug abuse (AODA)

Improved coordination and communication around disposition
- Give thorough hand-offs to either an inpatient receiving team or to a patient's outpatient care team
- Anticipate necessary components of a medical evaluation, as well as the need for medications to facilitate a safe patient transfer

Other hospital-centered approaches
- Improve and expand access to psychiatric services (e.g., telepsychiatry, integrated/patient flow)
- Hiring bed managers or case managers can aid with disposition issues and improve patient flow
- Collect and monitor data to make meaningful improvements

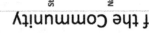

Role of the Community

Determine local needs
- Create taskforces made up of key stakeholders to systematically examine local circumstances leading to ED boarding (e.g., front-end, ED, and back-end precipitants)

Focus on diversion and coordination
- Divert patients to preferred resources facilitate the best system entry point for care (e.g., EMS triage system)—this requires access to a spectrum of non-emergency care environments in the community
- Support mobile crisis services to mitigate crisis situations before patients require an ED visit
- Coordinate between EDs, mobile crisis teams, and non-emergency community the resources needed for optimal outcomes
- Coordinate care within the ED to ensure adequate follow-up appointments to encourage ongoing management in the community

State involvement
- Focus on improving access to care (both in the ED setting as well as the community) via the closure of funding gaps, considering that state leaders allocate Medicaid funds and block grants
- Address any state legislation that decreases or restricts communication between healthcare teams (e.g., between ED staff and community mental health centers)

National involvement
- Collaborate with professional organizations (across specialties) to address shared concerns regarding patient care and access to appropriate services
- Address parity in reimbursement for psychiatric care with insurers
- Address fair reimbursement for psychiatric care, as the financial strain currently incurred by hospital systems disincentivizes hospitals to maintain psychiatric care units and/or other services
- Pursue more universal and standardized training around crisis intervention to ensure that physicians in any care setting have the appropriate tools to effectively address psychiatric crises

Figure 23.1 Potential solutions and best practice recommendations for ED boarding of psychiatric patients.
Adapted from Nordstrom et al.[17]

Box 23.1 Evidence-Based Advantages of Access to Psychiatry in the Emergency Department

---

Immediate/rapid initiation of medication regimens

Facilitate eventual discharge or ease the transfer process for patients[20]

Decreased length of stay

Resulting in saved "bed hours" and increased revenue due to more rapid bed turnover[20,21]

Improved diagnostic accuracy

Mitigation of "diagnostic overshadowing" (the misattribution of a patient's symptoms to mental illness)[22,23]

Improved treatment of medical illness in patients with psychiatric disease

Enriched formal training of emergency medicine residents

Core curricular content dedicated to psychiatry currently lacking[24]

Enhanced knowledge and confidence of ED staff in managing psychiatric patient presentations

Especially in cases involving both medical and psychiatric complexity, as well as the need for pharmacological management[9]

Reduction in substance use with trained teams able to effectively screen and provide brief interventions in the ED setting

Subsequent reduction in the negative consequences of use (e.g., injury) and a decline in repeat ED visits[25]

ED, emergency department.

Traditional Psychiatric Consultation to the General Emergency Department

There are many EDs without access to consulting mental health professionals in which emergency physicians are responsible for conducting a thorough evaluation of patients presenting with psychiatric concerns, often with a particular focus placed on the assessment of patients' risk of dangerousness and overall safety. In EDs with access to clinicians with psychiatric expertise, the traditional consult model follows a linear process whereby the emergency physician evaluates for any emergent or acute medical concerns (including necessary labs or imaging), the determination is made that the patient requires a psychiatric evaluation, and the psychiatric team (or individual mental health professional) is called to request an evaluation. The evaluations by the ED care team and psychiatric team or consultant are thus performed consecutively, with the ED team focusing on "medically clearing" the patient for further psychiatric care and the psychiatric consultant(s) evaluating the patient for level of care and disposition needs (if the consultant is a psychiatrist or other prescribing clinician, a pharmacological regimen or intervention will likely be recommended as a means of offering active treatment to the patient). The psychiatric consultant(s) is typically not on duty in the ED; rather, the consulting individual or team will arrive from elsewhere in the hospital or will be "on call" in the community. This model is inherently reactive and siloed, with ED and consulting teams working independently on their own areas of patient care focus rather than collaboratively, leading to delays in treatment and process inefficiencies that can extend ED

LOS.[26] This is likely the most utilized approach to providing emergency psychiatric care in the United States.[27]

There are a variety of mental health professionals with a vast array of training and credentials who are called upon to evaluate ED patients with psychiatric concerns. In addition to completing a full assessment of the patient's psychiatric concerns and clinical presentation, the services detailed in Table 23.2 are offered based on the consulting clinician's level of training, clinical expertise, and licensure.

Dedicated Psychiatric Patient Rooms/Area Within the General Emergency Department

Some EDs may have a specific area or pod of rooms dedicated to patients presenting with psychiatric concerns. These areas may be designed to provide more skilled, therapeutic care to patients, with trained staff and a quieter milieu. Because these areas are located in the ED, the patients' care is still managed primarily by ED physicians. Also, because these beds are allocated for use by patients with significant psychiatric concerns, clinical and operational workflows related to medically ill patients may continue unaffected. Staffing for these areas is variable: General ED staff may attend to these areas, or there may be specially trained psychiatric nurses, security, social workers, and in-house psychiatrists to provide expert care to this patient group.[27]

Embedded Psychiatry Services in General Emergency Departments

With the decades-long trend of increasing volumes of primary psychiatric patients presenting to EDs and worsening boarding problems in high-volume EDs, some EDs have explored creative arrangements that feature increased collaboration with/integration of psychiatric services. University of California, San Francisco launched an ED-psychiatry co-management model in which ED psychiatric patient care transitioned from a traditional consult model to an approach in which patient care was shared by the ED clinicians and the consultation-liaison (C-L) psychiatry service.[21] Following a consultation request, the C-L psychiatry service assumed full responsibility for providing direct psychiatric patient care (including the ordering of additional lab studies, medication, etc.) and regularly re-evaluating these patients until disposition was secured. With daily psychiatry faculty coverage in place, there was a significant reduction in ED LOS for both patients transferring to inpatient facilities and patients discharging to home after a brief period of reconstitution. In addition, ED revenue increased by $2.1 million, facilitating the hiring of 1.5 full-time equivalent psychiatrists and additional licensed clinical social workers.[21]

Similarly, a weekday psychiatry faculty rounds program was implemented at Wake Forest University to address ongoing care for patients boarding in the ED. Two psychiatry faculty members were given dedicated time to evaluate new ED psychiatric patients and to re-evaluate patients with prolonged stay Mondays–Fridays. The stated goals of this intervention included (1) initiation of medication regimens that could allow for the eventual discharge of patients to home, (2) daily reassessments that could lead to discharges rather than admission, and (3) improved care coordination with the

Table 23.2 Types of Mental Health Professionals Who May Offer Consultation to Emergency Departments

Clinician/Role	Educational Requirements	Licensure/Certification	Unique Patient Care Capabilities
Psychiatrist	Doctor of Medicine (MD) or Doctor of Osteopathic Medicine (DO)	Licensed physician, per state requirements. Board certification requires completion of a 4-year general adult psychiatry residency program (12,000 clinical hours). Psychiatrists may also opt to complete an additional 1- or 2-year fellowship program in a subspecialty area, including child and adolescent, addiction, consultation–liaison, or geriatric psychiatry.	Recommendation of pharmacological interventions Evaluation of high-risk patients Determination of decisional capacity Management of patients' psychiatric legal status Management of neuropsychiatric syndromes in medically complex patients Diagnostic clarification of complicated psychiatric presentations
Psychologist	Doctor of Philosophy (PhD) in a field of psychology or Doctor of Psychology (PsyD)	Licensure per state requirements	Conduction of in-depth neuropsychological evaluations Provision of specialized psychotherapeutic interventions (cognitive–behavioral therapy, dialectical behavior therapy, etc.)
Clinical social workers	Master's degree in social work (MSW)	Varies by specialty and state, with examples including Licensed Independent Social Worker (LICSW), Licensed Clinical Social Worker (LCSW)	Provision of case management services Connection of patients to advocacy services Connection of patients to community-based resources
Counselors/ therapists	Master's degree in a mental health–related field (psychology, counseling psychology, etc.)	Varies by specialty and state, with examples including Licensed Professional Counselor (LPC), Licensed Marriage and Family Therapist (LMFT)	Provision of therapies based on specific techniques
Psychiatric or mental health nurse practitioner	Master of Science (MS) or Doctor of Philosophy (PhD) in nursing, with 500 supervised clinical hours related to psychiatric patient care	Licensed nurse per state licensing board. The nurse practitioner (NP) license has different names in different states, including Advanced Practice Nurse Prescriber (APNP), and Advanced Registered Nurse Practitioner (ARNP).	Recommendation of pharmacological interventions
Certified peer specialists	Most states have a minimum requirement of a high school diploma or GED.	Formal training programs, delivered over a few days to a few weeks, are offered in most states to obtain state-specific certification.	Provision of support, mentorship, and guidance to patients based on lived experience with mental illness or a substance use disorder

Adapted from the National Alliance on Mental Illness.[28]

inpatient units that might accept patients. The team published their results in *Academic Emergency Medicine*, demonstrating a mean reduced ED LOS of 6.1 hours. During the 6-month post-implementation study period, this amounted to 3,123 "bed hours" saved, during which an additional 726 patients could be seen.[20] Other notable embedded ED-based psychiatric programs include the Psychiatric Fast Track Service piloted at the Morehouse School of Medicine in Georgia,[29] and the Division of Emergency Psychiatry with 24-7 psychiatry faculty coverage in the main ED at Prisma Health/University of South Carolina School of Medicine Greenville, with telepsychiatry coverage to the system's seven satellite EDs.[30] These programs, as the others detailed above, have reported success in reducing ED LOS and boarding, decreasing the volume of restraint episodes, and reducing patient LOS in restraints.

Despite these few models, there is not yet an extensive evidence base for a collaborative/integrated care approach in acute care settings, such as EDs. However, there is robust literature demonstrating superior outcomes when using a collaborative care approach in outpatient primary care settings.[31] There is also a growing body of literature around the substantial benefits of proactive, integrated psychiatric care in inpatient hospital settings.[26] The benefits demonstrated in the more extensive inpatient literature align with the positive results demonstrated by the few ED-based programs described in this section: decreased LOS, reduction in consultation latency (with more expedient interventions), and markedly improved staff satisfaction.[26]

Telepsychiatry

The evidence base for telepsychiatry in EDs is small but growing; given the rapid adoption of telemedicine during the COVID-19 pandemic, studies evaluating the efficacy and value of ED-based telepsychiatry will likely increase in number in the coming years. Note that the existing evidence base demonstrates comparable validity of assessments and clinical interactions when examining telepsychiatry versus face-to-face encounters, reduction in both ED LOS and psychiatric inpatient admissions when telepsychiatry is employed, and overall cost-effectiveness.[32] For further detail, see Chapter 5 in this volume.

Observation Units

A busy ED is designed to provide acute care for time-sensitive conditions over a period of approximately 6 hours maximum.[33] The evidence base supporting the use of ED observation units for medical conditions is robust; reductions in lengths of stay and admission rates have been demonstrated, in addition to improved cost-effectiveness and similar clinical outcomes as patients admitted to the general hospital.[34] For patients not well enough for immediate discharge from the ED but not sick enough to warrant full inpatient admission ("6-to-24-hour" patients), an observation unit allows the delivery of outpatient care provided in a hospital bed;[33] specifically, dedicated units with defined protocols have demonstrated shorter lengths of stay, lower probabilities of subsequent inpatient admission, and significant potential cost savings.[33]

Institutions that have implemented observation units dedicated to the care of psychiatric patients have noted reductions in ED boarding and ED LOS, decreased adverse events (e.g., the use of restraints, security staff), and improved system-wide flow.[35] Furthermore, the need for inpatient psychiatric admission has been decreased with the implementation of observation units, reducing unnecessary use of scarce inpatient psychiatric resources.[36] Dedicated psychiatric observation units offer acute, time-limited, and intensive care that would otherwise be challenging to provide in the physical environment of the ED.[35] Patient care benefits that have been cited include improved care coordination, enhanced medication management, prolonged evaluation with diagnostic clarification, and the provision of acute therapeutic interventions.[35] Staffing models include dedicated, consistent care team members versus ad hoc coverage by staff working in other areas of the hospital.

Future Directions

Emergency Departments have struggled to keep up with the growing demand of patients presenting seeking treatment for psychiatric disorders, and the strain on the system has been palpable. More than ever before, EDs and health systems are invested in seeking collaborative, creative solutions to these issues involving psychiatric patients, some of which have been explored in this chapter. Consider the following future directions that cross-specialty collaboration between EM and psychiatry might pursue:

- *Educational initiatives*: For EM trainees, the core curricular content dedicated to psychiatric disorders is not commensurate with the large and growing volume of psychiatric-related ED visits.[37] A 2003 survey of North American EM program directors revealed that 67% of respondents did not require their residents to undertake (nor did they provide) formal training in treating acute psychiatric emergencies.[24]
  - Create ED-based psychiatry rotation experiences specific to EM trainees.
  - Build formal curriculum for EM trainees relevant to the assessment and treatment of ED patients presenting with psychiatric emergencies. The American Association for Emergency Psychiatry published a model curriculum for consideration.[38]
  - Develop on-shift competency-based assessment tools related to the evaluation and treatment of psychiatric patients in the ED to build trainees' knowledge base and confidence levels.
  - Emergency psychiatry fellowship programs—mostly designed for psychiatry trainees, but newer programs are also open to EM trainees—are slowly growing in number nationwide.[39] Given a body of literature supporting superior patient outcomes when care is delivered by more experienced emergency psychiatrists, subspecialty fellowship training has been promoted as a transformative approach to improving the care of emergency psychiatric patients.
- *Clinical/patient care initiatives*: With integration of psychiatrists to provide specialty expertise and support to EM teams, opportunities abound to create innovative programming to enhance the care of psychiatric patients in EDs.
  - Consider implementing lethal means safety education and interventions in the ED. Lethal means safety is one of the most empirically supported interventions.[40] The distribution of gun locks and gun/medication safes, in addition to education of patients and ED staff, can be a life-saving intervention.

- "Caring contacts," or patient follow-up efforts post-discharge, have been shown to reduce subsequent suicide attempts and to improve rates of outpatient follow-up.[41] Implementation of systematic, protocolized follow-up contacts for patients discharged to lower levels of care is an empirically supported intervention.
- ED-based induction of patients presenting with opioid use disorder on suboxone has produced a growing evidence base demonstrating significantly superior treatment retention, reduction of illicit opioid use, decreased mortality rates, and cost-effectiveness.[42]
- *Informatics*: Electronic medical records (EMRs) that are increasingly sophisticated can be optimized to reflect and encourage best practice approaches to evaluating and treating psychiatric patients in the ED.
  - Consider the construction and implementation of order sets that mirror "best practice" clinical pathways for common psychiatric conditions (depression, anxiety, substance use, psychosis, etc.).
  - Consider optimizing the EMR to encourage the use of validated screening tools (suicide risk, substance use, etc.) and objective assessment scales (e.g., agitation, delirium, and substance use withdrawal) to guide interventions and treatment.
  - Leverage the EMR to collect and track data related to the evaluation and treatment of ED patients to drive continuous improvement efforts in the ED setting.
- *Systems- and community-based initiatives*: Cross-specialty collaboration between EM and psychiatry can produce larger-scale clinical and operational improvements.
  - Leveraging more robust access to psychiatrists at large, high-volume EDs with implementation of ED-based telepsychiatry can improve standardization of resources and clinical services across health system EDs.
  - Cross-specialty collaboration can produce more robust community-based partnerships, which can result in more streamlined pathways from the ED to different levels of psychiatric care within the community. Reducing barriers to access timely outpatient psychiatric care (including intensive outpatient programming, partial hospital programming, and office-based outpatient treatment) can further mitigate hospital-to-hospital transfers of psychiatric patients.

There has never been a more exciting time to be a psychiatrist working in close collaboration with our EM colleagues on ED-based patient care and systems-based initiatives.

References

1. HCUP fast stats. Healthcare Cost and Utilization Project, Agency for Healthcare Research and Quality. Published 2021. https://www.hcup-us.ahrq.gov/faststats/national/inpatienttrendsED.jsp
2. Theriault K, Rosenheck R, Rhee T. Increasing emergency department visits for mental health conditions in the United States. *J Clin Psychiatry*. 2020;81(5):20m13241.
3. Hooker EA, Mallow PJ, Oglesby MM. Characteristics and trends of emergency department visits in the United States (2010–2014). *J Emerg Med*. 2019;56(3):344–351.
4. Catalano R, McConnell W, Forster P, McFarland B, Thornton D. Psychiatric emergency services and the system of care. *Psychiatr Serv*. 2003;54(3):351–355.
5. Ding R, McCarthy M, Desmond J, Lee J, Aronsky D, Zeger S. Characterizing waiting room time, treatment time, and boarding time in the emergency room using quantile regression. *Acad Emerg Med*. 2010;17(8):813–823.

6. Costs of emergency department visits for mental health and substance use disorders. Healthcare Cost and Utilization Project, Agency for Healthcare Research and Quality. Published 2020. https://hcup-us.ahrq.gov/reports/statbriefs/sb257-ED-Costs-Mental-Substance-Use-Disorders-2017.jsp

7. Dombagolla M, Kant JA, Lai F, Hendarto A, Taylor DM. Barriers to providing optimal management of psychiatric patients in the emergency department (psychiatric patient management). *Australas Emerg Care.* 2019;22(1):8–12.

8. Weiland TJ, Mackinlay C, Hill N, Gerdtz MF, Jelinek GA. Optimal management of mental health patients in Australian emergency departments: Barriers and solutions. *Emerg Med Australas.* 2011;23(6):677–688.

9. Jelinek GA, Weiland T, Mackinlay C, Gerdtz M, Hill N. Knowledge and confidence of Australian emergency department clinicians in managing patients with mental health-related presentations: Findings from a national qualitative study. *Int J Emerg Med.* 2013;6(1):2.

10. Testa M, West S. Civil commitment in the United States. *Psychiatry.* 2010;7(10):30–40.

11. Yohanna D. Deinstutitionalization of people with mental illness: Causes and consequences. *Virtual Mentor.* 2013;15(10):886–891.

12. Cutler DL, Bevilacqua J, McFarland BH. Four decades of community mental health: A symphony in four movements. *Comm Ment Health J.* 2003;39(5):381–398.

13. Simon JR, Kraus CK, Basford JB, Clayborne EP, Kluesner N, Bookman K. *The Impact of Boarding Psychiatric Patients on the Emergency Department: Scope, Impact and Proposed Solutions: An Information Paper.* American College of Emergency Physicians; 2019.

14. American College of Emergency Physicians. (2014). Polling survey results.

15. Zeller S, Calma N, Stone A. Effects of a dedicated regional psychiatric emergency service on boarding of psychiatric patients in area emergency departments. *West J Emerg Med.* 2014;15(1):1–6.

16. Nicks BA, Manthey DM. The impact of psychiatric patient boarding in emergency departments. *Emerg Med Int.* 2012;2012:360308.

17. Nordstrom K, Berlin JS, Nash S, Shah SB, Schmeltzer NA, Worley LL. Boarding of mentally ill patients in emergency departments: American Psychiatric Association resource document. *West J Emerg Med.* 2019;20(5):690–695.

18. ACEP Emergency Medicine Practice Committee. *Care of the Psychiatric Patient in the Emergency Department: A Review of the Literature.* American College of Emergency Physicians; 2014.

19. Alleviating ED boarding of psychiatric patients. *Quick Safety.* The Joint Commission, Division of Health Care Improvement. Published 2015. https://www.jointcommission.org/-/media/tjc/documents/newsletters/quick_safety_issue_19_dec_2015l pdf.pdf

20. Blumstein H, Singleton AH, Suttenfield CW, Hiestand BC. Weekday psychiatry faculty rounds on emergency department psychiatric patients reduces length of stay. *Acad Emerg Med.* 2013;20(5):498–502.

21. Polevoi SK, Shim JJ, McCulloch CE, Grimes B, Govindarajan P. Marked reduction in length of stay for patients with psychiatric emergencies after implementation of a comanagement model. *Acad Emerg Med.* 2013;20(4):338–343.

22. Shefer G, Cross S, Howard LM, Murray J, Thornicroft G, Henderson C. Improving the diagnosis of physical illness in patients with mental illness who present in emergency departments: Consensus study. *J Psychosom Res.* 2015;78(4):346–351.

23. LaMantia MA, Messina FC, Hobgood CD, Miller DK. Screening for delirium in the emergency department: A systematic review. *Ann Emerg Med.* 2014;63(5):551–560.

24. Larkin GL, Beautrais AL, Spirito A, Kirrane BM, Lippmann MJ, Milzman DP. Mental health and emergency medicine: A research agenda. *Acad Emerg Med.* 2009;16(11):1110–1119.

25. Barata IA, Shandro JR, Montgomery M, et al. Effectiveness of SBIRT for alcohol use disorders in the emergency department: A systematic review. *West J Emerg Med.* 18(6):2017;1143–1152.

26. Oldham MA, Desan PH, Lee HB, et al. Proactive consultation–liaison psychiatry: American Psychiatric Association resource document. *J Acad Consultat Liaison Psychiatry.* 2021;62(2):169–185.

27. Glick RL, Zeller SL, Berlin JS. *Emergency Psychiatry: Principles and Practice.* Wolters Kluwer; 2021.

28. Types of mental health professionals. National Alliance on Mental Illness. Published 2020. https://www.nami.org/About-Mental-Illness/Treatments/Types-of-Mental-Health-Professionals

29. Okafor M, Wrenn G, Ede V, et al. Improving quality of emergency care through integration of mental health. *Community Ment Health J.* 2016;52(3):332–342.

30. Lommel K. *Transformation of behavioral health care in the ED.* National Update on Behavioral Emergencies; 2018.

31. American Psychiatric Association and Academy of Psychosomatic Medicine. *Dissemination of Integrated Care Within Adult Primary Care Settings: The Collaborative Care Model.* American Psychiatric Association; 2016.

32. Reinhardt I, Gouzoulis-Mayfrank E, Zielasek J. Use of telepsychiatry in emergency and crisis intervention: Current evidence. *Curr Psychiatry Rep.* 2019;21(8):1–8.

33. Ross MA, Hockenberry JM, Mutter R, Barrett M, Wheatley M, Pitts SR. Protocol-driven emergency department observation units offer savings, shorter stays, and reduced admissions. *Health Affairs.* 2013;32(12):2149–2156.

34. Baugh CW, Venkatesh AK, Bohan JS. Emergency department observation units: A clinical and financial benefit for hospitals. *Health Care Manage Rev.* 2011;36(1):28–37.

35. Cammell P. Emergency psychiatry: A product of circumstance or a growing sub-specialty field? *Australas Psychiatry.* 2017;25(1):53–55.

36. Bukhman AK, Baugh CW, Yun BJ. Alternative dispositions for emergency department patients. *Emerg Med Clin N Am.* 2020;38(3):647–661.

37. Pickett J, Calderone Haas MR, Fix ML, et al. Training in the management of psychobehavioral conditions: A needs assessment survey of emergency medicine residents. *AEM Educ Train.* 2019;3(4):365–374.

38. Brasch J, Glick R, Cobb TG, Richmond J. Residency training in emergency psychiatry: A model curriculum developed by the Education Committee of the American Association for Emergency Psychiatry. *Acad Psychiatry.* 2004;28:95–99.

39. Simpson S, Brooks V, DeMoss D, Lawrence R. The case for fellowship training in emergency psychiatry. *MedEdPublish.* 2020;9(1).

40. Mueller KL, Chirumbole D, Naganathan S. Counseling on access to lethal means in the emergency department: A script for improved comfort. *Community Ment Health J.* 2020;56(7):1366–1371.

41. Luxton DD, June JD, Comtois KA. Can postdischarge follow-up contacts prevent suicide and suicidal behavior? A review of the evidence. *Crisis.* 2013;34(1):32–41.

42. D'Onofrio G, O'Connor PG, Pantalon MV, et al. Emergency department–initiated buprenorphine/naloxone treatment for opioid dependence: A randomized clinical trial. *JAMA.* 2015;313(16):1636–1644.

24

Collaborations Beyond
the Emergency Department

Margaret E. Balfour and Matthew L. Goldman

Introduction

A lot happens outside of the emergency department (ED) that affects the outcome of a behavioral health (BH) emergency. Many ED visits originate with a call for help from someone in the community—the person in crisis, a family member, or a bystander. There is wide variability throughout the United States in how that call for help is handled. Some people experiencing mental health or substance use–related emergencies never make it to the ED, instead dying in police shootings or taken to jail instead of receiving the care they need. Fortunately, the new 988 mental health emergency number and police reform movements have highlighted the need to build BH crisis response systems that deliver the same quality and consistency of care as we expect for medical emergencies. ED psychiatrists will need to collaborate with the crisis system just as emergency medicine physicians collaborate with emergency medical services (EMS) and other prehospital programs.

Collaboration is important after the emergency as well. Linkage to aftercare is a critical component of successful discharge planning, and community-based resources such as peer wraparound services can help ensure this linkage is successful. Crisis observation units and crisis residential programs can serve as alternatives to inpatient admission and lessen the need for boarding. As crisis systems grow and evolve, collaborative partnerships will be critical for solving problems that have long burdened the ED, such as psychiatric boarding and the "revolving door" of repeat ED utilization.

Other chapters in this volume address the importance of collaboration with families, clinics, and other community-based supports in the standard evaluation and treatment of BH emergencies. This chapter instead focuses on the period immediately before and after the individual leaves the ED, with an emphasis on first responders and the continuum of community-based services that comprise a robust crisis system of care. Practical suggestions for collaboration are included throughout the chapter to spark ideas for action or quality improvement projects. Note that in this chapter, the term *behavioral health* (BH) is used to encompass both mental health (MH) and substance use disorders (SUD) and services, and the expectation is that all crisis services can address both.

Behavioral Health Emergencies and Intersection
with the Justice System

How a community responds to BH emergencies is both a health issue and a social justice issue. Former U.S. Congressman Patrick Kennedy, one of the co-authors of the Mental

Health Parity and Addiction Act, has lamented that people in need of mental health and substance use treatment often remain relegated to a separate and unequal system of care a decade-and-a-half later.[1] Nowhere is this disparity more apparent than in how mental health and substance use emergencies are handled, starting from the moment a person asks for help. Indeed, a 911 call for chest pain results in an ambulance response with emergency medicine technicians, but a call for suicidal ideation often triggers an armed law enforcement response. The 988 mental health emergency number (implemented in mid-2022) is intended to provide a more appropriate clinical response, but it will take time for communities to build the crisis systems that can provide the care that callers need.

As long as law enforcement remains the default first responder, a request for help places individuals in BH crisis at increased risk of incarceration and death. In the United States, people experiencing BH emergencies account for one-fourth of police shootings, half of which occur in the person's own home.[2] Training programs can provide law enforcement with tools to recognize and de-escalate persons experiencing BH emergencies, but officers often encounter barriers when trying to connect people to the treatment they need. For example, many EDs require officers to wait for hours while the person boards for hours or even days awaiting transfer to a psychiatric hospital. Without an easy way for law enforcement to connect the person to needed treatment, jail is often the last resort. Consequently, more than 2 million people with serious mental illness are booked into jail each year, often for nonviolent "nuisance" or "quality of life" offenses such as loitering or vagrancy, and the prevalence of mental illness and SUDs in jails and prisons is three or four times that of the general population.[3,4] These disparities are amplified for people of color. Black Americans are 2.6 times more likely to be killed by police compared to non-Hispanic Whites; for Black Americans with mental illness, the risk is nearly 10-fold.[2] For those struggling with SUDs, disparate sentencing penalties (e.g., harsher sentences for crack vs. powder cocaine) result in excessive imprisonment of Black Americans.[5] Is it surprising, then, that Black Americans are less likely to call 911 for help with a mental health crisis?[6]

Sequential Intercept Model and the Role of the Crisis Continuum

The sequential intercept model (Figure 24.1) is a conceptual model designed to help communities plan services and protocols aimed at preventing or decreasing criminal justice involvement for people with BH conditions.[7] It describes the typical pathway through the criminal justice system and identifies opportunities for the health care system to intervene. Intercept 1 focuses on programs that provide law enforcement and 911 call-takers with tools and processes to recognize BH emergencies and divert them to treatment. The upstream Intercept 0 was added in recognition that a well-coordinated and easily accessible crisis care continuum can potentially prevent the 911 call or police interaction. Collectively, Intercepts 0 and 1 are considered "pre-arrest diversion" because they connect individuals to treatment before the point of arrest and jail booking, which keeps them out of the justice system altogether. This differs from post-arrest diversion programs that focus on jail and court-based services such as mental health courts that occur after the individual has been arrested and taken to jail.

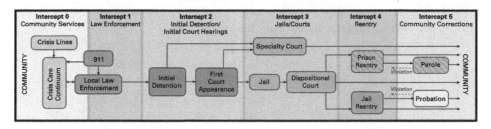

Figure 24.1 The sequential intercept model. Intercepts 0 and 1 focus on programs that prevent the arrest of people experiencing behavioral health emergencies and instead connecting them to the treatment they need.

Reproduced from Policy Research Associates.[7]

Law Enforcement Collaboration and Crisis Intervention Team Programs

Crisis Intervention Team (CIT) programs provide law enforcement with tools to recognize individuals experiencing a BH crisis, de-escalate them, and divert them to treatment instead of jail.[8] CIT began in the late 1980s in Memphis, Tennessee, in response to a police shooting involving a Black man with mental illness. Its centerpiece is a 40-hour training that involves scenario-based exercises and participation of community stakeholders including BH clinicians, treatment agencies, people with lived experience of mental illness, families, and advocacy groups. Volunteering to help with CIT training is an excellent way for psychiatrists to develop collaborative relationships with local law enforcement.

The National Council for Mental Wellbeing and CIT International both recommend that all of a department's uniformed patrol officers receive a basic 8-hour training such as Mental Health First Aid for Public Safety, whereas the 40-hour CIT training is voluntarily undertaken by a subset of officers large enough to ensure 24 hours a day, 7 days a week (24/7) availability of trained officers to respond to calls for service. 911 personnel should also receive training to help them dispatch CIT trained officers when needed. This approach ensures both a basic level of competency among all officers and 24/7 availability of a specialized CIT response.[9] (Mental Health First Aid has also developed a version of the training targeted to EMS workers.)

Although CIT is often thought of as a police training program, its creators continue to underscore that training is only one piece of a more comprehensive and community-based approach. Once officers are trained to identify a person in crisis and divert them to treatment, their first question is often "Divert to what?" Thus, the full CIT model recommends a crisis system with quick and easy access and 24/7 availability so that jail does not become the path of least resistance. In other words, the health care system should make it easy for officers to "do the right thing" and bring people to care instead of jail.

It is also important to track outcomes and stratify by race, ethnicity, and other demographic characteristics. Disparities in key law enforcement outcomes, such as use of force, arrest, and diversion to crisis care, can reveal implicit bias in policing.[10] Openly and transparently sharing such data with the public while working to address these issues is an effective way to improve community trust.

Collaboration Suggestions: Law Enforcement

- Does your local law enforcement agency have a CIT program?
  - Find out who the CIT coordinator is and invite them to participate in an in-service or grand rounds to learn about their perspective.
  - Volunteer to help with CIT training and/or serve on the local CIT steering committee.
- Find out the process for what happens when law enforcement brings an individual to the ED for BH care.
  - Do officers have to bring them through the main waiting area? Is there a faster and less stigmatizing alternative?
  - Do officers have to wait with individuals under an involuntary hold? Is there a way to transfer custody to the ED so that officers can get back on the street?
  - Can these processes be improved to make it easier? Consider regular meetings with law enforcement to improve the process. When searching for solutions, try to move beyond "we've always done it this way."

The Crisis Continuum: Community-Based Alternatives to Hospitals, Emergency Departments, and Jail

An oft-heard refrain in the ED is that boarding and access problems would be solved if only there were more psychiatric inpatient beds. However, this approach is contrary to the Supreme Court's *Olmstead* decision, which affirms the rights of people with mental health disabilities to receive the care they need in the most community-integrated (i.e., least-restrictive) setting possible.[11] Rather, a system of community-based care[12] is needed with services spanning a continuum of intensity and restrictiveness, as depicted in Figure 24.2 The more robust the continuum, the more options to meet the person's needs without resorting to EDs, hospitals, or jails, and the less competing demand for those who do need inpatient beds. Crisis systems should provide a "health first" response[13] that favors clinical interventions without the use of law enforcement unless absolutely necessary.[14] The continuum should include options for individuals most in need of specialized psychiatric care, such as people who are under involuntary commitment, highly agitated, or with co-occurring SUD needs, especially because people of color are more likely to fall into these categories. Stratifying outcomes by race, ethnicity, legal status, diagnosis, and other demographic characteristics can reveal inequities in access to quality care.

The Substance Abuse and Mental Health Services Administration (SAMHSA) defines a core crisis continuum consisting of three types of services: someone to talk to (crisis lines), someone to respond (mobile crisis), and somewhere to go (crisis facilities).[15] The report titled "Roadmap to the Ideal Crisis System" expands the continuum to include additional community-based programs to ensure the individual remains stable after the crisis or to prevent a developing crisis from escalating.[16]

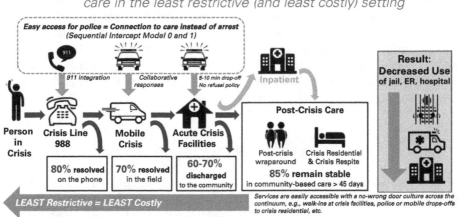

Alignment of crisis services toward common goals
care in the least restrictive (and least costly) setting

Figure 24.2 The crisis continuum. In a high-functioning crisis system, the individual services in the continuum work together to achieve a common goal—in this case, stabilization in the least restrictive (which is also the least costly) level of care. Crisis line resolved calls is the percentage of calls resolved without dispatching mobile crisis, law enforcement, or emergency medical services. Mobile crisis resolved cases is the percentage of face-to-face encounters resolved without the need for transport to a higher level of care. Crisis facilities community disposition is the percentage of discharges to levels of care other than hospital, ED, or jail. Continued stabilization is the percentage of individuals with a mobile crisis or crisis facility encounter who did not have a subsequent ED visit or hospitalization within 45 days. ED, emergency department.

Source: Data were provided by Arizona Complete Health/Centene and apply to the southern Arizona geographical service area for 2019 (Cochise, Graham, Greenlee, La Paz, Pima, Pinal, Santa Cruz, and Yuma counties).

Someone to Call: Crisis Lines, 988, and "Care Traffic Control"

Crisis lines are often the first entry point to crisis services, providing support 24/7 via phone, text, or chat. They vary widely in terms of scope, funding, and staffing. Suicide hotlines often include a mix of clinical professionals and/or volunteers, whereas "warm lines" focus on emotional support and are often staffed by peers who have lived experience of their own BH challenges. In some communities, crisis calls have been handled by nonemergency information lines such as 211 and 311 and can help with connection to services that address social determinants of health such as food banks and transportation.

The National Suicide Prevention Lifeline was created by the SAMHSA in 2005 to improve access by linking these local call centers via a single toll-free number (1-800-273-TALK) that routes the caller to the nearest available call center. The Lifeline has since grown to a network of nearly 200 centers that became the foundation for the universal three-digit crisis hotline number (988) in 2022, administered by SAMHSA and Vibrant Emotional Health. Studies of Lifeline call centers have found that callers have significantly decreased suicidality during the course of the call,[17] one-third are successfully connected with mental health referrals,[18] and less than one-fourth of calls result in law enforcement or EMS being sent without the caller's collaboration.[19] In addition to increased call volumes as public awareness grows and more crisis lines join the 988/ Lifeline network, many crisis lines are expanding their scope beyond suicide counseling to include "care traffic control" functions such as dispatching mobile crisis teams, making outpatient appointments, and bed placement. A growing number of communities are integrating their crisis lines into local 911 call centers so that BH calls can be diverted to the crisis line for a health-first response.

Someone to Respond: Mobile Crisis Teams

Mobile crisis teams (MCTs) are typically one- or two-person teams that meet the person where they are—at home, on the street, etc.—often eliminating the need to transport them to a more restrictive level of care for evaluation. In some communities, MCTs provide services to patients boarding in EDs who might not otherwise have access to a timely mental health assessment.

MCTs can be staffed by any combination of clinical staff, including master's-level clinicians, BH technicians, peers, nurses, paramedics, or emergency medical technicians. For this reason, they are sometimes called multidisciplinary response teams. In addition, a variety of "co-responder" models are emerging in which law enforcement officers respond to crisis calls with a clinician, peer, or other social services staff.

Some localities have established centralized dispatch for MCTs, often within crisis call centers, aided by technology such as Global Positioning System–enabled mobile apps for location tracking and transmission of clinical information. Studies of MCTs have demonstrated reduction of psychiatric hospitalization and ED utilization[20–23] and indicate that most people prefer clinician-staffed MCTs or co-responder teams to police-only teams.[24] In particular, they value responders with mental health knowledge and verbal de-escalation skills and a compassionate, empowering, and noncriminalizing approach.[25]

Somewhere to Go: Specialized Crisis Facilities

Crisis facilities can serve as a safe and therapeutic alternative to hospital EDs, inpatient psychiatric units, and jails. However, crisis programs vary widely in scope, capability, and populations served. Some are designed for low-acuity individuals who primarily need peer support and a safe place to spend the night, whereas others can treat the highest acuity individuals presenting with suicidal behaviors, acute agitation, and substance intoxication. A good working knowledge of and relationship with the programs available in the local community can open up new opportunities for safely discharging to less-restrictive community-based care instead of inpatient admission.

It is also essential to have a clear understanding of the level of acuity (in terms of agitation, dangerousness, etc.) and medical comorbidities that can be served in each facility. In addition, local processes for civil commitment may determine the types of crisis facilities available to individuals under emergency detention/involuntary commitment. Lack of a shared understanding of admission and exclusion criteria can lead to unsafe conditions (e.g., when a high-acuity individual is sent to a program unable to safely address their needs) and staff frustration (e.g., disputes over whether or not a program should accept a referral). Regular meetings between ED and crisis facility leadership can help address and prevent such disagreements.

The Level of Care Utilization System (LOCUS) is a useful standardized framework for determining the appropriate level of care. Need is assessed on six dimensions: (1) Risk of Harm; (2) Functional Status; (3) Medical, Addiction, and Psychiatric Co-Morbidity; (4) Recovery Environment—both level of stress and level of support; (5) Treatment and Recovery History; and (6) Engagement and Recovery Status.[26] The final assessment synthesizes all of these dimensions to guide decision-making. For example, someone who expresses suicidal ideation may be able to be managed in a crisis residential setting (LOCUS Level 5) if they are highly engaged, hopeful that treatment will be helpful, and nonviolent. Conversely, suicidal ideation may require a higher acuity setting such as 23-hour observation (LOCUS Level 6) if the person is poorly engaged, highly agitated, etc. Table 24.1 lists characteristic of common types of crisis facilities, including their LOCUS level of care.

High-intensity/high-acuity crisis programs (LOCUS Level 6) may be called by a variety of names, including 23-hour observation; crisis observation; crisis receiving centers; psychiatric emergency services; crisis stabilization units; and emergency psychiatric assessment, treatment, and healing units. They may be part of or adjacent to an ED, part of or adjacent to a psychiatric hospital, or freestanding. They accept any individual regardless of behavioral acuity or involuntary legal status, including those who may be actively suicidal, acutely agitated, intoxicated, or in withdrawal, arriving directly from the field via law enforcement. To incentivize the police to bring people for treatment, the center must have 24/7 availability, faster drop-off times than jail (10 minutes or less),[27] and a "no wrong door" policy of never turning officers away.[28] These units are typically staffed with an interdisciplinary team of psychiatrists and other psychiatric providers, nurses, social workers, BH technicians, and peers. They are not simply holding areas for boarding patients awaiting transfer to an inpatient unit but, rather, short-term intensive treatment programs. With rapid assessment, early intervention, and proactive discharge planning, most individuals can be stabilized and discharged to community-based care within 24 hours. This level of crisis care is associated with reduced rates of inpatient psychiatric hospitalization,[29] ED boarding,[30] and arrest.[31] EDs that do not have such a specialized unit on-site can minimize boarding by having a process to quickly identify individuals with BH emergencies, stabilize any medical concern, and transfer them to such a unit for the specialized care they need.

Subacute units (LOCUS Level 5 or 6) are inpatient-like units that are usually freestanding (i.e., separate from a hospital or ED). Acuity, intensity, and staffing vary depending on the program and state regulations. Subacute units can be good options for individuals who need more than 23 hours of stabilization but are too acute for the lower intensity programs described below.

Lower intensity/acuity programs (LOCUS Level 5) are typically unlocked residential settings that provide a safe, structured, and therapeutic environment without 24/7 nursing or physician coverage on-site. They can be good options for discharging individuals who need a more structured and safe recovery environment due to housing instability or a stressful home environment.

Living Rooms, detoxification centers, and sobering centers provide 24/7 alternatives for less acute needs and often accept police drop-offs for those who meet their admission criteria. They are typically unlocked and serve individuals who are voluntary, nonviolent, and

Table 24.1 Facility-Based Crisis Services[a]

Model	Description	Level of Care/ Service Intensity	Acuity of Individuals Served	Locked	Police Drops	Use of Peers
23-hourr. observation	Short-term (<24 hours) assessment and stabilization with hospital-level staffing and safety protocols; can be attached to hospital/ED or freestanding	LOCUS 6 "medically managed" with 24/ 7 nursing and medical coverage	Can take high acuity, including agitation, danger to self/other, intoxication, withdrawal	Yes	Yes	Yes
Subacute	Short- or intermediate-term (several days) inpatient-like care		Varies by program from high-acuity/locked to lower acuity/unlocked	Sometimes	Sometimes	Yes
Living Rooms	Short-term (<24 hours) stabilization in a home-like environment, often predominantly peer staffed	LOCUS 5/5A "medically monitored" with medical/ nursing staff available but not on-site 24/7	Lower acuity, not at imminent risk of harm to self/other, not agitated or violent	No	Sometimes	Yes
Sobering centers and "social detox"	Short-term (<24 hours) stabilization for individuals with substance use needs, typically not using meds			No	Sometimes	Yes
Crisis residential	Intermediate-term (days to a couple weeks) crisis stabilization in a residential setting			No	Usually not	Yes

[a]Examples of facility-based crisis services and how they differ in terms of intensity, population served, and LOCUS level of care. Until national standards are developed, any of these different programs might be called a "crisis stabilization unit," depending on state and local regulations. ED, emergency department.

motivated for help. Living Rooms offer a home-like environment with couches and art-work and are staffed predominantly by peer specialists, with limited coverage by a psychi-atrist or other provider. They are especially helpful if psychosocial stressors are the main precipitants of the crisis. Detoxification centers provide medically supervised detoxifica-tion services, whereas sobering centers employ primarily psychosocial and peer support.

Crisis residential, crisis respite, and peer respite facilities offer longer term (days to weeks) stabilization in a residential setting. They can be accessed directly or used as step-down from inpatient or acute crisis care. Some programs may accept lower acuity indi-viduals directly from law enforcement or mobile crisis teams.

Crisis clinics or mental health urgent care centers are outpatient programs that offer same-day or walk-in access for assessment, crisis counseling, medication management, care coordination, and bridge services until the person is connected to appropriate out-patient care. Including information about these programs in discharge instructions can help prevent repeat ED visits in the future.

After the Crisis: Post-Crisis Care

Linkage to aftercare is a key component of a successful discharge plan, with earlier appointments (within 3 days) associated with higher attendance and longer commu-nity tenure after discharge.[32] Once the person leaves the ED, however, many barriers conspire to keep them from successfully connecting with the services they need, such as transportation, difficulty navigating complex systems, or ongoing symptoms of the MH or SUD issue that contributed to their crisis in the first place. Good discharge pla-nning can foresee and mitigate some of these barriers, especially when combined with collaborations between the ED and community-based programs that can give the person extra support in the days or weeks following a crisis. Models include pre-discharge inter-ventions such as psychoeducation and structured discharge planning, post-discharge interventions such as follow-up phone calls and case management, and transitional interventions that engage with people prior to discharge and continue for some period of time after discharge. These interventions can be performed by ED-based staff or via collaborations with community-based agencies. For example, an ED might partner with a crisis line to perform follow-up phone calls or with a peer-run agency or community mental health clinic for post-crisis wraparound or case management services. Small study sizes and the wide variability in program elements, intensity, and duration make comparative research between different models difficult,[33] but best practices are emerg-ing. In particular, follow-up "caring contacts" such as phone calls and postcards have been studied as a suicide-prevention intervention with promising results in terms of effi-cacy[34] and cost-effectiveness.[35]

Peer Support: Engagement and Linkage to Community Resources

Peer support workers are people in recovery from mental illness or SUD who use their lived experience to help others with similar challenges. They are a rapidly growing part of the BH workforce and an important component of many of the community-based crisis programs described in this chapter. Some EDs are beginning to employ peers as well.

Although peers are a relatively new addition to the modern health care system, the value of peer support has long been recognized. The 18th-century French physician Philippe Pinel, who famously liberated the insane from their chains at the Bicêtre and Salpêtrière asylums, did so with the help of his colleague Jean-Baptiste Pussin, a former patient at Bicêtre who later became the administrator of its ward for incurable mental patients. The hiring of former patients was a cornerstone of their new "moral treatment," as Pussin observed that they were "better suited to this demanding work because they are usually more gentle, honest, and humane."[36] More recently, Alcoholics Anonymous was founded in the 1930s based on a model of fellowship and volunteer peer support. The modern concept of peer support grew from the self-help movement in the 1970s in which survivors of negative experiences in psychiatric hospitals began to organize and advocate for more consumer-driven and recovery-oriented models of care. In the early 2000s, peer support began to be recognized as a billable service. Today, peer support workers are often paid paraprofessionals with formal training and state certification.

Peer support provides a unique contribution to clinical care, and in particular superior engagement with "difficult to reach" individuals. The mechanism underlying this differential effect is hypothesized to be due to three factors: (1) instillation of hope through self-disclosure, (2) role modeling to include self-care of one's illness and firsthand experience navigating the system, and (3) enhanced empathy and conditional regard from having shared similar experiences.[37] Furthermore, the hiring of peers can help an organization improve diversity, equity, and inclusion by creating a workforce that more closely reflects the lived experience and demographics of the population served.[13,38]

Given the importance of engagement and linkage to aftercare in emergency psychiatric care, it is not surprising that peer support in ED and crisis settings is associated with positive outcomes, including reduced hospital admissions and ED visits[39] and improvements in engagement with high-risk populations,[40] provision of naloxone,[41] linkage to aftercare,[42] and primary care follow-up.[43] Families can benefit from peer support as well; in particular, the National Alliance on Mental Illness (NAMI) Family-to-Family program helps families increase acceptance, reduce distress, and improve problem-solving related to their loved one's mental illness.[44]

Collaboration Suggestions: Crisis Continuum

- Find out what crisis programs are available in your local community and what services they provide. Are these services being utilized to their full potential?
  - Could some admissions or repeat ED visits potentially be avoided by connecting the individual to a crisis program instead?
  - Are there barriers to accessing these services from the ED, such as lack of knowledge, confusion about admission/exclusionary criteria, or other process problems?
  - Consider inviting crisis programs to participate in an in-service or grand rounds for ED staff to learn about their program and/or regular meetings to work through process problems.
- Review the discharge process and patient-education materials for people with BH emergencies.

- Do discharge instructions contain options other than calling 911 in the event of another BH emergency? Consider including information about 988 and other local resources, such as warm lines, urgent care, and other crisis programs.
- What is your organization's process for requesting a "welfare check" for patients you are concerned about? Is it possible to use the crisis line and MCTs instead of the police?
- What follow-up do patients receive after their ED visit? Consider partnering with crisis programs to ensure patients get a follow-up phone call or access to post-crisis peer support.
- What information is given to families? Consider providing information about your local NAMI chapter.
- Review how peers are incorporated into BH emergency care at your organization.
  - If your ED does not employ peers, why not? Can peers from community-based programs come to the ED and meet with patients before discharge?
  - Consider inviting community-based peer programs to participate in an in-service or grand rounds to help ED staff learn about peer support.

Putting It All Together: Collaborative Approaches to "Familiar Faces"

Individuals who repeatedly present for emergency care can be frustrating for everyone involved, including the person seeking help. Treatment-as-usual clearly is not working for these "familiar faces." Successful solutions require an alternative approach and collaboration with multiple community partners.

Be a detective, not a bouncer. First, we must reframe our thinking about these individuals. It is easy to become frustrated and focus on why the person *should not* be accessing care in the ED. Instead, investigate why they are using the ED to get their needs met. What do they need and why haven't they been able to get it in the community? What is reinforcing their repeat visits? It is also important to remember that most people are doing best with what they have in terms of coping skills and social determinants of health. Try to put yourself in their shoes and imagine trying to navigate the system.

Find out who is responsible for the individual's care. Who is their psychiatrist, case manager, etc.? Who pays for their care? Payers do not want their members repeatedly visiting the ED any more than you do. Local BH authorities and managed care organizations (MCOs) can be powerful allies with the influence to help bring together multiple stakeholders and the ability to access specialized services on a case-by-case basis.

Convene relevant stakeholders such as clinics, group homes, family, and other natural supports, first responders (e.g., police or EMS for frequent 911 callers). Also include crisis programs that could be good alternatives to the ED. Explore the individual's needs and the barriers to getting them met. What precipitates their crisis and what can be done to proactively address it? Identify strengths to build upon by asking when was the last time they were doing well. What changed?

Develop a plan. It should list the responsibilities of each stakeholder and include what to do when the individual presents to the ED. The plan should have realistic goals adapted to the individual's stage of change. For example, "stop using substances" is not a realistic goal for someone precontemplative about their SUD. Instead, the plan should focus on engaging the person to help them move to the contemplative stage. A more realistic goal might be for them to agree to talk to a peer about their substance use. Small incremental steps that generate quick wins can be positively reinforced and improve the morale of both the individual and the ED staff. Review and adjust the plan if the person continues to come back to the ED.

Use a continuous quality improvement approach. Review and adjust individual plans if the person continues to come back to the ED. Aggregate data about crisis utilization can also be used to inform improvement efforts for the entire system. For example, one crisis center partnered with its MCO payer and discovered that a subset of schools were disproportionately sending adolescents to its youth crisis unit. The payer was able to target enhanced in-school mental health services to these outlier schools.[45]

Case Example

Ms. X frequently became anxious and overwhelmed when she felt lonely, resulting in multiple calls to 911 for suicidal thoughts. She had multiple visits to the crisis center and said she felt safe there and liked talking to the peers there. The team noted that her 911 calls were usually on evenings and weekends, so the warm line and her clinic scheduled outbound calls to check on her during these times. Building on the strength of her therapeutic relationship with the peers at the crisis center, her clinic assigned her a peer who would come to the crisis center to meet with her at every visit. She began reaching out to the clinic peer instead of calling 911. Her visits decreased from 17 within a 3-month period to just 1 during the same 3 months the following year.

Conclusion

Crisis care is a rapidly evolving field. Multiple factors have led to an infusion of interest in and funding for crisis care, including the implementation of 988, COVID's impact on mental health and associated relief packages, and momentum from social justice movements to remove law enforcement as the default first responder for BH calls. At the time of this writing, national standards have yet to be developed, and most communities do not have a crisis care system approaching that which exists for medical emergencies. New opportunities for psychiatrist leadership and advocacy are emerging.[46] It is an exciting time to get involved.

For those wanting to learn more:

- Read the "Roadmap to the Ideal Crisis System" report and associated resources at https://www.CrisisRoadmap.com.
- Join professional organizations involved in shaping crisis care, such as the American Association for Emergency Psychiatry, the American Association of Community Psychiatrists, the American Psychiatric Association, the National Association for Mental Wellbeing, and CIT International.
- Get involved with advocacy groups such as the National Alliance on Mental Illness, Mental Health America, and Fountain House.

- Find out who is working on crisis care in your local community and offer to help.
- Use the suggestions in this chapter to start a quality improvement project at your local institution.

References

1. Newman K. Patrick Kennedy: Parity still needed for mental health, addiction care. *US News & World Report*, December 7, 2018. https://www.usnews.com/news/health-news/articles/2018-12-07/patrick-kennedy-parity-needed-for-mental-health-addiction-treatment

2. Saleh AZ, Appelbaum PS, Liu X, Scott Stroup T, Wall M. Deaths of people with mental illness during interactions with law enforcement. *Int J Law Psychiatry*. 2018;58:110–116. doi:10.1016/j.ijlp.2018.03.003

3. Steadman HJ, Osher FC, Robbins PC. Prevalence of serious mental illness among jail inmates. *Psychiatr Serv*. 2009;60(6):761–765. doi:10.1176/ps.2009.60.6.761

4. Glaze LE, James DJ. Mental health problems of prison and jail inmates. Bureau of Justice Statistics, National Institute of Mental Health. Published 2006. https://www.nimh.nih.gov/health/statistics/index.shtml

5. Wildeman C, Wang EA. Mass incarceration, public health, and widening inequality in the USA. *Lancet*. 2017;389(10077):1464–1474. doi:10.1016/S0140-6736(17)30259-3

6. Kessell ER, Alvidrez J, McConnell WA, Shumway M. Effect of racial and ethnic composition of neighborhoods in San Francisco on rates of mental health-related 911 calls. *Psychiatr Serv*. 2009;60(10):1376–1378. doi:10.1176/ps.2009.60.10.1376

7. The sequential intercept model: Advancing community-based solutions for justice-involved people with mental and substance use disorders. Policy Research Associates. Published 2018. https://www.prainc.com/wp-content/uploads/2018/06/PRA-SIM-Letter-Paper-2018.pdf

8. Usher L, Watson AC, Bruno R, et al. Crisis Intervention Team (CIT) programs: A best practice guide for transforming community responses to mental health crises. Published 2019. https://www.citinternational.org/resources/Best%20Practice%20Guide/CIT%20guide%20desktop%20printing%202019_08_16%20(1).pdf

9. Margiotta N, Gibb B. Mental health first aid or CIT: What should law enforcement do? Published 2016. https://perma.cc/9TPC-DMHS

10. Police--mental health collaborations: A framework for implementing effective law enforcement responses for people who have mental health needs. Council of State Governments. Published 2019. https://csgjusticecenter.org/publications/police-mental-health-collaborations-a-framework-for-implementing-effective-law-enforcement-responses-for-people-who-have-mental-health-needs

11. Olmstead vs. LC: History and current status. Olmstead Rights. Accessed May 8, 2022. https://www.olmsteadrights.org/about-olmstead

12. Pinals DA, Fuller DA. Beyond beds: The vital role of a full continuum of psychiatric care. National Association of State Mental Health Program Directors. Published 2017. https://www.nasmhpd.org/sites/default/files/TAC.Paper_.1Beyond_Beds.pdf

13. From harm to health: Centering racial equity and lived experience in mental health crisis response. Fountain House. Published 2021. https://www.fountainhouse.org/assets/From-Harm-to-Health-2021.pdf

14. Balfour ME, Hahn Stephenson A, Delany-Brumsey A, Winsky J, Goldman ML. Cops, clinicians, or both? Collaborative approaches to responding to behavioral health emergencies. *Psychiatr Serv.* 2022;73(6):658–669. doi:10.1176/appi.ps.202000721

15. National guidelines for behavioral health crisis care—Best practice toolkit. Substance Abuse and Mental Health Services Administration. Published 2020. Accessed May 4, 2020. https://www.samhsa.gov/sites/default/files/national-guidelines-for-behavioral-health-crisis-care-02242020.pdf

16. Roadmap to the ideal crisis system: Essential elements. measurable standards and best practices for behavioral health crisis response. Group for the Advancement of Psychiatry. Published 2021. https://www.crisisroadmap.com

17. Gould MS, Kalafat J, Harrismunfakh JL, Kleinman M. An evaluation of crisis hotline outcomes: Part 2. Suicidal callers. *Suicide Life Threat Behav.* 2007;37(3):338–352.

18. Kalafat J, Gould MS, Munfakh JLH, Kleinman M. An evaluation of crisis hotline outcomes: Part 1. Nonsuicidal crisis callers. *Suicide Life Threat Behav.* 2007;37(3):322–337.

19. Gould MS, Lake AM, Munfakh JLH. Helping callers to the National Suicide Prevention Lifeline who are at imminent risk of suicide: Evaluation of caller risk profiles and interventions implemented. *Suicide Life Threat Behav.* 2016;46(2):172–190.

20. Scott RL. Evaluation of a mobile crisis program: Effectiveness, efficiency, and consumer satisfaction. *Psychiatr Serv.* 2000;51(9):1153–1156.

21. Guo S, Biegel DE, Johnsen JA, Dyches H. Assessing the impact of community-based mobile crisis services on preventing hospitalization. *Psychiatr Serv.* 2001;52(2):223–228. doi:10.1176/appi.ps.52.2.223

22. Fendrich M, Ives M, Kurz B, et al. Impact of mobile crisis services on emergency department use among youths with behavioral health service needs. *Psychiatr Serv.* 2019;70(10):881–888. doi:10.1176/appi.ps.201800450

23. Vakkalanka JP, Neuhas RA, Harland KK, Clemsen L, Himadi E, Lee S. Mobile crisis outreach and emergency department utilization: A propensity score-matched analysis. *West J Emerg Med Integrating Emerg Care Popul Health.* 2021;22(5):1086–1094. doi:10.5811/westjem.2021.6.52276

24. Boscarato K, Lee S, Kroschel J, Hollander Y, Brennan A, Warren N. Consumer experience of formal crisis-response services and preferred methods of crisis intervention. *Int J Ment Health Nurs.* 2014;23(4):287–295.

25. Lamanna D, Shapiro GK, Kirst M, Matheson FI, Nakhost A, Stergiopoulos V. Co-responding police–mental health programmes: Service user experiences and outcomes in a large urban centre. *Int J Ment Health Nurs.* 2018;27(2):891–900. doi:10.1111/inm.12384

26. Sowers W, Pumariega A, Huffine C, Fallon T. Best practices: Level-of-care decision making in behavioral health services: The LOCUS and the CALOCUS. *Psychiatr Serv.* 2003;54(11):1461–1463. doi:10.1176/appi.ps.54.11.1461

27. Balfour ME, Tanner K, Jurica PJ, Rhoads R, Carson CA. Crisis Reliability Indicators Supporting Emergency Services (CRISES): A framework for developing performance measures for behavioral health crisis and psychiatric emergency programs. *Community Ment Health J.* 2016;52(1):1–9. doi:10.1007/s10597-015-9954-5

28. Dupont R, Cochran S, Pillsbury S. Crisis Intervention Team core elements. University of Memphis School of Urban Affairs and Public Policy, Department of Criminology and Criminal; 2007.

29. Little-Upah P, Carson C, Williamson R, et al. The Banner psychiatric center: A model for providing psychiatric crisis care to the community while easing behavioral health holds in emergency departments. *Perm J.* 2013;17(1):45–49.

30. Zeller S, Calma N, Stone A. Effects of a dedicated regional psychiatric emergency service on boarding of psychiatric patients in area emergency departments. *West J Emerg Med.* 2014;15(1):1–6. doi:10.5811/westjem.2013.6.17848

31. Steadman HJ, Stainbrook KA, Griffin P, Draine J, Dupont R, Horey C. A specialized crisis response site as a core element of police-based diversion programs. *Psychiatr Serv.* 2001;52(2):219–222. doi:10.1176/appi.ps.52.2.219

32. McCullumsmith C, Clark B, Blair C, Cropsey K, Shelton R. Rapid follow-up for patients after psychiatric crisis. *Community Ment Health J.* 2015;51(2):139–144. doi:10.1007/s10597-014-9782-z

33. Bruffaerts R, Sabbe M, Demyttenaere K. Predicting community tenure in patients with recurrent utilization of a psychiatric emergency service. *Gen Hosp Psychiatry.* 2005;27(4):269–274.

34. Shand F, Woodward A, McGill K, et al. Suicide aftercare services: An evidence check rapid review. Sax Institute. Published October 2019. https://www.saxinstitute.org.au/wp-content/uploads/2019_Suicide-Aftercare-Services-Report.pdf

35. Hegedüs A, Kozel B, Richter D, Behrens J. Effectiveness of transitional interventions in improving patient outcomes and service use after discharge from psychiatric inpatient care: A systematic review and meta-analysis. *Front Psychiatry.* 2020;10:969.

36. Weiner DB. The apprenticeship of Philippe Pinel: A new document, "observations of Citizen Pussin on the insane." *Am J Psychiatry.* 1979;136(9):1128–1134. doi:10.1176/ajp.136.9.1128

37. Davidson L, Bellamy C, Guy K, Miller R. Peer support among persons with severe mental illnesses: A review of evidence and experience. *World Psychiatry.* 2012;11(2):123–128. doi:10.1016/j.wpsyc.2012.05.009

38. Beck J, Stagoff-Belfort A, de Bibiana JT. Civilian crisis response: A toolkit for equitable alternatives to police. n.d. https://www.vera.org/civilian-crisis-response-toolkit

39. Kaur M, Melville RH. Emergency department peer support specialist program. *Psychiatr Serv.* 2021;72(2):230. doi:10.1176/appi.ps.72102

40. Waye KM, Goyer J, Dettor D, et al. Implementing peer recovery services for overdose prevention in Rhode Island: An examination of two outreach-based approaches. *Addict Behav.* 2019;89:85–91. doi:10.1016/j.addbeh.2018.09.027

41. Samuels EA, Baird J, Yang ES, Mello MJ. Adoption and utilization of an emergency department naloxone distribution and peer recovery coach consultation program. *Acad Emerg Med.* 2019;26(2):160-173. doi:10.1111/acem.13545

42. Carey CW, Jones R, Yarborough H, Kahler Z, Moschella P, Lommel KM. 366 peer-to-peer addiction counseling initiated in the emergency department leads to high initial opioid recovery rates. *Ann Emerg Med.* 2018;72(4):S143–S144. doi:10.1016/j.annemergmed.2018.08.371

43. Griswold KS, Pastore PA, Homish GG, Henke A. Access to primary care: Are mental health peers effective in helping patients after a psychiatric emergency? *Prim Psychiatry.* 2010;17(6):42–45.

44. Dixon LB, Lucksted A, Medoff DR, et al. Outcomes of a randomized study of a peer-taught family-to-family education program for mental illness. *Psychiatr Serv.* 2011;62(6):591–597. doi:10.1176/ps.62.6.pss6206_0591

45. Balfour ME, Zinn TE, Cason K, et al. Provider–payer partnerships as an engine for continuous quality improvement. *Psychiatr Serv.* 2018;69(6):623–625. doi:10.1176/appi.ps.201700533

46. Psychiatric leadership in crisis systems: The role of the crisis services medical director. National Council for Mental Wellbeing. Published 2022. https://www.thenationalcouncil. org/wp-content/uploads/2022/01/22.01.25_MDI-Psychiatric-Leadership-in-Crisis-Syst ems-FINAL.pdf?daf=375ateTbd56

25

Quality Improvement in Psychiatric Emergency Settings

Making Care Safer and Better

Margaret E. Balfour and Richard Rhoads

Introduction

Quality improvement (QI) may seem like a dry topic reserved for health care administrators, but in fact all staff working in health care can and should participate in QI. QI is anything that improves the delivery, consistency, or outcome of care, ranging from large, multistep projects (e.g., changing the entire process for suicide assessment and triage) to small, seemingly minor improvements (e.g., updating a form or streamlining a process to make it more efficient). Frontline staff—including residents—are critical to successful QI efforts because they are often the first to notice processes that need improvement and can help develop practical solutions based on their real-world experience. And for improvement to be effective, the people doing the day-to-day work must have input and buy-in. Otherwise, changes will be incompletely or incorrectly adopted, and the hoped-for improvements will not materialize. This chapter gives those interested in improving quality the basic tools to get started.

Anyone working in health care needs to know that the care they provide is safe, effective, patient-centered, and compliant with established standards. But how is that measured? How do staff know that their department is providing value to patients and to their organization? How is it determined that health care provision is meeting regulatory requirements? How do staff know that improvement projects have made a difference? Before quality can be improved, it has to be *measured*. Choosing what to measure and how to measure it are also part of QI. As Lord Kelvin famously said, "If you cannot measure it, you cannot improve it." This chapter reviews how to select measurements to identify areas for improvement and chart progress.

Fundamentally, QI is about value. "Value" in this context has two meanings. The first is straightforward. Is the organization achieving the outcomes important to key customers and stakeholders? The second is more abstract, but no less important. Health care workers want to make a meaningful contribution to society and to their patients, and a health care organization's core values typically reflect this desire. The ability to measure adherence to core values affects both the health of the organization and the individuals working within it by ascribing meaning to the hard work put in every day. This chapter helps medical students, residents, and other health care workers become more directly involved in improving the organization's ability to live up to its core values.

Definitions

"Quality assurance," "compliance," "quality improvement," "performance improvement," and "quality management" are terms that are often used interchangeably. For the purposes of this chapter, the following definitions are used:

Quality assurance (QA) is the process of specifying quality and performance standards and then ensuring that those standards are met. These standards may be developed internally or via external professional or regulatory organizations. In the latter case, QA is closely tied to regulatory compliance. To ensure standards are met, QA activities employ tools such as chart audits, inspections, and data reports. When performance on a certain process is out of compliance, solutions focus on the individuals responsible for the process, via corrective action or education.

Performance improvement (PI) is the process of continuously studying and improving processes to improve outcomes and reduce errors. Performance targets may be set internally, via regulatory agencies, or by seeking input by customers and stakeholders. In contrast to the QA focus on individual performance, PI focuses on systemic problems and uses tools that help identify and improve processes that need fixing. When an error occurs, PI asks, Why *couldn't*—rather than why *didn't*—staff do their job? PI activities often seek input and participation of individual workers in improvement projects and thus can positively affect organizational culture as well.

QAPI and QI: An organization needs both QA and PI for a comprehensive approach to quality. The Centers for Medicaid and Medicare Services (CMS) defines the marriage of quality assurance and performance improvement (QAPI) as "the coordinated application of two mutually-reinforcing aspects of a quality management system: Quality Assurance and Performance Improvement. QAPI takes a systematic, comprehensive, and data-driven approach to maintaining and improving safety and quality while involving all caregivers in practical and creative problem solving."[1] Organizations with QAPI programs in early development often focus heavily on QA and compliance, whereas more mature organizations have distinct compliance, QA, and PI functions. The terms quality improvement or quality management are sometimes used as shorthand to refer to the full spectrum of QAPI activities. In this chapter, QAPI is referred to as quality improvement or QI.

A Brief History of Quality Improvement in Health Care

The scientific approach to QI in medicine can be traced as far back as Florence Nightingale's groundbreaking statistical analysis of the relationship between hygiene and mortality among soldiers wounded in the Crimean War in the 1850s.[2] However, the importance of QI did not come to the full attention of the U.S. health care industry until a series of landmark reports published in 2000–2001 by the Institute of Medicine (IOM; since renamed the National Academy of Medicine). *To Err Is Human*[3] exposed the troubling state of U.S. health care, specifically the 45,000–100,000 annual deaths linked to preventable medical errors. A follow-up report titled *Crossing the Quality Chasm*[4] concluded that health care lagged behind other industries in terms of quality and safety by at least a decade and stated that "fundamental, sweeping redesign of the entire health system"

Table 25.1 Defining Quality

The Institute of Medicine defined quality and safety and identified six aims to guide health care organizations in their improvement efforts.

Quality: The degree to which health services for individuals and populations increase the likelihood of desired health outcomes and are consistent with current professional knowledge.

Safety: Freedom from accidental injury when interacting in any way with the health care system.

Timely: Reducing waits and sometimes harmful delays for both those who receive and those who give care.

Six Goals for Improvement

1. *Safe*: Avoiding injuries to patients from the care that is intended to help them.
2. *Effective*: Providing services based on scientific knowledge to all who could benefit and refraining from providing services to those not likely to benefit.
3. *Patient-centered*: Providing care that is respectful of and responsive to individual patient preferences, needs, and values, and ensuring that patient values guide all clinical decisions.
4. *Timely*: Reducing waits and sometimes harmful delays for both those who receive and those who give care.
5. *Efficient*: Avoiding waste, including waste of equipment, supplies, ideas, and energy.
6. *Equitable*: Providing care that does not vary in quality because of personal characteristics such as gender, ethnicity, geographic location, and socioeconomic status.

was needed rather than incremental or piecemeal attempts at addressing the problem. Together, these works heralded a national call to action and laid out a framework for health care to begin to systematically approach quality and safety as a priority (Table 25.1).

Building on this work, the Institute for Healthcare Improvement (IHI) introduced the concept of the "triple aim," challenging health care systems to pursue three aspirational goals: improving the experience of care, improving the health of populations, and reducing per capita costs of health care.[5] More recently, it has been recognized that achievement of these aims requires a healthy and engaged workforce, resulting in the addition of a fourth aim focused on improving the work life of clinicians and staff (Box 25.1).[6] Subsequent work by IOM, IHI, and other key organizations such as CMS, the Joint Commission, and CARF International have further advanced the field of QI in health care. All have recognized a need to learn from and adapt advances in QI from other high-reliability fields such as manufacturing and aviation

Many of the QI methods used in health care settings are based on process improvement methods initially developed for the manufacturing industry in the early to

Box 25.1 Health Care's Quadruple Aim

1. Improving the patient's experience of care (including both patient satisfaction and clinical quality)
2. Improving the health of populations
3. Improving the per capita costs of health care
4. Improving the work life of clinicians and staff (including joy and meaning in work)

mid-20th century. Much of this work was pioneered by American statisticians Walter Shewhart and W. Edwards Deming. While working as an engineer at Bell Laboratories, Shewhart pioneered the concept of statistical process control,[7] in which performance is measured over time using "control charts" or "run charts" to indicate whether a process is working stably and reliably. Both Shewhart and Deming contributed to the development and dissemination of the now ubiquitous plan–do–study–act (PDSA) cycle.[8] This four-step process begins with identifying a problem and designing an improved process to address it (plan), followed by testing the new process (do), analyzing results to determine how well it worked (study), and deciding whether to continue with the new process (act) or start a new cycle. Deming went on to develop more advanced QI frameworks that have since been adapted to many industries.[9] He first introduced QI concepts to the Japanese manufacturing industry during post-World War II rebuilding efforts. During the next 50 years, these methods were widely adopted and further developed into quality management frameworks such as the Toyota Production System, Lean (the implementation of the Toyota Production System in the United States), and Six Sigma (developed by Motorola and further refined by General Electric).

Today, Lean and Six Sigma are used in many other industries, including health care settings,[10] and some QI frameworks have been specifically adapted for health care. For example, the FOCUS-PDSA framework (discussed later in this chapter) is an adaptation of Deming's PDSA cycle created in the 1980s by Paul Batalden at Hospital Corporation of America.[11]

Measuring Quality

As discussed in the Introduction, QI is an expression of value, and therefore the metrics chosen must represent the values important to the organization. One way to accomplish this is by using a quality improvement tool called a Critical-to-Quality (CTQ) tree.[10] This tool is designed to help an organization translate values and customer needs into discrete measures. Figure 25.1 shows how a CTQ tree was used create a measure set for crisis and emergency psychiatric facilities called Crisis Reliability Indicators Supporting Emergency Services (CRISES).[12] The first step is to define the overall aim the organization is trying to accomplish, in this case, "excellence in crisis services." The next step is to define the key attributes that comprise this value. In the CRISES example, these were defined as timely, safe, accessible least restrictive, effective, consumer/family centered, and partnership. The final step is to define discrete metrics that reflect each of the CTQ tree key attributes.

Whether building a CTQ tree or selecting metrics for a QI project, it is important to understand various types of measures and when their application is most effective to support improvement efforts. Avedis Donabedian—an early pioneer of quality measurement in health care—developed the commonly used structure–process–outcome model:[13]

> *Structure*—the environment in which care is delivered. Metrics may describe organizational structure, resources, or staffing (e.g., whether the emergency department [ED] is staffed with a psychiatrist on-site).
> *Process*—the techniques and processes used to deliver care. Metrics may describe the use of screening tools (e.g., percentage of ED patients screened for suicide risk) or how quickly a specific intervention is completed (e.g., door-to-doctor time).

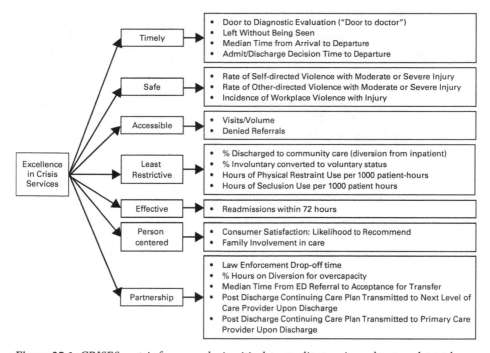

Figure 25.1 CRISES metric framework. A critical-to-quality tree is used to translate values into discrete metrics for mental health crisis services.

Modified from an earlier version previously published[12] by the chapter authors under the terms of the Creative Commons Attribution 4.0 International License (http://creativecommons.org/licenses/by/4.0).

Outcome—the result of the patient's interaction with the health care system (e.g., injury, death, quality of life, change in symptom rating scales, and readmissions).

Different types of measures are appropriate for different settings and purposes. Outcome measures are the most desirable. However, sometimes it is not feasible to collect outcome data, or it is not within the scope of an organization to change an outcome on its own; thus, a structure or process metric may be more appropriate.

Many frameworks exist to inform the selection and implementation of individual quality measures. A simple and straightforward approach was described by Hermann and Palmer[14] which requires that measures are meaningful, feasible, and actionable. The following are key considerations regarding each of these requirements:

Meaningful: Does the measure reflect a process that is clinically important? Is there evidence supporting the measure? Compared to other fields, there is a less robust evidence base for behavioral health measures, so we must often rely on face validity or adapt measures for which there is evidence in other settings. For example, the CRISES measures in the "timely" domain are adapted from existing core measures used for EDs. When possible, measures should be selected or adapted from measures that have been endorsed by organizations that set standards for quality measurement, such as the National Quality Forum, the CMS, the Joint Commission, the Agency for Healthcare Research and Quality, etc. Most of these organizations maintain online databases with measure definitions and specifications.

Feasible: Is it possible to collect the data needed for the measure? If so, can this be done accurately, quickly, and easily? Data must be produced within a short time-frame to be actionable. An organization's quality department staff should be able to spend most of its time addressing identified problems rather than performing time-consuming manual chart audits. With the advent of electronic health records (EHRs), it is now possible to design processes that support automated report-ing, making it feasible to quickly obtain data that were previously too complex or labor-intensive to collect via chart abstraction.

Actionable: Do the measures provide direction for future QI activities? Are there es-tablished benchmarks toward which to strive? Are the factors leading to subop-timal performance within the span of control of the organization to address? For example, a behavioral health crisis program is able to identify many problems in the community-wide system of care (e.g., lack of housing or ineffective outpatient follow-up after discharge). Crisis programs can be instrumental in collaborating with system partners to help fix these larger issues.[15] However, the crisis program's own core measures must be within its sphere of influence to improve; otherwise there is the tendency to blame problems on external factors rather than focus on the problems it can address.

Quality data can generate interest and enthusiasm among staff and should be shared regularly, presented in a format that makes it clear what is being measured and why. It is important to disseminate metrics in a way that is helpful to the end user. A QI com-mittee may need a detailed scorecard showing many different metrics, whereas executive leaders may prefer an abbreviated list of key performance indicators. Data posted for frontline staff might incorporate engaging graphs, charts, and infographics emphasizing how the data are linked to their everyday work.

Measurement and Standards in Emergency Psychiatry

There are few national standards for either the provision or measurement of emergency psychiatric or behavioral health crisis services. These services are primarily financed and regulated at the state level, and thus there is no national consensus on the defini-tions of various types of crisis services much less what their outcomes should be. Even when health care services are federally regulated, behavioral health is often overlooked in quality measurement systems. For example, the Hospital Consumer Assessment of Healthcare Providers and Systems, a patient satisfaction survey required by Medicare, excludes patients with psychiatric diagnoses. (This oversight presents a potential op-portunity for a resident QI project. How is patient experience measured for psychiatric emergency patients at your institution?)

Fortunately, there is increasing interest in developing the needed standards for these critical services. The nationwide implementation of a new 988 crisis line has bolstered federal interest in and funding for crisis and psychiatric emergency services. This pres-ents an unprecedented opportunity for a much-needed transformation in behavioral health crisis care, similar to how 911 catalyzed the development of emergency medical systems and trauma care. Recent progress has been made via the release of two seminal reports: "National Guidelines for Behavioral Health Crisis Care: A Best Practice Toolkit" by the Substance Abuse and Mental Health Services Administration[16] and "Roadmap to the Ideal Crisis System" by the National Council for Mental Wellbeing and the Group for the Advancement of Psychiatry.[17] Both reports incorporate the CRISES metrics framework and advocate for increased consistency and quality of care. Regulatory and professional organizations, including the American Association for Emergency Psychiatry, are continuing to work on guidelines and standards of care for patients in acute mental health or substance use crisis.

Improving Quality

The remainder of this chapter serves as a guide for anyone who wants to lead or participate in a QI project, including residents or medical students who are required to complete a QI project as part of their training.

Building a Quality Improvement Team

Quality improvement is meant to be performed in teams. Although it is important to note that *anyone* can participate in QI activities regardless of training, if possible, at least one member of the team should have training in QI methods and serve as facilitator. The other key roles do not require formal training and include clinical leaders, staff who work in the process of interest on a day-to-day basis, and a sponsor. The sponsor might not participate in all meetings but serves as a champion and liaison to higher level organizational leaders who can make policy decisions and allocate resources for the project. QI teams may also include a physician champion to provide medical expertise in the project design and implementation, represent the perspective of frontline physicians, and help achieve buy-in from the medical staff. Volunteering for this role is a good way for residents to become involved in QI. It is also possible to have multiple roles on the QI team; for example, a resident may facilitate a project as part of a training program in QI while also serving as the team's physician champion.

Writing the Aim Statement

The first task of any QI team is to determine the purpose of the project and write an aim statement. The aim statement is typically a brief (two or three sentences) paragraph that succinctly states the problem to be addressed and desired outcome of the project. It should address the following: (1) What is the problem? (2) Why is it important? (3) What measurable process/outcome are you going to improve? (4) By how much? (5) And by when?

The aim statement is as fundamental to a QI project as the hypothesis is to a research project, and it is well worth investing the time and effort to craft a good aim statement. Below are some considerations to help you craft an aim statement with a SMART goal—specific, measurable, actionable, realistic, and time-defined.[18]

Problem
A QI project is an opportunity to channel complaints into action. Think about what frustrates you or your patients, such as processes that take too long or are prone to error.

Or think about a patient population or treatment that interests you: Are best practices followed 100% of the time? Why is the problem important? How does it impact clinical outcomes, patient experience, safety, and cost?

Scope
Is the problem feasible to fix in the allotted time with the resources available? Projects fail when the scope is too broad or too vague. Focus on processes that your team has the authority and resources to change. Defining what/who your project does and does not include can help avoid "scope creep." For example, the team might focus on a specific part of a process with defined start and end points or a specific patient subpopulation.

Measurement
Choosing the right outcome metric is critical for determining whether the project achieved its goal. As discussed previously, the metric should be meaningful (reflect the problem), feasible (able to be collected before and after the intervention), and actionable (can be improved given the scope and parameters of the project). Then, the team must choose a target. The target could be a percentage (e.g., reduce by 20%) or a specified value (e.g., under 10 minutes). It is helpful when the metric is easily obtainable via reports pulled from the EHR, but this is not always possible. QI teams may use other methods, such as auditing a sample of charts, directly observing a process, keeping manual logs or tally sheets, etc. Then, if the project is successful, the EHR should be updated to support automated reporting.

Historical/Organizational Context
Learning more about the historical background is helpful in refining the aim statement. Have others tried to fix the problem? Did the process used to work better, and if so, why did it change? Are there regulatory requirements that must be considered? Be sure to ask staff outside your own discipline to get a more complete perspective.

Applying Quality Improvement Frameworks

Quality frameworks are systems used to understand and organize QI projects. The FOCUS-PDCA model[19] is a simple framework used in many health care organizations that is well-suited for beginners. It requires only a team, some basic data collection capabilities, and the desire to improve something. There are numerous online worksheets to help guide a team through the process. The basic elements are outlined below:

FOCUS on what to improve:

F = Find a process to improve.
O = Organize a team that knows the process. Be sure to include frontline staff who work in the process daily.
C = Clarify current knowledge of the process. Map the process to learn how it works in real life, and, importantly, determine how to measure whether it is working well.
U = Understand causes of variation in the process. Identify the root causes that keep the process from giving you the desired results.

S = Select the intervention. Develop an intervention to fix one of the root causes you identified in the previous step.

Use the PDSA cycle to perform a series of small pilots so that the intervention can be tested and adjusted before being implemented on a large scale:

P = Plan. Determine how you will implement the intervention and how you will measure the outcome. How will you know if you were successful?
- D = Do. Implement the intervention and collect outcome data.
- S = Study (sometimes called C for check.) Examine the results. Compare the actual outcome to the expected outcome. Summarize lessons learned.
- A = Act. Decide whether to adopt the change, abandon it, or tweak it by performing another PDSA cycle.

Lean and Six Sigma are more advanced frameworks that require specialized training. However, some of the tools associated with Lean and Six Sigma are widely used and can be used in FOCUS-PDSA projects. Six Sigma focuses on reducing variability and error, whereas Lean focuses on reducing waste.[10] Both emphasize the need for teamwork, participation of frontline staff in QI activities, standardized protocols, and data-driven decision-making. Lean's focus on reducing waste is naturally appealing to fast-paced health care settings and thus many implementations of Lean have been in EDs,[20] including crisis/psychiatric emergency settings.[21]

Quality Improvement Tools

The QI frameworks discussed above have generated hundreds of tools for use in QI projects, and many examples and templates are available online. Process mapping and root cause analysis are used in virtually all QI projects, and these two fundamental tools are discussed below.

Process mapping is a tool that helps the QI team understand the process it wants to change, and it involves making a flow diagram of each step and decision point. To ensure an accurate understanding, it is critical to include staff who do the daily work of the process to be mapped. It is not uncommon to discover differences in the way the process is "supposed" to be performed versus how it is performed, or that different staff perform the process differently. Value stream mapping[10] is an adaptation of process mapping used in Lean to identify and reduce waste. Waste is defined as anything "non-value added" to the customer, such as time spent waiting, duplicated work, unnecessary documentation, wasted motion, and not using staff to their full potential. Sources of waste are identified on the process map, and then a new process is created that eliminates or reduces these wasteful steps.

Root cause analysis is the study of a problem to determine its fundamental causes. The Ishikawa diagram[22] (also called a cause-and-effect diagram or "fishbone" diagram) is a commonly used tool that organizes causes into categories (people, environment, equipment, etc.). Ishikawa diagrams are a useful tool to help the QI team focus on a specific cause. Once a target cause is selected, the team can begin developing an intervention to address it.

Quality Improvement and Research

Although both QI and research employ many tools for data analysis and outcome measurement, they are distinct processes. Research expands the general body of knowledge regarding evidence-based care, and it is by necessity slow and methodical. In contrast, QI is rapid and iterative. QI focuses on applying what is already known to solve or improve complex real-world problems. Many interventions may be tried in rapid succession or at the same time. Results are measured quickly, and modifications are immediately applied and reanalyzed as needed. Both have value in improving health care, and both are publishable.

A question that often arises is whether a QI project requires approval by an institutional review board (IRB). Most do not, but some projects may require IRB review if they involve both research (versus QI as outlined above) and human subjects.[23] The intent to publish does not automatically classify a project as research, and publication of QI projects is becoming increasingly common. Most IRBs have information on their websites to help determine whether a project is QI or research. If there is any question, it is best to simply ask the IRB.

Additional Quality Training

There are many training programs in QI methods for those wishing to expand their knowledge. It is increasingly common for health care organizations to offer their own in-house training programs. Formal certifications for Lean/Six Sigma reflect increasing levels of expertise known as "belts" (e.g., green belt and black belt). The depth and quality of training programs (even the formal certifications) can vary widely. A good barometer of the quality and utility of a program is whether it requires the completion of a final QI project. The project gives the learner invaluable practical experience in applying QI concepts and tools in a real-world setting.

Putting It All Together: Example QI Project

We end this chapter with an example of a QI project that illustrates many of the concepts outlined above, using the FOCUS-PDSA model.

F = Find a process to improve.

Our real-world example focuses on reducing the time that police officers had to wait when bringing a patient for emergency psychiatric care at the Crisis Response Center (CRC) in Tucson, Arizona. This metric is part of the CRISES measure set (which was developed at the CRC) under the "partnership" domain. Police are an important partner because they are often the first responders to a behavioral health emergency. When police are required to wait with the patient for hours at the ED, it becomes quicker to take them to jail or leave them on the street without connecting them to the treatment they need. A fast turnaround time incentivizes police to bring individuals to the CRC for evaluation and treatment. This is a better outcome for the patient and part of the organization's core values of working with community partners to improve outcomes. Management staff saw that police wait times were above the target of 10 minutes. It was time for a QI project!

Aim Statement: Wait times for the police are longer than the target of 10 minutes, sometimes more than 20 minutes. This is important because a quick and easy drop-off process helps incentivize police to bring individuals with behavioral health emergencies to the CRC to receive the treatment they need. The goal of this project is to reduce the median police wait time (the time from when police enter the building to when staff release the officer) to under 10 minutes by the end of the month.

O = Organize a team that knows the process.

The QI team was composed of the Medical Director (physician champion), the Quality Manager (facilitator), the Vice President of Clinical Operations (sponsor), and representative staff from each of the disciplines involved in clinical care at the CRC: nurses, case managers, behavioral health techs, peers, and unit coordinators.

C = Clarify current knowledge of the process.

The Quality Manager observed the police drop-off process and interviewed frontline staff during all four weekly shifts (front-end days, front-end nights, back-end days, and back-end nights) and then created a process map documenting all of the steps in the process.

U = Understand causes of variation in the process.

The team identified where there was waste in the process (value stream mapping) and why (root cause analysis). The process involved assembling a multiperson team (unit coordinator, behavioral health technician, case manager, and nurse) to accept the patient and receive handoff from the police officer. While this team gathered, the officer had to wait. Often, the case manager and nurse were busy with other tasks, which increased the delay. The time staff spent waiting for the full team to assemble was identified as a major source of waste in the process.

S = Select the intervention.

The QI team reviewed these findings and reconsidered the assignment of the staff responsible for the intake. Who were the essential staff who needed to be present for the police drop-off? Which assessments and activities could be performed after police were excused? Which staff were generally available? The new process reduced the team to just two individuals—the unit coordinator and the behavioral health technician ("tech"). The unit coordinator opens the patient's chart, enters demographic information, and ensures any legal paperwork is in order. A structured questionnaire was developed for the tech to obtain information from the police officer regarding the situation leading to their arrival at the facility. After a brief verbal handoff, the tech releases the officer and moves the patient to an assessment room, where they are met by other clinical team members. It was important to retain the tech on the team because they are highly trained in de-escalation and behavioral management techniques, which may be necessary for patients who are highly agitated or aggressive.

PDSA cycle:

- *P = Plan*: The team planned for implementation by creating the new handoff form, training staff, and ensuring that the EHR reporting would measure the wait times correctly.
- *D = Do*: The team selected an implementation date and monitored the new process closely to address unforeseen problems and make minor adjustments.
- *S = Study*: After implementation, wait times significantly decreased from an average median value of 19.4 minutes to 4.0 minutes. Results are shown in Figure 25.2.

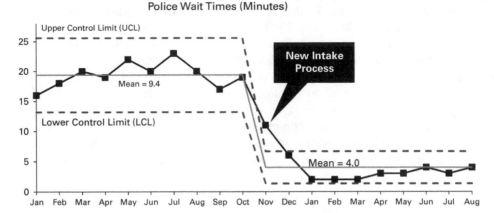

Figure 25.2 Statistical process control chart (Shewhart chart) illustrating a process before and after a quality improvement intervention. The graph depicts improvement in police wait times at the Crisis Response Center in Tucson, Arizona. Upper and lower control units are 3 standard deviations above and below the mean. After the intervention, the performance is significantly improved (consistently below the lower control limit), so updated control limits are set for the new process.

$A = Act$: The new process was adopted as standard procedure and incorporated into updated policies and training.

We hope that this introduction to quality measures, QI, and process improvement, along with some examples, has inspired you to try your hand at your own QI project. QI does not need to be formal or complicated. In fact, QI can be fun and rewarding—a real way to make a measurable and valuable difference.

References

1. QAPI description and background. Center for Medicare and Medicaid Services. Accessed October 11, 2021. https://www.cms.gov/Medicare/Provider-Enrollment-and-Certification/QAPI/qapidefinition

2. Kudzma EC. Florence Nightingale and healthcare reform. *Nurs Sci Q*. 2006;19(1):61–64. doi:10.1177/0894318405283556

3. Institute of Medicine. *To Err Is Human: Building a Safer Health System*. National Academies Press; 2000.

4. Institute of Medicine. *Crossing the Quality Chasm: A New Health System for the 21st Century*. National Academies Press; 2001.

5. Berwick DM, Nolan TW, Whittington J. The triple aim: Care, health, and cost. *Health Aff Proj Hope*. 2008;27(3):759–769. doi:10.1377/hlthaff.27.3.759

6. Bodenheimer T, Sinsky C. From triple to quadruple aim: Care of the patient requires care of the provider. *Ann Fam Med*. 2014;12(6):573–576. doi:10.1370/afm.1713

7. Shewhart WA, Deming WE. *Statistical Method from the Viewpoint of Quality Control*. Dover; 1986.

8. Deming WE. *Out of the Crisis*. Massachusetts Institute of Technology, Center for Advanced Engineering Study; 1986.

9. Womack JP, Jones DT. *Lean Thinking: Banish Waste and Create Wealth in Your Corporation*. Simon & Schuster; 1996.

10. Lighter DE, Lighter DE. *Basics of Health Care Performance Improvement: A Lean Six Sigma Approach*. Jones & Bartlett; 2013.

11. McLaughlin CP, Johnson JK, Sollecito WA. *Implementing Continuous Quality Improvement in Health Care: A Global Casebook*. Jones & Bartlett; 2012.

12. Balfour ME, Tanner K, Jurica PJ, Rhoads R, Carson CA. Crisis Reliability Indicators Supporting Emergency Services (CRISES): A framework for developing performance measures for behavioral health crisis and psychiatric emergency programs. *Community Ment Health J*. 2016;52(1):1–9. doi:10.1007/s10597-015-9954-5

13. Donabedian A. *An Introduction to Quality Assurance in Health Care*. Oxford University Press; 2003.

14. Hermann RC, Palmer RH. Common ground: A framework for selecting core quality measures for mental health and substance abuse care. *Psychiatr Serv*. 2002;53(3):281–287. doi:10.1176/appi.ps.53.3.281

15. Balfour ME, Zinn TE, Cason K, et al. Provider–payer partnerships as an engine for continuous quality improvement. *Psychiatr Serv*. 2018;69(6):623–625. doi:10.1176/appi.ps.201700533

16. National guidelines for behavioral health crisis care: Best practice toolkit. Substance Abuse and Mental Health Services Administration. Published 2020. https://www.samhsa.gov/sites/default/files/national-guidelines-for-behavioral-health-crisis-care-02242020.pdf

17. Roadmap to the ideal crisis system: Essential elements, best practices, and measurable standards for behavioral health crisis response. Group for the Advancement of Psychiatry and National Council for Mental Wellbeing. Published 2021. http://www.CrisisRoadmap.com

18. Dorian GT. There's a S.M.A.R.T. way to write management's goals and objectives. *Manage Rev*. 1981;70(11):35–36.

19. QI toolkit. American College of Cardiology. Accessed October 11, 2021. https://cvquality.acc.org/clinical-toolkits/qi-toolkit

20. D'Andreamatteo A, Ianni L, Lega F, Sargiacomo M. Lean in healthcare: A comprehensive review. *Health Policy Amst Neth*. 2015;119(9):1197–1209. doi:10.1016/j.healthpol.2015.02.002

21. Balfour ME, Tanner K, Jurica PJ, Llewellyn D, Williamson RG, Carson CA. Using lean to rapidly and sustainably transform a behavioral health crisis program: Impact on throughput and safety. *Jt Comm J Qual Patient Saf*. 2017;43(6):275–283. doi:10.1016/j.jcjq.2017.03.008

22. Ishikawa K. *Introduction to Quality Control*. 5th ed. 3A Corporation; 1997.

23. Bass PF, Maloy JW. How to determine if a project is human subjects research, a quality improvement project, or both. *Ochsner J*. 2020;20(1):56–61. doi:10.31486/toj.19.0087

Index

For the benefit of digital users, indexed terms that span two pages (e.g., 52–53) may, on occasion, appear on only one of those pages.

Tables, figures, and boxes are indicated by *t*, *f*, and *b* following the page number